ISBN 978-0-365-29596-9
PIBN 10000990

THE

DENTAL RECORD:

MONTHLY JOURNAL

OF

DENTAL SCIENCE, ART, AND LITERATURE.

DEVOTED TO THE INTERESTS OF THE PROFESSION.

VOL. X.

LONDON:

PUBLISHED BY

THE DENTAL MANUFACTURING COMPANY, LIMITED,

6 TO 10, LEXINGTON STREET, GOLDEN SQUARE,

LONDON, W.; AND

71A, GROSVENOR STREET, MANCHESTER.

LONDON:

PRINTED BY ADAMS BROS.,

MOOR LANE, E.C.

THE DENTAL RECORD.

VOL. X. JANUARY 1st, 1890. No. 1.

Original Communications.

SOME OF THE CAUSES OF DECAY IN CHILDREN'S TEETH AND THEIR TREATMENT.*

By R. DENISON PEDLEY, L.D.S. & F.R.C.S. Edin.

Dental Surgeon to the Evelina Hospital for Sick Children, Assistant Dental Surgeon to the National Dental Hospital.

WHATEVER interferes with the functions of the body or tends to retard its proper development, renders the body liable to become a prey to diseases which may affect it as a whole or only in part. Hence we have what may be described as *predisposing* causes of disease. Among the most important are, unhealthy parents, unwholesome food, and miserable homes.

Children brought up under such conditions have far less chance of being in possession of healthy bodies or retaining them, than those who are surrounded by every comfort. That this is true of the teeth, as of the body in general, there can be very little doubt; and we have learnt by experience that decay in teeth is more prevalent among the children of the poor than in any other class. *Inheritance* has an important influence on the teeth, both temporary and permanent, in many ways; but its direct influence is frequently obvious in the very defective structure of the temporary teeth, for their crowns are for the most part already calcified at birth.

Where we find the dentine and enamel pitted, ridged and honey-combed, in permanent teeth, it is usual to look for some constitutional or general disease in the child itself, as their calcification takes place after the child is born. Among the most important of such diseases influencing the teeth as a whole, are syphilis, rickets, and the eruptive fevers—as measles and scarlatina.

The predisposing and constitutional causes mentioned, with one

*A paper read before the Students' Society of the National Dental Hospital.

exception, must be left to the philanthropist and the physician; we are only called upon to treat their dental manifestations when they come before us.

The exception is *improper feeding*. This is a subject which should interest every dental surgeon. Having the care of children's teeth we are constantly brought in contact with it in hospital and private practice.

In the out-patient department of a hospital where those who are brought or seek for relief from dental troubles vary in age from twelve months to eight years, we frequently seek information of the parents as to the feeding of their children. They are people who live in one of our poorest districts. The impression we have gained is that it is not so much the lack of food as its mal-administration. Let me give you a case in point.

A child of two years was brought by its mother because it had a sore mouth and could not eat. On examination we found a carious molar on each side of the lower jaw. The margins of the gums were deeply ulcerated, exposing the necks of the teeth on each side, above and below. That portion of the mucous membrane of the cheek which came in contact with the gums was also ulcerated, showing a dirty yellowish ground, and from these surfaces came a thin, sanious discharge. The child's breath was very offensive, and the tongue thickly coated.

On enquiry as to diet, we found it consisted principally of bread-and-butter, tea, beer, and meat. The mother had a child in her arms, of six months old, poor and sickly, who was sucking vigorously at a dirty bottle containing milk, tea, and water. The woman was comfortably clad, and said they always had plenty of food.

Such cases are due to ignorance, not destitution, and it is our duty, wherever we find them, to point out that milk is the proper and natural diet for young children. For the first six or eight months it should be the only diet. All starchy foods are to be avoided. Later on good bread and oatmeal with milk, well cooked vegetables and gravy. Meat may be given, though in very small quantities, when the temporary molars are through, and it should not be forgotten that bones are as necessary for exercising the young teeth of children as they are for the dogs. There is any amount of variety in foods. I only wish to indicate some of the best and most nutritious. It is not so much diet tables we want as *nous*.

There are physiological reasons for insisting on a good diet which time will not permit me to enter into fully, but we will mention one of the consequences of improper feeding.

Rickets is essentially a diet disease, and manifests itself chiefly in the bones, which become enlarged at their ends and undergo a general softening. Eruption of the teeth is delayed, we have already stated that calcification of the temporary crowns is well advanced at birth, so their general structure is not much interfered with, though they are rapidly affected by disordered secretions of the mouth. The permanent teeth, especially the early molars and the incisors, are discoloured, pitted and ridged, their cusps are extremely pointed, and caries rapidly affects them. By signs such as these, we conclude that the blood is, or has been, deficient in lime salts, which it is the duty of the forming cells to abstract for their own nourishment, and for the building up of bones and teeth.

Uncleanliness is one of the principal local causes of early decay. When food is allowed to remain between or about the teeth, where the enamel is defective or the secretions are vitiated by stomach derangement, fermentation rapidly takes place, and the acids formed as a consequence soon start caries. Among the children of the poor a tooth brush is seldom known, among those of the middle classes it is not used. In the former it is due to the fact that the parents never cleanse their own teeth, among the latter because the habit is commenced too late. People seem to have an idea that it is unnecessary to teach a child to cleanse its teeth until they can teach it the reason why, or because they are only "sucking teeth." "I did not think my child was old enough" is the usual reply to a question on the matter. It is necessary to insist on the cleansing of a child's teeth just as soon as they have any. If any particular time is chosen let it be after the last meal at bedtime. This may appear a trivial matter, but you must remember that much of the mischief is done in the night.

Much as the public may recognise the value of conservative dentistry, it is astonishing what little care is taken of the temporary teeth. Seldom does the vigilant eye of a mother detect commencing caries, and advice is seldom sought until it is too late. This is invariably the case in hospital practice. When we remember how lasting are early impressions, it can scarcely be a matter of surprise that a child will avoid all future visits to one whom she or he considers an enemy.

So far we have dealt with the principal causes of decay and then general treatment. We will now speak of the special or *local treatment* of caries in young teeth. It is necessary to preserve a temporary tooth until the natural process of removal shall have taken place in the fangs; and whenever it is possible to take away the disintegrated tissue and insert a proper filling as a substitute, this should be done. There are many difficulties which will readily occur. The fears of the patient, the perpetual dribble of saliva, and the small size of the oral cavity, not the least among them. Whatever is done must be accomplished with rapidity, and with as little pain as possible. Should decay be very superficial, the use of a little caustic may suffice. We generally moisten a pledget of cotton wool, rub it on a stick of nitrate of silver, and pass it over the carious surface, then wash well with a little warm water. This, by-the bye, is good for old teeth as well as young. If that surface is kept clean, this simple application occasionally repeated, will often stop further trouble, and we have found it particularly useful round the necks of temporary teeth, and on their labial surfaces. When a filling is to be inserted, the same plan may be adopted where the whole of the carious portion of the tooth cannot be removed. A good gutta-percha and an amalgum (copper by choice) are the only fillings we recommend.

In our desire to retain temporary teeth, we must be careful not to keep them too long. Many have a great dread of removing temporary teeth "because the jaws contract and the permanent teeth cannot come through properly," are the usual reasons assigned. We have never seen any evidence of this. On the contrary large numbers of cases have come under notice where the temporary teeth have been lost very early, without any over-crowding of the permanent teeth.

Mr. C. TOMES,* who is our greatest authority on these matters enters into detail giving reasons for his belief that no contraction of the jaw takes place. The first thing to ascertain is the amount of pain the patient has suffered. If it has been severe enough to keep the child awake at night, we may expect that the nerve is exposed. If it has been only at meal times, or immediately after, caries has probably not yet reached the pulp chamber. On examination, should the tooth be loose in its socket, an evidence of periosteal inflammation, and we find that direct pressure causes pain, thereby

---

* Dental Surgery, p. 186, *et seq.*

preventing the child from eating with comfort, it is wiser to extract at once. Especially is this treatment necessary where in addition to the above symptoms, there is any sign of an abscess at the root, indicated by expansion of the alveolar plate and swelling of the gum, or a small sinus from which pus is oozing.

Where such teeth are retained, it not unfrequently happens that inflammation and suppuration spread to the permanent teeth. We have seen many cases where on extracting a temporary molar the dark discoloured cap of a bicuspid was found lying loose in the socket, showing very clearly that its formative pulp had been for some time destroyed. We have been asked "Is it advisable to destroy an exposed nerve and fill the root of a temporary tooth?" Such treatment cannot be recommended. What we generally call a dead tooth among permanent teeth, is not in reality a necrosed tooth, because the periosteum supplies nourishment to the cementum; but a temporary tooth, the nerve of which has been destroyed, becomes with rare exceptions, necrotic. The periosteum disappears, the alveolar process also, and the tooth is to all intents and purposes a piece of dead bone.

The absorption of the roots of temporary teeth is a vital process. It is accomplished by little papillæ or mounds of fibrous tissue, blood vessels and large many-nucleated cells called osteoclasts which gradually eat into the living roots of a temporary tooth until they disappear. When the pulp chamber is reached the nerve function is altered, the pulp and papillæ unite for the same purpose, and absorption still goes on until the crown is an eaten out shell and can be tilted off with the finger, when the papilla will be seen as a piece of gum underneath.

Absorption is not the only process carried on by the little mounds for they have the power of laying on fresh bone or cementum to a part of the tooth where absorption has already taken place.

As the roots of a tooth disappear fresh bone is thrown out to fill up their sockets, so that on one side of the soft tissue calcified structures are removed, while on the other new bone is formed.

If, in the course of its progress, the absorbing tissue comes in contact with a necrosed root, the former is destroyed and absorption ceases. This and the disappearance of periosteum with the bony socket from a necrosed root, are facts clearly demonstrated by their apices protruding through the gum at all angles, often piercing the sides of the cheeks. Even when the roots have gone and the papilla comes in contact with carious dentine in the crown, it will eat out all the living tissue surrounding it and leave the carious dentine standing alone.

Reports.

THE ODONTOLOGICAL SOCIETY OF GREAT BRITAIN.

THE ordinary monthly meeting of the above Society was held on the 2nd ultimo. The President, Mr. HENRY SEWILL, M.R.C.S., L.D.S., in the chair.

Mr. J. CHARTERS BIRCH (Leeds), was elected a member of the Society.

The LIBRARIAN (Mr. Ashley Gibbings) announced several additions to the library, including Dr. George Johnson's "Essay on Asphyxia."

Messrs. C. ROBBINS and C. D. DAVIS were appointed auditors for the year.

Mr. E. LLOYD-WILLIAMS read notes of two interesting cases. The first, originally diagnosed as sarcoma, was subsequently discovered to be one of myxoma. The particulars were as follows:—The patient, a woman, aged 23, in April 1888, began to suffer a good deal of pain in the upper jaw on the right side from the bicuspids forwards. The anterior division of the fifth nerve was evidently implicated, though it was interesting to note the posterior division was not affected. In April of the present year, suffering from intense neuralgia, she applied to the hospital for relief. Two or three teeth were extracted on the affected side, but finding that probably the mischief was of something more than dental origin, the case was referred to Mr. Bland Sutton, who diagnosed an antral tumour, and removed it by operation. Mr. Lloyd-Williams desired to call attention to one or two points as affecting dentists: first, the great desirability of not confining themselves entirely to the dental origin of mischief in cases of facial neuralgia, they were somewhat prone to blame their surgical bretheren for not attaching sufficient importance to the possibilities of dental origin, was it not equally necessary that they should themselves be on the alert for general symptoms. Secondly, the portion of the jaw removed had been skilfully replaced by a denture made by Mr. Schelling, one of the students of the Hospital. The patient being present the members would have an opportunity of seeing how efficient a substitute had been supplied. The second case was that of a man, aged 30, who contracted syphilis in April '87, and in August '88 perforation of the palate supervened upon periostitis. The case was a little remarkable for the short time between the primary stage and the tertiary perforation. The patient applied to the hospital in consequence of the great inconvenience caused by the passage of tobacco smoke, food and liquids through the palate into the nasal cavities. The question which arose was whether it was advisable to cover the opening with an obturator, or whether by so doing more harm than good would result from the possible injury that might be occasioned by the increased pressure of the obturator on the soft parts about the ulcer. A very carefully fitted obturator was made to cover the aperture so as not to exert undue pressure on the soft parts. After wearing the plate for some few months it was interesting to note that the perforation had all but healed and the patient could eat with perfect comfort.

Mr. Bland Sutton, in giving the clinical details of the first case, said that both pathologically and clinically it was one of great interest. The patient was sent to Middlesex Hospital complaining of neuralgia. Mr. Sutton observed some upward displacement of the right eye and feeling gently along the orbit could discover some resistance. On carefully testing for sensation with a pin he found that the soft parts supplied by the infra-orbital nerve were anæsthetic. A critical examination of the patient led to the diagnosis of a tumour, and removal of the jaw by operation was decided upon. Laryngotomy was performed and the larynx plugged, the lip was then divided and the cheek reflected; a lobulated tumour was found and removed with the upper jaw. The tumour upon dissection proved to be a myxoma involving the infra-orbital nerve, the nerve fibres being expanded over the growth which sprang from the intertubular fibrous tissue. Meckel's ganglion was exposed and also taken away. The fifth nerve was peculiarly susceptible to neuromatous growths, but, so far as Mr. Sutton was aware, this was the first instance of a growth of that nature invading the orbit and the antrum. The operation was completely successful, there being not the slightest recurrence of pain and Mr. Sutton did not think there would be.

The President remarked that in some points the case was unique, and as several hospital surgeons were present he hoped there would be a good discussion..

Mr. Storer Bennett, in connection with the first case, remembered one which came to the Middlesex Hospital while he was a dresser. It was that of a man over 70 years of age, who had for three or four years suffered intense neuralgia on the right side of the face affecting the eye and the cheek on that side. For treatment all the teeth of upper jaw were removed one after the other, but the pain still remained. It was then evident that something deeper than mere dental trouble existed. Mr. Henry Morris, in whose charge the case was, decided to stretch the infra-orbital nerve and cut away as much as he could. When exposed a number of small tubercular looking tumours could be seen on the nerve itself, springing from the neurilemma, and these pressing down on the hard bony canal had caused intolerable pain. After removing the nerve as far as it was possible to reach it no pain recurred. Unlike Mr. Sutton's case it did not grow into the antrum, and in that respect there was very great difference between them.

The PRESIDENT asked Mr. Sutton if he excised the whole of the jaw.

Mr. BLAND SUTTON said that that was so, but in future with the experience of this case before him he should not hesitate to enucleate the tumour. It was not until dissecting the tumour afterwards that he became aware of its nature. Having had no previous experience of a case of this kind, he thought it safest to perform the operation as he had described it.

The PRESIDENT, with regard to the second case, thought it unwise to interfere with a syphilitic sore while active ulceration was proceeding.

Mr. F. NEWLAND-PEDLEY, as a matter of routine, applied obturators in all cases where the bone had been removed, viz., in cases of necrosis from syphilis, or suicidal attempts ; looking upon the obturator as a natural splint.

The PRESIDENT asked if he understood Mr. Pedley to say that he would put an obturator while active ulceration was proceeding.

Mr. NEWLAND-PEDLEY replied that his statement was that in cases of perforation of the palate, whether from syphilitic or suicidal attempts, he would invariably employ an obturator.

Mr. W. A. HUNT (Yeovil), was rather struck with Mr. Pedley's remarks, and reiterated the President's question as to whether in cases of active syphilitic ulceration he considered it wise to employ an obturator ; he (Mr. Hunt) had always been taught the contrary.

The PRESIDENT observed that cases varied so infinitely that he thought it was impossible to generalize.

Mr. Newland-Pedley thought it important to bear in mind the variety of obturators. An obturator might be put through an opening or it might bridge it over to protect it from injury, and in such cases he found wounds and sores certainly healed much better. He thought openings in the palate would not become so large if obturators were introduced earlier in all cases of injury or suicide.

Mr. Hunt said his remarks were confined to cases where active syphilitic ulceration was going forward.

Mr. Newland-Pedley replied that in the case under consideration it was obvious that there was more bone to come away. After the bone has been removed and the first destructive change is over, the bone comes away and there is a cavity, one could not be wrong in bridging that over.

Mr. E. Lloyd-Williams professed himself quite of Mr. Pedley's opinion and would have been glad to hear opinions of other surgeons present. As he understood Mr. Pedley he would put in an obturator, not when syphilitic ulceration was at its highest pitch, but after that stage had been passed, and he quite agreed with him.

Mr. David Hepburn described a slide section tray which he had designed for the purpose of facilitating plaster impression taking, and to avoid dragging when a plastic modelling material is used. The special feature of the invention, is the division of the ordinary tray into two parts, the anterior external rim being detached and forming part of a moveable slide working on the handle. In order to take an impression in modelling composition, the slide is removed, the tray filled with compo and placed in the mouth; the anterior surface of the teeth is thus left exposed. A small roll of soft compo is then placed on the exposed surface and the slide pressed well home, which completes the impression. To remove the impression, both slide and tray are withdrawn and re-united outside the mouth, ready for casting. If a plaster impression is desired, the only variation in the process just described is the substitution of that material for the *posterior* surface of the teeth (the impression of the anterior surface is taken in modelling compo as before); should the plaster curl round the anterior portions of the teeth, when hard enough, it may be pared off. The tray, Mr. Hepburn thought, would be found useful in cases of marked erosion, irregularity, or cleft palate.

Mr. F. J. Vanderpant (Kingston on Thames) asked if there was not a difficulty in removing the front part of the tray in cases were patients had a long lip? In his own practice in one or two such cases, he had cut off the front part of the tray and replaced it by a piece of stent having first oiled or vaselined it to remove the suction.

Mr. W. A. Hunt, since he had been in practice, used nothing but plaster for modelling. He thought Mr. Hepburn's suggestion a most admirable one, but it seemed to him to be taking machinery where no machinery was required. With regard to undercuts of teeth large at the crown and small at the neck, many of his friends were attempting to draw them in stent, but it appeared to him an impossible thing to do so successfully. If drawn in plaster all the undercuts would be obtained. He contended that there was no model which could not be drawn better and more easily in plaster than in stent.

Mr. F. J. Bennett asked how Mr. Hepburn would find his tray answer in the case of a bar lower when the inner surface inclined inwards? He thought a model of the front surface of the teeth was not needed so much as the back.

Mr. D. Hepburn replying, said that matter was so simple and so easily understood in practice that he did not think much discussion was necessary. With reference to the point raised as to cases of long lip, that was a little difficulty, but the stent hardens so completely that in withdrawing the tray the lip yields and the stent passes over it. With regard to Mr. Hunt's remarks he was to be congratulated that he could combat all difficulties by confining himself to plaster as a material for taking models, but he (Mr. Hepburn) confessed he sometimes had cases in which he thought his tray would be of assistance.

Mr. G. Cunningham (Cambridge) showed several instruments and appliances, among them being (1) a root trimmer, the invention of Dr. Bing, to be used in ferrule crowning; (2) a specimen of removeable bridge work; (3) a novel crown, devised by Dr. Sachs, of Breslau, the special feature being that both the pin and the tube, which fitted into the root, were star-shaped, rotation being thereby avoided: the serrated pin was produced by a special star-shaped draw-plate; (4) models of Dr. Herbst's gold filling by the rotation method; (5) models illustrating glass filling.

Mr. J. Ackery read notes of a case of fracture of the superior maxilla and the nasal bones, under the care of himself and Mr. W. B. Paterson at St. Bartholomew's Hospital. The patient, a boy, aged 17, was struck on the left side of the face by a swing-boat and rendered unconscious. He was admitted to the hospital in March last. The face was much bruised and swollen, and marked crepitus was felt extending from the left molar region transversely across the face and over the nose. The orbital plate of superior maxilla was apparently not implicated. The tongue was lacerated in two places and much swollen. There was considerable displacement of the upper jaw, the left alveolar process and teeth being half an inch lower than the right. The left nasal bone protruded through a wound half an inch long over the bridge of the nose. Another wound, at the bottom of which was bare bone, extended transversely outwards from the left nostril an inch and a half. The left jaw could be moved *en masse* laterally. Mr. Ackery decided to put the fracture up, using the lower jaw as a splint. He was able to reduce the displacement fairly well under chloroform, though not without considerable force. A four-tailed bandage was applied, but owing to the damage to the nose, and the swollen condition of the tongue, the patient's breathing was difficult, and the bandage had to be loosened. The following day a piece of half-inch composition gas pipe was flattened and placed across the arch below the first molars, turned upward and backward, and secured by a bandage. Impressions of the jaws having been previously taken, a dental alloy plate was now struck up, fitting over the palate and teeth in the upper jaw. A socket was then cut and soldered along the upper and outer edge of the plate on either side. A piece of iron wire was then flattened at the end and fitted to the socket securely on each side and brought round in front of the angle of the mouth, being carried back to the ear with a hook at the end to which a bandage was made fast on either side and tied below the occiput; another bandage being passed under the bars on either side and tied on the top of the head. After this had been worn three days, it was decided to replace it with a Gunning's splint, but this gave rise to soreness, and failed to keep the jaws in position. The side wires of the splint were then removed, and a bite in wax taken on the plate; a vulcanite box was added to the plate on either side for the bicuspids and molars to bite into—in shaping the boxes a close fit was not aimed at. The splint arranged was fitted into the mouth (the same method being pursued as when taking the bite) and the lower teeth were made to close into the boxes, being fixed there by an external apparatus, consisting of a padded chin-piece with side straps, which were attached to a head-cap. After wearing the apparatus for a month the fracture became united and articulation of the teeth was perfect. Mr. Ackery replying to a question from the President, said the fracture commenced on the left side of the infra-orbital plate, passed transversely across the bridge of the nose and ended on the opposite side about half-an-inch above the alveolar border.

The PRESIDENT remarked the case was a very interesting one, and there were many members present steeped to their fingers in knowledge of diseases of the jaws, whom they would be glad to hear upon the subject.

Mr. WM. HERN said the fracture seemed to involve both antra; he should like to ask if there were any antral mischief on either side? He thought the case brought out two points of interest. First it proved the disadvantage of any splint which projected out of the mouth. Mr. Hern had a case at the Dental Hospital of London a few years ago in which he at first used a Kingsley's splint, but it was a constant annoyance to the patient, the arms getting in the way when the head rested on the pillow and tended rather to delay than assist recovery. The other point was the advisability of adopting a cap instead of bandages.

Mr. ACKERY in reply to Mr. Hern, said that with regard to any antral mischief none at present had shewn itself. With regard to the cap it was Mr. Paterson's idea. He might mention that the Kingsley splint was only on for three days, and in conjunction with Mr. Paterson he agreed that an internal splint should be used. Possibly Mr. Paterson's difficulty in putting in the splint about a week afterwards was due to the exudations having somewhat thickened.

The PRESIDENT announced that the next meeting would take place on the 13th January, 1890, when he would deliver his valedictory address, and a paper would be read by Dr. SCANES SPICER on "Nasal Obstruction and Mouth Breathing as Factors in the Etiology of Disorders of the Teeth." It would also be the occasion of the Annual General Meeting when officers for the ensuing year would be elected. The meeting then separated.

ODONTO-CHIRURGICAL SOCIETY OF SCOTLAND.

THE First General Meeting of the Session 1889-90 was held on the 14th November, Mr. JOHN A. BIGGS, L.D.S., President, in the chair.

At the conclusion of the formal business the PRESIDENT proceeded with his Inaugural Address.

GENTLEMEN,—After the remarks I made at our last annual meeting, when you did me the honour to confer upon me the office of President of this Society, I need hardly say that I feel proud of the position, and that I have great pleasure in being with you on this occasion in this distinguished capacity, but while thus frankly admitting to you so much, you will, I hope, bear with me while I also confess to you the misgivings I have of my own ability to fill the office creditably to myself and acceptably to you.

When I think of the roll of honourable and learned men who have filled the chair before me, you will own I have grave grounds for my fears. As you know, your choice fell first upon one whom, I am sure, we should all like to have seen filling this position, and who needs no praise from me to raise him in your estimation. He has never been sparing of either his time or money in the advancement of his profession in its ethical, practical, political, or its educational interests, and who, I am confident, would have held it with greater acceptance to us all.

You all know how ably Dr. Williamson has recently filled the the Presidential chair, and how difficult it will be to beat the record of his attendance, notwithstanding the distance he had to travel in order to be present, and the able and unbiassed manner in which he took part in the discussions. But I do want credit for something, and that is courage to accept the office just vacated by so worthy a predecessor, and declined by so distinguished a man as Mr. Macgregor. And now that I am in office, I mean to do my best with my poor abilities to maintain the honour and usefulness of this Society, and in whatsoever I may be found wanting it will not, at least, be in interest in its affairs. How many societies are heralded into existence in the course of a year with a flourish of trumpets, which never see the close of it; but this, The Odonto-Chirurgical Society, has not only survived a great number of years, but has been a power in Scottish dental affairs, having been one, if not the most important, means of banding the best dentists of the country together, and uniting them in a common cause. Before its existence there was a far greater amount of selfishness, petty jealousies, and prejudices rampant. Each man considered himself as good as another and a great deal better. If any important item of practical value came his way he endeavoured to conceal it from his professional brethren, and made what capital he could out of it for his own private interest He might be a man of a very sociable disposition to all around him, but not so to his fellow practitioner.

From the same sources as those from which our Society arose, sprang the Edinburgh Dental Hospital, than which I know of no more flourishing institution in the city, nor any more deserving of the liberal support of the citizens, and, compared with the cost of its maintenance, I feel sure it has no equal in relieving pain and giving comfort to the poor. Within its walls there is a staff of about twenty-four doctors and dentists, working together gratuitously for the relief of common humanity, and their kindly smiles and hearts are not reserved for their patients alone, but are there to welcome and to aid each other.

Then, again, we are indebted in the main to members of the Odontological and Odonto-Chirurgical Society for the passing of the Dental Act, giving us registration and the extension of the degrees we now hold; and then arose the British Dental Association, with all its power for good among us. There are a great many upon the Register still, who are, unfortunately, not a credit to the profession. The public cannot distinguish between such men as yet, but happily they soon will—not but what there are many good and trusty men who have yet no degree, but they are at liberty to declare their status by becoming members of the British Dental Association, and that will be a guide to the public in the near future.

While in Harrogate this year, a lady, knowing my profession, asked me—"Is So-and-so a good dentist?" I asked, "has he a degree?" She said, "no, but he is registered." I said, "do you know if he is a member of the British Dental Association?" She said, "I do not know." I said, "if he is, it is a voucher for his standing. If he be not a member, I cannot advise you further about him." The public is also fast finding out that men pretending to do dental work, and yet not daring to call themselves dentists, are not dentists at all, and are not to be trusted, and, no doubt, this is largely due to the publicity given to the transactions of the British Dental Association, and to the prosecutions under the Act. Now, gentlemen, if you have followed me, you will see I have been working up to a point in my address, and the point is, that we are largely indebted to this and kindred societies for the elevated platform on which we stand to-day, compared to that of thirty years ago. We must take upon ourselves the responsibilities of maintaining them in full vigour; and, to do that, it behoves every member to do his utmost to further its interests, and this may be done in so many ways that it is unnecessary to do more than briefly notice some of them. In the first place, an interest may be shown by the frequency of attendance, for that is the most essential of all, as it is most discouraging to those giving papers, showing specimens, and giving demonstrations to a limited audience. Then every member can, if he choose, give a paper on something or other which will afford food for reflection, and, no doubt, throw light upon his subject that will be useful to many, if not to us all. Some might be inclined to say that they are too busy to take anything like an active part in any society. My experience, however, is that only busy men ever do take an active part in these matters.

Then, again, many men declare they would readily give a paper, but that our literature is so prolific that it is out of their power to find a subject into which they could throw a sufficiency of originality to warrant them in delivering it. With that excuse I have some sympathy, as it has been my own experience. But where there is a will there also is a way.

Once I was asked to give a paper for a sister society, and declined on those grounds, but, being urged, I said, "give me a subject and I will do my best." A subject was proposed, I accepted, wrote and delivered it, and probably no one derived more benefit from the effort than myself. Now, if I may be allowed to suggest a few subjects for papers, I would first indicate anæsthetics, and that notwithstanding that we have had such able and instructive papers and discussions on the matter at Brighton last August. I am prepared to affirm that the subject is one than which no other can possibly be of greater interest, and my favourite mixture, of which I spoke last year—viz., nitrous oxide and chloroform—has not been included in the discussion, and, therefore, the subject has by no means been thrashed out. I would next suggest a paper on implantation, as one likely to be interesting and to lead to a lively discussion. Root-filling is also a good subject. Porcelain fillings might be repeated this year with advantage; and if some of our members would volunteer a demonstration on crown and bridge work, they might reckon with certainty on a large attendance of members.

Are micro-organisms the causes or effect of dental caries? would form a subject of interest for debate. What is the best known treatment for sensitive dentine? But demonstrations are at all times the most popular, and secure the most successful meetings. Cases of irregularity under treatment, and after, are good subjects, but it is useless to suggest. You all have your pet hobbies, and this is the place to trot them out and give them an airing. If I have trespassed upon your time by my detailed suggestions, I trust you will attribute it to my desire to have as flourishing and profitable a session during my term of office as any which preceded it, and with that explanation I conclude, thanking you all for your patient and indulgent hearing.

A vote of thanks to Mr. Biggs was proposed by Mr. ANDREW WILSON, seconded by Mr. REES PRICE, and carried by acclamation.

Mr. WATSON brought before the Society an interesting case of motor and sensory paralysis after tooth extraction. The patient, a lady, had two teeth, the second lower bicuspid and first molar extracted under the influence of nitrous oxide gas. On regaining consciousness she complained of a want of power and feeling in the lip of the side operated on. On examination it was found that a portion of the lip, about the size of a sixpence, in the neighbourhood of the mental foramen, was insensitive and somewhat powerless. The operation was performed last March, and at the present time, November, the part had not quite recovered itself. The accident was a somewhat uncommon one in connection with the removal of teeth so near the anterior portion of the jaw, and had been probably caused by stretching of the inferior dental nerve, which may have been adherent to or entangled in the roots of one or both of the extracted teeth.

Mr. CAMPBELL showed the model of a case of lupus of the soft and hard palates. The disease had removed all the palatal portion of the superior maxilla, the palatal bones, and most of the vomer and ethmoid. All that was left of the upper jaw was a portion of the alveolar process holding the six front teeth in position, the three molars on the right, and the last two molars on the left side. The roots of the molar teeth were very much denuded on the lingual side, but not at all on the buccal. The bicuspids were gone—in their place was a deep chasm.

Mr. Campbell supplied the defect with a hard vulcanite plate, which answers the purpose very well, and improves the man's speech greatly.

He also showed a model of a case where he had removed an upper central incisor, beneath which was an unerupted canine, which he also extracted. The patient was above forty years of age.

The peculiarity of this latter tooth was in the fact that, although beyond external influences, there was a cavity on the cutting edge. On examination the pulp was found to be in a very septic condition.

Mr. WATSON: In regard to Mr. Campbell's case of impacted canine with deep penetrating cavity at the apex of the cusp, having had an opportunity of examining it carefully, I conclude that there has been a deep fissure at this point, and that the relation of the tooth to the central incisor has caused the development of odontoclast cells (some of which are still seen at the margins of the cavity in the canine), which had proved destructive to the faulty enamel, and eventually to the pulp, on the death of which the swelling and tenderness ensued. The case is very interesting and unique.

Mr. PAGE: During my extraction of a number of teeth for a powerfully-built German gentleman, on grasping the right superior wisdom, I felt the tooth and its bony surroundings loosen. I immediately desisted, and on the patient recovering from the nitrous oxide anæsthesia, I had the disagreeable duty of informing him one of his offending members had not been extracted. Though persistent in his appeals to get me to extract the tooth, I merely left well alone, only painting with a weak solution of aconite and iodine, and requesting his attendance in a day or two. Several visits were made, and each one found the patient more persistent in his wish to have the tooth extracted—it being slightly painful to the touch, and so somewhat interfering with pleasurable mastication. Otherwise, the parts appeared quite healthy, and the fracture, at the end of three weeks, felt tolerably firm. At this time, in deference to the wish of my patient, I reluctantly extracted the tooth, and, in doing so, brought away the tuberosity, and the floor of the antrum immediately above the tooth. At once the patient presented an alarming appearance of syncope, blood flowing from mouth and nostril, features livid, and breathing slow. Restoratives were at once successfully applied, and the bleeding controlled, firstly, with ice, and, secondly, with hot Fletcher's carbolised resin plugged into the wound. In an hour the patient left for home, with instructions to sleep in a sitting posture, and to apply ice should hæmorrhage occur. I anxiously awaited his return next day, and was pleased to hear no bleeding occurred, no fluid passed into the antrum, and altogether he had felt little inconvenience.

Removing the greater part of the plug, a plaster impression was taken, and a black rubber case made, covering well the mucous membrane representing the tuberosity. Previous, however, to insertion the plug was removed, the cavity well washed with an antiseptic solution, and the wounded edges pared and brought together—not, however, in their entirety—an opening being left for drainage purposes. The wound was frequently washed with diluted carbolic acid, and the necessity of wearing the case impressed upon the patient.

A week after the tooth extraction, on passing a barbless Donaldson's bristle into the wound, resistance was felt, and, on wounding, a healthy-looking serous fluid, latterly tinged with blood, flowed from the cavity. Fluids then passed readily into the antrum.

To-day—eleven days after the operation—on removing the dentine, no fluid would pass readily into the antrum, and the wound had every appearance of health, and to the criticism of the subject I look for the prognosis of the case.

The fractured tuberosity embracing the roots of the wisdom tooth was exhibited. The cavity of the antrum had evidently passed further back into the substance of the maxilla than was usual, hollowing out the tuberosity to an extent which made its attachment to the body of the bone insecure, and liable to fracture on the application of any force.

Mr. MACGREGOR exhibited and presented to the museum the model of a lower jaw containing five incisors. Comment was made upon the comparative rarity of the specimen, but doubts were expressed as to whether it was actually as uncommon as it would appear to be, as if an extra incisor were to be erupted it would probably be removed almost at once, on the score of crowding, or it might even be extracted in mistake for a temporary tooth that had not been shed in due course.

Mr. CAMPBELL described the method he had adopted for making rubber bands for regulating purposes. He had been dissatisfied with those usually supplied for the purpose, as they so quickly lost their elasticity, due, he imagined, to the rubber from which they were made being adulterated. With different sized punches, such as those used by workers in leather, he cut out rings from rubberdam, using larger or smaller rings, and thick or thin rubber, according to the case for which they were required. He found they retained their elasticity well, and were far more serviceable.

The PRESIDENT announced that the next meeting would be held on Thursday, the 12th December, when Mr. Wilson had promised a paper on "The First Premolar in the Typical Dentition of the Placental Mammals."

DENTAL HOSPITAL AND SCHOOL OF LONDON.

THE Annual Dinner of the Staff and Past and Present Students of the Dental Hospital and School of London, was held in the Venetian Saloon of the Holborn Restaurant, on the 30th November, 1889.

Mr. CHRISTOPHER HEATH, F.R.C.S., &c., occupied the chair and was supported by Drs. Julius Pollock, Dudley Buxton, Hewitt, Stack, and Walker, and Messrs. J. Smith Turner, Woodhouse, Braine, Henry Sewill, Pearce Gould, Henry Morris, J. Bland Sutton, F. G. Hallett, Bowman McCleod, J. R. Brownlie, Sibley, Trimmer, Felix Weiss, Henri Weiss, and a large company of the staff, students, and friends.

The usual loyal toasts having been duly honoured, the CHAIRMAN gave "The Navy, Army and Reserve Forces," coupled with the name of Mr. A. O. MCKELLAR, Surgeon-in-Chief of the Metropolitan Police.

Mr. A. O. MCKELLAR, in responding said, he felt a peculiar pleasure in being associated with the proposer of the toast, when he remembered that they had both served in the Russian War together. Having referred to the Navy, Army and Reserve, he mentioned in conclusion that the medical branch held a larger percentage of Victoria Crosses than any other Branch of Her Majesty's services.

The CHAIRMAN then proposed the toast of the evening, viz., "The Past and Present Students," and in the course of his remarks said he was still a student himself although a teacher; he maintained that so soon as a teacher ceased to be a student he should cease to be a teacher. He had no doubt, therefore, that they would all remain students, for unless they did so they would make no progress, and he would add that he felt sure it would be admitted that the advance made in the dental profession in the past few years was in a great part due to the past and present students of the great institution in

Leicester Square. He urged them to keep abreast with the general advance of the day—speaking from a medical point of view, he knew how difficult it was for a busy man to do so, for knowledge was continually progressing, yet unless they could keep up with it they would find themselves dropping behind. So much for work. With reference to play, he thought one of the great advantages of being a student was that it brought men of similar tastes together, and association afforded opportunities for the development of their tastes in a manner both advantageous and pleasant to themselves and to others. In conclusion he coupled with the toast the name of Mr. J. R. Brownlie, of Glasgow (a past student), a very distinguished practitioner, a lecturer in dental surgery and one of the examiners on the Dental Board of the College of Physicians and Surgeons, Glasgow; and on behalf of the present students, Mr. Hoffman, who, he understood, was the best man of his year and had won the Saunder's Scholarship.

Mr. J. R. Brownlie, having expressed his thanks for the cordial reception given to the toast, spoke of the pleasure he had, which he felt sure was shared by all past students, in coming as occasion offered to the annual festival. He hardly knew of a more pleasant meeting, affording, as it did, opportunities of renewing old friendships and making new ones. They were glad to be able to enlarge their acquaintance by forming friendships under such agreeable conditions with those students who had not yet passed.

Mr. A. W. Hoffman having replied on behalf of the present students,

Mr. J. Smith-Turner proposed "The Dental Hospital of London and Staff." This was a toast that might almost go alone. With reference to the Hospital, there had been 13,000 cases of extraction last year, and nearly 10,000 cases of extraction under gas—a beneficient agent in connection with which he might say it was to the credit of the gentlemen who administered it that they rendered their services to the Hospital without remuneration. The Dental Hospital, he was happy to say, was fairly well supported by the public; he should only be too glad to be able to say it was better supported by them. Certainly, it was well supported by their own and the medical professions. And in referring to those who had supported it in their own profession it would be ungracious to forget the name of their great benefactor, Sir Edwin Saunders. With respect to the staff, it would be to paint the violet to enlarge upon their excellencies, but they had a most onerous duty to perform, if the profession was to be regenerated, if it was to obtain that position which it was entitled to among the learned professions, it could only be through education, and to the staff and lecturers was assigned the important duty of educating the dental student. He hoped that they would not only succeed in turning out educated gentlemen, but educated professional gentlemen—gentlemen above sounding their own praises or the praises of any particular system, who would base their reputation on being good all-round dentists, capable of supplying the wants and relieving the necessities of their patients in every direction. Having referred approvingly to the recent changes in the curriculum, he concluded by coupling the name of Mr. R. H. Woodhouse with the toast.

Mr. R. H. WOODHOUSE, replying, mentioned that he had been on the staff for twelve years, and that it was under Mr. Turner's care that he performed his first operation. As proof of the continued prosperity of the school, he stated that during the present year a larger number of freshmen had entered than in any single year previously. He claimed that the Dental Hospital of London had been the pioneer of all the Dental Hospitals in the United Kingdom.

Mr. HENRY MORRIS proposed "The London School of Dental Surgery." If there were one thing which could have afforded satisfaction to an after-dinner speaker, it was that he might convey a just meed of praise to those who thoroughly deserved it. If he might venture to outline what were, to his mind, the typical excellencies of a good lecturer, he would say that besides practical skill and scientific attainments, there should be lucidity of thought and expression, geniality and encouragement in manner, and kindly interest in the present success, and future welfare of those whose education was entrusted to his care. He was sure that it would be admitted that all those qualities were possessed by the present teaching body of the school. The clinics of the school required no personal recommendation ; its reputation was its own, the mention of its name, like the mention of some historic pile or national monument, reminded us that it had a history which was unquestioned and unquestionable. The success of the school must be considered unique, and with it the success of the hospital was bound up. With the toast he begged to associate the name of Mr. Morton Smale.

Mr. MORTON SMALE in responding, said it was with great pleasure he once more thanked them in the name of the Staff and Lecturers for the very kind way in which their name had been received, and he assured the students that it was a source of happiness to the staff to render them that assistance which enabled them to obtain their diploma and practice their profession. He would take this opportunity of reminding those who had passed, or were passing through the schools, that they were the salt of their profession and were looked to to savour their calling by honourable professional conduct. He warned them against quackery, charlatanism and chicanery, the various forms of which he pointed out, and exhorted them so to temper their bearing in their profession as to show by their conduct how much they disagreed in all unprofessional behaviour; to avoid even that semblance of advertising which is too common in a kindred profession, of writing testimonials for drugs, drinking waters, &c., and which the firm to which it is given advertises; to be content with the advertisement which comes from downright honest thoroughness in their work; content with the knowledge that if their incomes should be smaller they would have that satisfaction, which is far above reward, of having spent an honourable professional life, and served their profession as upright gentlemen.

Mr. A. S. Underwood proposed "The Visitors" to which Mr. E. Trimmer (Secretary Royal College of Surgeons) responded.

Dr. Dudley Buxton gave the "Health of the Chairman," and in the course of his remarks said, about twenty-one years ago Mr. Heath won the Jacksonian prize by his essay on "Injuries and Diseases of the Jaws," the publication of which at once placed him in a position of authority on that branch of surgery, and brought him closely in touch with the dental profession. Among his many excellent qualities the tact with which he had presided over them would specially recommend the toast; he had avoided alike the brusqueness which paralyses eloquence, and the prolixity which might be termed the disease of the jaws, from which after-dinner speakers not infrequently suffered.

The Chairman in acknowledging the toast said that his sympathy with the dental profession began long before the Jacksonian Essay, both his grandfather and his father, and also three uncles had been dentists, and it was only by the merest accident that he was not a dentist himself.

"The Musicians," a toast not on the list, was proposed by the Chairman and responded to by Mr. David Hepburn.

The proceedings were enlivened by vocal and instrumental music given by the Musical Society of the Hospital, assisted by Mr. H. L. FULKERSON, and directed by Mr. PERCY JACKMAN.

DENTAL HOSPITAL OF LONDON STUDENTS' SOCIETY.

THE Ordinary General Meeting was held on Monday, December 9th, 1889, at 8 p.m. WM. HERN, Esq., President, in the chair.

The minutes of the previous meeting were read and confirmed.

Messrs. Blaine, Goddard and Carter signed the Obligation Book, and were formally admitted to the membership of the Society.

Messrs. Vanderpant and Blaaberg were proposed members of the Society.

The PRESIDENT then read the list of gentlemen recommended by the Council as officers for the ensuing year.

Messrs. READING and GASK were appointed to audit the Society's accounts for the past year.

On *Casual Communications* being called for, Mr. D. CORMACK presented a left lower wisdom tooth, with a supplemental cusp and four patent nerve canals.

Mr. HARRISON exhibited a new appliance for putting on the rubber dam.

Mr. W. MAY presented a supernumerary tooth, which he had removed from the region behind the central and lateral. This tooth after having been in position for five years, had suddenly given pain. After removal he found that the root was partly absorbed, though there had been no pressure on the tooth when in position.

Mr. HARSANT showed a piece of bridge-work, to which the following history was attached. The patient's upper incisor teeth had been very prominent and unsightly so she determined to have them replaced by an artificial set. Accordingly the four incisors were extracted, and the crowns of the canines cut off. A bridge plate was then put in, supported by a gold cap, over the second molar on each side, and a cap and pivot over each canine root. The piece shortly after became loose and was refixed. A few months subsequently, she had the misfortune to break off two teeth from the gold bar. Learning that the piece would have to be removed in order to be repaired, and being by this time tired of the American method, she then consulted Mr. Harding. The roots being tender and slightly loose, he advised her to have them all extracted and a new plate fitted. Mr. Harsant then saw her and endeavoured to remove the piece previous to extracting the roots, but found that it was so firmly fixed, that he was eventually obliged to saw the bar through in three places. The patient was then given an anæsthetic, and teeth and plate removed together. Mr. Matheson recorded a somewhat similar case which had occurred in his own practice. Mr. Hern and Mr. Dolamore also commented on this case.

The PRESIDENT then called on Mr. D. CORMACK for his paper on

THE TREATMENT OF PULPLESS TEETH.

The discussion was opened by Mr. WRIGHTON. His mode of treating dead teeth was first to syringe out the cavity and pulp chamber with some weak antiseptic, and then to treat the roots by the dry method. For this purpose he found a solution of iodoform in ether very useful, since the ether quickly evaporated and left the root. He believed that dressings of wax and iodoform were more permanent than was stated by Mr. Cormack. He had found them unaltered after two years. A rapid and economical method of opening up large cavities was to cut through the enamel with a corundum disc and then to drill through the softer dentine with a steel bur.

Mr. MARSHALL narrated a case of a tooth he was called upon to extract because of severe alveolar periostitis, consequent on, he believed, the passage of perchloride of mercury through the apical foramen. He advocated the treatment of abscessed teeth by drilling through the alveolus above the roots.

Mr. RILOT differed from Mr. Cormack, as to the rarity of septic matter passing through the foramen, and congratulated him on his apparent exemption from that untoward accident. These unfortunate cases came when we least expected them and were congratulating ourselves that all was well. He also differed as to the order of procedure in the treatment, for he himself would prefer to use the antiseptics first and then drill out after. It was very important to open up the cavity well, so as to get the drill in the direct line of the root. He also had found wax and iodoform dressings to last longer than was supposed. He had seen them last unimpaired for six years. We should choose our root filling in accordance with the requirements of each individual case. Very recently at the hospital Mr. Bennett had removed a plain wool dressing from a tooth and to his surprise found the dressing perfectly sweet though it had been in the root for four years.

Mr. SCHELLING preferred, when he had filled the ends of the pulp canals with iodoform and wax, to cap this with osteo or some similar material, so as to obviate any possibility of the iodoform leaking into the mouth.

Mr. PORTER thought that every man should have a knowledge of the phenomena of inflammation in order to be able to treat dead teeth scientifically. The pulps of teeth often died as the result of a blow. A patient had lately appeared at the hospital with a dead central. The cause of the lesion was very obscure, until she admitted that she walked in her sleep, and, on one occasion had knocked her face against the mantelpiece. The best way to remove a dentalized pulp was to pass up a Donaldson's bristle slightly bent at the end. When rotated this would sweep round the canal and often brought away the pulp entire.

Mr. GASK asked Mr. Cormack why he had omitted to treat of Rhizodontrophy in his paper?

Mr. KNOWLES had found the nerve-destroying fibre sold at the depôts more effective than the plain arsenious acid. The best way to remove a broken piece of drill from the nerve canal was to seal in a little hydrochloric acid.

Mr. PREEDY had recently extracted a tooth which had been filled for some time, but which, though firm, had given constant pain. He found the root well filled, there being neither perforation, exostosis, nor absorption. He thought some septic matter must have been forced through the apex, setting up chronic inflammation. He objected to Rhizodontrophy, since the breath was apt to become tainted thereby.

Mr. MAY advocated the use of as large a drill as possible so as to remove all the infiltrated dentine round the canal.

Mr. BRIAULT asked in reference to lead fillings for roots, whether the metal had any antiseptic properties?

Mr. HERN was surprised that Mr. Cormack had not divided the subject into at least two divisions, treating first—of teeth, the pulps of which had been destroyed by the operator, and, secondly, of those which had died previous to treatment. The after treatment differed widely in each case. He laid stress on the importance of opening up the cavity and funnelling out the orifices of the canals. The object of treatment was to get as near asepticity as possible, though a perfectly aseptic condition was unattainable. In the early stages of treatment only naked instruments should be used, and no cotton wool wrapped round them.

Mr. CORMACK then briefly replied, after which a vote of thanks was accorded to him and to the gentlemen which had brought forwarded *Casual Communications*.

The PRESIDENT then announced that the next meeting would be on January 20th, 1890. This would be the Annual General Meeting, when Mr. E. Preedy would read a paper on "Replantation, Implantation and Transplantation of Teeth."

The proceedings then terminated.

THE NATIONAL DENTAL HOSPITAL STUDENTS' SOCIETY.

A SMOKING Concert was held on the 11th ultimo, at the "Horse Shoe" Hotel, under the presidency of Mr. Charles W. Glassington, M.R.C.S., L.D.S., and, as usual, proved very enjoyable. The greatest attractions perhaps were Mr. Ernest Genet's Recitation, "The Penny Showman," and Mr. Horsfall's Comic Song, a parody on "The Caller Herrin."

Dental News.

QUEEN'S BENCH.

PARTRIDGE *v.* THE GENERAL COUNCIL OF MEDICAL EDUCATION AND REGISTRATION OF THE UNITED KINGDOM.—In this action the plaintiff sued the defendants, who are a quasi-judicial body taking their powers under the Medical Act (21 and 22 Vic., chap. 90), to recover damages, alleging that they had wrongfully and maliciously caused his name to be taken off the Register in June, 1886, and to remain off until ordered by writ of *mandamus* to reinstate it in September, 1887, and that during that period a number of his customers had refused to pay their accounts on the ground that under the Dentists' Act, 1878 (41 and 42 Vict., chap. 33), the plaintiff's name not being upon the Register, he could not at law recover his fees. The defence was in substance that the defendants, as a judicial body, had had certain matters connected with the plaintiff's professional conduct brought before them to decide, and that although the Court of Appeal had decided that their decision had been wrong, yet it was arrived at *bonâ fide* and without malice, and that, therefore, they were not liable in damages to the plaintiff for their mistake in exercising their discretion.

Mr. WADDY, Q.C., and Mr. LYON were for the plaintiff; and Mr. R. T. REID, Q.C., and Mr. MUIR MACKENZIE appeared for the defendants.

Mr. WADDY opened the case, and called the plaintiff, Mr. H. F. PARTRIDGE, who said he practised as a dentist at Sussex House, Sussex-place, Old Brompton-road, and had done so for twenty years. In 1878 the Dentists' Act was passed compelling registration, and so he wished to become a Licentiate in Dental Surgery of the Royal College of Surgeons in Ireland. Witness went to Dublin, and passed the required examinations, and received a diploma, at the same time signing a declaration that while he held it he would not advertise in order to benefit his practice as a dentist, under the penalty of having the diploma cancelled. In February, 1882, he had gone to bed quite well in health, and awoke the next morning totally blind, and he had been so ever since. In order to obtain a living he had formed the South Kensington Ladies' Dental Institute. He had, in fact, advertised that institution. He had found it necessary to do so. He had received a copy of the resolution of the Council for Ireland in July, 1885, and a notification that they had again had under their consideration the fact of his advertising his institution, and that his diploma was cancelled. On July 11th, witness replied to that. On June 8th, 1886, he received a letter from the General Medical Council of Education in England informing him that a meeting of that Council "after due and careful consideration, had decided that his name should be removed from the Register." Witness applied to the Court thereupon for a *mandamus* questioning that decision, and in the result the Court of Appeal ordered his name to be restored, and it was, in September, 1887. During the time that his name was off the Register, he had been unable to sue for or recover any fees. During that time a number of his patients refused to pay him his fees. His out-of-pocket expenses over the whole matter, including his solicitor's costs, had been £36 odd.

Cross-examined by Mr. R. T. REID, Q.C.: The institution was wholly his own business, and all its profits his. From 1882 until now witness had constantly and largely advertised, and had advertised himself as an "L.D.S.," as described in the certificate to his diploma. He meant by that to describe himself as connected with the Irish Royal College of Surgeons. He was aware that by his diploma he had undertaken not to advertise. In 1883 the Dublin College complained of his doing so, and in effect he had promised not to do so any longer. Nevertheless he continued to so advertise. He thought that he had a right to use the title of L.D.S., after his diploma had been cancelled. Since he had been struck off the Register he had still advertised as L.D.S. He could not help himself. He did put L.D.S., on his "plate," but with the word "late" before the L.D.S.

Mr. Baron HUDDLESTON: When was it you put the word "late before the L.D.S.?

Witness: Oh, a few weeks ago.

Cross-examination continued.—During the period you were off the Register was it not a fact that your income had increased?—Yes, that is so, but I ascribe it to the fact that I largely advertised during that period.

Mr. WALTER OLDHAM said he was the plaintiff's secretary since June, 1886. There were only one or two cases where refusals to pay accounts were based on the fact that the plaintiff's name was off the Register.

Cross-examined.—The plaintiff's income increased during the time his name was off the Register.

Mr. R. T. REID then said that as there was no evidence of malice here, this action could not be maintained.

Mr. WADDY, for the plaintiff, argued that the defendants had gone entirely beyond the powers given them by the Legislature, and were therefore liable in damages, there being in fact legal or constructive malice.

Mr. Baron HUDDLESTON said he might say at once that he was prepared to decide that this action would not lie unless malice were proved, and he would therefore suggest that the jury should be discharged and it be left for his decision, in which event either party could go direct to the Court of Appeal.

Mr. WADDY said his client wished the matter to go to the jury.

Mr. Baron HUDDLESTON: But I will not permit it. I have told you I am going to decide the matter at once.

Mr. WADDY: Then I can say no more, my lord.

Mr. Baron HUDDLESTON then gave judgment for the defendants, holding that there was no evidence of malice on the part of the defendants, and that therefore the action did not lie. In reviewing the facts, the learned Baron observed that the defendants, when the matter of the plaintiff's conduct in respect of the violation of his agreement not to advertise was brought to their notice, had taken his name off the Register, and subsequently, by order of the Court of Appeal, they had to reinstate it. But for this were the defendants liable to an action? He did not think it required authority to establish that where persons in a quasi-judicial capacity exercised their discretion wrongly no action could be maintained against them for such a decision unless it could be shown that they arrived at their decision maliciously. Here there was no evidence at all of malice, and the plaintiff must therefore be non-suited and judgment entered for the defendants.

TENTH INTERNATIONAL MEDICAL CONGRESS, BERLIN, 1890.

Regulations and Programme.

I. The Tenth International Medical Congress will be opened in Berlin on Monday, August 4th, 1890, and will be closed on Saturday, August 9th.

II. The Congress shall consist of legally qualified medical men who have inscribed themselves as Members, and have paid for their Card of Membership. Other men of science who interest themselves in the work of the Congress, may be admitted as Extraordinary Members.

Those who take part in the Congress shall pay a subscription of 20 Marks (£1 sterling or 5 dollars), on being enrolled as Members. For this sum they shall receive a copy of the Transactions, as soon as they appear. The enrolment shall take place at the beginning of the Congress. Gentlemen may, however, be enrolled as members by sending the amount of the subscription to the Treasurer,* with their name, professional status, and residence appended.

III. The object of the Congress is an exclusively scientific one.

IV. The work of the Congress will be discharged by eighteen different Sections. The members shall declare upon enrolment, to which Section or Sections they intend more particularly to attach themselves.

---

* Treasurer's Address: Dr. M. Bartels, Berlin SW., Leipzigerstrasse 75. Please to enclose a visiting-card.

V. The Committee of Organisation shall at the opening sitting of the Congress, suggest the Election of a definite Committee (or Bureau) which shall consist of a President, three Vice-Presidents, and of a number—as yet undetermined—of Honorary Presidents and Secretaries.

At the first meeting of each Section a President and certain member of Hon. Presidents shall be elected; these latter shall conduct the business of the Sections in turn with the Presidents.

On account of the different languages employed, a suitable numbers of Secretaries shall be chosen from among the foreign Members. The duties of the foreign Secretaries shall be confined to the sittings of the Congress.

After the termination of the Congress the editing of the Transactions shall be carried out by a Committee, specially appointed for this purpose.

VI. The Congress will assemble daily, either for a General Meeting or for the labours of the different sections.

The General Meetings will be held between 11 and 2 o'clock. Three such meetings will take place.

The time for the sittings of the various sections will be fixed by the special committee of each section, it being understood, however, that no such sittings are to take place during the hours allotted to the General Meetings.

Joint sittings of two or more sections may be held, provided that the Bureau of the Congress can offer suitable rooms for such sittings.

VII. The General Meetings shall be devoted to :—

a. Transactions connected with the work and general management of the Congress.

b. Speeches and communications of general interest.

VIII. Addresses in the general sittings, as well as in any extraordinary meetings which may be determined upon can only be given by those who have been specially requested by the Committee of Organisation.

Proposals relative to the future management of the Congress must be announced to the Committee of Organisation before July 1st, 1890. The Committee shall decide whether these proposals are suitable to be introduced for discussion.

IX. In the sittings of the sections, questions and problems will be discussed, which have been agreed upon by the special Committees of Organisation. The communications of those appointed by the

Committee to report on a subject, shall form the basis of discussion. As far as time.. allows, other communications or proposals, proceeding from members and sanctioned by the Committee of Organisation may also be introduced for discussion. The Bureau of each section decides as to the acceptance of such offered communications, and as to the order in which they shall come before the meeting, always provided that this point has not been already determined in the sitting itself by a decree of the section.

Scientific questions shall not be put to the vote.

X. Introductory addresses in the Sections must as a rule not exceed *twenty minutes in length.* In the discussions no more than *ten minutes* are allowed to each speaker.

XI. All addresses and papers in the general and sectional meetings must be handed over to the Secretaries, in writing, before the end of the sitting. The Editorial-Committee shall decide whether—and to what extent—these written contributions shall be included in the printed Transactions of the Congress. The Members who have taken part in the discussions, will be requested to hand over to the Secretaries, before the end of the day, in writing, the substance of their remarks.

XII. The official languages of all the sittings shall be German, English, and French. The Regulations, the Programme and the Agenda for the day will be printed in all three languages.

It will, however, be allowable to make use of other languages than the above for brief remarks, always provided that one of the Members present is ready to translate the gist of such remarks into one of the official languages.

XIII. The acting president shall conduct the business of each meeting according to the parliamentary rules generally accepted in deliberative assemblies.

XIV. Medical Students and other persons, ladies and gentlemen, who are not physicians but who take a special interest in the work of a particular sitting, may be invited by the President or be allowed to attend the sitting by special permission.

XV. Communications or enquiries regarding the business of separate sections, must be addresssed to the managing members thereof. All other communications and enquiries must be directed to the General Secretary, Dr. Lassar, Berlin NW., 19 Karlstrasse.

The officers of the XIV. Section, that devoted to Diseases of the Teeth are:—Busch, Berlin NW., Alexander-Ufer 6; Calais, Hamburg; Hesse, Leipzig; Fricke, Kiel; Holländer, Halle.

EXTRACTS.

TOXIC SYMPTOMS PRODUCED BY HANDLING PRIMULA OBCONICA.

I HAVE been much perplexed for some months by a series of cases of a most obstinate rash, which looked to me, as well as to some others, very much like urticaria, but which others, again, designated eczema. The cause of it was quite a puzzle to me, and so, indeed, was its effective treatment. I noticed, however, that it usually occurred on exposed parts only—the hands, wrists, and face—and nearly always, so far as my experience went, in well-to-do people who spent much time in greenhouses.

I am much indebted to a lady for showing me a letter in the *Gardener's Chronicle* of August 3rd last, who has herself been a sufferer for more than eighteen months from this rash, accompanied with dyspeptic symptoms. She has paid great attention to diet, and tried many medicinal remedies, local and general, but could obtain no relief except by going away. On her return home, however, the rash invariably reappeared. She spends very much time in her greenhouse, and has been in the habit of often handling the primula obconica. Since reading the letter in the *Gardener's Chronicle* she has left off touching the plant, except by way of experiment, and has been free from her trouble; but by way of experiment she has handled the plant a few times, which has always resulted in the return of the rash and the dyspeptic symptoms. Further, two of her nephews, who have been staying with her, have handled the plant to test its effect upon them, and have suffered from the rash in the same way.

In one case, which I have recently seen, the irritation of the skin was intense, and there was extreme swelling of the face, with much œdema of the eyelids, so as to cause a horrible temporary disfigurement. The cause, therefore, seems very clearly indicated, it being obvious that the primula obconica must be let alone, unless one wishes to be stung; but it may be well that these effects should have been observed that they may not be confounded with eczema or other diseases of obscure origin.—CHARLES E. OLDACRES, M.R.C.S. in *British Medical Journal.*

RESECTION OF THE INFERIOR DENTAL NERVE.

Service of T. L. Gilmer, M.D., D.D.S.

This case calls for surgical interference, namely, resection of the inferior dental nerve. This gentleman, the patient, is thirty-seven years old. He has suffered from facial neuralgia for over nine years. He tells me that when he first noticed the pain it was situated in the body of the inferior maxillary bone, at a point corresponding to the roots of the second bicuspid tooth on the right side, and still remains most prominently here. Later on he has had a slight pain in the gum on the lingual side of the jaw, but this pain is not always felt as is the one deeply seated in the bone. If it was, or if the pain at this point was independent of the other, we should feel doubtful if action of the inferior dental nerve anterior to the point where the mylohyoid branch (which supplies the gum where the pain is located) is given off would afford relief, as it would indicate that the lesion was posterior to this division. The probabilities are that the deep-seated pain felt in the jaw, and which is easily excited by a touch on the lip over the mental foramen, or by a draught of cold air on this side of the face, indicates the location of the lesion, and that the pain felt in the gum is reflected from this point, and that it will pass away with the removal of a section of the inferior dental nerve. The patient has been treated medicinally by skilful physicians with but temporary relief, and has had two sound teeth extracted with no benefit. Before section of a nerve for neuralgia, the mouth should be thoroughly examined to determine whether there may not be some peripheral irritation, which may cause the pain. In this case we find none, and I conclude the operation for section of the inferior dental nerve indicated. We will perform the operation known as Garretson's operation. We wish to perform it as nearly aseptically as possible, so that we will have adhesion of the soft parts by first intention, or cicatrization without suppuration. To this end, with the exception of the hand-piece of the dental engine, we sterilize the instruments to be used by placing them in boiling water for a few minutes. The hand-piece we dip in a 50 per cent. solution of carbolic acid in glycerine. The hands are thoroughly cleansed with soap and warm water, afterwards washed in 1-4000 bichloride solution. The instruments, after sterilization, are laid on and covered by a towel wrung out of a 1-2000 bichloride solution. The face, having been shaved, is washed in the 1-2000 bichloride. Among the more prominent precautions to be observed in performing this operation, are, first, not to sever the facial artery, and, second, if possible not to sever the inferior dental artery.

The facial artery is easily found, since it passes over the base of the jaw in the notch just anterior to the angle. Placing the thumb of the left hand on the artery, the soft tissues are severed on the base of the bone from the thumb forward, to a point slightly in advance of the mental foramen. The incision is made at the base of the jaw in preference to one higher up, that the scar may be as nearly hidden from view as possible. The soft tissues are now turned up so that the inferior dental canal may be reached. We now seek out the mental foramen which we find greatly constricted. This constriction may be the secret of the trouble, but as I am not certain that the cause lies here, I will remove a section of the nerve posterior to the foramen. With this circular saw I will make two parallel incisions in the bone about three-sixteenths of an inch apart, extending from the mental foramen immediately over the dental canal nearly as far back as the cut in the soft tissues. The two incisions in the bone are connected posteriorly by this small trephine. With an excavator the narrow strip of the outer plate of the bone is easily turned out exposing the vessels. The nerve is taken up with this small tenaculum and raised from its bed, care being exercised not to injure the dental artery. That part of the nerve posterior to the opening in the bone is thoroughly stretched and then partly cut and partly torn off just back of the incision in the bone; that part anterior to this is removed from its bed and severed at the mental foramen. The edges of the bone are now nicely rounded and the particles of tooth syringed away with the bichloride solution, and the wound thoroughly washed, first with ether to remove the fat which might interfere with the healing process, then with alcohol to further remove fat and for its antiseptic qualities. The wound is now closed by carbolized silk sutures and the parts washed with the carbolic acid solution in glycerine. The line of incision is covered with Lister protective taken direct from the bichloride solution and on this the moist lint antiseptic dressing is placed, the whole being covered with gutta-percha film. The bandage supports the parts. Unless there are indications of suppuration this dressing will not be disturbed under five or six days, when if the case progresses favorably, the sutures may be removed.—*Dental Review*.

COLD WATER IN FACIAL NEURALGIA.

Dr. E. Orvin Barker writes:—"What I have to say on this subject will perhaps not be new to many readers of the *Brief*, while to very many it will no doubt be.

Some two years ago I was called in to see a patient who was being treated by Dr. G., of this place, for facial neuralgia. The doctor being absent at the time, I found the patient—a large, muscular man, about thirty years of age—suffering excruciating pain in one side of the face, with eye almost swollen shut. I gave him a large dose of sulph. morphia, hypodermically, assured him that it would relieve him, and left. Perhaps two hours after, I met Dr. G., and told him what I had done and that perhaps he had better call and see the man. He requested me to stop with him, and on going in we found patient suffering very much, and the family applying hot applications to the face, which they had been doing from the beginning of the attack.

Dr. G. had them remove the hot applications and replace them with cold; and in one minute the patient was easy and had no more trouble in controlling the attack.

Some time after this I called one morning to see a Mr. H., a large stout man of about fifty, and found him suffering great pain in one side of the face, and his wife constantly applying hot applications. Remembering the case above referred to, I ordered the hot applications removed and replaced by cold, and almost immediately the whole muscular system seemed to relax, and the patient cried out that he was gone, that he was dying, and called his wife and son to him and bade them good-bye. Of course they were greatly frightened, and I was accused of killing him. But a glance at the patient was sufficient to tell me that he was not dying. However, I told them to remove the cold cloth and in a very few seconds he was painfully reminded that he was not a corpse by any means. A hypodermic injection of morphia sulph. soon relieved the pain.

Not long ago I was called to see a lady, perhaps thirty years of age, who was subject to, and suffering at the time with a severe attack of the same trouble, and was treating it with hot applications. This patient thought that she could not take morphia, so I concluded to try the effect of cold water. Accordingly, I applied a cloth wet with cold water, and very soon the patient remarked that she felt so queer, and then cried out that she was sinking, and called her husband to her and seemed to think that she was actually dying. As in the other case the cloth was removed and the pain soon returned, and had to be relieved by the use of other remedies.

Now, what was the cause of the strange feelings? Was it all owing to the shock to the nervous system, caused by the sudden change from hot to cold? Or was it partially due to a sort of an ecstasy resulting from the instant relief from such great pain?

I am inclined to think that in both cases, as it did in the first, it would have resulted in a cure had the cold been retained.

Have any of the brethren had a similiar experience?—*Medical Brief.*

BIRMINGHAM DENTAL HOSPITAL.

The number of patients treated during the month of October was 443—Males, 119; Females, 170; Children under ten years of age, 154. The operations were as follows:—Extractions, 460; gold fillings, 11; other fillings, 65; miscellaneous and advice, 96. Anæsthetics were administered in 21 cases.—FRED. R. HOWARD, *House Surgeon.*

MONTHLY STATEMENT of operations performed at the two Dental Hospitals in London, and at the Dental Hospital, Manchester, from October 31st, to November 30th 1889:—

		London.	National	Victoria.
Number of Patients attended		——	1820	1191
Extractions	Children under 14 ...	342	316	748
	Adults	927	452	
	Under Nitrous Oxide ...	923	798	136
Gold Stoppings		455	98	44
Other Stoppings...		1420	466	151
Advice		——	434	——
Irregularities of the Teeth		80	70	——
Miscellaneous and Dressings		755	115	430
Total		4,902	2,749	1 509

THE DENTAL RECORD, LONDON: JAN. 1, 1890.

THE DENTAL YEAR.

In very many respects the year 1889 will be remembered as a noticeable one. There have been signs not a few of progress, both within and without the dental fold. One of the matters which have engaged the most attention has been the question of dental education. Alike among those who lead and those who are led has education been widely discussed, nor has the matter ended with words, distinct steps have been taken which will modify the careers of the future members of the profession. By the recent enactment of the Royal College of Surgeons the curriculum is considerably modified and approximated in scope to that which obtains for the general medical student. Again, with the view of expanding the teaching of the general hospital to meet the requirements of the dental student, a fully equipped dental school has been inaugurated at Guy's Hospital, and quite recently a dental laboratory has been added. A staff of dentists, lecturers, and anæsthetists occupy the school, and are prepared to teach students the special subjects germane to the domain of dentistry. The Guy's Hospital Dental Department has, we believe, received the recognition of the College of Surgeons.

Special efforts have also been made at the dental hospitals by means of demonstrations to give additional facilities for the acquisition of modern modes of treatment, such as cannot be as yet included in the formal lectures or work of the stopping-room. A fresh departure has been made, also, in the direction of teaching simple facts about the physiology, hygiene, and pathology of the the teeth to popular audiences, with a view to checking the thoughtless disregard of the uneducated for matters connected with the preservation of the teeth. The benefits accruing to the indigent poor by the increase of hospital accommodation have been increased during the year, notably by the opening of the Dublin Dental Hospital, and erection of the new buildings for the Edinburgh Dental Hospital and School. The societies have not been idle. The Odontological Society has introduced some valuable papers, and held discussions upon eminently practical and useful subjects. Among the papers we may specially note the careful utterances of Mr. Jonathan Hutchinson, F.R.S., dealing with Pyorrhœa alveolaris and other dental matters, and the incisive contribution ot Dr. Ferrier, who, in dealing with reflex neuroses referable to the fifth pair of cranial nerves, applied to these curious affections the recent researches of Gaskell upon the sympathetic system. Again, the utility of the papers and discussions upon electricity applied to dentistry, antisepticism and the mechanical restoration of lost parts about the mouth and face, and of the peculiarly instructive evenings devoted to mechanical dentistry and, cases in practice, can hardly be overestimated. Kindred discussions have marked the meetings of the Odonto-Chirurgical Society of Scotland and the Odontological Society of Manchester, as well as those of the provincial branches of the British Dental Association.

Among the noticeable events of the year has been the Annual General Meeting of the Association at Brighton, one of the most successful gatherings of English dentists. Much interest was centred in the discussion upon general anæsthetics, in which Mr. Bailey, Dr. Dudley Buxton, Dr. Cruise, Dr. Hewitt and Mr. Bowman Macleod took part.

Another event connected with anæsthetics was the unfortunate death of Lady Milne in Edinburgh, but which seems to have been only indirectly, if at all, attributable to the action of nitrous oxide gas. The incident naturally gave rise to much comment.

Cocaine has during the year received much attention, and a considerable number of cases have been reported in which toxic symptoms manifested themselves. Added to these, instances of addiction to the "cocaine-habit," and a terrible list of its attendant sufferings have been brought to light. While more insidious than morphinomania, the cocaine-habit seems less curable and more easily acquired.

Besides the general meeting at Brighton, the British Dental Association has been active in other directions, and has brought to a successful issue more than one prosecution instituted by it under the enactments of the Dentists' Act.

During the summer, Paris being *en fête* with her splendid exhibition, the opportunity was taken to hold a congress of dentists to discuss professional subjects, the English section being under the presidency of Sir John Tomes, F.R.S. A congress was also held by German dentists in Hamburg to deliberate upon the best means of consolidating the profession in Germany.

Perhaps the subjects which have during the year received the most wide discussion, if we omit dental education, are advertising by dentists, and dental designations. Many suggestions have been offered to facilitate discrimination by the public between dentists and unregistered practitioners, one, which, however, met with but slight support, being to adopt the word "dentist" as a prefix to the name as is the use in the case of medical men who are called "doctor." Among the most noteworthy legal items of the year was the case in which a plaintiff was nonsuited while attempting to obtain damages from Messrs. Cottam for an alleged unskilled dental operation. The evidence showed that the dentist had used all reasonable skill, and that the claimant had, upon the onset of hæmorrhage, made no attempt to obtain advice from the dentist.

Death has been busy during the year, besides numerous members of the profession who have passed away, we have had to chronicle the loss of Mr. Spence Bate, F.R.S., at once a dentist and scientist, and that of Dr. John Wreford Langmore, so long associated, to its benefit, with dental literature, alike as sub-editor of the *Transactions* of the Odontological Society of Great Britain and of the *Journal* of the British Dental Association.

Dentistry, as an art, has not stood still. Its technical progress has been great in the direction of the application of gold crowns to broken-down teeth. Porcelain facings and inlays (by How's method) have received some support, and Bar and Bridge Work has been brought more upon its trial in this country. The consensus of opinion seeming to be, that provided the cases are carefully selected, these procedures are distinctly of value.

It is hoped that the DENTAL RECORD has passed through the year with advantage to its readers; it has developed in what it is deemed are several useful directions, not only affording increased space for original articles from members of the profession, but through its correspondence columns and under the novel heading of "Notes and Queries," offering a wide field for individual effort from those dentists who, while without time for lengthy papers, have yet leisure sufficient to give their fellow workers brief hints in manipulative procedure or new methods. It is to be observed that the value of these columns becomes greatly enhanced when all unite to contribute some note, however brief, or suggest some pertinent question likely to elicit useful replies.

STUDENTS' SOCIETY OF THE DENTAL HOSPITAL OF LONDON SMOKING CONCERT.—On the 11th of December the second of the series of smoking concerts took place. Dr. Dudley Buxton occupied the chair. Thanks to the energy of the honorary secretary, Mr. Forsyth, a most successful and pleasant evening was spent. The programme was got through in good time, and consisted of some excellent singing and equally good recitations. Among the singers, Mr. Wheatley and Mr. Giles rendered their very diverse songs with great effect, while Mr. Garcia won great plaudits for his recitations. The Dental Hospital Musical Society sang some glees with much feeling, and were loudly applauded.

ANNOUNCEMENT.

ODONTOLOGICAL SOCIETY OF GREAT BRITAIN.

THE Annual General Meeting of this Society takes place on January 13th, at 8 p.m., at 40 Leicester Square. *Business*—Election of officers. President's Valedictory Address. *Paper by* Dr. Scanes Spicer on "Nasal Obstruction and Mouth Breathing as Factors in the Etiology of Diseases of the Teeth."

APPOINTMENTS.

ANDERSON, GEORGE H., has been appointed Dental Surgeon to the Exeter and District Medical Association (first appointment).

BRIGGS, H. FIELDER., L.D.S., D.D.S. (Mich.), has been appointed House Surgeon to the Liverpool Dental Hospital.

BAINES, ARTHUR, L.D.S.I., of Hanley, has been elected Honorary Dental Surgeon to the North Staffordshire Infirmary, Stoke-upon-Trent, *vice* W. Bartlett, M.R.C.S., L.D.S., resigned.

KEKWICK, I. F., L.D.S.I., has been appointed Honorary Dental Surgeon to the Cumberland Infirmary, Carlisle, *vice* Warwick Hele, L.D.S., resigned.

GOSSIP.

IN another column will be found an interesting account of the toxic systems which may be produced by handling the *primula obconica*. A patient of our own has suffered precisely in the way described, and has been free from what her doctor called "gouty eczema" since she discarded her favourite flower, which she liked to have in her bedroom.

SOME little time since a correspondence took place in the columns of a medical contemporary anent "maggots as a cause of dental caries." The following letter of Mr. L. B. Brunton, of Commercial Road, E., revives the matter :—"Henbane seeds are still not uncommonly used for toothache, under the impresssion that the ailment is caused by worms in the decayed teeth. A penny is made hot in the fire, and immediately on removal a pinch of the seeds is dropped on it, and the whole covered at once with a wineglass, which becomes filled with thick fumes. The glass is then applied to the mouth and the smoke inhaled, when the worms are supposed to be expelled. I called one morning to see a patient who had just used the remedy, and I naturally essayed to correct his notion of the cause of his malady; but he smiled in a superior manner, and said that he had not only seen the worms on two or three occasions, but could show me three in the glass he had recently used. There, sure enough, were three little brown-headed larvæ—or, at all events, they looked exactly like larvæ to the naked eye—but on examining them at home under a 2-inch glass, their true nature was explained. They were simply the embryos of three seeds which had been forcibly expelled on the rupture of their seed-coats and had adhered to the moist side of the glass, and thus escaped the destruction which had overtaken the rest. Science was triumphant; my patient confessed his defeat, and remarked that he had long known that we must not believe all we *hear*, but found also that we must not believe all we *see*."

THE *Dental Record*, the official journal of the Students' Society of the New York College of Dentistry, has completed its first volume. The *Dental Record* (N. Y. C. D.) is the first journal started by dental students in America, and the volume just completed shows considerable merit and plenty of promise of better things to come.

WERE not the matter too serious a one with which to joke, it might be suggested that in Dublin with its Dental Hospital and very active *corps dentaire*, there were simpler methods of curing toothache than killing oneself, yet poor Dinnage seems not to have known of them. For recently an inquest was held before Mr. R. Blagden, at Monk's Common, Nuthurst, touching the death of a young man, aged eighteen, named William Dinnage. It appeared from the evidence that the poor fellow suffered the most excruciating torture from the toothache for the last four or five months, during which time he was observed to cry, day by day, for hours together. The jury found that the deceased committed suicide while laboring under temporary insanity, induced, the coroner stated, by the torture to which he was subjected.

CORRESPONDENCE.

[We do not hold ourselves irresponsible in any way for the opinions expressed by our correspondents.]

NITROUS OXIDE AS AN ANÆSTHETIC.—A REPLY.

To the Editor of the DENTAL RECORD.

SIR,—I have neither time nor inclination for a prolonged personal controversy with Dr. Dudley Buxton on the action of nitrous oxide gas. With the assistance of my colleagues in the physiological laboratory of King's College I am engaged in a series of observations and experiments on the operation of various gases, the details of which will in due course be published, with the result of proving not only that nitrous oxide is a rapidly asphyxiating gas, but that its anæsthetic action is a simple result of its deoxidising influence. Meanwhile, Dr. Dudley Buxton's paper in the last number of the DENTAL RECORD contains some statements upon which I feel called upon to offer a few brief comments.

I deny the accuracy of what Dr. Dudley Buxton is pleased to call a "logical analysis" of my explanation of nitrous oxide anæsthesia, from which it would appear that my knowledge of the asphyxial phenomena of nitrous oxide inhalation has been mainly obtained "*In conversation* with friends."

In his attempt to prove that nitrous oxide is "not an asphyxiant," Dr. Dudley Buxton says that "it produces anæsthesia before it kills, whereas animals simply asphyxiated (rendered apnœic) are not anæsthetic until moribund, if then." No one of course would deny the first proposition; and in my letter in your October number I say that "nitrous oxide may induce anæsthesia without complete asphyxia," but to deny that anæsthesia may result from simple apnœa is to ignore the numerous cases of recovery from suspended animation (anæsthesia) by drowning, and other forms of apnœa, and the narcosis which precedes death in many cases of asphyxiating pulmonary and cardiac disease.

Dr. Dudley Buxton says, "the wild conscious convulsions which obtain, when death is brought about by asphyxia, find no place in the procession of events under laughing gas." In this sentence no distinction is made between the *conscious strugglings* which occur immediately after the exclusion of the air and the *unconscious convulsions* which are of constant occurrence in the final stage of asphyxia. That similar unconscious convulsions invariably occur when nitrous oxide inhalation is carried beyond a certain point will scarcely be denied even by Dr. Dudley Buxton, for in his book on "Anæsthetics" he says (p. 37) "In giving nitrous oxide to children the face-piece should be removed with the very first sign of jactitation, otherwise their small bodies become so convulsed that it is difficult to keep them still for operation, and valuable time is lost in the attempt to place them in a convenient position for operation." That these convulsions are identical with those which occur in the last stage of asphyxia (apnœa), and that they are of an epileptiform character will, I think, be admitted by every competent pathologist.

I am well aware that Dr. Snow had no knowledge of nitrous oxide as an anæsthetic, but I venture to say that if he had lived long enough to study the action of the gas he would have looked upon it as affording additional evidence in support of his theory that the common action of all anæsthetics is to impede the oxidation of the nervous tissues. Dr. Dudley Buxton charges me with "ignorance, or a curious ignoring" of Paul Bert's researches upon a mixture of nitrous oxide and oxygen. Having long since had the advantage of studying Dr. Dudley Buxton's able treatise on anæsthetics, I cannot plead ignorance of Paul Bert's experiments with the compressed gases in Fontaine's chamber. But Dr. Dudley Buxton admits that "the large and expensive chamber and apparatus render its use, except in hospitals, almost impossible," and in my letter to you I referred only to what I had seen of Dr. Frederic Hewitt's simpler and more practicable method—a method which has the advantage of preventing the occurrence of cyanosis and other asphyxial phenomena, to conceal which the late Mr. Clover, who will be admitted to have been an experienced and skilful administrator of the gas, was in the habit of covering the patient's face with a handkerchief.

I am, Sir, Yours, &c.,

GEORGE JOHNSON, M.D., F.R.S.,

Emeritus Professor of Clinical Medicine.
Physician Extraordinary to H.M. the Queen

Savile Row, *December* 17*th*, 1889.

GROVES & THORPS CHEMICAL TECHNOLOGY.

To the Editor of the DENTAL RECORD.

SIR,—The writer of the part of this work referring to coal gas has made use of my name pretty freely, but apparently the bulk of his quotations are from old trade lists which are not usually the sources from which theory and calculations are likely to be obtained for a work on Chemical Technology, and this is probably the reason why the article in question is so very deficient in necessary information. On page 431 it is stated "there exists no information as to the influence exerted by the shape and dimensions of the gas nozzle, and of the delivery tube for the mixture of gas and air" . . . . "there is no rule to guide in fixing the proportion." Any one who is at all conversant with the subject, is fully aware that this matter was worked out by myself, and that the full details of the theoretical construction of burners are given in the *Transactions* of the Gas Institute for 1883. Another serious error is the analogy the writer attempts to draw between light and heat from coal gas, the conditions as regards pressures and other matters being in many cases exactly the reverse of each other.

It is well known that the practice of heating by gas is in a state of rapid transition and evolution; this is too much for the writer of the article, who specifies a pattern four years old and quite superseded, as the "newest." On page 401, I am made to say "that gas fires cost from 1d. to 4d. per hour;" this might have been true years ago, but it is very far indeed from the truth now. Out of sixty modern gas fires tested by myself, the maximum consumption of the largest was 40 cubic feet per hour at $\frac{8}{10}$ pressure, which at 2s. 1d. per 1,000 cubic feet, is exactly one penny per hour; the minimum consumption of the smallest is seven feet per hour, being about one penny for six hours.

The writer makes several remarks about absence of proof and figures for certain statements made in trade lists, whilst his own statements as to the relative radiation of coal fires and gas fires are not only vague, but are on the face of them absolutely incorrect and incapable of proof, and states that he does not know why I call a gas stove a gas fire. As I never did such a thing, I should be curious to know where he got his information from.

It is not at all necessary to evolve a new theory as to the general antipathy to stove or convected heat being "prejudice or rays of less refrangibility:" even "old trade lists" would have explained that with convected heat the lower part of the room is always the coldest, and cold feet and heated upper extremities are not conducive to comfort. If the writer had copied the American habit of lifting his feet out of the colder air near the floor level he would have understood that no new theory was required, and that the cause was very well known.

I am, Yours &c.,

THOS. FLETCHER, F.C.S.

AUSTRALIAN DENTISTS.

To the Editor of the DENTAL RECORD.

SIR,—For the past three years I have been (through your agents, Gordon & Gotch, Brisbane) a subscriber to your journal, but have never yet met with any contributions to its pages from Australian dentists. What is the reason of this? It cannot be want of subject matter to write about, nor can it be that their whole attention is devoted to local journalism, for there is not a single paper devoted to dentistry in the colonies. I have noticed in my travels about Australia that very few members of the profession subscribe to a Dental Magazine. Not long since, I visited a dentist in Brisbane, and remarked to him the absence of dental works in his bookcase. "Oh!" said he, "books and journals are all rot; I don't believe in book learning." "Then," said I, "how do you keep pace with the times in your knowledge of the profession." "I learned my *trade* when a boy, and I flatter myself that I am a better workman than any of your men with college degrees" was his reply. I fear he is not the only Australian dentist who rejoices in the same opinion of himself. Unfortunately, the Dental Act has not yet found its way to our shores, and judging by the state of Medical and Pharmacy Acts generally, and the difficulties the members of the medical profession have to contend with, opposed and baffled in every direction by an army of quacks, who may make post-mortem examinations and give certificates of deaths, it will be some time before the L.D.S., or any other dental qualification, can look for protection by Act of Parliament in Australia. Most of the large towns teem with dentists (?) more especially Sydney, and no wonder. The only qualification necessary to enable, I cannot say entitle, one to practice dentistry in Australia, is plenty (to use a slang term) of good, unblushing Australian cheek, without which even the F.R.C.S., L.D.S., &c., would fail to secure patronage. Some short time ago I wrote to a firm of dentists in one of our capital towns, asking them to do some gold work for me, in reply to which they suggested I should call on them, pay them £50, for which sum they guaranteed to teach me the *trade* in a few months, and mentioning several young men whom they had turned out of their establishment in three months, full fledged dentists, as practical illustrations of their ability to do so. What a chance for the village barber to become a barber-dentist again. It is most amusing to see the various modes of advertising that some of these professional (?) men adopt. When in Sydney, some short time ago, I saw a lad parading the street clothed in the uniform of the 1st Life Guards, with the following advertisement painted on his cuirass, "Teeth painlessly extracted, 1s.; artificial teeth, 5s. each; full sets, £5. Fit and workmanship guaranteed. N_2.O. Gas administered daily. No extra charge. Roll up and give —— & Co., the Dental Artists, a turn. No. —— Street." Another exhibits wax figures in his window showing various operations. Another employs a boy to stand at his front door and distribute gem photos of the dental artist upstairs. In North Queensland we are well supplied with dentists. In this little town of about 1,500 inhabitants, there are three struggling for a living. This colony will, when we have a Land Act suitable to the nature of the country, that will enable the white man to make a living on the land, become a good field for the dentist who has had a thorough training, but at present there is not sufficient population to support one in a permanent practice. Children born and brought up in this Northern colony as a rule lose their temporary teeth a few months after cutting them. Disease usually attacks the upper incisors first, then the lower molars. It is quite a common thing to see a young lad at fourteen years of age without a sound tooth in his mouth, yet with the Aboriginals and Chinese half-casts it is quite the reverse. I should think specimens of Aboriginal dentition, showing first and second, or any irregularities, would be interesting to dental students who have not had the opportunity of studying the anatomy of the head or neck of the untamed native of Northern Queensland. If you can suggest a safe mode of forwarding such a parcel to your office, I should be happy to comply with any reasonable request, and supply you with specimens. Trusting that I am not encroaching upon your valuable space, and that I may shortly be able to communicate something of interest to the profession, such perhaps as "Dentistry as Practised by the Queensland Blackfellow,"

I am, Yours &c.,

20th October, 1889. YANNA MEENA.

GAS OPERATIONS.

To the Editor of the DENTAL RECORD.

SIR,—The letter of your correspondent "Mr. George Seymour," cannot but prove interesting, especially to the junior practitioner, and as one recently qualified, I ask leave by criticism, to add matter that may further the discussion. The little I know anent the methods pursued in England, necessarily confines my remarks to the north, where the veritable heads of our profession administer gas, and operate without assistance.

Naturally, with such examples before me, I must disagree with the strictures of your correspondent, when he considers my teachers "quite dishonest" in their gas operations. That their method is open to grave criticism I cannot deny, but is it not going too far, to stamp one dishonest, because he follows the method adopted in his own particular country? Were I to refuse the administration of gas, without the presence of a medical gentleman, I know my dental brethren, and indeed many medical practitioners, would consider I had no confidence in myself.

As it is, I never operate under gas without the presence of an assistant who is trained to be of service should any untoward incident occur. Again, I believe I have read all matter published anent the subject; have intimately studied the lungs, the heart, and their diseases, and am therefore justified in thinking I, at least am not dishonest, and that my patients may have every confidence in any operation I may undertake.

In a limited extent I agree with Mr. Seymour, and look upon the question of gas as the root of the evil he so dogmatically brings before your readers. At least, so far as many of our junior L.D.S.'s are concerned, they operate with no assistance whatever, at all hours, and accept fees that the most rampant charlatan could not but consider miserable.

This condition of things must ere long bring disgrace on an honourable profession, and all of us will gladly welcome any practical suggestion to lessen the evil. Enclosing my card,

I am, Sir, Yours most sincerely,

Edinburgh, *December 26th*, 1889. A RECENT L.D.S.

THE DENTAL RECORD.

VOL. X. FEBRUARY 1ST, 1890. No. 2.

Original Communications.

THE USE AND ABUSE OF THE DENTAL ENGINE.

By WILLIAM RUSHTON, L.D.S.

AT the present time there are very few dentists who do not use, and find the benefit of, the dental engine, though some practitioners look upon it as totally unnecessary, besides being a barbarous instrument and a terror to their patients. These gentlemen—the small minority—maintain that they can do their work by the aid of chisels, hand-drills, excavators, and files, in a manner perfectly satisfactory to their patients and themselves, and that to introduce the dental engine extensively, or even at all, into their practice, would be detrimental to their interests, and would frighten their patients away.

The minority certainly have a right to be heard, and we must confess that, to a certain extent, they have good cause for their abstinence from the use of the dental engine. We have all encountered the patient who exclaims in a tone, more in sorrow than in anger, "Oh! are you going to use that dreadful thing?" and we who have experienced the sensation of the swiftly rotating burr on our own sensitive dentine (and every dentist ought) know there is good cause for the terror often evinced by our nervous patients when they see us fixing a burr and placing our foot on the treadle.

I said the other day to a brother dentist, whom I much respect, "How is it you cannot get your patients to stand your using the engine?" He said, "My dear sir, I can; my patients will let me do what I like, if I tell them it is necessary; but they will like it none the better, and will seize the first opportunity of leaving me." I afterwards watched this gentleman prepare and fill a cavity with hand instruments, using them with great skill, and though I thought that the violence with which he had sometimes to use his chisels and excavators compared unfavourably with the action of the dental engine on similar hard tissues, and though his edges were not as perfect as if he had gone round them with a finishing burr, yet the work was good, and had every appearance of lasting, and showed what could be done in a somewhat awkward cavity in a short time by hand instruments only.

But although the work was good, it was not as good as if the cavity had been prepared with the aid of the dental engine; although the operator was rapid he took a longer time than if he had used the engine, and, as I have remarked before, his chisels and excavators were used with such violence, that it seemed to my mind that a sharp burr on the engine would have been far preferable. Therefore, I say, granting that I am correct in these statements, it seems to me a mistake in these gentlemen, from a notion of not frightening their patients, to discard an instrument capable of doing so much.

But, on the other hand, I am quite certain the engine has got itself disliked by the public, owing, to a great extent, to its abuse. We know perfectly well that we cannot do honest dentistry without giving occasional pain, however careful we may be, and "painless dentistry" is well known to be synonymous with "arrant quackery." Now, the dental engine not only gives physical pain, but what is often far worse, gives mental pain and great nervous strain. It is not always so much the actual pain the instrument may give, but it is the dread in the patient's mind of what it may do if it slips. The appearance, too, of the instrument is not in its favour. It is not like the young man "whose appearance was the best testimonial to character." Patients hate the sight of it, even the jar of the burr on the teeth (especially when a coarse cut burr or a corundum stone is used) is unbearable to many persons, and when this is accompanied by the thought "what if that thing should slip and fly wildly round my mouth" (a thought ever present to the minds of some patients) we can easily understand how they dislike its use.

The chief practical points seem to me to be, firstly, only use the engine when necessary. I once had some conversation with a gentleman, who told me his trouble was to get an assistant "who was not wedded to the dental engine," as he found this matrimonial alliance not followed by the propagation of more patients, but on the contrary, a diminution of his practice. Very often a well directed sweep of the chisel or excavator will do all that is required, and as Opie mixed his colours "with brains" so we ought to mix a little common sense in the use of our tools, and not proceed by stereotyped rules, as no two patients are alike. I have seen dentists use the dental engine to clear out disintegrated and softened dentine from a cavity; there would be quite as much sense in cutting a cream cheese with a steam saw. On the other hand, in shaping up the cavity the engine is invaluable; in making retaining points, undercuts, and trimming edges, we must all acknowledge its use, as also for finishing off fillings, polishing with discs, corundums, &c. Of course all this can be done by hand, but who would take the time and trouble to walk to Brighton if he can go Pullman express.

Secondly, our burrs must be sharp, and all our gear in good order. A blunt burr gives far more trouble to us and pain to our patient than a sharp one, yet how many dentists there are who neglect this important point (the same remarks apply to excavators), and the dental engine gets the credit of the extra pain and trouble. Some dentists sharpen their own burrs, but the usual way is to send them to be sharpened to the depôts, and by having two sets, one can always be in use while the other is being sharpened or kept in reserve. The engine, too, should be well oiled, taking care to use no oil which smells, better have an oil which clogs than one which offends your patient's olfactory sense. The cord of the engine should not be too tight or too loose, as it slipping, or the engine stopping, or the burr catching in the rubber dam, all may give your patient a shock, and help to earn the engine a bad name.

Thirdly, use the utmost discretion in using the engine, about guarding against the hand slipping, &c.

There are some patients, children, invalids, and highly neurotic subjects, in whose case it is sometimes advisable not to think of using the engine. You may not in such cases put in as good work as you would like, but better put in work of a temporary character than frighten these subjects away from the ministration of the dentist, and perhaps let irremediable mischief be done.

Children who have not been previously frightened, as a rule will not mind the engine *if you do not hurt them*, and children up to, say twelve years old, should not be hurt if possible, as they conceive a dislike to visiting the dentist, and therefore conceal tooth mischief from their parents. It is a good plan to use the dental engine with a child, even if you do next to nothing with it, as it accustoms the child to its use, and on a future occasion it will not rebel against its being used.

Choose a suitable burr, and do not plunge *in medias res* at once, but touch the tooth with the burr, constantly taking it off and putting it on again, till you see how your patient bears it; and even in good patients I think it is advisable never to keep the burr on the tooth for more than two or three seconds at a time, as it gives them relief from that nerve tension they all suffer from during its application.

Always steady your finger or thumb on a neighbouring tooth (the same remark applies to the chisels and excavators) so that if your burr happens to slip it cannot slip far, and if you find your patient starts, make it slip again in the same way two or three times *on purpose* and they begin to see it was a mistake for them to think your hand was not steady, and that you are doing it for some special reason.

The burr need never be pressed very hard upon the tooth; if the burr is sharp it will not require that, if it is blunt, reject it. I have heard of dentists taking the temper out of a burr by pressure and swift rotation, I should think it would also take the temper out of the patient.

In summing up these few thoughts, I think we may say that those who use the engine too much, and those who use it too little or not at all, are equally unwise, that it has found a lasting and honoured place in our dental armoury, and that it remains for us, by a wise and prudent use of it, to get its full services without unduly martyrising our patients, teaching them that it is a beneficent and time saving friend not only for the operator, but for the patient.

IMMEDIATE TORSION.

By W. Scott Thomson, M.R.C.S., L.D.S.

A case of a nature by no means uncommon, but very troublesome to treat, presented itself to me some few months ago. A girl 15 years of age having the superior lateral incisors twisted through a segment of a circle, the lingual surface looking towards the central incisors as is usual in these cases. The teeth were small and the necks of nearly cylindrical form. A vulcanite plate was constructed, having four pieces of piano-wire attached, two lingual and two buccal, so as to impinge upon the misplaced teeth, and in the course of two months considerable improvement was evident, they being very nearly in correct position. The patient then leaving England for educational purposes, a retaining plate was made, and I proposed to complete the treatment when she should return—in three months. However, whilst she was away the plate became loose and uncomfortable, and, although a dentist was consulted where she was staying, nothing was done, so the plate was laid aside, and when she again presented herself to me the teeth were *in statu quo*. The parents were very anxious that something should be done but had only a few weeks to remain in town. The laterals were slightly less firm than the contiguous teeth, due, I surmised, to the sockets having become somewhat enlarged from the previous treatment, and, as I have before said, the teeth were small and conical, I therefore decided to try immediate or forcible torsion. Previous to the operation an impression was taken, and the right lateral sawn off the plaster model and replaced in the desired position in the arch, and a vulcanite frame with a gold cap to fit over this tooth was constructed; gas being administered, the right lateral was grasped with forceps and rotated, but considerable force had to be used, the tooth becoming elongated and loose. The plate was at once adjusted. Not thinking it advisable to operate on the other side until I saw the result of this, and yet, not wishing to lose time, I commenced to treat the other mechanically. Without going into details, suffice it to say, that in three weeks the left lateral was only a quarter of a circle out of position, and the tooth operated on firmer, neither painful or tender. A second operation *easily* brought the left lateral into good position, and a retaining plate with caps for both teeth was at once applied. The patient was seen two months later when passing through town, and the right lateral was still a little long, but firmer, its colour as good as its neighbours, and it was translucent by electric trans-illumination; the left was almost normal in every way. The points which seem to me noteworthy in this case are: first, the age at which the operation was undertaken, it being laid down as a rule, that it should only be performed between the ages of eight and ten, that is before the roots and sockets are fully developed, although, in this respect, it is not a unique case; and secondly, the difficulty of the first as contrasted with the second torsion, the ease of the latter being doubtless due to the three weeks mechanical treatment having enlarged the socket. Upon looking up the literature of the subject

I have been able to find but little. Tomes, in his Manual,* describes the method of the operation, the precautions to be taken, and points out the dangers necessarily incurred of rupturing the vessels, entering the pulp and fracturing the tooth, and does not advise the operation after the age of ten years, although he has himself successfully twisted a central incisor in a patient of fifteen. Coleman, in his Manual,† protests against the operation on the ground of the frequency of cases of necrosis of the tooth following. Kingsley, in his "Oral Deformities," does not mention it, although he quotes Tomes' paragraph on torsion by mechanical means. Talbot's "Irregularities" is silent on the subject, and Guildford, in the American System of Dentistry, only speaks of it to condemn it. Balkwill, in a paper on‡ "Rotating Teeth," was opposed to the operative treatment, and mentioned, as a curious accident occurring afterwards, a case of a child who fell down and knocked out the loosened tooth. On the other hand, accounts of two successful cases have been published in recent years. R. H. Woodhouse ‖ recorded a case of immediate torsion of a central incisor in a girl eight years of age, and Morton Smale§ a similar case in a boy aged also eight. My own view is that the operation of immediate torsion should only be undertaken as a *dernier ressort.*

VALEDICTORY ADDRESS.

Delivered before the Students' Society National Dental Hospital, January 10th.

By Sidney Spokes, M.R.C.S., L.D.S.Edin.

Gentlemen,—The time has now arrived for me to deliver what is termed a "Valedictory Address," and as I was anxious that while occupying your time and attention I might be of some service, it seemed possible that I might make use of the Third Edition of "Tomes' Dental Anatomy," a perusal of which I enjoyed at Christmas. To those of us interested in Dental Anatomy its publication is welcome, and the student who makes a first acquaintance with the subject must, to a large extent, rely upon this standard text-book.

---

* Third Edition, p. 202 *et seq.* † p. 50. ‡ *British Journal of Dental Science,* 1881, 1125. ‖ *Journal British Dental Association,* 1886, 27. § *British Journal of Dental Science,* 1886, 1067.

There are some fifty pages of new matter and about twenty additional illustrations. In many places there is a re-arrangement of paragraphs and the new classifications and some of the animals introduced in the latter half of the book will be familiar to those students who have attended the courses of lectures at this school.

In Chapter I. there are fresh remarks upon horny teeth and a reference to the horny plates of Ornithorhynchus. With regard to the forms of teeth there is a further reference to the true calcified teeth of Ornithorhynchus, and it is pointed out that most Mesozoic mammals had the full typical number of teeth. Specialisation usually takes the form of a shortening in the length of the jaws with consequent change in number and form of teeth. The argument in favour of man's missing incisors being the second and not the third is also set out.

Chapter II. The only additional point worth noticing is where the author refers to the fact that as the shape of the face largely depends upon the form of the maxillary bones, and as these again are largely influenced by the teeth and the muscles which bring them into play, it follows that the face of an animal largely depends upon its dentition.

In Chapter III. comes a description of the horny teeth of Ornithorhynchus, the lamprey and Myxine. In the latter beneath the horny cone there appears to be an attempt at the formation of the more ordinary dental tissues. Mr. Tomes still considers that the enamel organ is probably present at an early age in tooth germs, even if no enamel is ultimately formed. Enamel is compared with the shell of Pinna and other mollusks found amongst invertebrata, but these latter have not so large a proportion of lime salts.

Enamel is also penetrated by dentinal tubes in some deep sea fishes. One wishes it might be described as tubular enamel in all such cases, as many are puzzled to understand the prolongation of a dentinal tube, as such, outside its own matrix. At all events a junction between a dentinal tube and an enamel tube is more easily to be appreciated, and the acceptance of calcification by conversion provides a way of escape. With regard to the "Sheaths of Neumann" the opinion is held that they can only be demonstrated after partial destruction of the dentine; they are therefore to some extent artificial and may not have any real existence until after the action of re-agents. The term "areolar dentine" applied to the outline of old interglobular spaces is stated to be falling into disuse.

The foot-note of Fig. 49, still describes the tooth of Lamna as containing *vaso*-dentine, thus contradicting the text and the figure itself.

Mr. Mummery's specimens of tooth pulp, prepared *in situ*, show an appearance of bands from the matrix running into the dentine something like Sharpey's fibres. This may be due to the dentine being only half-formed. The number of lamellæ in cementum is said to be about the same in all parts of the tooth, but they are thin at the neck and thick at the apex;. and Black is quoted as saying that cementum may possibly be regarded as growing at intervals through the the life of the individual. The older a tooth is the thicker the cementum. The actual attachment of the alveolo-dental periosteum takes place by means of connective tissue fibres, which pass right into the bone and cementum as Sharpey's fibres. Malassez thinks it should be considered as a ligament, rather than a periosteal membrane, and that it is homologous with the fibrous bands which hold some fishes' teeth in place. There is a free anastomosis between vessels from the pulp, gum and bone, and close to the cementum there is a rich capillary plexus. Some observers have described cells more like epithelium than osteoblasts, which have been found on the surface of the cementum, deep in the socket, and Von Brunn claims that the original enamel organ is co-extensive with the dentine and therefore intervenes between this and the cement-forming tissue, the connective tissue bundles from which divide up what is left of the enamel organ into small areas found in the adult alveolo-dental periosteum. Dr. Black describes other cells as lining lymph canals which are always found close to cementum, and says he has traced pus along them.

Chapter IV. deals with the development of teeth. The vascularity of the enamel organ is confirmed by Professor Howes and Mr. Poulton, but Dr. Sudduth disagrees on this point, and also denies the existence of papillary projections of the dental sacculus into the external epithelium of the enamel organ during the active period.

Fig. 69 represents a section, by Mr. J. Andrew, of a human fœtal jaw, and shows the origin of the germ of the first permanent molar to be derived from the second temporary molar, instead of from the original epithelial inflection as stated in the last edition, and as appears till in Magitôt's table on p. 154.

In describing Kölliker's view of the formation of enamel, there is a comparison made with the manufacture of the shell in the mollusk by the mantle, which can be separated, and which probably secretes something which is afterwards hardened by lime salts.

The term ameloblast is substituted for the adamantoblast of the last edition.

With regard to formation of dentine Mr. Tomes thinks there is still room for doubt and conjecture. If the appearances noticed by Mr. Mummery, and those, after macerating dentine in glycerine, by Mr. Bennett are not due to methods used in preparing the specimens, there is still something to be explained.

With regard to Mr. Hopewell Smith's suggestion, that the odontoblasts are purely sensory, and that the matrix of dentine is formed by cells beneath, Mr. Tomes is of opinion that comparative anatomy shows that many vaso-dentines, which are destitute of both tubes and fibrils, are formed by a layer of cells like ordinary odontoblasts.

Chapter V. contains a reference to Mr. Bland Sutton's paper on the "Development of the Lower Jaw." Albrecht thinks that each intermaxillary bone is developed from two centres, and divides it into an "endognathion" and an "exognathion."

The section on Eruption of Teeth concludes with a list showing the ages at which the roots of human teeth are completed.

Dealing with the attachment of teeth, it is pointed out that a large number of fish have a sort of annular ligament, allowing slight motion of the teeth upon the bony pedestal on which they are placed, and this condition points the way to the more specialised arrangement in hinged teeth.

On page 214 it appears that the inner and shorter teeth of the Hake are anchylosed. This needs a double correction which can be found on p. 245.

Fig. 91 illustrates the hinged tooth of Odontostomus, with a barbed point and tubular enamel. Another fish mentioned is Bathysaurus ferox, with teeth attached by ligamentous hinges. Both these are predatory fish obtained by the *Challenger* from great depths.

Fig. 95 illustrates the peculiar arrangement of the bone of attachment in the mackerel.

Chapter VI. contains a later classification under which the Elasmobranchs and Ganoids are included in Palæichthyes. The horny teeth of the Cyclostomata are described, the tooth of Bdellostoma, Fig. 96, being very interesting in its structure. There is a cap of thick strong yellow horn fitted into an epithelial groove at its base. Beneath this is a layer of epithelium, like an enamel organ covering a calcified cap which contains dentinal tubes and vascular canals, derived from an odontoblast layer of the pulp. These buried teeth ask the question, "Did the ancestors of these Cyclostomes have jaws carrying teeth." Another question "Have the Chelonians obtained the horny covering to their jaws, and the birds their bills, by a fusion of horny teeth?" has been raised by the condition found in the lingual teeth of the Myxine. The Sword-fish and Chauliodus also claim attention, and fig. 105 shows the edge of jaw in Pseudoscarus with the denticles arranged as a row of hollow cones covering other cones.

Chapter VII. A description is given of the salivary glands in Heloderma, the only poisonous lizard known. The ducts seem to perforate the lower jaw, and open between the lips and the teeth.* In the Python, although the ducts open in the same way, they do not perforate the bone, and the secretion is not poisonous.

Under birds there is no reference to the Berlin specimen of Archæopteryx, in which the head is very well preserved, and a drawing of which shows fourteen teeth apparently implanted in distinct sockets, and smooth, pointed and coated with enamel.

Mr. Tomes thinks it possible an extended research might reveal rudimentary surviving teeth beneath the functional horny bill in birds, or even above it, as in Ornithorhynchus.

In Chapter VIII. the last line on p. 284 should be read as the first. Mammalia are now divided into three groups, Prototheria, Metatheria, and Eutheria, and it is more probable to suppose that some early and unknown mammalian forms have given rise to these stems than that they are derived from one another. Under Prototheria the dental armament of Ornithorhynchus is fully described as was to be expected. Figs. 119, 120, 121, 122. In the young animal there are twelve functional calcified teeth, two on each side being much larger than the third. The upper teeth have broad-topped crowns with two long cusps on the inner edge and a crenated border along the outer edge with many small cusps; in the lower this is reversed. The internal structure would suggest that these teeth have degenerated; there are many interglobular spaces in the crown and tubular dentine is absent in the roots. These teeth are replaced in the mature animal by the horny plates with which we are all acquainted. These are not to be regarded as horny teeth but simply hardened epithelium which at first surrounds the teeth and is perforated by

* This is well shown in a specimen in the lizard case at South Kensington.

their short roots, the former position of which can be traced on the surface of the completed horny plate.

The classification of Eutheria adopted by Professor Flower in the *Encyclop. Brit.* is followed. Ungulata includes Hyrax and the Proboscidea, as well as Amblypoda which contains many extinct animals. A new order, Tillodontia, is added, comprising other extinct animals with affinities to Rodentia, Carnivora and Ungulata.

It is now found that the variations occuring in individuals and which afford material upon which natural selection can work, need not be so small as was formerly thought, and a quotation from Mr. Wallace with regard to the jaws in the Wolf is introduced. As examples of rudimentary teeth, those of Mystacoceti, the teeth under the horny plate of the Dugong and the larval teeth of the Sturgeon are instanced. To these may be added those on the under surface of the snout of the Sword-fish mentioned on a previous page.

A reference is made as to the possibility of high feeding producing early formation and eruption of the teeth and thus interfering with their reliability as a test of age. This question has recently been raised again. Professor Brown does not believe in this theory and, in a revised edition of his pamphlet,* does not hesitate to say that no change has been observed in the rate of development during the last forty years.

The generalised members of the Mesozoic mammals, grouped by Professor Marsh in a new order Pantotheria, were perhaps the ancestors of the modern specialised Insectivora. The usual pattern of the tooth was tricuspid, the central cusp greatly preponderating.

Mr. Oldfield Thomas proposes to write out the dentition of an animal in full, in order that it may easily appear which teeth, if any, are missing from a series.

Virchow suggests that multicuspid teeth may have been formed by the coalescence of several separate teeth of the homodont parent dentition.

Dr. H. F. Osborn thinks that Mesozoic mammals show three primary cusps on each molar, the triangle of cusps in the lower closing in front of that of the upper, and he believes that the majority of recent molar types have diverged from the trituberculate molar by the addition, modification, and reduction of cusps. He proposes six names to distinguish the three primary cusps and three supplementary ones.

* "Dentition" 1889.

With regard to the milk dentition, it is a possible hypothesis that the normal mammalian dentition is Diphyodont, and that the Monophyodonts have wholly lost their milk dentition, while it is still present, as in Tatusia peba, in full strength, or gradually dying out, as in the seals. Mr. Tomes thinks that an explanation of the fact that there is no succession of teeth in the molar region may perhaps be found, when we remember that this portion of the jaw is not formed until after the time for milk teeth has passed.

Oscar Schmidt suggests that as the facial region became shortened, there was not room for all the tooth-germs inherited to lie in order, so that some of these were pushed on the top and became developed first, as milk teeth.

In Chapter IX. the Orycteropus is mentioned as having some thirty-six teeth instead of, as formerly, twenty-six, the anterior ones being shed before the posterior ones are erupted.

The Cetaceans are now divided into Odontoceti and Mystacoceti, as was to be expected, and an additional member of the Archæoceti in the shape of Zeuglodon is introduced. Fig. 142 accompanies a good account of the peculiar tooth of Mesoplodon, described by Sir W. Turner and Professor Lankester.

Chapter X. The Insectivora are now regarded as ancient and somewhat generalised mammals, perhaps not differing much from the parent forms of other mammalia, and it is said that it would not be difficult to imagine how the teeth of all other Diphyodonts might be evolved from them. They can be divided into two groups, one in which the molars present a **W** pattern, and the other a **V** pattern.

With regard to the Chiroptera it is pointed out that the milk dentition of the majority does not at all resemble the permanent successors.

Under the heading of Proboscidea there are additional remarks on mammoth ivory, and a figure of Dinotherium, with which some of us are already acquainted.

In Ungulata the dentition of Rhinoceros is omitted, except for a reference to the pattern of the molars. An explanation of the Palæotherium tooth is introduced and the ancestry of the Horse, from the American point of view, is illustrated by a page of figures showing the changes in the fore-foot and molars from Orohippus in the Eocene up to Equus. The eruption of the incisors of the horse and the changes in the "mark" are differently described, the present statement agreeing with that in Professor Brown's pamphlet.

The Artiodactyles are divided into Bunodont and Selenodont, the latter including Anoplotheridæ.

In Carnivora there is a list of modifications which Professor Cope has traced through a series of extinct Cats. There is still a misprint in the dental formula of Hyæna.

In Primates, Mr. Tomes states that he has collected eighteen examples of the first lower bicuspid in man where there is an attempt at the formation of a second smaller anterior root, such as is found existing in the anthropoid apes. Fig. 202 shows the enormous length of roots found in the Orang. There is an explanation of Professor Flower's "Dental Index" and some further remarks on the missing incisors of man.

Chapter XI. deals with the Marsupialia and contains many important and interesting additions. It is now thought that the original numbers of premolars was four, and that it is the second one which is missing. Mr. Oldfield Thomas' suggestions as to the explanation of the milk dentition must also be studied as well as Professor Cope's "Haplodont" tooth.

But the many quotations from this third Edition which I have given you, will, I am sure, be sufficient to stimulate you to read this welcome book with the attention it deserves. Besides those mentioned above there are many other animals, not appearing in the last edition. Fig. 61 is still upside down, and the apparent contradiction with reference to the canine tooth in the female musk deer can still be found on pp. 299, 412. The canines should also be inserted in the dental formula of Desmodus.

Reports.

THE ODONTOLOGICAL SOCIETY OF GREAT BRITAIN.

THE Annual General Meeting of the above Society was held on Monday, the 13th ultimo, at 40, Leicester Square. The President, Mr. HENRY SEWILL, M.R.C.S., L.D.S., in the chair.

The following officers were elected for the ensuing year :—

PRESIDENT : Felix Weiss.

VICE-PRESIDENTS: (Resident), F. Canton, J. Stocken, David Hepburn; (Non-Resident), J. Cornelius Wheeler (Southsea), W. Bowman Macleod (Edinburgh), J. H. Redman (Brighton).

TREASURER: Thomas Arnold Rogers.

LIBRARIAN: Ashley Gibbings.

CURATOR: Storer Bennett.

EDITOR OF THE TRANSACTIONS: Walter Coffin.

HONORARY SECRETARIES: E. G. Betts *(Council)*, J. Ackery *(Society)*, W. A. Maggs (*for Foreign Correspondence*).

COUNCILLORS: (Resident), R. H. Woodhouse, L. Matheson, W. Scott Thomson, C. S. Tomes, F.R.S., Willoughby Weiss, W. H. Woodruff, W. Hern, F. Newland-Pedley, C. J. Boyd Wallis; (Non-resident), T. C. Parson (Clifton), R. T. Stack (Dublin), F. J. Vanderpant (Kingston-on-Thames), M de C. Dickinson (St. Leonards-on-Sea), A. A de Lessert (Aberbeen), Alex. Fothergill (Darlington), W. B. Bacon (Tunbridge Wells), H. B. Mason (Exeter), Mordaunt A. de C. B. Stevens (Paris).

Messrs. HARRY BALDWIN and W. B. PATERSON were the Scrutineers.

Mr. ALFRED COLEMAN was recommended by the Council for honorary membership and was elected by acclamation.

The TREASURER (Mr. Arnold Rogers), in presenting his report, said he was pleased to be able to state that the year had been more prosperous than its predecessor, the receipts being £2 more and the expenses £35 less.

The LIBRARIAN (Mr. Ashley Gibbins), in the course of his report mentioned, amongst several other books, they had acquired the new edition of Tomes's "Dental Anatomy and Physiology," Mr. Bland Sutton's book on "Dermoids," and one by Dr. Magitôt on "Cysts of the Superior Maxilla." He took the opportunity to point out that the usefulness of the library would be increased if members would return books promptly when done with. He also reminded them that a suggestion book was always kept in the library, and trusted they would use it freely. In conclusion, he stated that the list of new members would be published in the *Transactions*, arranged, for the first time, both topographically and alphabetically.

The CURATOR (Mr. Storer Bennett) having briefly made his annual report, proceeded to say that some two months ago Dr. Talbot, of Chicago, presented seven cases of models to the museum illustrating various abnormalities in children's jaws. Dr. Talbot considered that there are two principal peculiarities in the method of development of the upper jaw in children, which he classified as "V-shaped" and "saddled shaped," these he sub-divided into half V-shaped and half saddled shaped. The description of his models would be found in his paper reported in the *Dental Cosmos*, October, 1889, a *résumé* of which he had kindly sent to the library. Mr. Storer Bennett also mentioned the gift by the President of a lower jaw found amongst some remains of pottery in Algiers, it seemed to be a perfectly authentic specimen. The left six-year-old molar was lost long antecedent to the death of the person.

Dr. SCANES SPICER, M.D.Lond., B.Sc., then read a paper on

NASAL OBSTRUCTION AND MOUTH BREATHING AS FACTORS IN THE ETIOLOGY OF CARIES OF THE TEETH, AND IN THE DEVELOPMENT OF THE VAULTED PALATE,

of which the following are the leading points.

As a consequence of a routine examination of the teeth, he had been specially struck with two things: first, the great prevalence of caries in the teeth of patients who had nasal obstruction, and were consequently by necessity mouth breathers. Secondly, the large number of his younger patients, from the ages of eleven years upwards, having the well recognised symptoms of nasal obstruction, who had at the same time palates of a highly vaulted character, much contraction of the dental arch, and decided irregularities of teeth: he thought that there were sufficient reasons for at least tentatively supporting the position that a genetic relation existed between nasal obstruction and the dental and maxillary conditions referred to. As to how we should normally breathe, the experiments of all the leading authorities abundantly answered, through the nose, in which, and its accessory cavities, almost all the warming, moistening, and filtering of inspired air is done. All the higher animals, primitive tribes, and practically all children at birth, breathe through the nose. Civilized man, too often with the first catarrh, takes to mouth breathing, which should only be resorted to in circumstances of special stress. Having described the various forms of nasal obstruction, which were much more common than would generally be supposed, he gave several reasons for coming to the conclusion that it was an affection far more frequently met with in civilized than uncivilized mankind. Could any exciting cause in his environment account for this? Dr. Spicer thought that it could, and suggested that the artificial and partial way in which houses are heated, the rash way in which individuals expose themselves to extreme, sudden, and frequent changes of temperature, were such causes. In this way, the nasal mucous membrane would get into a state of inferior vitality and irritable weakness, inducing nasal obstruction.

Turning from the rhinological to the dental aspect of the subject, Dr. Spicer quoted from Tomes's "System of Dental Surgery," Dr. Magitôt, and Mr. Mummery, to show that the frequency of caries bears a tolerably close relation to the habits of luxury which civilization engenders. Referring next to the contracted jaw, vaulted palate, and irregular teeth, he relied upon the authority of Mr. Mummery that among savage races they are as rare as destructive attrition is common, while precisely the contrary is true of civilized races. Summing up the phenomena to which he had drawn attention, Dr. Spicer said that, speaking generally, savage modes of life, comparative freedom from catarrh, nose straight breathing nasal septums, good palate and jaws, regular teeth free from caries, were correlated conditions; whereas, with the advance of civilization and luxury were associated tendency to catarrh, nasal obstructions, mouth breathing, vaulted palates, contracted jaw, irregular and carious teeth. It seemed legitimate to enquire how far nasal obstruction and consequent mouth breathing were related to dental and maxillary variations as cause and effect. In the numerous text books on dental surgery and papers which he had consulted, no detailed examination of the question seemed to have been made. Nevertheless, Catlin, a shrewd observer, though a layman, in his little book "Shut your Mouth" referred to "the saliva flooding every part of the mouth while it is shut, and carrying off the extraneous matter which would otherwise accumulate, communicate disease to the teeth, and taint the breath"; he further alludes to the teeth, as immersed in protecting fluid and with powers of existing in the open air long enough for the various purposes for which they are designed, but beyond that abuse begins, and they soon turn to decay." It is the suppression of saliva with dryness of the mouth, and any unnatural current of cold air across the teeth and gums during the hours of sleep, that produces malformation of the teeth, toothache and ticdoloureux, with premature decay, and loss of teeth so lamentably prevalent in the civilised world." ' Among the brute creation that never open their mouths except for taking their food and drink, their teeth are protected from the air both day and night, and seldom decay; but with man, who is a talking and laughing animal, exposing his teeth to the air a great portion of the day, and oftentimes during the whole of the night, the results are widely different—he is sometimes toothless at 40." Though some of the foregoing facts and opinions were erroneous and extravagant, others Dr. Spicer thought well worth attention. He further quoted from Tomes' "Dental Surgery" and Sewill's "Dental Caries" as to the predisposing causes of that disease, and proceeded, that it would probably be readily agreed, that the condition of the teeth and gums during normal respiration, *i.e.*, through the nose with the mouth shut, is as follows:—(1) They are kept at a uniform temperature, practically that of the normal body temperature, and are protected from sudden change by the thick non-conducting tissues of the lips and cheeks; (2) They are perpetually bathed in the warm alkaline salivary fluid which wells up between them and washes away any mucus or food tending to stagnate or decompose, as well as any micro-organisms which may have gained access to the mouth; (3) they are being constantly scoured with the alkaline saliva by the almost incessant action of the lips, cheeks, and tongue, so as to ensure the complete removal of *débris* from their surface and interstices. Whereas, if the subject is lying on his back indulging in wide open mouth breathing, the teeth and gums would be exposed to a current of air at 50° F. (taking that as the temperature of an unheated bedroom) after they had enjoyed one of 98·4 during the day. Congestion and inflammation of the mouth and pharynx would sooner or later result, leading to the increased secretion of strongly acid mucus. The air being dry, must absorb moisture, and thus tend to inspissate the mucus, rendering it liable to stagnate and act as a nidus for micro-organisms, whose arrest is also favoured by the spongy state of the gums produced in catarrh. There could be little doubt, that the sour taste in the mouth, of the thick clammy paste in the morning, after a night of mouth breathing, found an explanation here. Again, in mouth breathing during sleep, the mouth would be parched and dry, and the teeth consequently not properly flushed: that the absence of a constant flow of saliva is an important factor in deterring caries is seen in the tendency to that disease in patients suffering from rheumatism, diabetes, and the other diseases which induced aptylism. Further, in the same conditions, the teeth are not properly scoured, the accumulation of *débris* is favoured, and the excess of fresh oxygen breathed being highly charged with micro-organisms, putrefaction is encouraged in every way. Moreover, it could not be doubted that chronic mouth breathing during the period of the growth and evolution of the permanent teeth would influence the tooth sacs and lead to an inferior quality of enamel and dentine.

Dr. Spicer next examined in some detail the relative incidence of caries on the different groups of teeth, making use of Dr. Hitchcock's and Magitôt's tables for that purpose. In connection with this branch of the subject, it would be interesting to know if the relative incidence of caries in nose breathing nations did or did not agree with those tables; further, if animals showed a tendency to have disease of the most used teeth; also, if caries, when it attacked the upper molars, preferred the labial or lingual aspect. Information on these points would afford tests on some of the points he had raised. Dealing lastly with vaulted palate, contracted arch, and irregularities of the teeth in relation to chronic nasal obstruction and mouth breathing, Dr. Spicer quoted Sir John Tomes, Dr. Greville MacDonald, and other authorities in support of the fact that these nasal and oral conditions existed concurrently. This association admitted of a rational explanation on the hypothesis that prolonged disuse of the nasal channels for their natural functions during the growth of the organisms leads to stunted evolution of the nasal framework. The septum and sphenoidal sinuses partake in this, and fail to rush down the palatine processes of the maxillæ, while the rest of the face, including the freely used alveoli, continue to grow. The median line of the hard palate along the attachment of the vomer tends to retain its infantile position. The weight of the lower jaw—which drops to allow of mouth breathing—acts through the tissues of the cheeks and presses on the superior maxillary alveoli, flattening each curved lateral half, so as to diminish the space available for the eruption of the canines and other teeth, which therefore are compelled to assume irregular positions.

Should further investigation prove the views enunciated correct, it followed that the restoration of the breathing channels and the treatment of the teeth of palate should be carried out *pari passu* by the rhinologist and dentist respectively.

DISCUSSION.

The PRESIDENT said in the first place he would express his opinion without hesitation and in the strongest terms that the nature of caries is demonstrated. That there is no difference of opinion as to the essential nature of caries in the mind of any individual who has any claim to speak with authority on dental pathology. The predisposing causes which Dr. Spicer had mentioned are the only predisposing causes, that is to say, it is proved that caries is entirely due to external agents. The question whether the enamel can undergo any change predisposing it to caries seemed to him demonstrated. The enamel does not contain the physiological elements necessary to carry on a physiological process. That the formation and development of the jaws may be due to mouth breathing had been held by a great number of observers some of whom Dr. Spicer had quoted. Dr. Spicer had with perfect clearness put before the Society a number of facts, some hypotheses and some speculations which were very interesting and might form the subject of a well developed debate.

Mr. R. H. Woodhouse: With regard to the theory which Dr. Spicer had advanced that caries resulted from the changes of temperature occurring in the mouths of mouth breathers, if the theory were a true one, surely decay would take place more on the inner surfaces of the teeth, on those surfaces which according to his theory it would first come in contact. He thought the circulation of the blood in the teeth was so rapid that the temperature of the teeth was maintained at its normal point even if cold air passed into the mouth in very great quantities. Another matter with regard to mouth breathing, they were told it was the cause of the shape of the jaws. Now he thought the shape of the arch depended very much on the individual, so much so that the build of a person would to a great extent indicate the shape of his jaw, thus a tall thin person would have a jaw in proportion. In Dr. Spicer's paper they seemed to have a new theory. With reference to caries, it was known that in uncivilized races the teeth are not only better but their character is different—even if they *did* practise mouth breathing, Mr. Woodhouse was of opinion they would not have caries.

Mr. Henri Weiss was inclined to take the question of oxygenation in the production of caries. It was a question how far, in the case of mouth breathers, the free current of air with the contained micro-organisms passing over the teeth enter into the production of caries.

Mr. Storer Bennett pointed out to the author of the paper that there are several animals—notable, the wolf and the dog, which in taking exercise breathe through the mouth, but except as the result of civilization, caries was unknown in the dog.

Mr. W. E. HUXLEY (Birmingham) said the same thing had occurred to his mind, but on thinking it over he was inclined to say that in the case of the dog, the fact of the absence of caries is more than accounted for by the extra flow of saliva and the activity of the tongue affording a greater protection to the teeth.

Dr. WILLIAM HILL had devoted a good deal of attention to the subject, and had come to the conclusion that the vitiated condition of the buccal secretions played an important part in the production of caries. Would Dr. Spicer say that the mouth breather is always a dry breather? He (Dr. Hill) could imagine that the mucus would be of a very much higher specific gravity, and in that condition it would be proved to undergo acid fermentation. Acid, he believed, is a factor in caries, and on this view, caries of the teeth is the result of mouth breathing and modification of the buccal secretions. With regard to V-shaped arches, he was struck with the number of them among idiots, and was inclined to regard it as brought about by mouth breathing.

Dr. GEORGE CUNNINGHAM thought that not only the paper, but also the discussion, demonstrated how little was known as to the cause of caries With regard to the clinical aspect of the disease, there were a series of observations about to be made under the auspices of the British Dental Association, on the teeth of children, and he thought it would be a fit opportunity for a collective investigation on many points that had been raised. The frequency of caries in mouth breathers he took to be practically undetermined. So far as the chemical action of the secretions is concerned, he was of opinion that an investigation of the secretions would be an important point upon which they were lacking information. Possibly they might now look forward to getting some definite information with regard to the secretions. With reference to the mechanical aspect, he thought dentists would endorse the reader's views. Altogether, he thought the result of the paper, of the opportunity they had had of discussing it, would lead to a collaboration which would result beneficially in extending their knowledge on this interesting subject.

Dr. SPICER having briefly replied, the President then delivered his

VALEDICTORY ADDRESS.

The PRESIDENT in delivering his Valedictory Address said: The time had now arrived when he must give up the trust which had been placed in his hands a year ago. It had been the custom hitherto for the President of this Society to deliver a valedictory address, possibly it was a custom which at some future time might be more honoured in the breach than the observance. Instead of retiring in silence he should like to take stock of the past year's progress and if he could not adorn a tale he might yet be able prehaps to point a moral.

They had heard from the officers the general condition of the Society; their library was an extremely good one, the Museum was excellent—perhaps the best dental museum in existence; the financial position of the Society was good: there was only one complaint to make, viz., as to the smallness of their numbers, they barely maintained their roll, the deaths and new elections giving only one member to the good. It seemed strange that members of their profession did not join their Society and the British Dental Association in numbers such as they might have hoped they would.

During the year they regretted to have to record the loss of several members, some young, some full of years; among them Matthew Finlayson of Edinburgh, M. Brasseur of Paris, Dr. J. W. Langmore, an honorary member, Mr. Palmer of Peterboro', Mr. Charles Spence Bate, F.R.S. of Plymouth. Most of these members had had obituary notices in the journals and he need not attempt to add to the loss that had been sustained. Mr. Spence Bate must undoubtedly be looked upon as one of the most distinguished; he was one of the few members of their profession who held the blue ribbon of science, the fellowship of the Royal Society. His work lay far out of dental science, for his name would be chiefly associated with the science of entomology which he enriched by his observations and researches, his work having been referred to as an authority by the late Charles Darwin—and here it might be remarked that nothing in the vast range of nature is so insignificant as to be unworthy of the attention of the observer and investigator, it is impossible to establish a fact concerning even the humblest beetle without adding to the mass of evidence to be used again by future investigators and without that fact ultimately dropping into its proper place in the gradual unfolding of nature's plan. With regard to Mr. Spence Bate's personal character, the President thought he could not do better than quote from a letter from Sir John Tomes in which he said, "Speaking of Spence Bate, I regarded him as a thoroughly good fellow," now, if when the time came for their epitaphs to be written it could be said of each of them by so discerning a judge of character as Sir John Tomes "he was a thoroughly good fellow" they would need nothing else.

The Odontological Society was a scientific society, and the question always was what had they done during the year to advance or contribute to science? They had listened to a great number of contributions from members, the time of each meeting had been fully occupied, and the papers had covered the whole range of subjects connected with their profession. Antisepticism in Dental Surgery was ably dealt with by Mr. R. H. Woodhouse. Mr. Amos Kirby had given them the advantage of his experience on the subject of electricity in connection with dentistry. Mr. Hepburn's papers treated upon useful and practical subjects, and from Dr. Cunningham they had the fragment of what promised to be an interesting and new research, viz., the occurrence of a crystal forming micro-organism in the mouth; unfortunately want of time deprived them of the opportunity of hearing the whole of the paper, but they hoped to do so at some future time. They had also had a number of useful *Casual Communications*, and the Curator, Mr. Storer Bennett's descriptions of the contributions to the museum, though they were often passed over without discussion, always contained interesting facts, and exhibited a knowledge which they highly appreciated.

With reference to the papers of non-members and visitors, it was, he thought, a thing to be proud of that the Odontological Society commanded the very foremost men of science; it was no new thing for them to be their guests. This year they had had Mr. Jonathan Hutchinson, who stood in the very front rank of philosophical surgery; his paper was a very valuable one, but it was not very fully discussed, minor points were seized upon and more important ones were passed over. Mr. Hutchinson mentioned that he had observed an occasional injurious influence upon the tongue and mouth generally of amalgam stoppings. His statements had been criticised, but he (the President) felt quite sure that Mr. Hutchinson would not publish facts which had not come under his own personal observation, and did not think he intended to associate ulceration of the mouth and amalgam stoppings in the relation of cause and effect. Mr. Hutchinson's remarks on Pyorrhœa Alveolaris were extremely important, as directing the mind to scientific investigation on that subject, and out of the vast number of observations he made, he gave them a fact, for the first time published, viz , that patients with honeycomb teeth are more susceptible to the action of mercury than others; now that was a very practical fact which should be of great importance to the dentist. Alluding to Mr. Bland Sutton's highly interesting and valuable contributions, the President remarked upon the distinguished and leading position which Mr. Sutton had attained though still quite a young man. Mr. Sewill next referred to Dr. Ferrier's paper, which, he said, handled an extremely complex subject in a most lucid and incisive manner. There was one suggestive point made prominent to which importance should be attached, viz., the possible relation, in many cases, of facial neuralgia and visceral disease, and *vice versâ*. Dr. Semon in an unassuming, but very able way, had collated the various authorities on Empyema of the Antrum, making his paper one of great usefulness.

With reference to the presence from time to time of eminent scientists, the point which he wished to bring home to them was this, seeing the reputation the Odontological Society had attained as a scientific society, they should very carefully guard against opening the door to those whose scientific competence was at all in question, or those who might be willing to use the society for personal and ambitious ends.

It was quite evident that no society of a limited specialty like dentistry, or even the wider sphere of surgery, could go on for ever discussing the incidents of everyday practice, therefore if societies were to exist, they must go further afield to the basis of science; though they ought not to forget the practical, still they must go to science and widely to science, if they were to fill their meetings and take their proper share in the scientific work of the day. While, however, they went to the basis of things, they should remember that subjects not germane to their specialty were outside their province. It was not difficult to give illustrations of what he meant: for instance, they might discuss a tumour of the brain interfering with the dental nerves, but they could not discuss a tumour of the brain which affected the brain only. It was right to deal with the circulation of the blood as circulating through the dental periosteum, but they ought not to wander off to discuss the pulse or the beat of the heart. In a paper on the teeth, one might refer to their effect upon speech, but if one wandered off into the psychology and physiology of speech, it might occasion a feeling of regret that speech was ever invented; but these things would not occur if they freely criticised papers. With regard to criticism, he was bound to say they were not quite what they should be, and here he would like to lecture the younger members but that he had hardly attained the age which conferred the privilege to do so. He did not think the younger members did their duty in the matter of criticism. The excuse was made that the subject was new, and they could not discuss it, but he did not know that that was always a valid excuse; there were always fundamental facts of science in all papers with which the youngest should be acquainted and upon which questions might be based or information elicited. No really scientific man was afraid of criticism, on the contrary he desired it; criticism need not be bitter or personal but it should be free and fearless, and so far as the reputation of the Odontolgical Society was concerned the more thoroughly they attacked the papers the better would be their success in drawing the best men to them. Scientific men would always go where they could get the best criticism, and therefore, he would repeat, if they wanted to sustain and enhance the reputation of the Society as a scientific body they must be sharp in their criticism. He was addressing himself to the younger members —the older men hesitated to show their wisdom—and he trusted they would improve the critical element and so help forward the reputation of the Society and of the profession. It must be remembered that the reputation of a profession was the aggregate reputation of its individual members, and he would urge young men while they were yet young to cultivate a taste for, and interest in, science. He who attained the most happiness was he who did the most for mankind. The only hope for a man dealing with human weakness and human suffering was to cultivate a philosophic mind and that could only be done while he was young. If he came into the profession with the determination only to make money, the profession had very little to give in that way, and when he reached the age when the disappointments of life came upon him he would find he had neither wealth nor the satisfaction of having done good. Therefore if he had any eloquence he would use it in impressing the value, from the moral point of view, of cultivating scientific tastes upon their younger members.

Mr. Henri Weiss in a few appropriate sentences proposed the usual vote of thanks to the President and Officers which Mr. W. A. Maggs seconded.

The PRESIDENT announced that the next meeting would be held on the 3rd of February, when the President would give his inaugural address, and papers would be read by Dr. Cunningham and Dr. Mitchell.

The proceedings then terminated.

ODONTO-CHIRURGICAL SOCIETY OF SCOTLAND.

THE Second Ordinary Meeting of the Session 1889-90 was held in the Rooms of the Society, 5 Lauriston Lane, on Thursday, the 12th December—the President, Mr. J. AUSTEN BIGGS, L.D.S., in the chair.

At the conclusion of the formal business, the following gentlemen were balloted for and admitted Members of the Society :—Herbert Bycroft Ezard, L.D.S.Edin., 32, Buccleuch Place, Edinburgh; Frederick Page, L.D.S.Edin., 6, Hope Street, Edinburgh; John Turner, L.D.S.Edin., 60, Lauriston Place, Edinburgh; John Girdwood, L.D.S.Edin., Patriothall House, Hamilton Place, Edinburgh; Gordon Reid Shiach, L.D.S.Edin., 1, N. Guildry Street, Elgin; David Monroe, L.D.S.Edin., 3, Howe, Street, Edinburgh; James Leslie Fraser, L.D.S. Edin., 5, Castle Street, Inverness; John Stewart, L.D.S.Edin., 65, Queen Street, Edinburgh; John Crostwhaite Macnamara, L.D.S.Edin., 1, Rankeillor Street, Edinburgh.

Mr. MACLEOD gives notice that at next Annual Meeting he will move that Law II., defining the qualification of Membership, be altered.

The Law as it at present stands reads thus :—

The Society shall consist of Ordinary, Honorary, and Corresponding Members.

The Ordinary Members shall consist of Gentlemen practising as Dentists in Great Britain, and of Medical or Surgical Practitioners interested in Dental Surgery.

The Honorary and Corresponding Members shall consist of Gentlemen practising Dentistry in Great Britain, in the Colonies, or in Foreign countries, and of retired Dental Practitioners in Britain, as well as such Medical or generally Scientific Men as may have distinguished themselves in connection with Dental Surgery.

The Ordinary Members shall have vested in them the government of the Society, and all cases not otherwise specified shall be decided by them, by a majority of votes, by ballot, if required.

Mr. Macleod will move that it shall in future read :—

II. Ordinary, Honorary, and Corresponding Members.

The Society shall consist of Ordinary, Honorary, and Corresponding Members.

(*a*.) Ordinary Members.—Gentlemen shall be eligible for Ordinary Membership who hold the Licentiate in Dental Surgery of any of the Licensing Bodies of Great Britain or Ireland, or a Colonial or Foreign qualification recognised by the General Medical Council entitling them to practise Dentistry in Great Britian.

(*b*.) Honorary Members.—Gentlemen [practising or retired] who hold a qualification recognised by the General Medical Council, or Foreign or Colonial Dentists holding a qualification recognised in their own country, who may have distinguished themselves in the practice of, or in connection with Dentistry, and Medical or Scientific Men who may have distinguished themselves in connection with Dentistry shall be eligible as Honorary Members.

(*c*.) Corresponding Members.—Gentlemen resident in the Colonies or Foreign Countries holding qualifications recognised in their respective countries shall be eligible as Corresponding Members.

The Ordinary Members shall have vested in them the government of the Society, and all cases not otherwise specified shall be decided by them, by a majority of votes, by ballot, if required.

The following Paper by Dr. Booth Pearsall was, in the absence of the author, read by Mr. W. Bowman Macleod, and was illustrated by diagrams, metal casts and dies, and appliances :—

The sand-moulding flask I have the honour of showing to you to-night has been designed to meet some of the many defects we find in zinc discs as they are commonly made by dentists. This design has been the subject of a good deal of thought for many years, if one can be said to think out a design never put into practice, and I think anything that will aid us in our workroom labour by shortening labour—meaning tensile strength and decreasing waste—is worthy of attention. The sand-moulding flask before you was invented about eighteen months ago, as an experiment to see how far the Bayley flask and die could be improved upon, and has been in constant use in my workroom ever since it was made. During this time of constant use, the only improvement has been to have two patterns of moulding-plates, one with the cone-shaped aperture somewhat larger than the pattern before you, so as to suit very large jaws. The flask is made of two parts—a moulding-plate and an iron sand-ring made to fit the plate.

The moulding-plate is circular; the upper surface has four concentric grooves on its surface and four projectors or tabs; the grooves are for holding the sand in such a way that the grooves make so many dykes or obstructions to prevent the hot metal running out between the moulding-plate and the surface of the sand surrounding the mould. The concentric grooves have another object, namely, to guide the workman in correctly centering or ex-centering the position of the model, so that the cone or striking part of the die will come where it may be wished to have most strength in the die—in other words, where the heaviest hammering is to be done. On the under side of the moulding-plate are to be found four webs or feet running from the circumference of the plate to the aperture in the middle, which moulds the truncated cone for hammering upon, the object being to make the moulding-plate strong enough to stand rough usage, of sufficient weight to prevent the moulding-plate from floating off the sand mould by the weight of the melted metal as it is poured into the mould, as well as to form steady feet for the plate to rest on in the sand-moulding trough. The iron sand-ring is made of strong hoop iron in the usual way, and it should fit easily and truly on the grooved surface of the moulding-plate next to the projectors or tabs.

When sand-moulding is to be done, the moulding-plate is placed in the sand-trough grooved side *upwards*, and on it the shallow plaster model (from $\frac{3}{4}$ to 1 inch deep, as may be desired). The model is either correctly centred by the aid of the grooves, or it may be put out of the centre so as to bring the cone-shaped aperture wherever it may be desired. The position of the plaster model having been determined, the iron sand-ring is put on the moulding-plate surrounding the plaster model. The sand is then packed in the usual way, and when the packing is finished, the iron ring full of sand and the moulding-plate are turned upside down, the moulding-plate removed, exposing the plaster model, which is then removed by the aid of a point and a hammer in the usual way.

The mould having been examined and any loose particles of sand blown out of it, the melted zinc can be poured into the sand-mould and the moulding-plate put over the mould, and the remaining zinc poured in to make the coned end of the die. If the sand-mould is not quite filled with zinc, there will not be any difficulty in placing the moulding-plate on the sand-mould, but if the metal is poured in a slovenly way, there is no doubt that a difficulty will occur, the overflow of metal preventing the moulding-plate from going into its place. With skilful workmen and ordinary care, the pouring of this die is just as easy as any other form.

In use, the swaging of a plate will be found more certain and accurate because of the ease with which heavy blows can be struck on the truncated cone, and if the section of a die be examined, the hollow formed by the cooling of the zinc in the centre is really a source of strength, so far as the construction is concerned.

The cone-shaped end, with the model projecting over it, enables the die to be held in a vice in such a way that blows struck on the palate or teeth of the model will not cause it to slip in the jaws of the vice, but has a steady bearing, forming a great contrast to the slippery and uncertain hold of the ordinary form of die when placed in a vice to be filed or hammered, and it can be easily turned round when the jaws of the vice are opened, and instantly tightened again in the desired position, whereas the Bayley or ordinary form of die cannot be secured with the same certainty, precision, or rapidity in a vice. You will also notice the ease with which blows can be struck outside of the cone, on the shoulder formed by the projection of the mould under the cone, and such blows are often of the greatest service in certain cases, the instances of which will readily occur to practical minds.

The advantages may be summed up as follows :—

1st. Saving in the amount of metal to be melted, as zinc deteriorates by constant melting; this is important, as the usual supply of zinc ought to go farther in the constant use of smaller dies.

2nd. The ease with which a shallow plaster model can be removed from the sand as compared with a deep one.

3rd. The great increase of strength, owing to the improved construction of the die, aided by the cooling of the zinc.

4th. The ease and rapidity with which the new form of die can be held in the ordinary vice.

5th. The certainty of blow secured by the use of cone-shaped end of the die.

6th. The choice offered to the workman in placing the strength or blow-resisting cone where it is needed to resist heavy hammering.

7th. The ease with which the hammer surface of the die can be struck with a heavy hammer.

8th. Simplicity of method, the details being nearly the same as those used in the dental work-room.

In diagram No. 5 you have sections of the same model used as a die in my method, the usual method, and that invented by Bayley. I have to inform you that manufacturers, so far, cannot see any advantage in my method, and one firm have generously offered to *connect my name with the invention* if I will place my invention in their hands without any remuneration for the cost of experiment and wear and tear of brain substance, and they have also informed me that I shall have great difficulty in converting dentists to the use of my form of die. That there is great scope still to be found in the improvement and increased efficiency of work-room tools, I have no doubt, and I hope from this time forward to do something to make our work-room places where work shall be an enjoyment, not a sorrow. Whatever may be said about American inventions, and the appreciation shown whenever any good and practical invention is placed in the hands of our profession, I do not think the British dental manufacturer can lay any claim to any credit in promoting or fostering inventions of any kind amongst us until the demand for the newer and more efficient appliances of the men of progress has become so marked on the part of dentists that they cannot avoid "going with the times." I do not think the difficulties and inconveniences found in connection with the forms of metal dies have been sufficiently studied by practical dentists; and I trust you will find, by practical experiment, that I have done something towards making dies something less of a worry and something more of a pleasure than they have been found in the past.*

The President called on Mr. ANDREW WILSON for his paper on :—

THE FIRST PREMOLAR IN THE TYPICAL DENTITION OF THE PLACENTAL MAMMALS.

The number of species in which there are, in the adult, four teeth separating the canine from the molars, is considerable, but in very

* Mr. Macleod has, since the meeting, tested this method of making dies, and finds it much more simple and useful than the reading of the paper would lead one to expect.

few of these cases are anatomists or naturalists agreed in regarding the one next to the canine as a premolar.

These are those in which the typical four milk molars are succeeded vertically by four permanent teeth, and, so far as observed, they are very few indeed. As examples in recent species we have the tapirs, and, according to Mr. Spence Bate, the mole.

In the vast majority this tooth has neither had a predecessor nor will have a successor; and, while regarded by some as the first premolar, it is by others held to belong to the milk series, thus giving rise to considerable confusion, which is not lessened by its being occasionally counted in both.

As showing this confusion, I will quote a few extracts from great authorities. Professor Huxley,* writing of the Horse, says, "The tooth here counted as a first premolar may be a milk tooth, as it appears to have neither a predecessor nor successor, and soon disappears."

Of the Rhinoceri † "of the four milk molars, the first, as in the Horse, is smaller than the others, and is not replaced."

I may notice, in passing, that in some extinct Rhinoceri there was both a MM.^{1} and a PM.^{1} in the upper jaw at least.

Speaking of the Tapirs, ‡ he says, "In the anterior premolar (or milk molar ?)"

In this genus it is now known that there is in the upper jaw both a MM.^{1} and a PM.,^{1} as is well shown in the beautiful preparations lately added to the Science and Art Museum in this City. These consist of the crania of types of the several mammalian orders, having the milk series of teeth "in situ," while, the outer wall of the alveolar process having been removed, the permanent teeth are seen lying in their crypts.

I would strongly recommend members to inspect this most interesting and instructive collection.

Of the Pig,§ on one page he gives the adult formula as having PM then a couple of pages further on, and after giving the milk dentition as having MM, he says, "The first permanent molar is the first tooth of the permanent set which comes into place (at about six months after birth) and the permanent dentition is completed in the third year, at which time the first deciduous molar, which is

---

* Anat. Vert. Animals, p. 295.
† *Idem.*, p. 309.
‡ *Idem.*, p. 311.
§ *Idem.*, pp. 3R3. 317.

not replaced, falls out," and he then gives the permanent formula as having PM$\frac{3}{3}$.

Of the Hippopotamus,* after giving the milk molars as $\frac{4}{4}$, he says, "The first deciduous molar persists a long time, and seems not to be replaced."

Treating of the Camel,† he says, "There are not more than five grinding teeth, in a continuous series, above and below," but he ignores the presence of the caniniform PM.^{1} in the upper jaw, which is separated from PM.^{3} by a diastema, PM.^{2} being suppressed.

One more quotation from him. Of the Dog,‡ he says of the anterior three premolars, "These teeth are two fanged," when in reality the first is single rooted, and almost rudimentary in form.

Again, "The first premolar of the adult dentition, having no deciduous predecessor, so that in this, as in so many other cases, it is doubtful whether it should be counted in the milk, or in the adult dentition." "The so-called 'first premolar' of the adult, and anterior molars appear before any of the deciduous molars are shed."

Professor Owen, in his Odontography (pages 477, 484), says of the Dog :—"The first permanent premolar comes into place before any of the deciduous teeth are shed, its germinal predecessor disappearing before birth," and, of the Hyæna, "The figure of the skull of the young *Hyæna Crocuta* . . . shows that stage when the correspondence with the formula of the genus *Felis* is completed by the appearance, in the upper jaw, of a small premolar in the interspace between the canine and the first molar of the deciduous series; but this appearance is due to the apex of the first permanent premolar, which cuts the gum before any of the normal deciduous teeth are shed; whether it is preceded, as in the dog, by a deciduous germ tooth in the fœtus, I know not."

Mr. C. S. Tomes in his Manual is very unsatisfactory in his treatment of this tooth, in some cases speaking of it as a temporary tooth, in others as a permanent one, and even the figures and text contradict each other.

Lastly, in a footnote to the first page of the Introduction to vol. iv. of the Cat. Fos. Mam., Brit. Mus., 1886, we find it stated, "The author is inclined to believe that the first cheek-tooth in the Perissodactyla—which in *Tapirus* is always replaced by a vertical successor, in *Rhinocerus* is occasionally so replaced, but in *Equus*

---

* Anat. Vert. Animals, p. 328. † *Idem.*, p 319. ‡ *Idem.*, pp. 356-357.

never had any successor, and is frequently absent—belongs to the milk molar rather than to the premolar series." No notice being taken of the homologous tooth in either the Artiodactyla or the Carnivora, although any decision regarding the one must be equally applicable to the others.

Turning now to the reasons given in support of its being regarded as a milk molar, these are two—first, its not having had a predecessor, and, second, its being soon shed.

Having in the Mammalia many instances of the absorption of milk teeth in various stages of development "in utero," and seeing the contradictory statements made regarding the presence of such a tooth in the fœtal dog, as evidenced in the quotations given from Owen and Huxley, much importance cannot be attached to the first reason. But, even supposing that there is no predecessor, we may put this reason aside, as we find that the same authorities who hesitate to recognise this tooth as one of the permanent series, recognise as an established fact that in the marsupials all the premolars, excepting the last, have had no predecessors, and that in some species, even of the last one, it is doubtful or not proven, so far as present knowledge goes.

Turning now to the second reason, its being in many cases soon lost, we find that while in some it is so, in many more it is long retained—the more surprising, seeing that it seldom is a functional tooth. A more important point would be the period of its eruption, compared with that of the undoubted milk molars, as also with that of the first permanent molar. Supposing it to be a milk molar, we have the anomaly of its eruption being preceded by that of the second, third, and fourth milk molars, and coincident with, if not slightly after, that of the first permanent molar. Now this, which would be remarkable if a milk tooth, would not be so if a permanent one; its early eruption, compared to that of the other premolars, could be explained by the fact of its having had no predecessor.

In man we frequently, I may say usually, find that when a milk tooth has had to be removed very early in life, its successor appears much sooner than would have been the case had it been normally shed. Still more to the point, in the only case in man in which I have met with a front permanent tooth, which had no temporary predecessor, it erupted long before any of the other permanent teeth, but after all the temporary ones. It did duty with the temporary series, and now, years after they have disappeared, it is doing so with its permanent colleagues. As to the periods, when what I claim to be the first premolar is shed, there is unfortunately, very little data on record. In the carnivora we have it in place along with the full adult dentition, and in the bears it is in place long after the second and third premolars have been lost.

In showing the inconsistency of those objecting, on the first ground, I referred to their treatment of the marsupials premolars; and, as doing the same for the second, I point to a special tooth in the same group—namely, the penultimate premolar, as seen in the larger species of *Macropus* (kangaroos). This tooth is erupted very early in life—a young skull in my collection, in which the third upper incisor is just erupting, shows two cheek-teeth in place, the first, the tooth in question, with, to its distal side, the temporary molar. The first is shed, and its socket obliterated, in advance of the shedding of the temporary tooth.

In these species, its being so shed is thus not due to the eruption of a large last premolar (the reason given by Mr. C. S. Tomes in his Manual), but to the same cause, which, as the animal ages, leads to the shedding of all the permanent cheek-teeth, except the third and fourth molars. Still there is now no hesitation in recognising this tooth as a premolar, although Owen regarded it as one of the temporary series.

In conclusion, I will just bring under your notice a remarkable peculiarity, occasionally met with in the first premolars, but seemingly rarely—namely, its being duplicated, that is, we have, besides the second, third, and fourth premolars, *two* first. This occurrence, I suspect, is not so rare as records would lead us to believe, as there are two in my own collection—one in the upper jaw of a Dingo, the other in the lower jaw of a Bear. In both it is on the left side only, and in both the one next to the canine is the larger, and I venture to throw out the suggestion, may this smaller tooth not be the first milk molar, which is normally suppressed.

The SECRETARY said, Mr. H. H. Edwards, whose name we are rapidly learning to associate with the question of the Missing Incisors in Man, has again sent to us drawings of models he has taken, illustrative of the subject. It will be remembered that, four years ago, he sent us a valuable communication on this topic, with nine pen and ink sketches, which were reproduced in the Society's *Transactions*. Mr. Edwards in some recent correspondence, says :—

That, as far as his field for investigation is concerned, he much regrets that he is principally engaged in a family practice, and is unassociated with any hospitals, and that therefore his opportunities of observation are necessarily limited, but those that occur he does not pass by—examines every tooth he removes, to see if there is anything abnormal to be detected, and, where possible, taking impressions of a mouth which shows any peculiarities. In his practice he saw mainly the same people year after year, the children presenting the same characteristics as their parents or grand-parents ; and it was that gave him the idea he expressed, four years ago, of the theory of inheritance as evidenced in those organs over which we have the special care. It would take years to produce a basis on which to found even a theory ; therefore, in the meantime, it behoves us all to contribute authenticated drawings or models of those cases that come directly under our notice. One swallow does not constitute a summer ; but if we could produce thousands of swallows, we should, at all events, be entitled to a consideration. Therefore he would again urge upon his fellow-members to exert themselves, and, in the words of the title-page of a well-known journal, "Observe, compare, reflect, record." It is to our seniors to whom we would especially look for enlightenment, who, having made a competency —with time at their disposal, and with minds ripened by long experience—are better fitted to pass an opinion on the pabulum with which we younger men should make every effort to supply them

Mr. Edwards is becoming rather of the opinion that the supernumerary tooth is a freak of nature ; but respecting the lateral incisors, he sees but little, no doubt, in the theory that they are becoming suppressed, and that if nothing were put on record on the subject, future generations might fall into the error that we possessed no lateral incisors at all, or that in the case of a supernumerary tooth presenting itself, its original position might be argued to all eternity.

Fig. 10. Male, adult.—Common phase of suppression of upper lateral incisors, centrals slightly spaced.

Fig. 11. Female, adult.—Upper jaw. A redundant right lateral situated within the arch, behind, and similar in shape and size to the normal tooth.

Fig. 12. Male, adult.—Model of upper jaw. Centrals much spaced; right canine next to central; temporary canine still standing, and supernumerary tooth between it and left central.

Fig. 13. Male, adult.—Upper jaw. Canines next to centrals, and slightly overlapping them, and on the left side a supernumerary or dwarfed lateral, and also the root of the left temporary canine still remaining.

Fig. 14. Male, adult (figured below).—This is perhaps the most interesting of the number. It is the model of an upper jaw, with two supernumerary molars in place, behind the third molars, or rather behind the roots of them, as the crowns have been lost by decay. The left lateral is suppressed.

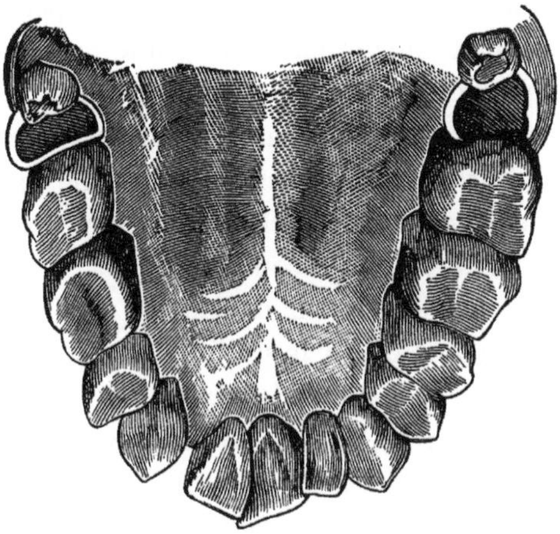

The suggestion that naturally presents itself is, were the teeth not removed, either in mistake for temporary teeth (in the lower jaw), or, in either case, for purposes of regulating on the score of crowding? Mr. Edwards thinks this is not the case, the patient assuring him that no teeth had been removed from either of these positions indicated, and if the latter hypothesis were correct, their removal was very ill advised, as the teeth are leaning in too much, and additional teeth would rather have been required to have kept their inclination at the normal angle, and the gentleman in question had been under the hands of his predecessor and ante-predecessor (carrying him back some thirty years), and he is not inclined to believe they would have accorded him such mistaken treatment.

Mr. Walker (Dundee) exhibited a cap which he had constructed to fit over the exhalation valve of the "gas" face-piece, constructed somewhat on the principle of the ventilation shafts with reversible heads, which usually form a very prominent feature on the deck of a steamer, the object aimed at being to direct the respiratory exhalations away from the face of the operator. Mr. Walker said :—

Allowing that the face-pieces supplied to us by the depôts are, wonderfully perfect, as far as the safety of our patients is concerned he would venture to think they were not so as regards the operator, on account of the present open shield on the expiration valve.

The exhaled air and gas is often expelled with unusual force in the face of the operator, and there is no way of avoiding this extreme danger except by getting into rhythmical breathing with the patient. He would say extreme danger advisedly, because of the possible risks encountered with patients in the first stages of phthisis ; but leaving these out of the question, he would condemn the open shield on the minor principle of the escape of fetid breath and oral gases, especially where there had been much previous inflammation. The operator, very watchful of facial symptoms and respiratory surroundings, is too often forgetful of this, and, in bending over the patient, is often quite close to the exhalation valve, thus presenting, to our minds, a picture far from pleasant, even in contemplation.

With the aim of avoiding such danger, he exhibited a safety or melioration cap, composed of a "bysel" or ferrule, to fit the existing valve-chamber, with $\frac{1}{8}$ inch outside flange, to form an enlarged cylinder chamber $\frac{1}{4}$ inch in height. The dish rises only to touch upon two stop pegs, fixed on to the bottom of the cylinder cover, which equalises the air passage leading to a right-angle funnel, made to revolve so that germs of disease may pass into the room, and not be expelled directly into the face of the operator. The face-piece had also a small chain and catch attached, by which it was secured to a light bracket arm, similar to that used with the water-motor engine, and could thus be rapidly swung out of the way when sufficient gas had been administered to the patient.

Mr. J. Graham Munro exhibited a very ingenious binder for lathe bands. It consisted of a spiral steel spring of about 2 inches in length, with a bore sufficiently large to admit the ends of the "gut." The free ends of the wire were bent up, so that after the band was admitted the wire, on being pressed down, passed diametrically across the opening through the centre of the cord, firmly securing it in position.

Mr. Munro also exhibited a model of the lower jaw of a youth of 16. Two of the incisors were missing, and a temporary incisor still retained. The boy had never any of his lower incisors extracted and his grandmother had the same teeth missing, and had also retained the temporary tooth.

Dental News.

TENTH INTERNATIONAL MEDICAL CONGRESS, BERLIN, 1890.

As stated in our last issue, the proceedings of the Tenth International Medical Congress to be held in Berlin will begin on Monday, August 4th, and will terminate on Sunday, August 10th, 1890.

The principal work of the Congress will be conducted in eighteen different Sections. The following additional information concerning Section 14, which will be devoted to Dental and Oral Surgery may be of interest, especially as we may hope it will maintain the prestige achieved by its predecessors at the Congresses of London and Washington, more especially as the constitution of the Committee of Organisation is in itself a sufficient guarantee of efficiency.

This Committee consists of the following well-known members of the dental profession :—Professor Dr. Busch, Berlin, Chairman ; Dr. Calais, Hamburg ; Dr. Friek, Kiel ; Professor Dr. Hesse, Leipzig ; Professor Dr. Hollander, Halle ; Professor Dr. Miller, Berlin ; Dr. Paetsch, Breslau ; Dr. Weil, Munich. The General Secretary is Dr. Lasser, Karlstrasse 19, Berlin, N.W. Germany.

It is proposed to elect three Honorary Presidents and a Secretary to represent Great Britain.

The statutes of the Congress require all members to be legally qualified practitioners of the country of which they are subjects.

The work of the Section will be divided as follows :—

(1) Discussions on three general subjects, each of these discussions will be introduced in one of the three official languages of the Congress, viz. : German, French and English. The German subject will be Bromaethyl, but the others have not yet been decided.

(2) Reading of Papers, of which a short extract or table of contents must be sent in beforehand.

(3) Practical Demonstrations in all departments of Dentistry.

(4) A Museum of Exhibits.

In order to facilitate arrangements, correspondence on the Dental

Section may be addressed as follows:—In German to Professor Busch; in French to Dr. Calais, Hamburg; and in English to Professor Dr. Miller, W. Vosstrasse 32, Berlin.

GOSSIP.

DEATH IN THE TOOTHPICK.—The *Boston Herald* announces upon the authority of a physician whose name, however, does not transpire, that among the ills to which flesh is heir, not the least is the wooden toothpick! Doctrinaires of this instrument become addicted to chewing it, some even go so far as to swallow it, if the Boston physician is not exaggerating, and as the rough splinters are sucked or bitten off they cause irritation about the gums, force their way into crevices, and set up gastric ulceration by scraping and tearing the delicate mucous membrane lining the stomach. Although not classed under "death from toothpicks," fatalities are stated to have resulted from this toothpick-chewing habit, and altogether its lethal effects are sufficiently evident to make us feel the danger is real. To carefully cleanse the teeth with a quill or metal instrument, and then wash the mouth with a weak boric acid solution, is a fit and proper precaution, but to plough up the gums and sow splinters of wood with badly made and unpolished rough wooden toothpicks is a dangerous and thoughtless habit to be contemned and discouraged.

A DENTAL LABORATORY FOR GUY'S HOSPITAL DENTAL DEPARTMENT.—A dental laboratory is being built on a site immediately fronting the conservation room, and it is expected that it will soon be ready for use. The room will be more than 22 feet long, and will be lit from the front by four windows already prepared, and from above by small "sky-lights" over the lathe, the casting bench, and the plaster bench. In front of the windows jeweller's benches will be arranged, at which about twelve students can work at the same time. There will be all the necessary appliances for casting in metals and in plaster of Paris, vulcanizing, plate making, gilding, and the numerous arts included under "Dental Mechanics," which every student is supposed to have learnt during his three years of pupilage before entering hospital. Students will thus be able to construct for their own use "Correction plates," necessary for the treatment of dental irregularities and oral deformities. Demonstrations will from time to time be given on the construction of metal and vulcanite splints used in the treatment of fractures of the maxilla and in the preparation of obturators and vela. The laboratory will afford the means of supplementing the lectures on Dental Mechanics by practical instruction.

ONE of Germany's greatest surgeons, Volkmann, has passed away. His colleague, Von Bergmann, speaking in loving regard for his departed friend says :—"About twenty-five years have elapsed since Volkmann began his academic career. He was one of the first surgeons who 'domesticated' Lister's antiseptic method in Germany, and the brilliant successes which he gained by it went far to confirm it and to gain its acceptance. Another part of his work was the study of cancerous tumours, and it occupied him till the last days of his life. His great excellence as a clinical teacher and as a military surgeon during the last campaigns is sufficiently known. But it is not only in his capacity as a scientist and an operator, but also as a man, that we owe him our admiration, for he was in every respect so true a character, so sincere a man, ever mindful of his great and serious duties. He was a poet too, and a fresh breeze blows through his 'Songs from the Vale of the Sarle'; but especially his widely known and popular 'Reveries at French Firesides' are a proof of his poetic endowment, and a memorial of that time of the great war of 1870-71 which was so glorious for Germany. In him a man has departed who succeeded in gaining a name such as few possess, and who in full measure deserves that his memory be warmly cherished by men of science and by the nation."

MONTHLY STATEMENT of operations performed at the two Dental Hospitals in London, and at the Dental Hospital, Manchester, from November 30th to December 31st, 1889 :—

		London.	National	Victoria.
Number of Patients attended		—	1338	749
Extractions	Children under 14 ...	315	205	438
	Adults	915	356	
	Under Nitrous Oxide ...	1035	600	79
Gold Stoppings		293	39	24
Other Stoppings...		1039	206	141
Advice		—	295	—
Irregularities of the Teeth		75	57	—
Miscellaneous and Dressings		402	61	311
Total		4,074	1,819	993

THE DENTAL RECORD, LONDON: FEB. 1, 1890.

Epidemic Influenza.

SINCE the cultivation of what may be called meteorological medicine, and which of course includes epidemiology, the belief has gained ground that atmospheric conditions are largely accountable for the inception, progress and dissemination of disease. The alarming spread of the new disease, which for want of a better name has been termed "Influenza" has drawn considerable attention to the question of the spread of disease by atmospheric and telluric influences. "Influenza" so-called, has an interest not only for dentists, *qua* as being more or less medical men, but in so far as it has brought to the fore a number of those exceedingly obscure forms of neuralgia which sooner or later drift to the dental surgeon. But not only has la grippe, pseudo dengue, or Epidemic Influenza been rampant in our midst, but there has been a most curious intensification of the symptoms of ordinary maladies throughout the last few weeks. It may safely be said that for every hundred maladies attributed to Epidemic Influenza, not more than one can justly be accounted a genuine case. Colds in the head, of greater or lesser intensity are prevalent as a matter of course at this time of year, and in these days "fashion in suffering," as in doctors, is acute and consolatory. But a sudden onset commonly with a chill or rigor, often with nausea and vomiting, intense frontal headache, and pains in the limbs, recalling the grim invention of Louis the Eleventh's minister, Cardinal Balue, at once inventor and victim of the restless chamber, associated with the most intense muscular prostration, mental lassitude and inaptitude for physical exertion, with or without albuminuria and obstinate insomnia, and we have a picture of so-called Epidemic Influenza.

It is beside the present question to discuss the treatment of this disease. Antipyrin is useful in allaying the temperature, and quinine, although of little value during the acute stage, is distinctly serviceable as the attack is passing off. But to the average dental practitioner two questions ot interest arise in connection with Epidemic Influenza. Of these, the first is, how best to avoid contagion amongst his patients; and the second, how to recognise the epidemic neuralgia which follows in the train or replaces the disease itself. It has been demonstrated that thorough ventilation and free air interchange are the best prophylaxis against infection. Warmth of waiting rooms is very different from stuffiness, and where stoves are employed, frequent refilling of water containing vessels should be practised. Epidemic neuralgia as at present prevalent does not offer any very special symptoms worthy of comment. In some cases it is associated with pains in the temporal fascia of possibly a rheumatic origin. Too often these cases come under the care of the family doctor, who arriving at the diagnosis of toothache, passes on his patient to the dentist who may for the nonce be puzzled. The langour, muscular prostration and general feeling of being good-for-nothing, will give him a valuable clue for diagnosis, and suggest as a line of treatment supporting diet, stimulating food, and tissue forming medicine.

The Hyderabad Chloroform Commission.

THE first instalment of the Report tendered by this Commission has been placed in the hands of the profession. It would be premature to offer any criticism until the whole of the report is before us and the details of the experiments have been carefully overhauled by the experts. It may not be inopportune at the present juncture to remind our readers of a fact which seems to have been lost sight of by several of our contemporaries, especially in the lay press, that the Hyderabad Commission on Chloroform is by no means a first commission which has undertaken to decide the question whether or no chloroform is a safe or a deadly anæsthetic. Up to the present the answer has been unfavourable to chloroform, and unless we are mistaken, it will require a very strong line of argument to convince people that because monkeys, dogs, horses and rabbits die in Hyderabad through failure of respiration, while human beings succumb in Europe with all the symptoms of heart failure, that chloroform is safe if it be only given after the manner of Simpson and Syme.

The International Medical Congress.

In our present issue we add particulars to those which appeared in the January journal. Few will contest that when properly managed International Congresses subserve a useful end. Although the meeting at Berlin is a Medical Congress, it is none the less one for dentists. Section 14—the Dentists' Section—includes as officers the names of men who are capable enough of carrying out a really international representative programme of dental work. It only remains for English dentists to, for once, take the trouble to show the world that dentistry as an art and as a science is not *effete*, but is up to date, fairly lively, and about able to take care of itself in the matter of work done, although somewhat behind its neighbours in plethoric outpourings of verbiage. It is hoped that in view of the really good work which was done at the 1881 Congress in the Dental Section, that a great effort will be made to ensure a satisfactory representation of England at the Berlin meeting.

Valedictory Addresses.—At the Annual General Meeting of the Odontological Society of Great Britain, Mr. Henry Sewill, the retiring President, concluded with, we think, considerable show of sense, that a Valedictory Address was not a thing to be lightly foregone. It does not often fall to the lot of ordinary men to talk to a number of their fellows, and yet feel safe against nasty carping critics. Yet such is the way with those who make Valedictory Addresses. We remember listening to a lecture descriptive of the passion and languishings of Clarissa Harlowe given by a learned member of the British bar. The Lord

Chief Justice of England presided, and quite a number of Q.C.'s and barristers, minus silk, assisted as audience. At the close of some very flattering remarks eulogistic of the lecturer, that gentleman replied that he felt very grateful for the pretty things which had been said about him, but even more for the forbearance, which his experience made it hard for him to credit, which had induced so many members of the *Bar*, including the Lord Chief Justice, to listen to him for a whole hour without once *interrupting* him! Mr. Sewill did not occupy his audience for an hour, but he uttered a good deal of common sense and sound advice. He told his audience that the man who lived for himself threw his life away, but he who adopted a cosmopolitan interest—science—would find happiness for himself, and utility for the human race.

CORRESPONDENCE.

[We do not hold ourselves irresponsible in any way for the opinions expressed by our correspondents.]

To the Editor of the DENTAL RECORD.

SIR,—I obtained the enclosed formula from a medical man who first used it at my house in the case of his own daughter, but it contained as I thought too small an amount of cocaine to be of real service when applied locally.

He got the formula itself, I believe, from Mr. ——, one of a large firm of manufacturing chemists.

When he gave it to me, I laughed, and thanked him, and laid it by. However, one day I had it made up, doubling the quantity of cocaine, as in the present prescription. I confess I began to use it with little or no faith whatever, but my cases have seemed to show that operations are, at least, greatly lessened in severity by its careful application.

No better case have I had than that of a very sensitive young lady who had gas first for the removal of some teeth, but on her mother's representations tried to do without an anæsthetic for further operations.

Here I brought in cocaine. The last operations illustrate well what I mean, and show that it was no child's play for the patient.

The second left lower molar was gone below gum, and the instrument had to be well pressed down long tough roots, but ending satisfactorily. Second left lower molar still more gone. I tried to remove with forceps, but the crown simply crumbled. I then took my elevator and removed first one long root and then the other, and the patient said that all sensation had been deadened except at the very bottom of the socket, and considered cocaine a wonderful remedy.

My method is to soak two rolls of cotton wool well with the solution, holding them in position for about two minutes, then operate with warm instruments. I do *not* like the risk attending hypodermic injections.

Another case, that of the wife of a retired medical man, an old lady of 70, highly nervous (and her husband almost more so about his wife), came to me to have a set of teeth, and I had to remove six tough roots and teeth.

Her husband would not allow gas or chloroform. I removed three roots in the front and side at each sitting, and she went away saying "how beautifully I extracted teeth," that the pain had been only nominal, and so forth. I pointed to the cocaine, and she said it was wonderful stuff.

Now, Sir, how much of all this is due to the patient's imagination, I cannot say, but if *they* are satisfied, and if we can do our operations without risk of any sort by so simple an application as this, it surely is well to use it instead of applying the *cold* steel, about which there is no mistake if no anæsthetic is used.

R Cocaine Mur.	... ...	gr. 50
Acid Boracic...	.. ...	gr. ii.
Liq. Hyd. Bichlor	.. ...	m. 40
Aquæ Destil ad.	... ...	m. 250

To be applied locally as directed.

E. M. Tod.

GAS OPERATIONS.

To the Editor of the Dental Record.

Sir,—I must thank a "Recent L.D.S.," for his criticism of my remarks on gas operations. I am extremely sorry to apply the word "dishonest" to anyone; but my feelings upon the gas question are very strong, and if I have expressed myself too strongly, I trust your readers will not take it in bad part.

I am surprised to hear that the "Veritable heads of our profession in the North administer their own gas and operate too without assistance." "A Recent L.D.S.," himself admits that their method is open to grave criticism. I should rather think it was.

Dr. Dudley Buxton says in his useful little book on "Anæsthetics," "It cannot be doubted that to give any individual an anæsthetic subjecting him to a minimum of danger is all one person can do and can only be accomplished by those specially instructed and experienced in anæsthetics."

Mr. A. S. Underwood in his little book on "Anæsthetics" says, "A patient has been known to die during the extraction of a tooth without the operator knowing it."

"A Recent L.D.S.," consequently leaves the life of his patient practically speaking in the hands of an unqualified assistant, for he cannot be giving his undivided attention to getting out the teeth and at the same time be studying the condition of the patient's heart and respiration himself. He may look up one day and find his patient is no more. It makes little difference even if "A Recent L.D.S." were an M.D. *He* may possess a most thorough knowledge of the whole body, yet the patient's life is in the hands of the assistant, and since that assistant is not qualified to give gas I do not consider it right.

Even if the "Veritable heads of the profession in the North" do wrong, is that a justifiable reason why a recent L.D.S. should follow in their footsteps when he himself admits that their method is open to grave criticism?

Then your correspondent says that his dental brethren and many medical practitioners would consider that he had no confidence in himself if he refused to jeopardise his patient's lives. I rather disagree with him, and I think he would find that people would have a much greater confidence in him.

The medical men I think would rather side with him, knowing that he was acting in an upright spirit and showing that he respected the lives of his patients rather more than the opinions of some who give their own gas, operate, too, and take the double fee. He says he thinks this condition of things must ere long bring disgrace on an honourable profession; then why does he do it and why does he not set a better example to his professional brethren?

The veritable heads of our profession in London do not give gas themselves and operate at the same time, why should we? The only excuse that can with any justice be brought forward is that of fees.

If a man has to have a leg off does one surgeon give the anæsthetic and operate too? Certainly not; then do you suppose that the medical profession would point the finger of scorn at us because we want an anæsthetist while we perform our operation?

I think that always having a medical man for gas would tend to bring the medical and dental professions into a closer bond of friendship than ever, instead of causing the one to despise the other and say they had no confidence in themselves.

Again, sir, "A Recent L.D.S.," may gas his own patients for 999 times without trouble, but the 1000th may be a case in which he would give anything for a medical man to be by his side and lend him an *intelligent* helping hand. I may be dogmatic, but am I not right?

I trust that "A Recent L.D.S.," will again think the matter over and decide to act up to that which is right and have sufficient moral courage to stand a little chaff from some of his *confrères*, who will before very long, I hope, be calling in a medical themselves. Many will of course still give their own gas till the law (which is at present asleep) steps in to correct the present sad state of things.

I am, Sir, yours, &c.,

103, Sandgate Road, Folkestone, GEORGE SEYMOUR.

January 22nd, 1890.

NITROUS OXIDE AS AN ANÆSTHETIC.

To the Editor of the DENTAL RECORD.

SIR,—Kindly allow me space for a few sentences, explanatory of matters which apparently have not been made clear, and with these must retire from the discussion. Dr. George Johnson's researches proving that nitrous oxide is a rapidly asphyxiating gas" have not at present, he tells us, been published, so it is impossible for me to accept or refuse them credence. To prevent mistakes we must note that by "asphyxiating" Dr. George Johnson means "deprivation of air" (*see* "An Essay on Asphyxia," p. 7, line 7, *et seq.*). My contention has always been, and I submit has at present not been disproved, that nitrous oxide produces anæsthesia by a specific action upon the nerve centres; that the concurrent deprivation of air rendered necessary would eventually cause apnœa no one will deny. Dr. George Johnson reminds me that cases of recovery from suspended animation by drowning and the cases of persons who grow comatose as a result of suffocative pulmonary and cardiac disease are conditions in which deprivation of oxygen brings about a state of stupor which Dr. George Johnson calls "anæsthesia." How far the phrase is correct I need not wait to enquire, most persons would I submit regard it as far-fetched. My contention however is this, that animals suddenly deprived of oxygen do not become insensitive to pain; but even this is an unnecessary length for me to go, since I have simply to refer to experiments made and published to show that animals in one series obliged to inhale nitrous oxide for a given time, in another deprived of oxygen only for an equivalent time, are in the one case (when nitrous oxide is taken) rendered anæsthetic, but in the other remain conscious of painful stimuli.

Dr. George Johnson says he learnt from my little manual *On Anæsthetics* what he knows about Paul Bert's experiments with mixtures of oxygen and nitrous oxide, and further quotes me to make me admit Paul Bert's method of giving the gases is "almost impossible." As a matter of fact I referred in my paper which appeared in your December issue not to Paul Bert's method and experiments with nitrous oxide and oxygen *under pressure*, but to other experiments of his (not mentioned in my book) with simple mixtures of oxygen and nitrous oxide administered as they are now given both in Germany and this country. The practical point is then that the fact remains that nitrous oxide, if properly administered, due care being taken to get rid of once breathed air or gas, will produce anæsthesia and can be stopped before any true asphyxial (apnœic) symptoms occur. In its use for practical anæsthesia we do stop short of this point.

I am, Sir, your obedient servant,

DUDLEY W. BUXTON, M.D., B.S.,

Instructor in Anæsthetics in University College Hospital,

Anæsthetist to Dental Hospital of London.

Mortimer Street, W.

IRISH DENTISTS.

To the Editor of the DENTAL RECORD.

SIR,—I notice in your issue of January 1st, a letter signed "Yanna Meena" by an Australian correspondent. Will you kindly allow me space for a few lines on Irish dentists? Our brother in the Antipodes thinks if he had a Dentists' Act that it would save him that revulsion of feeling which he has on seeing the "1st Life Guardsman" of the "Dental Artist" or the advertisement which announces "Teeth, each 5s., sets £5, painless extraction 1s." Well, I beg to say that, although we have a Dentists' Act here, we have also some of the most outrageous specimens of quack advs. to be found in any country in the world. True we have not yet arrived at sending forth our warrior friend, but in some of the large towns the people are deluged with circulars from the Blank Dental Company, setting forth the merits of their own and demerits of their rival's the Dash Dental Co.'s system of dentistry? Of course the Dash Co. is as well up in the art as the Blank Co. and his man (I say his because there is only one in the Co.) is quite as energetic. How would "Teeth, each 2s. 6d., stopping with gold amalgam and enamel, 2s. 6d., sets £1" compare with the "Dental Artist"? Why, his fees are whât I would term "fancy" compared with the home grown article. Again, your correspondent mentions cheek, we could "knock him out (to use a pugilistic phrase) in no time if he had the pluck to come over here. Our circulars state that we are all able to put "L.D.S., R.C.S.I., D.D.S., R.D.S.," and every letter in the alphabet after our names if we were so disposed. "We get all our teeth and materials from *our own* manufactory *in New York* from which place we have just arrived." Just one other eye-opener for "Yanna Meena" which, if not as elaborate as the "Dental Artist's" six-footer in guards' uniform, is just as disgusting to the members of our profession who carry on their practises in a professional manner. These men cover every available space announcing their coming with posters having every letter six inches long. I beg to assure "Yanna Meena" that, although we have a Dentists' Act, people can practice here with impunity without being on the register. Ireland is the El Dorado for the charlatan because the law is never put in force, a state of things quite different in England where they are prosecuted, but all they have to do is come over here and announce themselves as the Dash Dental Co. and all is safe for them.

This will certainly strike "Yanna Meena" as preposterous when it catches his eye, but I assure him that I have not exaggerated, on the contrary, I could cite other instances in support of what I say. The question naturally arises, in what way would Colonials benefit by a Dentists' Act, and in what way do we benefit by our Act? I trust I have not asked you, Mr. Editor, to overtax your valuable space, but must plead as excuse that this is a matter intimately connected with the interests of the profession as well as the general public.

I am sure a great many readers will be always delighted to hear the Australian news which "Yanna Meena" promises. For my part I shall look forward to his next with pleasurable anticipation.

I am, Sir, Yours, &c.,

January 20th, 1890. "NIL ADMIRARI."

THE DENTAL RECORD.

VOL. X. MARCH 1st, 1890. No. 3.

Original Communications.

CLINICS: THEIR VALUE AND EFFECT UPON DENTAL SOCIETIES.

By WILLIAM MITCHELL, D.D.S. (Mich.)

THE value of clinics cannot easily be overestimated, owing to their far-reaching influence, and it is to this fact that no one should remain disinterested, or treat the subject with apathy, for they are a practical means to a very tangible and practical end ; and in the subject under consideration I am sure you all will agree with me, that in this case the end justifies the means. In societies where things must necessarily go in their order, it follows with clinics from the committee, so on down the line of those connected with them, either actively or passively ; even to the active and busy practitioner, who may only have a few minutes to spare to drop in "just to see what is going on," the effect is beneficial.

For the committee, in arranging the programme, will endeavour to secure those to demonstrate for them whose methods are considered reliable, and whose special methods of practice have merited attention, and if any are carrying on investigations in any advanced line of practice the opportunity is here afforded to demonstrate its availability in competent hands, while it will also be in the best place for friendly criticism, as to the merits or demerits of the methods, means, or appliances then being considered.

There are those who may have made research in new fields of treatment, or with new filling materials, or instruments for their application, or adjuncts to better facilitate our labour in the operating room or laboratory; here then is the place to best accomplish what might possibly take years under a solitary and selfish *régime.*

Dentistry the world over is looked upon by people who do their own thinking as an advanced and liberal profession; this impression will prove lasting or otherwise only in proportion as we prove our right to that designation; this end is best secured by a liberal exchange of ideas, and can only be fully lived up to where a due appreciation of the heading of this paper is entertained.

We owe it to ourselves and to those about us, to do our best to promote and further our professional interests, and through our members to conserve those of the public, and any of us who do less than that are placing ourselves in a false position.

There is no one so great that is not subject to influence ; there is no one so wise but might possess more wisdom ; so it is as regards our professional attainments, we all might be better dentists than we are, and we no doubt would be, were there a more healthy friction of practical ideas ; and I claim if any of us neglect any means of further perfecting ourselves in our calling, we are dishonest to ourselves, and dishonest towards our patients, for they come to us, and place themselves in our care, in full confidence that they will receive the best possible attention at our hands ; they pay for it, consequently they are in honour bound to receive it.

The personal effect of clinics is good ; it tends to break down very many of those little selfish ideas that the average specimen of humanity—and dentists in particular— are possessed of ; it broadens the mind, teaches us self-reliance, and what is much better, makes us more tolerant of the peculiarities and failings of our fellow-men ; and it is only by this contact of demonstration that this can be accomplished.

If a man is inclined to be cynical and circumscribed in his ideas, clinics afford the best means of modifying, if not curing, this unfortunate condition, and prepare him to receive impressions that will eventually manifest themselves in his future methods of practice.

There are many in our profession who may have evolved ideas and methods, and who, if having had the opportunity to demonstrate their utility, might have developed into an inestimable boon to our profession and to the public, but being debarred from this congenial influence the reverse of this has resulted in the idea being selfishly embraced and blighted by the sordid and mercenary caresses of the mind that conceived it, and the world has been cheated of its dues, if an unknown grave has not.

We are subjects of dependence ; no matter how unwilling we may be to admit it, the fact remains the same. A great many—if not most—of our best ideas are adaptations of those of others ;

therefore, should not we as individuals contribute our mite towards the common weal, and in that way, to a certain extent at least, repay the debt we owe our profession? I think there is but little chance for two opinions on this point.

The value of clinics to the young and rising members of our profession should not be undervalued. The student leaving the halls of learning, with his theoretical groundwork as near perfect as possible for his able instructors to make it, may have only had a very ordinary opportunity of developing his practical capacity. This being the case, to what extent will his theoretical knowledge assist him when he is called upon to contend with a case that presents itself for completion at one sitting? It may be only a simple operation, if so, so much the better for him; but should it prove a complicated case, and should he not possess the capacity of putting his theory to a practical test, his patient will not be long in making that discovery, and he will not have far to go to find the reason for his patients making their first and last visit at the same time.

When a student leaves college, he is just in the position to commence studying intelligently; he is then enabled to study cause and effect, and the relation of means to ends from a practical standpoint. It is from this standpoint that clinics are a benefit to the young practitioner, because he has the exceptional or complex operations performed, which, when analysed, assist him to the better performance of the every day practice that he has to contend with.

To those of a riper experience the clinic is a form of post-graduate course that they can ill afford to do without, for here they find that some of their much-cherished courses of practice have been superseded by easier and more satisfactory methods, that recent investigations and inventions have enabled them to more easily cope with difficulties that had been to them a source of consternation and dismay; and here it may be worthy of mention, the support afforded the projectors of the late post-graduate courses by the older members of the profession plainly shows that "Ephraim is joined to his idols." This in contradistinction to the younger members, who seemed imbued with the progress of the age, evincing a desire for knowledge that redounds greatly to their credit. It is to the wideawake active members of the profession that I especially direct my remarks—men who by their enthusiasm and presence make dental meetings a desirable place to attend on account of the practical professional advantages to be derived from contact with kindred spirits, the convivial side of the programme only securing a perfunctory attention at their hands. What is possible elsewhere is possible here. We read of meetings and clinics attended by hundreds, some of whom have travelled thousands of miles to demonstrate their methods, and we have looked with interest and profit upon the operations of our transatlantic brethren who have shown us their interesting modes of practice here; this is the spirit that should prevail to advance the best interests of a profession that has been second to none in its rapid strides towards perfection.

In those cases where clinics have been held but imperfect arrangements have been made to best utilise the time of those who have kindly consented to demonstrate, this is a matter that requires careful consideration at the hands of committees. As operations promote the keenest interest in conjunction with the lectures of the class-room, so do clinics enhance the interest attached to meetings, cause papers and clinics to become coexistent, and conventions for discussions will develop a vitality hitherto unknown. Gentlemen let us have more clinics.

INAUGURAL ADDRESS.

By Leonard Matheson, L.D.S.

Delivered before the Students' Society of the London Dental Hospital.

Gentlemen,—Little did I think, when as a member of this Society some fourteen years ago, I stood up with fear and trembling to read the paper of the evening, that I should one day rise to address its members from this chair. I am very proud to occupy this position, and I beg very sincerely to thank you for the honour you have done me in electing me to be your President.

The honour is a twofold one. In the first place, I am occupying an office which has been successively filled by men whom it is a distinction to follow; men whose names are "familiar in our mouths as household words," because of the good work they have done and are doing—both in connection with this Society and outside of it. In the second place, I am brought at once by my election to this chair, into a closer intimacy—than it is possible for me otherwise to enjoy—with you gentlemen, the present active members of the Society. It is a privilege which I assure you, I value very highly—to find myself brought once more closely in touch with the energetic, enquiring, progressive spirit which is so characteristic of the student mind, and which acts like a tonic and a stimulant on the mind of those, who though still looking upon themselves as students in a very real sense, have, it may be, but very little time to learn and study much else than that which is taught them in the practical school of daily experience.

And this twofold honour I appreciate none the less because the Society is now in a sound and flourishing condition. No one now thinks, or even dreams, of proposing its dissolution on account of lack of interest and support on the part of its Members. It was not always so. In early days this Society had a hard struggle for existence. Originally established in the year 1863, five years after the opening of the Hospital, in Soho Square, when the number of students was very small, it was vigorously supported by a small handful of men, amongst whom may be mentioned the names of, Mr. Harry Harding, Mr. Warwick Hele, the first presidents. But as the student days of the original members came to an end, it appears that interest in the Society's doings dwindled, the new generation of students did not take up the work of their predecessors, and in 1865 the meetings ceased to take place.

Not till 1871 was the Society again set afloat. It was successfully launched under the Presidency of Mr. Samuel Cartwright, supported by a strong council, and a goodly list of members. From that day to this, although its vigour has at times flagged, yet as the number of students attending the Hospital has increased, so the Society has also steadily grown, both in the number of its members, and in the energy and interest of its Meetings. Comparing the days when the average attendance was something under ten, with the present time when the average is, I understand, somewhere about four times that number, we may, I think, congratulate ourselves that our day finds the Society in such a prosperous condition.

Do not, however, let me be misunderstood. I would not have it thought that I gauged the value of a Society like this merely by its age, and the number of its members. On the contrary, such a Society has to be on its guard, as it becomes firmly established by time and fullness of membership, against two evils. On the other hand as it acquires the dignity of age so it may also acquire the slowness and formality not seldom characteristic of that venerable period of life; it may exchange the buoyancy and eagerness of early life for the dullness and indifference of second childhood ; it may grow stiff in the joints, depend too much on the staff of custom and routine, and find the ruts of use and wont better suited to its ambling pace than the rough, cross-country excursions in the fields of science and the breezy uplands of discussion and debate, that it loved so fondly in the days of its youth. On the other hand as a Society gains in standing and importance, and its roll of members is swelled by many who only join it because they understand that it is the proper thing to do, and not because of any real interest they take in its proceedings—so its proceedings, influenced by such members, may tend to become trifling and childish. Whilst these two dangers are far from being imaginary ones our Society has so far been, and in the nature of things we may hope will always be, preserved from the first of them, because its individual members do not have a chance of growing old together—worse luck say some of you,—and of grinding along the groove of mere usage, until we become so fitted to it that we cannot with comfort move along any other path ; whilst the second we may hope effectually to escape by the exercise of good sense and right feeling.

Perhaps to this end I may be allowed for a moment to remind you of the objects for which the Society exists.

What meaning does our title convey ? "The Students' Society." There is a story told of an old lady in some out of the way country parish, who, having or being supposed to have an inveterate taste for literature, was for ever borrowing books from her clergyman, until at last she had read through all his library, and there was nothing left but the dictionary. Still the old dame clamoured for more intellectual food, so in despair the vicar lent her his Johnson, and calling upon her a few days later, was informed that the volume was a most interesting one, although the thread of the narrative was not very clear. Taking up that narrative at the word Society, I find the worthy doctor defining it as "the union of many in one general interest." We, as individuals, having many and diverse interests, find a bond of union here in one interest which is common to us all—our work.

What are the ways in which that interest is served by the meetings of this Society?

In the first place, no one can attend meetings with any degree of regularity without making appreciable additions to the stock of knowledge, which is an important part of his stock in trade

Lectures, text books, and hospital practice teach us much no doubt; but, all important as they are, they are not all comprehensive, and I am sure that those of you who are best acquainted with the doings of the Society will fully bear me out when I say that in the papers and communications brought before it, and in the discussions which take place here, there is constantly to be found valuable information which is not easily to be met with elsewhere.

But the acquisition of knowledge, important as it is, is by no means the only end that we attain. Honest interchange of thought, opinion and experience, such as we here enjoy, cannot take place without those who make the exchange experiencing mutual stimulus and encouragement. A member relates an unusual case, and the relation brings to the mind of another a similar case, which he had almost forgotten, but which proves of the greatest interest when set by the side of the first; a difficult case described elicits remarks, and suggestions as to diagnosis and treatment which is often times most valuable; an appliance is shown, which, in its very ingenuity and fitness for its purpose, stimulates invention in some other direction; we hear a method of practice graphically described, and see models and specimens in illustration, and we are so attracted, that forthwith we adopt it as we never should have done had we not listened to a personal narration; or a point of ethics comes up for discussion, and we realise, perhaps for the first time, and if so with some astonishment and a salutary enlargement of our mental horizon, how differently different minds judge of the same action or motive—how diverse in short are men's views of life.

And so we give and take; we act and react upon each other. The ardent man fires his quiet neighbour; the accurate man checks the careless; the plodder shows what can be done by steady work; and because man is an imitative and gregarious animal, we both learn from each other, and are moved by fellowship of feeling to follow a good lead, where as individuals, we might, not improbably, have remained unimpressed.

Again, as to the value of our meetings in revealing and in exercising powers of mind and originality of thought which might otherwise have remained unsuspected, and have slumbered on in dormant inactivity as to the lifelong friendships which these occasions help to strengthen, if not to originate—much might be said.

Nor is this all; besides the enlargement of our store of knowledge, besides the mental stimulus springing from the mutual contact of mind with mind, besides the quickening of our *ésprit de corps* and the deepening of personal friendships, there is the further advantage in belonging to this Society, namely, that we may during our membership acquire, if we will, no little experience in the art of public speaking. There are happy individuals who feel as much at home in speaking before a room full of auditors as if they were only holding forth to a friend of their own fireside, but the average man not blest with the gift of ready speech, if he has anything to say which necessitates his getting on his feet before a number of others, experiences the most extraordinary sensations, and displays the most distressing symptoms when he makes his first attempt as an orator. His pulse goes up in the most alarming manner, his respiration becomes accelerated and irregular; his forehead, bedewed with cold perspiration, suggests a prescription containing all the most powerful sudorifics in the Pharmacopœia; and his words sticking in his throat suggests a recent study of that scene in Richard III. where Gloucester says to Buckingham:—

> "Come cousin, canst thou quake, and change thy colour,
> Murder thy breath in the middle of a word,
> And then begin again, and stop again,
> As if thou wert distraught and mad with terror?"

Am I drawing a fancy picture, and laying on the colours a little thickly? All I can say is, that I know myself what it is to undergo pretty much what I have described, and, whilst entirely sympathising with any who suffers in the same way, I would press upon them the fact, that to overcome the miserable sense of self-consciousness, and the unreasonable dread of hearing one's own voice in public, which are so difficult to control, the only way is to take such opportunities as are offered here, and to force one's self to speak again and again.

There is yet another, and a very valuable purpose which these meetings serve.

We acquire here that habit of mind which is one of the distinctive marks of a professional man—I mean the readiness to communicate to others an advance in thought, any improvement in practice which it may be our good fortune to initiate or test. Believe me, he who shuts himself up to his own thoughts and ways of doing things, not only has a very dull time of it, but he fails to fulfil his duties, and to enjoy his privileges as a member of a liberal profession.

By learning as we do here, to appreciate and value what others have to give us, and by accustoming ourselves to give in return, we prepare ourselves for taking part with interest and pleasure in the doings of other societies and associations, with which we may throw in our lot, when our hospital days are over we find ourselves—as many of us must do—severed by long distances from old haunts and friends. Besides the Odontological Society of Great Britain, which still holds its own as our leading scientific body, there are now similiar societies in several of the larger towns throughout the country; whilst the British Dental Association is spreading its ramifications in every direction. I have such a strong faith in the value of association in matters professional, and I have seen so much good done by it, in the way of mutual education, and in the removal of isolation and prejudice, those bars to scientific and social intercourse, that I look forward eagerly to the time when a man will consider the enrolment of his name as a member of the British Dental Association, at the very least, as a matter coming only second in importance and time to his acquisition of a diploma, and his registration as a qualified dentist.

There are other points I might touch upon did time permit, and did I wish to discover the breaking strain of your patience, I might dwell upon the advantages accruing not only to the hearers but to the writers of papers, pointing out for instance how their preparation is an incentive to the careful study of the subjects dealt with, and how the writing itself is valuable practice in the expression and orderly arrangement of facts which are in one's mind, but which one cannot easily marshal in due method and sequence. I might urge upon all students of the Hospital who are not yet members the good to them and to us of their joining our ranks. I might utter a protest against the short-sightedness of those who suppose that it is the same thing to read our transactions as to take a personal part in them.

But I must bring my remarks to an end. I asked just now what we understood as the meaning of the word "Society," applied to us as dental students. I ask, as a parting shot another question—what is a dental student?

Is he to be described as an individual who is seeking to acquire, at the least possible amount of trouble to himself, just sufficient knowledge and skill to enable him to scrape through an examination which he looks upon as the portal leading to a satisfactory income; or is he one, who, studying to make himself a worthy member of an honourable profession, throws himself eagerly into the necessary training—who studying to render himself worthy of his patients' confidence by making *their* interests and welfare, so far as they lie in his hands, his chief aim,—works with an alert mind, a willing hand, and a conscientious determination to overcome the difficulties in his path, and finds that there is abundant interest in his work, interest which is never found by the man who merely sees in his work the means of making money.

Do we, I ask, throw ourselves with a hearty good will into the study of those things which are to engage our time and faculties for many a year, or do we save our best energies for interest outside our work, looking upon the latter simply as a means whereby we can obtain the wherewithal to indulge in other and more congenial pursuits?

I do not presume to answer these questions. I can only say, that, in my opinion the man is to be deeply pitied who has no enthusiasm for his work. He who looks upon his daily occupation as an unpleasant thing, to be got through and forgotten as quickly as possible, must always find it a wretched drudgery,—and wearily performing it as such, he will never do it well,—for the man who is indifferent to his work, can do it in no other way but indifferently. And this is certain, that so surely as any one of us makes money getting his one object, so will he gradually become careless and slipshod in his work,—until some day, something shows with him with a start, how miserable his work is, as compared with that done in the days when his one thought was how to do it well. Is this cant? I believe it to be the truth.

I have occasionally heard men say, "What chance has the honest man who conducts his practice in a professional manner, against the quackery, still so rife, in high as well in low places, against those whose maxims and principles, or want of principles, would disgrace a petty tradesman?" To such questioners, I would offer two remarks. First, I would ask them to look back only a few years and see, as they may see, what headway *has* been made against the evils we all deplore. Secondly, I would urge what I believe to be an undoubted fact, that the public *are* beginning, are more than beginning, to appreciate and understand good dentistry, and that the one the only way, effectually and finally to stem the tide of flaunting falsehood, is to show by one's own life and practice, what education and honesty can do. An honourable career is, and always will be, a stronger argument, even in the eyes of a gullable British public, than any Act of Parliament, or any number of prosecutions. And I would further say, show me a man who is a good and a conscientious operator, who, along with the special knowledge acquired at the hospitals, possesses and uses a tolerable stock of common sense and discrimination, and who is a gentleman—by which term I mean a man who is refined and considerate, not only in manner, but in feeling—show me such a man I say (and I do not think the demand is an extravagant one), and I will show you a man who is certain to succeed.

You ask what do I mean by success. Do I mean an enormous income? No, I do not; conscientious, honest dentistry only under exceptional circumstances produces that. By success I mean, as much work as one can faithfully do; a tolerable income, enabling one to live comfortably, if not luxuriously, and last though by no means least, the regard and appreciation of one's patients, increasing as time goes on and the value of one's work becomes more and more apparent. I put it to you whether such success is not worth working, and even waiting for? Or shall we prefer and choose that cheap so-called success which makes a miserable failure of a man's life, and which can be bought by anyone—at what cost? Only at the cost of truth and manhood—a birthright for a mess of pottage.

Gentlemen, I will not detain you any longer. I thank you for listening to me so patiently; I thank you once more for the honour you have done me in electing me to be your President; and as I have yet done nothing to deserve it, I can only say that I shall endeavour to prove worthy of your trust by striving during my year of office to promote, so far as in me lies, the welfare of the Students' Society of the Dental Hospital of London.

CASES OF INTEREST IN DENTAL PRACTICE.

By J. F. Colyer, M.R.C.S., L.R.C.P., L.D.S.

CASE OF OPEN BITE.

Miss M——, aet. 15, was brought by her mother, who complained that during the last three years her daughter's teeth had been gradually growing apart.

An examination of the patient found her to be tall, of rather spare build, with a tendency to a "strumous" aspect.

Examination of the mouth revealed the fact that the teeth, with the exception of the first permanent molars, were fairly sound; that the arch was considerably contracted, and that the only teeth which

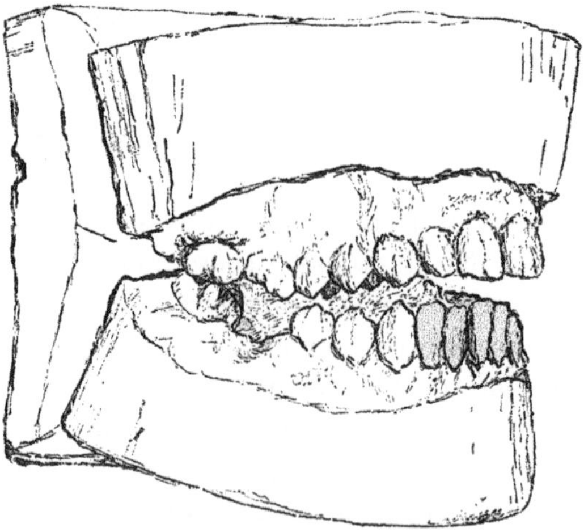

FIG. 1.—Before Treatment.

articulated were the second permanent molars (as shown by Fig. 1) Examination of the throat showed that chronic enlargement of both tonsils existed.

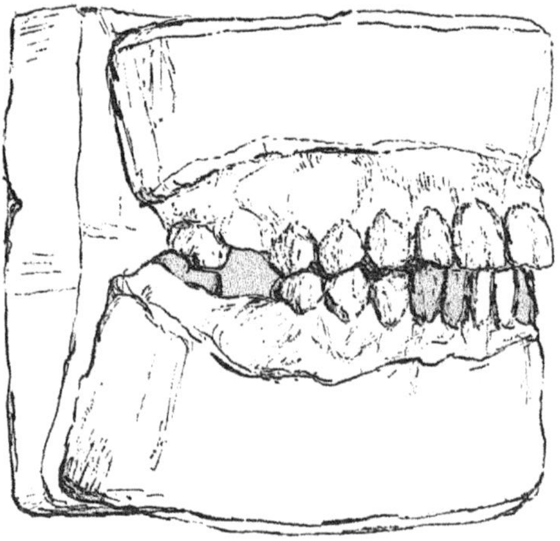

FIG. 2.—After Treatment.

The treatment adopted was as follows:—

(1) Removal of the stumps of the first permanent molars

(2) Cutting in the bite.

(3) Treatment of the tonsils.

"Cutting in the bite" was accomplished by means of small stump wheels (corundum) on the dental engine, and the method adopted was exactly similar to that pursued when "cutting in the bite" of an artificial case. This step occupied three sittings, and at the termination, the surfaces of the teeth were carefully polished by means of arkansas stones and rubber discs.

In order to allay the sensitiveness caused by grinding the teeth, the following was prescribed:

℞ Spr. Ammon. Aromat... ... ... ℥j
Spr. Vini Rect. .. .. ℥iij
Misce. Ft. applicatio.

To be mixed with equal parts of water and applied on cotton wool to the teeth frequently.

"Treatment of the tonsils" consisted in their removal by the guillotine followed by a general tonic treatment.

The result of treatment is shown in Fig. 2.

Remarks.—This case is useful as illustrating a method by which one is enabled to cope fairly successfully with some varieties of this most troublesome irregularity. In many of these cases a "chronic enlargement of the tonsils" is found, and in some cases may be the cause, hence an examination of the throat should not be omitted, and if found necessary, the tonsils should be removed or otherwise treated.

In that part of the treatment, which consists in "cutting in the bite," a point to be observed is this, "not to do too much" at one sitting; if this is carefully observed, the patient will be saved to a great extent the discomfort caused by the sensitiveness of the teeth.

With regard to the damage done to the teeth, this will be practically "nil" if care is taken to thoroughly polish them at the conclusion of the operation.

CASES OF EPULIS.

J. J., aet. 30, applied for advice concerning a small growth in mouth. Examination revealed a small, painless fibrous tumour in the region of the right upper lateral and canine teeth, which had been growing during the previous three years.

Treatment:—Cocaine (gr. ½ dissolved in 7m. distilled water) was injected, and the growth removed by means of a small scalpel, the bone between the teeth from which the growth sprung being cut away by small enamel chisels and coarse cut burrs on the dental engine.

The wound thus made was carefully syringed with carbolic acid (1 in 40), and crystals of chloride of zinc applied. The patient being directed to use the following as a mouth wash :—

℞ Acidi Carbolici (glacialis) ... ... } āā ʒ ii
Liq. Potassæ ... ... }
Aquam. ... ... ad. ℥ ii
M Fiat Lotio.

One teaspoonful in half a tumbler of water to be used frequently.

The wound healed in the course of fourteen days. When last seen, which was eighteen months since removal, there were no signs of any recurrence.

CASE II.

Miss F. B., aet. 13, applied at the hospital in February, 1888, with regard to a small growth in the region of the right lower canine and lateral.

The history was briefly as follows :—About five years previously, patient noticed a swelling which continued slowly to increase in size ; this persisted for nearly three years, when she went to a doctor who removed it, but it recommenced to grow immediately afterwards, and was again removed a year previously to her applying at the hospital.

When seen, the growth appeared to be springing from the septum between the teeth named. Mr. Claude Rogers, under whose care the patient was, recommended the removal of the lateral, and the cutting away of bone around the canine.

This operation was carried out under ether, the bone being removed in the same manner as stated in the previous case and the same after treatment adopted.

When last seen, which is now nearly two years since the operation, there appeared no signs of any recurrence.

Remarks.—These two cases which in themselves present nothing remarkable, are, however, useful, since they show the two courses which are open in the treatment of epulis, viz. (1), by removing the growth and retaining the tooth, and (2), by removing the growth and tooth as well. Many hold that for the successful treatment of epulis the tooth should be removed in all cases ; that this is not absolutely necessary I feel sure, the majority of cases met with in dental practice being able to be treated as successfully by retaining the tooth, as by removing it.

The lines of treatment should, I think, be, to first remove the growth and retain the tooth, then if this fails, resort to the extraction of the tooth as well.

If it is decided to retain the tooth, then success depends on the thoroughness with which the bone is removed, and this can always be accomplished with enamel chisels and coarse cut conical burrs. With regard to the treatment of the wound caused by the removal nothing seems to promote the formation of healthy granulations better than chloride of zinc, and this should be applied to the wound at intervals of about three to four days, (two applications being generally sufficient), and during those periods the mouth kept clean by means of an antiseptic mouth wash.

To Mr. A. W. Hoffmann I am indebted for the excellent drawings from which the engravings have been made.

Reports.

THE ODONTOLOGICAL SOCIETY OF GREAT BRITAIN.

THE Ordinary Monthly Meeting of the above Society was held on the 3rd ultimo. The President, Mr. FELIX WEISS, L.D.S.Eng. in the chair.

The LIBRARIAN (Mr. Ashley Gibbings), announced the receipt of the usual journals, and also the presentation of Mr. P. Dubois' "Aide-Memoire du Chirurgien-Dentiste" to the library.

The CURATOR (Mr. Storer Bennett), mentioned the addition to the museum of sections of the skull of a Collared Peccary, which he described, and stated that the dentition of the Peccary differed from the true pig tribe, such as the wild boar, in that it had only thirty-eight teeth instead of forty-four.

Mr. WILLIAM HERN read notes on a case of buried lower molar in the lower jaw, of which the chief points are the following: the patient, a woman, aged 38, was troubled early in 1888, with a small swelling on the border of the body of the lower maxilla on the right side. The swelling occasionally got larger and then the side of the face would become swollen up to the ear. There was also at times some neuralgic pain and stiffness under the jaw. Examination showed some thickness of the alveolar portion of the jaw, but no obliteration of the sulcus between the jaw and the cheek existed. There were only two molars on that side, but the patient could not remember whether a tooth had been extracted. There was no appearance of caries in the maxilla. The second bicuspid being loose and apparently dead, was regarded as the probable cause of the swelling, and the house-surgeon of the Dental Hospital was requested to remove it. In doing so, greatly owing to the dense resisting nature of the alveolar border, the tooth was fractured. Mr. Hern subsequently saw the case, and having failed in a first attempt to remove the remaining fragment of tooth (owing to the patient's very rapid recovery from anæsthesia), he advised postponing further operation on finding that the fragment was deeply imbedded and that the surrounding bone was so dense. Six months later, the patient again presented herself, and Mr. Hern probed the socket of the bicuspid tooth, when he was surprised to get a sound like the ring of enamel against the probe at the posterior and deepest part of the socket. After further visits and examination, a buried tooth was distinctly diagnosed. Mr. R. H. Woodhouse, who then saw the case, recommended the removal of the superjacent molar (which had no antagonist) in the hope that the buried tooth might rise, and that the gums, which were at that time freely discharging on the cheek, might heal. Mr. Hern therefore removed the molar under gas. In February of last year Mr. Hern attempted to remove the buried tooth with a curved elevator, but finding it required more force than was advisable to apply to the weakened jaw, Mr. Pearce Gould, of Middlesex Hospital, was consulted and requested to take the patient under his care, which he kindly consented to do. In the succeeding month, the patient was placed under chloroform, and Mr. Gould then carefully retracted the soft tissues overlaying the bone, and proceeded to cut away the outer wall of the bone with a dental engine, until, with a curved elevator and a pair of forceps, the tooth could be coaxed out of its bed and grasped with the latter instrument. Very little blood was lost in the operation, and the patient left the hospital next day. Mr. Hern showed models which he said conveyed a better idea of the position of the tooth than any description could do.

Mr. Pearce Gould being invited by the President to remark upon the case, said that he could add very little to Mr. Hern's interesting account. The part he played was to enlarge the opening in the body of the jaw and remove the buried molar, which he did by making an incision along the side of the jaw, and with an ordinary surgical elevator strip off the soft parts of the periosteum, taking care to preserve as much of the periosteum as possible. Then with a dental engine (which enabled him to perform the operation with an ease and success otherwise impossible) and some burrs specially designed by Mr. Hern, the outer wall of the alveolus and a small portion of the lower jaw were removed. The patient made an excellent recovery. One interesting point was the complete restoration of the body of the jaw (but probably none of the alveolus), showing that after removal of a tooth there is absorption of the alveolus and no tendency to its regeneration. Another interesting point was, that owing to the smallness of the jaw and the large size of the tooth, the inferior dental nerve must, had it followed its normal course, have been seen during the operation, and run the risk of being damaged, possibly in dipped down.

Mr. GEORGE CUNNINGHAM (Cambridge), followed with a paper on

INTERNATIONAL DENTAL NOTATION.

The object of the paper was to demonstrate the advisability of a system of Dental Notation which could be used in common by all nationalities, and to suggest a method by which it could be accomplished. A Commission, consisting of MM. Grosheintz, Dubois, Schwartz, Trallero, and George Cunningham, had considered the subject. The Commission in the first place decided that figures rather than letters were desirable to designate the various teeth, and resolved, that numbering by 32 being inconvenient and difficult to memorise, the systems of 8 and 16 were the only ones worth entertaining. The system of 8 was warmly advocated by the Commission, the unanimous opinion being that it was the easiest to comprehend and to memorise. It consisted of four groups of eight numerals starting from the median line, the respective teeth of the upper or lower jaw being indicated by the position of the numerals above or below the horizontal line, and their situation relative to the median line being shown by a vertical line on the median line side of the figures. Mons. Dubois' was the only system of 16 considered, and though slightly more difficult than the system of 8, it was yet thought sufficiently easy, and had the advantage of ingeniously avoiding the necessity of any vertical line before or after the numerals. It was decided to retain the horizontal line to denote the teeth in the lower jaw by placing the line above the numerals, the teeth in the upper jaw being distinguished by the absence of the line. The even numbers were recommended for indicating the right upper and lower teeth, and the odd ones for denoting the left upper and lower teeth. The following is the system ultimately recommended by the Commission for numbering the permanent teeth :—

RIGHT.

Upper ...	16	14	12	10	8	6	4	2
	—	—	—	—	—	—	—	—
Lower ...	16	14	12	10	8	6	4	2

LEFT.

Upper ...	1	3	5	7	9	11	13	15
	—	—	—	—	—	—	—	—
Lower ...	1	3	5	7	9	11	13	15

For the temporary teeth it was decided to adopt the numbers 1 to 10 on the same principle as the permanent teeth, merely distinguishing the former from the latter by a decimal point in front of the numeral.

With reference to the symbols to indicate the surfaces of the teeth, it was decided to adopt those employed in the system which Mr. Cunningham had published. The only difficulty that arose, was with regard to the symbol to represent the crown, there being no equivalent in the various languages; neither "crown" nor "coronal," being used in France. "T" as the corresponding mnemonic contraction for triturating surface was therefore substituted for "C." Labial and buccal practically being only synonymous it, was decided to employ only "L." In like manner, palatal and lingual applying to the same surface, "P" was the only symbol adopted. "M" was chosen to represent mesial, and "D" distal. The segment of a circle was agreed upon as the symbol to express cervical, lending itself as it does by accentuating the curve, to graphically indicate the precise extent to which a tooth might be involved.

By means of the first five signs and their obvious combinations, such as mesio-palatal and so forth, it would be easy to sufficiently define even any irregularly disposed carious cavity, *e.g.*, a cavity extending from the mesial over the crown to the distal surface would be sufficiently indicated by the letters *m. t. d.* If instead of a single compound cavity, it was desired to represent three separate cavities, the use of the colon would distinguish the difference thus, *m : t : d :*,

The colon was solely employed to define the localization and the operative terms, and so prevent confusion with any adjacent symbols. For the present it was not thought advisable to suggest any further abbreviations, and it was agreed that some mnemonic system was more likely to lead to satisfactory results than a system of arbitrary signs such as commonly used in America.

The foregoing mode of notation, recommended by the commission, was unanimously adopted by the Congress in its final session. Mr. Cunningham said, in conclusion, that although previously much attention had not been given to the subject, it seemed unnecessary to dilate upon the very obvious advantages of the uniform system of notation so as to be able to produce order from chaos in the dental literature of England, America, France and Germany. He recommended a trial of this International Dental Notation as being easily acquired, time-saving, and eminently practical. Its value to the individual in keeping a record of his work, and in corresponding with another practitioner, was evident. But he would urge its value to science, as affording a help in transforming the crude commercial entries of the day-book or ledger into the carefully recorded facts of the case book, the tabulation of which would certainly do much to remove the endless records of vague, unverifiable conclusions with which scientific dental literature abounded.

The PRESIDENT having invited discussion, Mr. H. BALDWIN said that while he thought it desirable to settle upon some definite plan, it seemed to him that the old notation was preferable to the so called "International Notation." To make the angle on the right or left side came quite naturally, whereas there seemed an element of caprice in the International System.

Mr. WALTER H. COFFIN thought there was also an element of confusion which would not unfrequently arise. If one wished to write down the left superior central and lateral by the figures one, three, that would be thirteen, which designated the second molar on that side. Or, if the central and canine were noted, the figures one five, might be. mistaken for fifteen, which would designate the wisdom tooth on that side. By the old notation, one could designate quite generally a class of tooth, such as first bicuspid, by the proper figure only, without any other sign.

Mr. GEORGE CUNNINGHAM, in reply, said that it must not be imagined that the points raised had been lost sight of by the commission, on the contrary they had been fully considered. It was essential in attempting to devise a system to be used internationally, that a spirit of give and take should be exercised With regard to Mr. Baldwin's preference for the old notation, as a matter of fact, the printers could not print it without special type. With reference to Mr. Coffin's criticism, if a comma were used—as it should be used—to separate the one and the three, they could not be mistaken for thirteen.

The President's health not permitting him to deliver his Inaugural Address himself, it was read for him by Mr. ACKERY (one of the secretaries). The following is a summary:—

Not the least difficult task of one occupying the Presidential chair for the first time was fitly to acknowledge the honour conferred upon him. However much the world's friction might make one callous of the world's opinion, the esteem of those with whom we had toiled, and step by step advanced in professional life, must carry with it a lasting interest. To him the occasion was the more memorable, for it marked the generous way in which good intentions, more than achievements of a distinguished nature, were acknowledged. To the younger members of the Odontological Society his elevation to the chair presented a lesson which should never be forgotten, for it told them how willingly the heads of their profession were ready to recognize patient industry and a contempt for charlatan practices. Having given some interesting reminiscences of the reform movement in the early days of the profession, and borne testimony—which as an office bearer of many years standing he was able to do—to the zeal, fairness, and efficiency with which the council of the Society did its work, he took "heredity" as the text of his address. The strength of the law which determines the transmission of character from parent to child still far from received the attention it merited, and was unquestionably, even in the present enlightened days, but little understood. A somewhat eccentric author, named Alexander Walker, wrote years ago very fully on the subject, and tried to prove that each parent communicated a distinct series of organs; that the male and the female on the average exercised an equal influence in the form and the mental characteristics of the progeny. "That where the father was young and vigorous he gave the locomotive system and the back portion of the head, the mother conferring the forehead and the vital system." Dr. Walker further observed "that the educational capacity of children for learning will depend upon the educational aptitude of the parents, for the natural dulness of children born of uneducated parents is proverbial." Sir Henry Holland had very happily remarked that the real subject for surprise was, not that any peculiarity should be inherited, but that any should fail to be inherited ; and Darwin had said that the most correct way of viewing the whole subject would be to look at the inheritance of every characteristic as the rule and non-inheritance as the anomaly. The President proceeded to give some singular instances of the transmission of general peculiarities, mentioning among others the case of Lambert, "the Porcupine man," whose warty projections (which were periodically moulted) were transmitted through two generations. Also that of a family in France, the leading representative of which could, when a young man, pitch several books from his head by the movement of his scalp alone. This peculiarity descended through several generations, even to a cousin in the seventh degree, who being asked if he possessed the same faculty, immediately exhibited his power.

Similar instances, the President said, could be quoted *ad infinitum*, but he would pass on to those organs which admitted of a more careful examination and classification, viz., the teeth. He desired more particularly to confine himself to hereditary peculiarities in the teeth, and their position in the mouth generally. Peculiarities in shape were very common. For many years he attended to a gentleman, all of whose superior molars had a well defined cusp on the lingual side. Such a form of tooth was not unusual, but the cusp in this instance sprang from the lingual face of the tooth and looked like a small canine attached to its side. He (the President) had had six of the children under his care and four of the boys had similar cusps springing from the same molar. A very peculiar fact in connection with the case was that two of the younger children in the same family, a boy and a girl, under six years of age, had this characteristic spur of enamel growing from the lingual side of the temporary molars also, and he had on more than one occasion noticed peculiarities of the deciduous teeth imitated in the permanent set.

It was not unusual to see peg-shaped teeth taking the place of the lateral incisors. Irregularities in position, both in the upper and lower jaw, but more frequently in the lower, were commonly transmitted from parent to child. Hereditary variations in the position of the jaws themselves commonly occur, the lower teeth in some cases crossing the plane of the upper. The "underhung" jaw was an equally frequent irregularity. As a good illustration of strongly marked hereditary transmission, the President mentioned a family in which the father had a powerful square looking jaw, boldly in advance of the upper circle, and teeth of moderate size. The mouth of the mother was perfectly regular, both jaws and teeth being well placed. The eldest son had the same projecting jaw, teeth, and facial expression as the father. The second child, a girl, also resembled the father. The third and fourth children, boys, had perfectly regular teeth like those of the mother. The fifth and sixth, both girls, precisely resembled the father. With reference to the hereditary transmission of caries, if capable of proof at all—and it was very difficult, owing to the necessity of detecting its inception at about the same period of life in both parent and child, which involved an extremely careful record of every case by the dental surgeon—it could only be demonstrated after years of patient research, and its consideration should be entered upon with the greatest caution, for that which might be regarded as conclusive might simply be a coincidence. As an example of inherited caries, Mr. Weiss gave the history of two of his own patients, mother and daughter, who each lost the four bicuspids from that disease at about the same age. After quoting further instances of the transmission of other dental diseases, such as facial neuralgia and honeycombed teeth, the President said in conclusion, that a careful study of the subject left no doubt in his mind that the following inferences might safely be made: that the teeth distinctly take after one parent or the other, as well in health as in disease; that the intemperance of parents led to some form or other of degeneracy, commonly idiocy, frequently caries and other defects of the bony structure. Diseases were known to remain latent in the system for years—why should it not be the same with the teeth?

Mr. James Smith Turner proposed, and Mr. Morton Smale seconded, the usual vote of thanks to the President for his address and the resolution was carried by acclamation.

The next meeting was announced for March 3rd, when Messrs. Bland Sutton and Charters White will read a paper on "Ovarian Teeth." Mr. Storer Bennett will report on Mr. Harding's case of impacted fracture of a tooth, and "Casual Communications" will be made by Messrs. W. F. Henry, F. J. Vanderpant, and J. Ackery.

The meeting then separated.

ODONTO-CHIRURGICAL SOCIETY OF SCOTLAND.

The Third Ordinary Meeting of the Session of 1889-90 was held in the Rooms at the Dental Hospital, Lauriston Lane, Edinburgh, on January 9th—Mr. J. Austen Biggs, L.D.S., President in the chair.

After the usual business the following paper was read by Johnson Symington, M.D., F.R.S.E., on the

DESCRIPTION OF A SPECIMEN OF CLEFT PALATE.

This specimen was met with in a male subject, aged 70, dissected in my rooms last summer session. The cleft was obviously congenital, and extended through both the hard and the soft palates and the right alveolar arch. It opened above into the right nasal cavity.

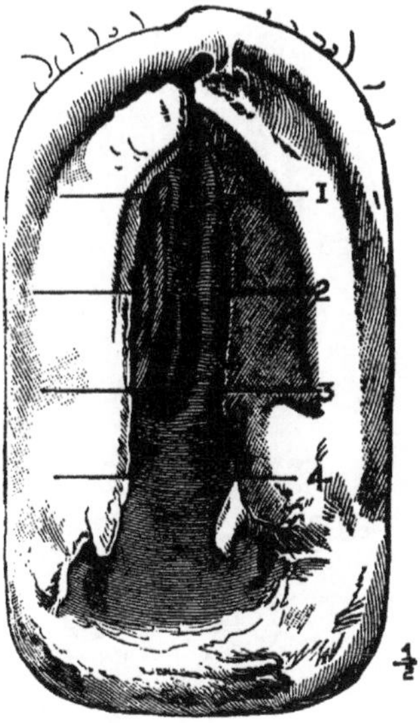

Fig. 1.

The upper jaw was practically edentulous, so that it was not possible to determine the relation of the cleft to the incisor teeth. It may be noticed, however, that the cleft passed through the alveolar arch barely a quarter of an inch external to the frænum of the upper lip, so that on the right side there was obviously not room internal to the cleft for more than the central incisor tooth.

Mr. Bowman Macleod kindly made a cast of the deformity for me, and I then froze the specimen, and made a series of transverse vertical sections through the palate, nasal cavities, and maxillary sinuses. Sections of this kind are very useful for the demonstration of the relations of the palate and nasal cavities, and Zuckerkandl* has employed th s method very extensively for the illustration of diseased conditions of the nasal cavities. I have, however, been unable to find any published drawings of similiar sections in cases of cleft palate. Indeed, the illustrations of this condition appear to be practically confined to representatives of the cleft as seen from the mouth These figures which are generally diagrammatic, merely represent what can be readily seen on an examination of the deformity in the living body, and give a very incomplete view of the condition of the palate and nasal cavities.

Fig. 1 is a drawing of the cleft in my specimen, as seen from the oral aspect. There is a cicatrix in the upper lip below the right nostril, and it looks as though there had been a hare-lip on that side

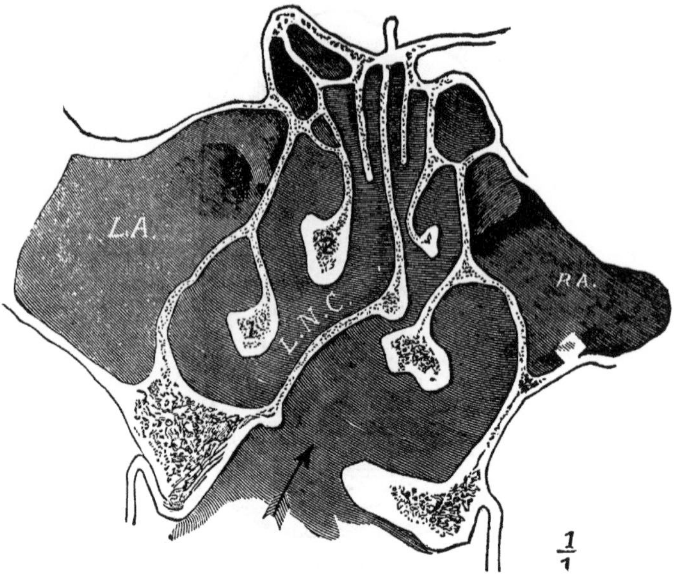

FIG. 2.

which had been operated on. The anterior part of the alveolar arch to the left of the cleft projects lower down and overlaps somewhat the thickened and warty-like mucous membrane attached to the alveolar arch on the right side of the cleft. The left alveolar arch gradually becomes less prominent as it passes backwards. The fissure extends through both hard and soft palates, and there are two distinct uvulæ.

Four transverse vertical cuts were made with a saw, so as to

* Normale und Pathologische Anatomie der Nasenhöhle. Wien. 1882.

divide the specimen into five pieces. The two anterior cuts went through the nasal cavities, and the two posterior ones through the naso-pharynx. The transverse lines on Fig. 1, numbered 1, 2, 3, and 4, indicate the position in which the sections were made.

Fig. 2 is from a tracing of the posterior cut surface of the anterior slab. The ethmoidal sinuses and superior and middle turbinated processes are fairly symmetrical, except that the right middle turbinated process is distinctly smaller than that of the left. The septum nasi passes downwards, and slightly to the right, for $1\frac{1}{4}$ inches. At this point it is thickened, and then makes a very marked bend downwards and to the left, to join the left palatine process.

It will be seen that the fissure, although opening into the right nostril, is situated to the left of the mesial plane, and the closure of

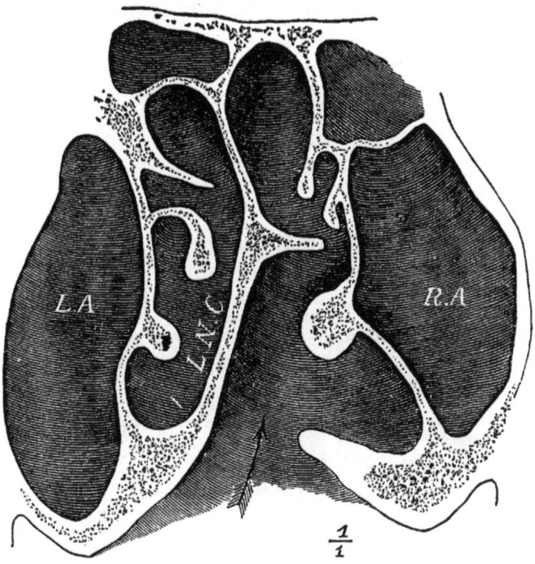

FIG. 3.

the left nasal cavity is not associated with any marked development of the palatine process on that side, but depends upon the deflection of the septum nasi to the left. The vertical thickness of the left alveolar arch is decidedly greater than that of the right, but it lies farther from the mesial plane. The antrum of Highmore is larger on the left than on the right side. The openings from the antra into the infundibula are anterior to the section, and there are no apertures leading directly from the antra into the middle meatuses.

Fig. 3 shows the posterior surface of the second slab. It will be observed that in this plane the septum has a very prominent ridge projecting from its right side into the space between the superior and middle turbinated processes. Below this ridge the septum inclines downwards and slightly to the left. The antrum extends much lower down on the left side than on the right.

Fig. 4 is taken from the posterior surface of the fourth slab. The body of the sphenoid is divided nearly half an inch behind the posterior clinoid processes. The left sphenoidal sinus is opened, but the right one does not extend so far back. The section is a little behind the pterygoid processes, and corresponds to the pharyngeal ends of the Eustachian tubes. Each Eustachian tube is bounded internally and above by its cartilage, the outer wall being membranous. The two halves of the soft palate are of about the same thickness. Below the Eustachian orifices they are about three-quarters of an inch thick, but become rather thinner as they

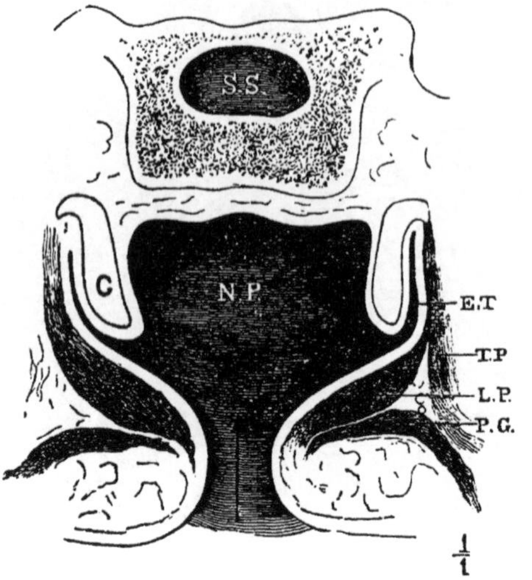

FIG. 4.

approach the mesial plane. This section shows extremely well the relations of the palatal muscles. The levator palati forms a well-defined mass of muscular tissues, which lies just beneath the mucous membrane, covering the upper surface of the soft palate. The tensor palati appears as a thin sheet of fibres lying external to the Eustachian tube. On the right side, after removing a little fat, its tendon was easily traced to the hamular process of the internal pterygoid plate. A small bundle of fibres connected internally with the lower part of the levator palati, and passing outwards and downwards, belongs to the palato-glossus. The section is immediately in front of the tonsils, and consequently anterior to the palato-pharyngeus.

The muscles of the soft palate are separated from the mucous membrane on the oral surface of the palate, by a thick layer of glandular tissue and fat. It is scarcely necessary to point out how clearly this specimen demonstrates the relations of the muscles of the soft palate, as described by Sir William Ferguson. It also shows that the levator palati lies much nearer the upper than the lower surface of the soft palate, and, therefore, can be most readily divided by Ferguson's method.

Mr. Macleod exhibited the dies and models which should have accompanied the reading of Mr. Booth Pearsall's paper at last meeting. They enabled one to gauge exactly the difference between the old-fashioned die and the Pearsall die, in every respect to the advantage of the latter. Those who gave the Pearsall method a trial would discard the clumsy old-fashioned die for ever. The Bayley flask for die and counter-die was a great advance on the old method Pearsall's was a still further advance, but he thought a still further improvement might be made by the adaptation of the Bayley counter-flask to the Pearsall cone-die. These two methods, however, separately or combined, gave a most effective and *handy* swaging tool.

Mr. Stirling in giving a demonstration on root filling with oxychloride of zinc (using for the purpose teeth out of the mouth), said that he had read a paper on this subject before the Society some four or five years ago, but it had occurred to him that if he were to show how it was done it might induce a more extensive adoption of this method of filling roots. As far as he could learn, the filling of roots with oxychloride of zinc is practised by very few dentists in Scotland, although he thought it was otherwise in the United States; and he remembered reading, not long ago, of an American dentist who had visited this country and expressed as his opinion that we we were far behind in root filling He would recommend those who did not already make use of this method to try it. If they began with easy cases, after considerable practice he thought they would be able to fill roots which at present they might consider impossible to be filled. Mr. Stirling said he would not say anything about the treatment of roots before filling, as that had been given in the paper to which he had already referred. He then showed his instruments for filling roots, steel bristles made of piano wire and fixed in a penholder, some of them so fine as to be able to go to the apex of the narrowest of nerve canals. He then put carbonate of soda, moistened with a drop of water, into the cavity of a tooth, and, with the bristles, forced it into the canals, working the bristle well up and down to cleanse them thoroughly, afterwards syringing out with water. Then, to force carbolic acid in he took a small pledget of cotton-wool, well saturated with the acid, put it in the cavity of decay, and, passing a bristle in by the side of the cotton into a nerve canal, worked it well up and down each one to pump up the carbolic acid. A weak solution of bichloride of mercury was then forced up in the same manner. Then, on a glass slab he mixed some of Fletcher's white enamel, in order to show the necessary consistence. He was indebted to Mr. Fletcher, of Warrington, for the information that borax retards the setting of oxychloride stopping. Previous to that he had found that sugar delayed it, but borax was rather better. An exceedingly small quantity of powdered borax, added to the liquid on the slab, previous to mixing with the powder, will cause the oxychloride stopping to remain liquid for about two hours before it begins to set. This could be capped over with a quick setting cement and the cavity of tooth filled at once, in any manner the operator pleased. Mr. Stirling then filled the cavity of decay with oxychloride, and pumped it with bristles into the canals. In cases where the nerve has been but recently devitalised, Mr. Stirling treats them with carbolic acid only, before filling; but in other cases he uses soda first, then sometimes permanganate of potash, then bichloride of mercury, and then, always lastly, carbolic acid.

Mr. WILSON exhibited a peculiarly formed supernumerary tooth which he had lately extracted. It was the largest he had met with, and its removal involved the application of some force. The crown was hemi-spheroidal, $\frac{3}{10}$-inch in diameter, and the root increased in dimension steadily from the neck to near the apex, where it became rather abruptly truncated and showed signs of absorption. The root was $\frac{11}{20}$-inch in length, its greatest diameter $\frac{10}{20}$, and its transverse diameter $\frac{7}{20}$, thus giving the whole tooth a decidedly almond form. The position of the tooth was inside the arch between the central and lateral of the left side, and there was another supernumerary, somewhat larger than usual, but having the usual sharp conoid crown, in the corresponding position on the right side. Strange to say, the arch was very little disfigured by their presençe. He purposed making a transverse section ôf the larger tooth.* He also exhibited a case of dilaceration in an upper bicuspid. The crown had been moved on the root, so as almost to expose the pulp cavity, which seemed to have been afterwards protected by a secondary formation of cementum. The pulp had not become calcified. As to the history, he learned that the patient had, when about three years old, met with a fall, knocking out the upper incisors. Although, latterly, the pulp cavity had become exposed and the pulp dead, the patient had never complained of its giving pain.

Mr. WATSON gave details of a case of necrosis of the palate bone, as a result of an abscess in the second superior bicuspid. The patient, a gentleman, some three years ago had an abscess, arising from a second upper bicuspid, which caused him very great pain, a sinus eventually forming in the median line of the palate, not far from the junction of the soft and hard palates, and from which there was a constant discharge of pus. The tooth was removed some three months after this, but the sinus had continued discharging. On examination he found there was necrosed bone, part of which was removed and the patient was told to syringe daily with antiseptic solution. About a month after, finding that the discharge was still going on, the sinus was slit up and all the necrosed bone removed. The case was interesting from the fact that it was very uncommon for abscessed upper bicuspids to open on the palate, the tooth which more particularly has a tendency to do so being the lateral incisor.

Mr. STIRLING asked if any of the members had ever cut the frænum of the upper lip, where, from its unusually dependent position, it interfered with the security of upper suction cases. He had done so once or twice, and he thought, with beneficial result.

Mr. WATSON had never done so with that object in view, but he had cut it in young subjects, where it was abnormally developed, and was hindering the approximation of the two central incisors.

The CHAIRMAN announced that the next meeting would be held

* On section the root was found to be composed of a shell of ordinary dentine, having an irregular edging of secondary dentine, there being several nodules of osteodentine in their line of junction. The centre was a mass of osteodentine, having only a few, and these slight, connections with the outer shell, almost the whole pulp having become calcified. The osteodentine, which formed fully half the root, showed traces of vessels, and in many places extensive groups of bone lacunæ, with well marked canaliculi.

on the 13th February, and would be a conversational one. The subjects for discussion would be one on antiseptics, opened by Mr. Watson, and one on combination fillings, commenced by Dr. Williamson.

EXTRACTS.

HISTORY AND USES OF THE PROTECTED SURGICAL ELECTRIC LAMP.

By N. Stevenson, M.R.C.S., L.D.S.

In 1883 I designed an electric light for dental work. The lamp was made expressly by the Swan Electric Light Company. It was fitted into an ivory socket firmly screwed to a metal tube like a No. 8 catheter, and covered with a glass shade, so as to allow sufficient air space, to prevent contact at any point between the two. The tube passed through a suitable wooden handle, and being open at each end, allowed the air to circulate freely. It was described at the time in the medical journals, and exhibited at the Pathological and Odontological Societies of London and Edinburgh, but the difficulty in getting the lamps and unsatisfactory working of the batteries made me abandon the use of it; now, however, that better lamps can be easily obtained and that the batteries are immensely superior to the old ones, I have taken to use them again and adapted them to other surgical purposes besides my own.

I find this lamp useful for any kind of examination where light is required without undue heat. It may be used in contact with any part of the body, if it is not kept lighted too long; for this reason I prefer to let the patient control it if possible, for then it can be lit at pleasure, and confidence is established. It is valuable in most operations of dental surgery, but especially so in preparing difficult cavities for fillings, or for working out nerve canals and in detecting exposure of the pulp. In cases of closure of the jaws from spasm or other cause, it gives enough light through a gap in the teeth to enable one to see perfectly the whole cavity of the mouth. It may be put into one nostril to examine the other by lighting it up through the septum. It is useful also (with a slight alteration in the bend of the stem) for gynæcology, and in abdominal surgery specially valuable.

In another application chiefly useful for scaling long teeth sloping inwards, the lamp is fixed by the air tube to a flat silver ring, which is surrounded with gutta-percha, so that it may be conveniently held in position by passing the forefinger through it. Whilst the lamp lights the whole floor of the mouth, it also keeps the tongue out of the way, and the ring prevents the mouth from closing and protects the finger from the teeth.

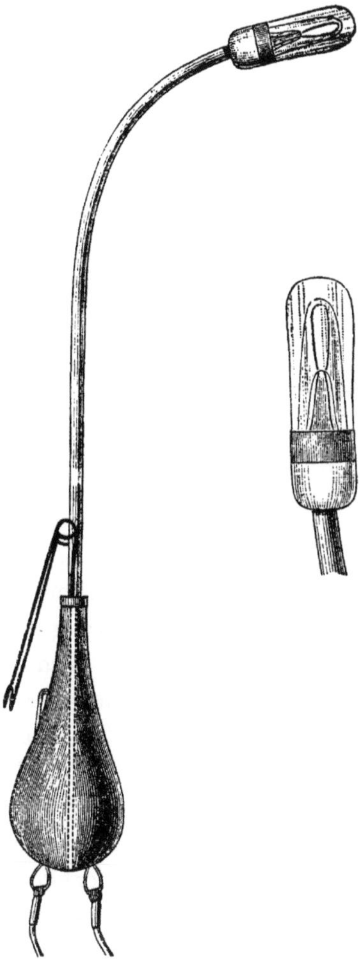

I fitted another into the tongue plate of Mr. Smith's gag for cleft palate operations; with this the surgeon gets a perfect light, and is relieved from the nuisance of having constantly to dodge his own shadows; this, indeed, is one of the chief advantages in all these lights. The necessary air tube here is carried in a groove in one side of the lower limb of the gag, and emerges into the open air near the hinge. The operator regulates both these instruments by pressing with his foot or knee a specially arranged switch for the purpose If a constant light is wanted for a long operation, air would have to be forced through one tube and out at another by means of a similar arrangement to that used for diffusing spray, but although this would be less complicated than the hydraulic plan, it is quite unnecessary for ordinary purposes.

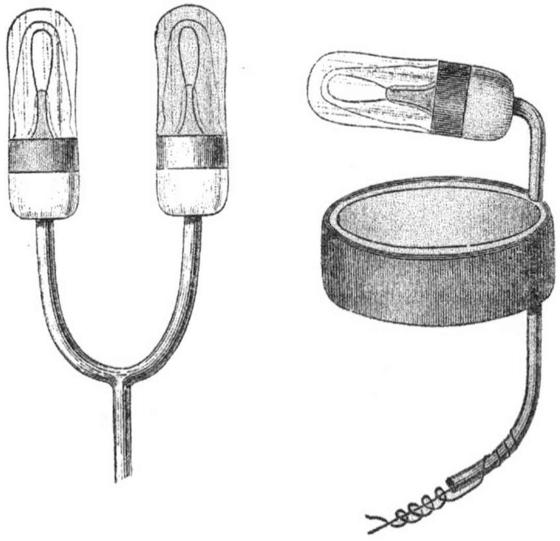

Dr. Felix Semon suggested that I should try the experiment first employed by the late Professor Heryng to diagnose empyema of the antrum. He used a five-volt lamp fixed to a tongue depressor, and in a perfectly dark room, lighted the bones of the face from the mouth. I have repeated this with two five-volt protected lamps on one stem, and have further modified it by introducing them into the nostrils. The bright red in the facial cavities and the lurid glare of the soft tissues gives the face a ghastly aspect, the practical value of which is that if either antrum is diseased or filled with pus, it will be less luminous than the other, and the abnormal condition will be detected. Of course, a naked lamp cannot be used in the nostrils, as the heat would be unbearable. I cannot estimate the practical value to others of these instruments, but I think there must be many who will find them as I do of great service. I have myself made or mounted all those I have referred to, and if anyone wishes to do the same, I may as well mention that the lamps are from the Edison and Swan Electric Light Company, and are called five-volt pencil-shaped micros. In mounting the most important points are to have the lamps without other attachment than the conducting wires, and to hermetically seal the glass cover to the socket. Those who do not care to make them can obtain them with the batteries from Mr. Schall, Wigmore Street. The carbons are so delicate that the instruments must be handled with great care; a drop of three inches on anything hard will probably break them. I always try to place them gently on something soft, like blotting paper or velvet. —*British Medical Journal.*

A STUDY OF ELECTRICITY, WITH THE VIEW OF COMPREHENDING ITS APPLICATION IN DENTISTRY*.

By HOWARD E. ROBERTS, D.D.S., PHILADELPHIA.

IN preparing this paper for your consideration I have found it difficult to express my ideas without defeating the object for which it is written. To those who have given the subject much study, or who are practical electricians, my paper will be of little interest, but as it is to those who are not so well posted in the subject that I wish to address my remarks, I trust you will pardon me if I repeat what you are already familiar with. It is difficult to understand and remember if we do not know and see the reason why; therefore, I will try to explain some of the laws and define some of the terms used, making use of as few technical terms as possible, and defining those I have to use.

In many ways electricity may be compared to a stream of water, and, as we can see and measure the water, it makes it easier to understand and appreciate the laws which govern the electrical current. One difficulty which many have in trying to understand many of the terms used in connection with electricity comes from the impossibility of being able to see and handle,—you might say there is nothing tangible to work from.

In order to speak intelligently about electric currents, there are three terms or words the meaning of which it is necessary to understand. They are the Volt, the Ohm, and the Ampère, and they are so related that by Ohm's law, if any two are known we can determine the third. The volt is the unit of pressure, the ohm is the unit of resistance, and the ampère is the unit of volume or quantity.

---

* Read at the twenty-first annual meeting of the Pennsylvania State Dental Society, held at Cresson, Pa., July 30, 1889.

In defining these terms I will first take the unit of resistance. If it were water or steam we were considering, we could say that the unit of resistance would be the resistance offered by a pound weight, and with water flowing through a pipe the resistance would be the friction of the water against the sides, which would be represented by so many pounds. Every wire or conductor, or non-conductor either, offers a certain resistance to the passage of a current of electricity, and the resistance which is offered by a column of pure mercury 106 centimetres long by one square millimetre cross-section at 0° C. has been accepted as the unit of resisance, and has been called the ohm. One mile of ordinary telegraph wire has about 13 ohms resistance. As we have a unit of resistance, we must have a unit of pressure to overcome that resistance, and it is called the volt. One volt will overcome a resistance of one ohm. With water we would say there was a pressure of so many pounds, and with electricity it is a pressure of so many volts; in either case it is a pressure to overcome a resistance. The ampère is the unit of volume or quantity: with water it would be the gallon, but we cannot measure electricity as we would water, though we can measure the effect that a given current will produce in depositing a given metal from its salt held in solution, and the deposition is directly proportional to the current.

The quantity of electricity that will pass in one second through a resistance of one ohm when the pressure is one volt has been taken as the unit of quantity, and is called the ampère. One ampère will deposit $\frac{17,253}{1,000,000}$ of one grain of silver in one second. It is said that one volt will overcome a resistance of one ohm, and it is a little difficult to understand or catch the exact meaning of it. I think a pipe carrying water will help us to understand. Suppose we have 1000 feet of pipe which we can lay perfectly level; now turn up both ends and fill the pipe with water; if either end is elevated, say one inch, the water will flow slowly from the other. An elevation of one inch would represent a pressure of about $\frac{1}{24}$ of one pound; now increase the elevation of that end to two feet, which will give about one pound pressure, and we will find the water to flow about twenty-four times faster. If, on measuring the water flowing from the pipe, we found one gallon to flow in one second, we would say that one pound would overcome the resistance of the pipe, so that one gallon of water will be discharged in one second, and one volt will overcome the resistance of one ohm, so that one ampère will be discharged or flow in one second, which is one way of writing "Ohm's law."

If we increase the voltage while the resistance is kept constant, we will increase the number of ampères, or, if the resistance is increased with a constant voltage, the number of ampères will be decreased, and the increase or decrease will be in direct proportion. Divide the volts by the ohms,—that is, the pressure by the resistance,—and the quotient will be the ampères.

By the "difference of potential" is meant the difference of pressure or level, and the earth is taken as zero potential in the same way that the ocean is the zero for water level, the current flows from the higher to the lower potential; we say there is a difference in potential of so many volts.

I have not given as much attention to the galvanic battery as I have to some other parts of the subject; however, I may be able to give you some ideas that may help you to explain some things which you do not now quite understand.

I believe there are two theories about the generation of electricity with the battery. One is that it is due to chemical action, and the other is that it is simply the contact of different metals or substances, and that it is the contact which produces the chemical action. The plates of a battery are supposed to be of different potentials, and, as the current falls from one to the other through the external circuit, the battery fluid serves the purpose of a pump, as it were, to raise it from the lower to the higher potential, so that it can again fall, and thus keep up a continuous circulation.

How much power can be gotten out of a battery, and how is the best way to arrange the cells, are questions frequently asked. The power of one horse is supposed to be able to lift thirty-three thousand pounds one foot in one minute, or five hundred and fifty pounds in one second. The electrical equivalent of the horse-power is seven hundred and forty-six watts. A watt is one volt multiplied by one ampère,— a volt ampère, as it is called,—and any combination of volts and ampères which when multiplied will give seven hundred and forty-six will represent one horse-power.

For instance, the horse-power may be one ampère and seven hundred and forty-six volts, or it may be one volt and seven hundred and forty-six ampères, and one volt and one ampère will be $\frac{1}{746}$ of one horse-power.

Ohm's law is one of the most important of electrical laws, and is the key to the distribution and use of electricity. The law is, "The strength of a current in a wire or conductor is in direct proportion to the difference of potential between its ends, and inversely proportional to its resistance," and the units are so chosen that one volt will overcome the resistance of one ohm, so that one ampère will flow in one second. You may divide or multiply and split your current and conductor as you please, but the law will hold good.

Let us now consider the power of a battery-cell. Take a simple plunge-battery having two carbon plates and one zinc, it will give about two volts and, we will say, ten ampères on short circuit,—that is, with no external resistance. Multiply two by ten and we have twenty watts; divide 746 by 20, and we have $\frac{1}{37\cdot3}$ of one horse-power. But before we can use that power, we have to introduce a transformer, say a motor or mallet, which will have some resistance, say one ohm.

The cell that will give ten ampères with two volts must have an internal resistance of $\frac{1}{5}$ ohm, for the volts divided by the ampères will give the resistance. If we add the external and internal resistance, we get $1\frac{1}{5}$ ohm; divide the two volts by that, and we have $1\frac{2}{3}$ ampères, which is multiplied by the two volts, giving $3\frac{1}{3}$ watts, which is a very small part of a horse-power, being only $\frac{1}{223}$.

We will now take six cells of the same kind and arrange them in series,—that is, with the carbon of one cell joined to the zinc of the next, &c. The external resistance is the same, but the internal is six times as great, or $1\frac{1}{5}$ ohms; add the external and internal resistance (= $2\frac{1}{5}$ ohms), and divide the volts, which would be 12, by it, and we have $5\frac{5}{11}$ ampères of current; multiply 12 volts by $5\frac{5}{11}$ ampères, and we get $65\frac{5}{11}$ watts; divide 746 by that, and we get a little less than $\frac{1}{11}$ horse-power.

In connecting the cells in series you increase the voltage, but the ampères remain the same; while with the cells in parallel,—that is, all the carbons connected to one pole and the zincs to the other,—you increase the ampères by decreasing the internal resistance, but the voltage is the same as for one cell. Though the watts of the battery would be the same on short circuits in either case, the power through the resistance of one ohm with the cells in parallel would be but little better than for the single cell.

In regard to the arrangement of the cells to give the best results: it is said, to so arrange them that the internal and external resistance shall be the same will enable you to get the greater amount of work from the battery, and therefore that should be the best and most economical arrangement. The idea is that, as the resistances are equal, there would be an equal amount of heat used in either circuit, or fifty per cent. of the total energy, and that with a perfect transformer of power you could never realize more than half the power developed by the battery. If you want to do the greatest amount of work in the shortest time, I believe that arrangement of cells will do it, but I think it is not the most economical arrangement.

In every case where electrical energy is converted into mechanical there is generated what is called a counter-electromotive force. If this counter-electromotive force equals the electromotive force of the battery, there would be no current flowing; consequently there would be no heating, and no work would be done. Electromotive force means the pressure of the current, or the number of volts given by the battery, and is generally written an E. M. F. of so many volts. The heating of the circuit is in proportion to the square of the current. The counter-electromotive force acts as a resistance, inasmuch as it reduces the current, and it should be as great as possible, to allow enough current to flow to do the work. Make the internal resistance of the battery as small as possible,—that is to say, use large carbon and zinc surfaces. The heat in the cells is wasted; you can only use the current in the external circuit.

In the calculation of the battery power, it is the electrical and not the mechanical power you get; there is always a loss in the conversion of energy.

In converting the heat energy of coal into mechanical, in the best and largest engines we cannot recover more than twenty per cent., while the locomotive engine, I believe, uses about eight per cent. With a good motor about ninety per cent. of the electrical may be converted into mechanical energy.

In regard to the storage battery and its care I feel that I know little, but as there may be some here who know less, I will try to define it.

Take two plates of lead and place them in dilute sulphuric acid (ten per cent. solution), and pass a current from two or more cells through them for a short time; upon disconnecting the cells and connecting the lead-plates you will get a current in the opposite direction, which will only last for a short time, though it may be of large volume; if the plates are charged and discharged a great many times in opposite directions, which is called forming the plates, they get a spongy surface upon them, when they are capable of receiving a large amount of electricity and returning a large portion of it. (Planta.) The forming process took several weeks, and was very tedious. Now the plates are generally coated or filled with oxide of lead in some manner, so that once charging forms the plates.

The storage-cell gives about 2·25 volts when freshly charged, which soon falls to 2, and is held at that for the greater part of the discharge. You cannot recover all of the electricity which is put into the cell in charging, but you can recover in a useful form a current which would be too small to use either with a lamp, cautery or motor. The storage-cell may be charged with a battery of gravity-cells which would give a very small current. But it would take many hours' charging to get one hour's work, and the rate of discharge will depend upon the resistance of the circuit.

Before considering the use of the electric-light current in our offices, I think it would be well to understand a little about the generators of the current or the dynamos.

Professor S. P. Thompson's definition of a dynamo-electric machine is, "A machine for converting energy in the form of mechanical power into energy in the form of electric currents, or *vice versa*, by the operation of setting conductors to rotate in a magnetic field, or by varying a magnetic field in the presence of conductors." The generators may be divided into two classes,—that is, those giving a continuous current, or a current flowing in one direction; and those giving an alternating current,—that is, the current that flows first in one direction and then in the other, the alternations being very rapid.

The alternating current is not adapted to run the mallet, neither are there motors for that circuit very well adapted for our use; therefore I will not consider that current or its generators further.

The continuous current generators may be again roughly divided into those giving currents of high and those of low potential or voltage, though this is a comparative division. The dynamo to give a high potential current has many turns of rather fine wire on its armature, and is intended to give a current of small volume and great pressure, while the low potential dynamo gives a large current at low pressure, and has few turns of large wire or copper bars on its armature. One generator may give 10 ampères at 1000 volts, or 10,000 watts, and another would give 100 ampères at 100 volts, which also would be 10,000 watts, requiring the same power to drive them, and giving out the same power. The dynamo giving 100 volts would be called a low potential machine, and you can handel the wires without danger and with but little care, while a shock from the 1000-volt machine would probably prove fatal; the wires would be dangerous things to fool with, and they must be handled with great care.

The question is naturally asked, Why is one machine, or the current from one machine, dangerous, and the other harmless, when they both represent the same power? The answer comes from Ohm's law in this way. The resistance of the body from hand to hand with a dry skin is something like 3000 ohms, with the skin wet and making good contact, it will be in the neighbourhood of 1500 ohms. If we have 100 volts with a resistance of 3000 ohms, we would only get one-thirtieth of an ampère through the body, while with 1000 volts there would be ten times as much, or one-third of an ampère. It is the ampères which do the work, and the volts are only necessary to overcome the resistance of the circuit, so that the required number of ampères can flow. You can take a spark from a Holtz machine which may be 1,000,000 volts without danger, because the current is infinitesimal.

The dynamo does not generate electricity, but it does generate a difference of potential; the amount of electricity flowing will depend entirely upon the resistance of the circuit, if the difference of potential is kept constant.

The arc light is generally placed on a circuit of high potential, while the incandescent is used with a low potential. The arc-light current, or the current of high potential, should *never* be introduced into the dentist's office for the purpose of using it to run the engine or mallet, or for any other purpose where the conductors have to be handled or brought in contact with either the patient or operator. The current could be handled and used all right if it were possible to be certain that the insulation of the wires would never fail, but, as that is an impossibility, no one has a right to expose himself, and particularly his patient, to a possible injury.

The incandescent current of 110 volts is higher than we want but it is impossible to hurt your patients with it without making a special effort, and even then it would be very difficult to do more than burn them. In using the incandescent current to run the engine an electric motor is used, which is so constructed that the full current can pass through without any external resistance being introduced, when the motor will run at its maximum speed; it will also generate a counter E.M.F. nearly equal to the E.M.F. of the dynamo.

To regulate the speed, there is used what is called a resistance-box, in which is wound a number of coils of German silver wire, and by pressing a lever with the foot more or less of the wire is thrown into the circuit, and in that way regulating the amount of current passing through the motor, and consequently the speed. It is theoretically possible to get a better method of regulating the speed of the engine, but whether it is practical, I have not yet determined.

If a motor wound for use with a battery were put in an incandescent circuit without any external resistance there would be so much current pass through, on account of its low resistance, that it would be burned out; and if resistance were added until only the number of ampères for which the motor was wound could pass, there would be a great many watts wasted; and if the watts were reduced to the watts of the battery, the motor would probably not go at all. The motor has to be wound for the number of volts of the circuit on which it is to be used.

In using the incandescent circuit for running the mallet there has to be a very decided change in the potential,—that is, it must be reduced.

Where there is a potential difference of about 30 volts, it is possible to produce an electric arc, and when the arc is formed the current is not broken. As the action of the mallet depends upon the interruption or breaking of the current, the mallet would not work where there was a potential difference of 30 volts, because an arc would be formed at the interrupter.

I believe the mallet will work best with from 4 to 6 volts, or say three cells, so that the volts ought to be reduced to about that number. Adding resistance will reduce the current, but not the volts; therefore some other means has to be found.

In the apparatus gotten out by S.S. White Dental Manufacturing Company, resistance is introduced in the form of three lamps, so as to reduce the current to about two ampères; the current is then divided, part passing through the mallet, and the rest through a variable resistance which is less than the resistance of the mallet, so that most of the current passes through the variable resistance. The mallet works nicely, the arrangement is simple, and there is very little to get out of order. The current used represents about one-third of a horse-power, a small part only of which is used in the mallet. When the current is measured by meter and charged for accordingly, one-third of a horse-power costs less than three cents an hour. A motor of sufficient power to drive the engine should not cost as much per hour.

The electric motor is the reverse of the dynamo, and depends for its power upon magnetic attraction and repulsion, or upon the attraction and repulsion of a magnet for a conductor carrying an electric current, or both.

The amount of magnetism induced in an iron bar will depend upon the number of ampères passing around it, and is independent of the volts. With a given bar of iron the magnetism will be the same if 100 ampères is passed once, or 1 ampère 100 times around it.

Any one who wishes to use the incandescent current in connection with dentistry should always remember Ohm's law, should give study enough to the subject to understand the principle upon which the appliance they use is founded, and understand its construction. The use of electricity in dentistry is in its infancy, and there is room for improvement in the existing appliances and for new ones.

I think there are few who, having used the incandescent current and understanding its use, would be willing to give it up.—*The International Dental Journal.*

HYPNOTISM IN DENTISTRY.

Dr. Hugenschmidt, of Paris, writing in the *Dental Review* says:—It is a well recognised fact, by all those who have carefully studied the subject of hypnotism, that certain persons can hypnotize *themselves*, without the aid or presence of a second person.

The hypnotic state being obtained, insensibility of a certain part of the body can be easily produced, just by the verbal statement of the operator, who simply says: "This or that part has become insensible to pain." At this moment the operation can be performed painlessly.

In certain cases the patient, as soon as hypnotized, is in a general anæsthetic condition.

I have now studied this method for over seven years in general medical practice, but have only once employed it in dentistry, this being in a general hospital. I object to using this method in our office, on account of the general superstition still attached to this subject of hypnotism or magnetism by a majority of patients, who believe that one who occupies himself with hypnotism is endowed with a "supernatural power," rendering him capable of doing anything with a patient who places herself or himself into his hands. It is needless to say that this is an erroneous idea; yet, as in our speciality, we are most of the time alone in our office with a patient, I have preferred to keep on the safe side, and, to prevent any disagreeable allusion, I have always positively refused to employ hypnotic sleep in our office for a dental operation, although I am absolutely convinced that this method would be of the greatest value in our specialty, especially in painful or very long operations.

M. Godon, in a communication read before the Odontological Society of Paris, in May, 1888 (*Odontologie*, July, 1888), speaks on the use of hypnotism in dental surgery, mentioning the fact that this method was then being used at the Paris Dental School for the painless extraction of teeth. M. Godon also reported a case in which he used, on several occasions, mental suggestion on the same person for the purpose of excavating sensitive dentine on a highly nervous patient with complete success.

The only time I used this method in our specialty, as stated above, was in a military hospital of Paris, in 1882, on a soldier who was suffering severely from an exposed pulp in a superior bicuspid.

Before hypnotizing the patient I slightly touched the pulp with a needle. The way in which the patient expressed his delight in regard to my proceeding proved to me that the pulp was by far not a dead one. The man was then hypnotized. When he was placed in that condition I was able to touch the pulp, to pinch it, to tear it. I introduced a needle in the middle of its substance; it bled, but not the slightest indication of sensation could be denoted on the patient's countenance. He was then again restored to consciousness—to his normal state—and the needle was again introduced into the pulp canal. A formidable cry, accompanied by a good, solid profane word, was highly expressive of the variation of sensibility of our patient's pulp.

THE DENTAL RECORD, LONDON: MAR. 1, 1890.

Electrical Appliances in Dentistry.

WE have the opportunity of issuing in the current number of the RECORD more than one interesting paper connected with Electricity as adapted to the purposes of dentistry. Few changes involving such saving of time and energy have occurred which compare favourably with the use of electricity. At present the practical application of that great force in the arts and manufactures is in its infancy, and in dentistry, although much progress has been achieved, there is still a great deal to be done. Mr. Amos Kirby's paper on "Motors" attracted attention to that most important branch of the subject, and left the impression that at present there does not exist any very satisfactory arrangement of batteries for dental purposes. Since that time, however, some have come to the front, and the latest development of the Cuttriss Motor has greatly improved matters. Manipulative skill and adaptive invention are indispensable traits in the *personel* of the successful dentist, so that it may be hoped with a fair amount of confidence that some more accurate and reliable appliance will before long find its way into dental work-rooms. But recently an attempt has been made to bring the aid of electricity more prominently into requisition as a therapeutic agent, and in this connection, if the results justify the sanguine estimates entertained, electricity will become a most important curative agent in the hands of dental surgeons. Dr. Apostoli suggested, and largely practiced, treating uterine tumours by means of a powerful electric constant current. These tumours being composed of muscle and fibrous tissue possess more or less analogy with the fibrous outgrowths of the gums, which, as commonly treated by the knife, cause such troublesome hæmorrhage, and necessitate a most undesirable degree of cauterisation. Tonsils again have shown themselves tractable to such treatment. Following on Apostoli, we have a proposal to eradicate cancerous growths by very powerful currents, and

Dr. Inglis Parsons appears to have had success in his treatment of cases. How far dentists will feel inclined to deal with small epitheliomas and epulides without outside aid must remain at present in doubt, but it cannot be a matter of indifference to them to learn that such growths appear peculiarly favourable to the treatment suggested. The energies of the younger men in the profession may well be turned in the direction of perfecting appliances, and no wider field presents itself than that of electricity. Those who are interested in the matter will find much interesting reading in some singularly lucid and full papers by Mr. Boyd Wallis, which appeared in the RECORD four or five years back.

Clinics at Dental Societies.

The value of demonstrations of the practical methods of dentistry needs no emphasising, and yet with the exception of post graduate classes, which cannot from their very nature appeal to more than quite a small number of men, the annual meeting and some branch meetings of the British Dental Association, there are no opportunities for their exhibition. We all know of "one song" men and "one poem Wolfe," and we also know of many one method men who although unable to demonstrate all along the line can show how to do one thing well, a no mean accomplishment, by the way. We publish a paper which strongly advocates the establishment of evening meetings for "clinics" and we think the suggestion is a good one and certainly well worth considering, pro and con. We would suggest that those of our readers who are interested about the matter should write and offer their reasons for and against holding such meetings, and further, give us any suggestions how they could be arranged. Whether, for example, the present societies afford the opportunity required, and if not, whether modifications of their laws may not be advisable. An alternative scheme worthy of consideration might be the establishment of a Dental Clinics Society for the express purpose of promoting such meetings. It is, however, always a most undesirable thing to multiply societies if existing ones are inclined to co-operate and render such a step unnecessary, and we think a full and careful discussion of this point may decide the question.

NEW INVENTIONS, APPLIANCES AND REMEDIES.

We invite *all manufacturers* to send us anything useful and novel, which we shall be pleased to report upon.

A New Separator.

We have received for inspection a new separator, the invention of Mr. Blandy of Nottingham, which has been manufactured and introduced by the Dental Manufacturing Company, Limited.

It has several distinct advantages over other separators in use.

1st. It is capable of universal application to force any teeth apart in either jaw and on either side.

2nd. The vertical portion standing half-an-inch away from the wedging points allows ample room for the operation of stopping, filling-up and polishing.

3rd. It is strongly made, and not liable to break or get out of order.

4th. This strength is further secured by the connection between the two opposing halves being made by a box-joint, and not by a spring.

5th. It has only one screw for applying tension, which cannot lock as when two are used, and the milled nut is sufficiently large to admit of easy turning by the thumb and finger; but for back teeth, or very tight ones, a key is supplied to assist in turning it.

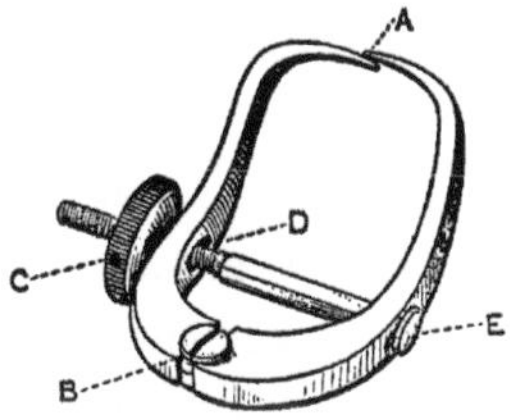

The advantages of a separator are very great to the gold filler when he comes to deal with approximal cavities—or cavities in which it would be inexpedient to cut away enamel—either to open up and get to the cavity, or by so doing to lose a possible retaining surface, while a space as wide as a sixpence, or even a shilling, can be gradually gained in a few minutes after applying the rubber dam. This effectually does away with the painful and slow process of wedging teeth apart by continuous application of cotton wool or driving in wooden pegs.

The separator supports the teeth while being stopped, and being at the same operation applied and withdrawn, periostitis has no time to be set up or tenderness excited.

Mr. Blandy's separator was exhibited at the meeting of the Midland Branch of the British Dental Association at Liverpool, and also at Brighton, and was well thought of.

Cork Points and Discs.

THE Dental Manufacturing Company have sent us samples of Cork Points and Discs made by them at the suggestion of Mr. J. Stewart, Edinburgh. These Discs promise to be of great service for polishing fillings and finishing after scaling; they carry powder well and are not much affected by moisture.

REVIEW.

A Practical Treatise on Artificial Crown and Bridge-Work. By George Evans. Second Edition. Philadelphia: S. S. White. 1889.

THAT a second edition of Mr. Evans' book on crown and bridge-work should be required so soon after the appearance of the first, speaks well for the popularity of the work. On perusing the new edition, we must confess to being a little disappointed at finding that comparatively little has been added to the old subject matter; there are, however, thirty-three additional pages, including several illustrations, and we are pleased to notice that the quality of the paper has been considerably improved. A parsimonious regard for economy in the quality of paper is scarcely compatible with the usefulness of a book of reference. Part iv. still remains meagre and poverty-stricken; surely the subject of "materials and processes" used in the manipulations described, deserves more space than seven-and-a-half pages. The subject of *soldering*, is dismissed in a very unceremonious fashion, and fuller directions will be missed by the younger student. Dr. Knapps' blow-pipe is indeed very briefly described, principally it would appear, as an apology for introducing a large advertisment woodcut, but the oxy-hydrogen blow-pipe is not even mentioned. If the author should be tempted in the future to bring out another edition, we look for improvements in the direction indicated, and an efficient index would by no means be unacceptable. If Mr. Evans can also "throw in," some little amelioration in the matter of spelling, and dispense with such atrocities as "vise" and "*fulfill*," he will be conferring a distinct benefit not only upon "Britishers," but also on his own countrymen who admire the literary style of such men as Dr. Oliver Wendell Holmes.

GOSSIP.

DUBLIN DENTAL HOSPITAL BAZAAR:—Royal College of Surgeons, 14th February, 1890.—Raffle for Old Silver. 20 Prizes. 1st—5251 T. F. Pigot, 41, Upper Mount-street, Dublin; 2nd—8797 G. H. Boughton, West House, Compton Hill Road, London; 3rd—A11612 J. H. C. Murray, Ashfield, Beau Parc, co. Meath; 4th—979 B. F. Fleming, 3, Uxbridge-terrace, Dartmouth-road, Dublin; 5th—606 Mrs. M. Burke, 107, Baggot-street, Dublin; 6th—11692 Mrs. Townsend, Harrow House, Ballybrack, co. Dublin; 7th—22544 Mrs. Cherry, 36, South-street, New Ross; 8th—367 W. Geale-Wybrants, Esq., 45, Raglan-road, Dublin; 9th—603 Miss F. Wingfield, 2, Eaton-square, Monkstown, co. Dublin; 10th—3009 E. H. Kelly, Grosvenor Hotel, Dublin; 11th—B269 Rev. R. Atkinson; 12th—10492 Adam L. Blood, 6, Longford-terrace, Monkstown, co. Dublin; 13th—A6039 Robert Whitehead, Greenside Lodge, Woodhouse, Milthorpe, Westmoreland; 14th—8901 Mrs. J. E. Vernon, Castle Park, Kingstown, co. Dublin; 15th—30085 H. Williams, 32, Ship Quay-street, Derry; 16th—30405 W. H. Woodhouse, 10, Melcombe-place, Dorset-sq., London, N.W; 17th—15003 A. Cane, Esq., 12, St. James'-terrace, Clonskeagh, Dublin; 18th—616 T. Purcell, Esq., 71, Harcourt-street, Dublin; 19th—9048 Miss Hannan, 130, Lower Baggot-street, Dublin; 20th—8171 H. Verner, Esq., Churchill, Moy, co. Armagh. Percy R. Grace, Bart., *Chairman*; Geo. Drury, *Secretary*. These winning numbers were published in the *Daily Express*, *Irish Times*, and *Freeman's Journal*, in Dublin, on Monday, 17th February, 1890. The *London T.mes* stated at the last moment that it was against their rules to publish them.

TO CORRESPONDENTS.—Owing to pressure on our space we are obliged to postpone several answers to correspondents until our next issue.

TEACHING OF MECHANICAL DENTISTRY IN THE DENTAL HOSPITAL OF LONDON.—We understand that a scheme has been matured and practically determined upon, whereby the mechanical teaching in this school will undergo great extension and development. Under its provisions the *bonâ fide* necessitous poor may be supplied with artificial dentures. In this way the students of the hospital will become familiarised with taking impressions and fitting and adapting dentures in the mouth.

RETIREMENT OF MR. E. LLOYD-WILLIAMS —We have to report that Mr. Lloyd-Williams, under whose able guidance the DENTAL RECORD was piloted through the last year, has been compelled by the increased demands upon his time, to vacate the editorial chair. An Editor never dies, still all will regret the loss of Mr. Lloyd-Williams, but as he has promised that the RECORD shall from time to time "hear from him," the feeling of severence is less.

APPOINTMENTS.

ROBERTS, REGINALD W., L.D.S., Honorary Assistant Dental Surgeon, to the Birmingham Dental Hospital, has been appointed Dental Surgeon to the Hammerwich and District Hospital.

RYMER, JAMES F., M.R.C.S., and L.D.S.Eng., of Maidstone, has been appointed Honorary Dental Surgeon to the West Kent General Hospital.

LIVERPOOL DENTAL HOSPITAL.

The number of patients treated during the month of January was 1,986—Males, 987; Females, 999. Gold Fillings, 35; Plastic Fillings, 92; Extractions, 2,267; Under Anæsthetics, 149; Miscellaneous Cases and Advcie, 66; Total 2,609.—H. FIELDEN BRIGGS, D.D.S. and C. B. DOPSON, L.D.S., *House Surgeons.*

MONTHLY STATEMENT of operations performed at the two Dental Hospitals in London, and at the Dental Hospital, Manchester, from December 31st, 1889 to January 31st, 1890:—

	London.	National	Victoria.
Number of Patients attended	—	1634	1098
Extractions: Children under 14 ...	833	294	795
Extractions: Adults	355	443	
Extractions: Under Nitrous Oxide ...	747	551	132
Gold Stoppings	307	56	33
Other Stoppings...	994	313	180
Advice	—	183	—
Irregularities of the Teeth	43	58	—
Miscellaneous and Dressings	360	109	302
Total	3,639	2,007	1,442

THE DENTAL RECORD.

VOL. X. APRIL 1ST, 1890. No. 4.

Original Communications.

THE NEW CURRICULUM FOR DENTAL STUDENTS.

By MORTON SMALE, M.R.C.S., L.S.A., L.D.S.

Dean of the Faculty, London School of Dental Surgery.

THE recent alterations in the Dental Curriculum distinctly mark an advance in the right direction with regard to dental education. The College of Surgeons have seen from their experience, as an examining body, the necessity for some such changes as those recently chronicled; moreover, they have recognised the fact that dentists are specialists of the medical profession just as much as ophthalmologists, aurists, or laryngologists, and that the same general knowledge with regard to anatomy, physiology, and surgery, is requisite for the one as the other.

In what sense are the teeth different to the eyes or ears? They are each special organs and are each supplied with blood and nerves from the main arterial and nervous organism, and each gives rise to morbid symptoms that are serious and of importance to the general economy. Let us compare ophthalmic surgery and dental surgery: wherein is the difference? The treatment of the diseases of the teeth is as difficult, and some will maintain as important, as that of the diseases of the eye. The removal of an eye is nearly as simple an operation and in many cases more simple than the removal of a tooth. In each case serious complications may arise and sequelæ follow, which make it important that the operator should be well grounded in general surgery to meet such complications. It is also of importance in each case that the operator shall be skilled in, and duly and properly taught, his specialty.

True, there is this difference: the dental surgeon is a skilled mechanic in the matter of replacing the organs he may remove; it has yet to be proved that ophthalmic surgeons would be losers had they learned how to manufacture artificial eyes, or to grind lenses and make spectacles; indeed, had they done so, it seems highly probable that part of their science would have advanced in something like the same ratio as the kindred department in the dental education. Again, had the aurists devoted themselves to the mechanical side of their department, it seems highly probable that ere now some means would have been found to meet the numerous cases of deafness due to perforation of the membrana tympani. There is no adequate reason therefore why the education of dentists should differ from that of medical men, save that they should receive the special training in dental surgery and mechanics that is necessary to make them good, useful practitioners of their calling. This is provided for by the Dental Curriculum and Examination, and in this matter the dentists are far ahead of their *confrères* who treat the eye and the ear.

How then is it best to meet the requirements of those gentlemen who intend to follow the dental profession? There are two suggestions that may be made:—(1) That the dental hospitals should remain open all day to give the students greater opportunities for dental practice; this can be provided for by a double staff, one for the morning another for the afternoon. (2) A mechanical department should be attached to each dental hospital under a skilled mechanic, and special instructions be given in the manufacture and fitting in of artificial teeth. This latter is surrounded with many difficulties, not altogether insurmountable.

Our advice then to intending students, for we must be practical, is during the three years apprenticeship to receive instructions from a doctor, a pharmaceutical chemist, or some other teacher in chemistry, theoretical and practical, materia medica and pharmacy; and as soon as he enters at a general hospital to pass the examination in these subjects held at the Examination Hall. At the same time that he enters at a general hospital he should enter at a dental hospital and pursue his studies at both institutions simultaneously. At the end of his first winter session he may pass the examination in elementary anatomy and physiology; at the end of his second winter that on anatomy and physiology proper; and at the expiration of two years the examination for the L.D.S. The subjects for the final examination may then be taken as he pleases, either all together, or one subject at a time, spreading the examination over a period of years if need be.

Under the new regulations the mechanical instruction and

teaching in chemistry, materia medica, and pharmacy, may be taken before the preliminary examination has been passed.

Those gentlemen who will follow this advice will never regret the extra devotion to work that it will entail, and such a course will do far more than anything else to place the dental profession in that position which on all grounds it deserves to occupy, viz., that of being numbered amongst the learned professions.

Each dental student should endeavour, for the general welfare of his profession, to improve his general culture by devoting his spare time to art, literature, science, and philanthropy.

There is one danger against which all have to be on their guard, viz., the temptation to become mere money makers for selfish ends. Every dentist, no matter where situated, should be able to give some time to the general welfare of his profession.

NOTES ON A CASE OF SYPHILITIC CLEFT PALATE, WITH ITS TREATMENT.

By E. LLOYD-WILLIAMS, L.R.C.P.Lond., M.R.C.S., L.D.S.Eng.

Assistant Dental Surgeon to the Dental Hospital of London.

A WOMAN, 37 years of age, applied at the Dental Hospital of London for relief under the following circumstances. About seventeen years ago she had acquired syphilis, which in its tertiary stage had caused severe ulceration in the mouth and throat. Upon examination, all active ulceration appeared to have ceased, the soft tissues being firm and healthy. The hard palate was extensively cleft from a point immediately behind the anterior palatine canal, a large quantity of bone having been removed as a result of the syphilitic periostitis; there was also a large gap in the alveolar border anterior to the cleft. The mucous membrane covering the hard palate was intact with the exception of an opening the size of a goose-quill at about the middle of the palate, and one somewhat larger, anterior to it. The soft palate was very slightly split from below, through, and as far as the base of the uvula, while the free edges were glued to the walls of the pharynx. The nose was thus completely cut off from the pharynx posteriorly, with the exception of a small opening where the soft palate was fissured. One sound bicuspid remained, all the rest of the teeth being either absent, or represented by loose and unhealthy stumps. The loose stumps having been removed, and the alveolar tissues brought into a healthy condition, the question remained as to what might be done to relieve the patient in speaking, eating, and drinking. It was doubtless desirable, in order to improve the vocal articulation, as well as to make swallowing more easy, that the soft palate should, if possible, be freed from its attachment to the pharynx; and on this point I obtained the opinion of Mr. Bland Sutton, who thought that there was very little chance of successful interference.

It was then decided to afford what relief was possible by mechanical means. An impression was attempted in plaster of Paris, with most disastrous results; and as the accident was a somewhat uncommon one, an account of it may be of some slight value as a warning to others. The tray was an extemporised one, formed by cutting out a wax impression in an ordinary tray; into this the plaster was poured and pressed into place. When the impression was removed, it was found that the plaster had run through the two openings in the palate, and becoming confluent, formed a fairly large mass which was retained within the nose. The mass was split up as well as possible into small fragments, and by means of forceps, syringe, &c., several pieces were removed. The patient departed, and when next seen, complained of considerable inconvenience from a foreign body in the nose. On examination it was found that a tolerably large lump of plaster still remained imprisoned. As it was difficult to seize and crush, it was decided to divide the soft tissues between the two openings, thus forming one larger orifice. This was done, but the bony edges of the cleft prevented the escape of the plaster. Crushing was then resorted to, followed by syringing strong streams of water in all directions. Tampons of cotton-wool were eventually passed through the narrow pharyngeal opening, in both directions, but all to no avail with regard to one piece which evaded all our ingenuity; so the patient, being thoroughly exhausted, was once more dismissed. Four days later a happy solution of the difficulty occurred by the patient finding the piece of plaster in her mouth. I need scarcely add that nothing will induce me in the future to use plaster for impressions of this description.

Ultimately an impression was taken in composition, and a very light vulcanite denture made, which not only acted as an obturator, but also proved of great comfort both in speaking and eating. At the part where the loss of alveolus was most pronounced, the plate was made hollow; and as this method of lightening vulcanite dentures is useful in a large number of ordinary cases, the *modus operandi* may be described for the benefit of those who may not be acquainted with it.

The plaster model is carefully dried, but the oral surface, untouched by stearine or any other hardening agent, must be kept clean and free from dirt or grease. The case is now built up in the ordinary way in wax, and flasked in *three parts*—the only safe method with which I am acquainted—the original model in the lower part, the teeth and labial aspect of gum, embraced by the middle part, and the palate covered in by the third part of the flask or *plug*. In other words, this method of flasking is the *contour* method *plus* the splitting up of the first part of the investment into two operations. Almost any ordinary roomy flask may be made available, if the lid be drilled and a good strong tag riveted on to it. Having boiled out the wax and dried thoroughly, the pink gum is carefully packed all round the teeth in the *second* part of the flask, and put away to keep just warm. The first part is now taken and the model painted with a solution of the rubber to be used in methylated chloroform. At the spot where the hollow chamber is desired a thin layer of rubber is pressed over the surface with the fingers, and then with hot smooth oval-surfaced packer shaped into a deep saucer-like cavity, the surface being made sure by a layer of rubber solution. The first and second parts of the flask are now brought together in a vice, and secured by pins or wedges. The remainder of the packing is now done from the palate, the contouring being complete except the lid of the hollow chamber. Having cut an overplus channel at the heel of the plug, paint the surface of the plug *opposite* the lid of the chamber with rubber solution, and press on one thickness of rubber. Place two or three drops of water in the cavity; put in the plug, avoiding pressure; keep in an upright position whilst placing in vulcanizer; and screw home when the gauge stands at 25 lbs. If these steps are carefully taken various chambers of different shapes may be made in ordinary edentulous cases, when the matter of weight—and sometimes porosity of rubber—become a serious consideration. The method of flasking and packing described is in my opinion the only one for general purposes which is absolutely reliable. Properly carried out it becomes impossible to raise the bite, or to produce that *piebald* appearance of gum caused by the erratic wanderings of rubber, which is *not* artistic although common, and which patients unfortunately sometimes take exception to. I know it is dangerous—especially in mechanical matters—to appear to dogmatise on a subject to experienced persons, but perhaps some of the younger students who read this may care to try a method of flasking which will save them a good deal of heart-burning in the future days of busy practice.

A BRIEF DESCRIPTION OF THE MICHIGAN UNIVERSITY DENTAL COLLEGE, AND ITS COURSE OF INSTRUCTION.

By H. FIELDEN BRIGGS, D.D.S.(Mich.), L.D.S.

House Surgeon to the Liverpool Dental Hospital.

ANN ARBOR, the seat of the University, situated on the river Huron, about 35 miles west of Detroit and 600 west of New York, has a population of 10,000 including 2,000 students, over a hundred of whom are dental. It is a pretty town, the streets are laid in squares, and trees run down each on either side of the road.

The University buildings, seventeen in number, including a library, museum, and hospitals, stand on the "Campus;" this campus being a square of a-quarter of a mile sides, and nicely laid out with walks, trees &c., thus the hospitals, medical college, anatomical laboratory, chemical building and dental college being in close proximity, on the same ground, is very convenient for dental students.

The dental college consists of two operating rooms containing over forty chairs, two mechanical laboratories, with seventy benches, museum, waiting room, and lecture room.

The course is one of three years' residence at the University. There are no dormitories connected with the college, but the students find rooms and board in the town, the population of which mainly exists by catering in some way for the students.

On the student's arrival at the dental department, he presents himself for the preliminary examination, unless exempted by showing a certificate of having passed an equivalent one. He must then settle down to put in three courses of nine months each, this being the only dental college where three courses are made compulsory.

His first lecture commences at 8.30 a.m. He has four each morning till 12.30, when he gets dinner and returns for practical work from 1.30 till 5. He then has another lecture from 5 till 6, and then supper. After this his time is at his own disposal, to read, &c. There is no work at the college on Saturday afternoons. In practical work he takes in his first year mechanical work and dissection; in the second year chemical laboratory and mechanical work, including cases for patients, and crown and bridge work; in the third year histological laboratory, and operating. The theoretical work includes general anatomy, dental anatomy, chemistry, physiology, surgery, medicine, materia medica, oral pathology and surgery, prosthetic dentistry, dental surgery, histology and hygiene.

The method of testing the student's knowledge is by oral, written, and practical examination, and by a system of "quizzes" during the course—the lecturer delivering a couple of lectures, and at the third questioning on the subject matter of the two former, marking the student according to his answers: these marks go towards his total required for graduation.

In the practical courses, the professors record the work done, and these marks also go towards his total for diploma.

In the third year the practical work is mainly crowning and gold filling, only few plastics being inserted: this gives the student a splendid opportunity of learning to fill difficult cavities with gold. There are abundance of good class patients, many having to wait two or even three weeks for an appointment. Patients pay for materials used, except student's instruments, and so the place is more than self-supporting.

The L.D.S. courses of the United Kingdom are recognized, so that the L.D.S., after putting in his two courses at a hospital at home, can get the D.D.S. by one year's residence in the University and passing the required examinations. In carrying out such a plan, his views become more generous and broadened by seeing other people's methods, by the travelling, &c., in the same manner that a foreigner "learns a few things" by living in England.

There are plenty of amusements at the College, football, skating and toboganning all the winter, besides shooting, and fishing: and for indoor recreation are the different societies, a glee club, dramatic club, and so forth.

I look back with pleasure to my residence at the Michigan University Dental College.

Reports.

THE ODONTOLOGICAL SOCIETY OF GREAT BRITAIN.

THE above Society held its ordinary monthly meeting on the 3rd ult., the President, Mr. FELIX WEISS, L.D.S.Eng., being in the chair.

Messrs. Charles F. Rilot, J. Brookield, R. Wynne Rouw, J. F. Colyer and J. O. Butcher were nominated for membership. Messrs. M. J. Bloom, R. E. Wood and J. H. Reinhardt were ballotted for, and duly elected.

The LIBRARIAN mentioned various additions to the library.

The CURATOR (Mr. Storer Bennett) reported that Mr. Morton Smale had presented an extremely interesting odontome to the society. It had formed in the upper right wisdom tooth of a lady aged 35. Mr. Hutchinson had sent the skull of a mummified cat said to be 4,000 years old. With regard to the last specimen, Mr. Storer Bennett had not had an opportunity of making more than a casual examination of the teeth, but they seemed to be quite perfect, a slight mechanical abrasion on the canines being all that was observable.

Mr. BLAND SUTTON having examined the odontome, regarded it as one of great interest; he knew of none like it. He suggested that it should be cut into two parts and figured in the *Transactions*. The cat's skull, he would suggest, should be macerated, the muscles removed, and the Curator asked to compare it with the modern cat.

Mr. DAVID HEPBURN intimated the opinion that the odontome was a left, and not a right wisdom tooth. He was led to that conclusion when, sometime previously, Mr. Morton Smale showed the tooth to him, partly from the curvature of the fangs, and partly because he had a case of a lady suffering from severe facial neuralgia for many months, and on examination of the mouth, this peculiar left lower wisdom tooth had a little accessory denticle on its buccal aspect. On probing it the whole surface yielded, and the denticle seemed to collapse, showing exposed nerve. He cut off the denticle with an enamel chisel, and filled the cavity with gutta percha stopping, upon which the neuralgic pain disappeared. One fact seemed to be suggested; that these little denticles had abnormally large pulp cavities; and therefore he would endorse Mr. Bland Sutton's suggestion.

Mr. Storer Bennett wished to be allowed to say, that he stated the tooth to be a right lower wisdom on the authority of Mr. Morton Smale, who extracted it, and not as the result of his own personal examination. As he had already mentioned, the tooth was a very interesting one, and he might add that some three years ago he presented one like it in character, though smaller in size, to the museum.

Mr. David Hepburn remarked that in addition to the fact that the fangs were tending in a direction which suggested the tooth came from the left side, Mr. Morton Smale originally agreed with him that it was a left and not a right tooth, and therefore his later description was probably an inadvertent slip.

Mr. W. F. Henry mentioned the subject of "shell corners" for restoring defective teeth, remarking that he did so more with a view to eliciting the opinion of the members and inviting the attention of manufacturers, than for the purpose of making any definite assertions with regard to them. Many patients, it would be agreed, had a great objection to contour fillings in gold. Could not shell corners be made which would be an advantageous substitute? He had been under the impression that porcelain corners were made by the manufacturers, but this impression was incorrect. He thought the idea was quite practicable, and showed plaster models embodying his suggestions. The corners might be fixed on with white cement, and strengthened, if necessary, with wire, as in the case of gold fillings.

The President remembered that many years ago Mr. Robinson introduced something of the same kind. He did not think there would be much difficulty in making the corners; the chief difficulty he apprehended would be to get them to be permanent. The suggestion seemed a useful one.

Mr. Henry was glad to hear the President's remarks. A firm of manufacturers to whom he had mentioned the matter, considered that the sale would not be sufficiently large to compensate for the initial expense.

Mr. James Stocken stated that he had on more than one occasion taken a portion of an ordinary porcelain tooth, and fitted it into its place with osteo stopping. He found the plan answer exceedingly well; it was impossible to detect where the substitution had been made. And as to its durability, he had recently seen one of the corners which he had fitted some three or four years previously and there were no signs of a necessity for renewing it.

Mr. F. J. VANDERPANT (Kingston-on-Thames), brought forward what he described as a somewhat singular case of non-eruption of upper laterals and lower centrals. The models shown were taken from the mouth of a boy aged fourteen. In the lower jaw the central incisors, permanent canines and posterior bicuspids were absent; one temporary incisor was standing. In the upper jaw, both permanent lateral incisors were wanting, and the deciduous canine stood distally to the permanent canine—that he also considered somewhat singular. He had pleasure in presenting the models to the museum.

Mr. CHARTERS WHITE observed that the case was a very interesting one. Occasionally such cases of delayed eruption were met with in children, and the parents were concerned to know what was likely to happen; the only comfort one could give was, that the teeth were somewhere, and in all probability would ultimately come down. A short time ago a lady patient of his, aged 50, wearing an artificial denture, erupted a canine of very irregular shape under the palate.

Mr. J. ACKERY related a similar case, suggested by that detailed by Mr. Vanderpant. It was some years since he had seen the patients and taken the models exhibited. The eldest girl in the family, aged 17, had only two lower incisors and the eye teeth were perfectly regular and normal. The second member of the family had three lower incisors between the canine. The abnormality in the third child, also a girl, was of the same type as in the eldest daughter; she had only two incisors. The mother, an observant and highly intelligent lady, knew of no dental peculiarity of the same nature in her husband, nor in other branches of their family, but, feeling an interest in the subject, at a later date she examined her husband's mouth and discovered that he had only three lower incisors. With regard to the fact of the missing incisors in the lower jaw, there seemed to be no such abnormality in the museum, except in cases where many teeth were absent. As far as the children were concerned, they had been under his care for some time, and there was no ground for suspecting that any of the laterals had at any time been extracted.

Mr. F. J. VANDERPANT asked if there were any peculiarity in the upper jaw?

Mr. ACKERY: None. He should mention one peculiarity, the canines in the lower jaw partook of the same character as the incisors.

A paper, the joint production of Mr. T. CHARTERS WHITE, and Mr. J. BLAND SUTTON, F.R.C.S., was delivered by Mr. Sutton, entitled

OBSERVATIONS ON THE STRUCTURE AND DEVELOPMENT OF OVARIAN TEETH.

The subject hitherto had not been investigated in a manner commensurate with its interest, and it was thought by Mr. White and himself that it would be of value to place before the society some facts in connection with this subject. They were unable to state the age at which these teeth developed, for they found children of five, seven, and ten years of age having dermoids with teeth fully erupted. Quite recently they had the opportunity of observing an ovarian in a girl aged seven, and this contained teeth well developed, with fangs; the ovarian also contained a lock of hair thirty inches in length. Dermoid cysts in adults and old women would frequently be found, on examination, to contain no teeth. They were equally unable to state the age at which ovarian teeth are shed. Now they knew that the hair in ovaries becomes grey, and the cysts become literally bald, but an edentulous dermoid, in the sense that the teeth have been shed, had yet to be demonstrated. The number of teeth in dermoids varied greatly, in many—probably half, perhaps more—none were detected; when present they were frequently overlooked, and so statistics were unreliable. Two, three, or four teeth is a common number, but if they contain twenty they might be described as numerous. Ovarians have been met with containing 300 or 400 teeth, one on the table contained 350 teeth, a large multilocular dermoid. The structure of these teeth had not previously been carefully described. Only two papers of any importance had been written, one was by Mr. Salter, published in *Guy's Hospital Report*, 1863, and the other by Mr. Coleman, published in the *Transactions* of this Society. But neither went into the matter with any thoroughness. Now, in so far as these ovarian teeth consist of enamel and dentine they correspond with ordinary teeth. They are lodged in bony sockets, and these are lined with periosteum. The bones in which they are lodged are developed afterwards, because in many instances such teeth are lodged in the soft tissues of the tumour; sometimes they are embedded in a piece of bone and look like so many pieces of nails projecting from a piece of wood; and then again, in their early stages they are unassociated with any cartilage. They really correspond to the alveolar process of the jaw, and this was a matter of some importance, because it had given rise to the theory that they are instances of a retained fœtus; the skin and the hair attaching to them gives apparent support to the theory. The fact of the bone being developed round the teeth makes them look very like the alveolus of the upper jaw, and it was perfectly wrong to describe them as due to a retained fœtus. These teeth agree with normal teeth, inasmuch as they consist of enamel and dentine, that is to say, they would find a body of teeth all formed of dentine radiating regularly enough so far as the crown of the teeth is concerned from a central pulp chamber. In the multi-cuspidate teeth they had this regular dentine, and on the top of that a lot of rough hummocky enamel. The other forms of teeth are like bicuspids. There was a remarkable relation of the enamel to the normal enamel on definite pulp chamber; between the dentine and the enamel, there are the usual interglobular spaces such as are seen in the normal teeth. Attention should also be drawn to the fact that in some of the teeth these hummocks of enamel have very deep clefts, or ravines between them, which in a later stage are filled up with fibrous tissue. In the case of the enamel, the fibres run in all sorts of directions, and although enamel, dentine, and cementum would be found in apparent normal relation, there was in reality the utmost disorder. The amount of cementum is variable, in many teeth it is absent, in some teeth it would be found coating only one side of the fang, but the dentine and enamel are constant. In all these teeth there was only one fang; so far as Mr. Sutton was aware no observer had seen an ovarian tooth with more than one fang. In the cuspidate teeth there was what botanists would call a "tap root." The bicuspids, incisors, and canines had much longer fangs than the multicuspidate teeth. When the crown is long, the fang is short, and inversely when the fang is long the crown is short. What was more remarkable, these teeth had no pulp-chamber: this was noticed by Salter and also by Coleman. In the multicuspidate teeth sometimes pulp would be found, and sometimes not; in some the pulp is ossified. In some specimens the whole of the pulp is replaced by fat globules and blood. The existence of nerves in the pulp has been demonstrated by Salter, in the paper of 1863 referred to, and Mr. White and Mr. Sutton had been at considerable pains to see if they could get some nerves in pulps, for Salter's observations had never been confirmed, and as yet they had met with no trustworthy specimens. Quite lately two specimens had come into their possession which seemed to give some indications in support of Salter's view, but their appearance under the microscope was too uncertain to warrant any definite conclusions and so for the present that part of the investigation required more work, though ultimately they expected to be able to demonstrate the presence of nerves. That nerves do exist in dermoids was beyond question, because one of the authors of the paper had had opportunities of experimentally showing this; for instance, the patient in these cases is often able to localize the pricks of a pin with the same certainty as in other parts of the body. Furthermore, there is a peculiarity in the character of the pain arising from dermoids, so that it had been possible to suggest the nature of the tumour from the description of the pain.

So much for the structure; now for the development. So far as Mr. Sutton was aware, no previous observers had described, or figured, or given any satisfactory evidence, as to the modes in which these teeth are developed. Recently Mr. White and himself had been able to trace their development. In dermoids, bodies composed of cells named epithelial pearls are found. The cells are large, but become compressed as they approach the peripheral part of the pearl, and ultimately become lost in the environing capsule. After their enclosure such pearls may increase in size from the growth of the enclosed cells. The epithelial pearls are worthy of close study, for they are allied to enamel organs, and indeed may be regarded as enamel organs, for in one of the illustrations one of them might be seen descending upon a dental papilla beneath like an avalanche. One involved the head of a papilla like a normal enamel germ. These germs lack a definite follicular wall which might possibly explain the deficiency and occasional absence of cementum to the fang. As yet they had not succeeded in detecting any evidence of germs of secondary teeth. It is remarkable that these pearls may remain cellular or give rise to enamel. The relationship of epithelial pearls is of interest in another direction; the pearls had been most closely studied in the median line of the hard and soft palate, as a rule they are small in size but occasionally act as tumour germs, and give rise to neoplasms known as palatine adenomata. It had recently been pointed out that such pearls are occasionally associated with papillæ in the meso-palatine suture, and gave rise to a not uncommon phenomenon, viz., a meso-palatine tooth. In conclusion, much remained to be investigated in ovarian teeth, especially with regard to their character when growing in the ovaries of other mammals.

Mr. CHARTERS WHITE, commenting upon the microscopic specimens which he had prepared, said the forms which had been supplied to him might be assigned to the molars and bicuspids, but were not of the form of normally developed teeth. The molars were stunted in their growth and finished abruptly at their necks in some cases, while in others the root extended as a single tap root brought suddenly to a close. The most striking feature about the molars was their well pronounced and numerous cusps separated from each other by deep fissures. The bicuspids might in many instances have been taken for multiform canines, the apical foramina in some cases were quite absent. The enamel presented a sodden appearance and was perforated with holes resembling those met with in any worm-eaten wood. On cutting sections with a dental engine and diamond disc or wet piercing saw, the perforations before noticed on the enamel entered and traversed the enamel in tortuous tubes, as if bored by some annelides. The enamel prisms presented every degree of granularity, and were frequently marked by those cross striations usually found in imperfectly developed enamel. The most marked irregularity was perhaps observed in the dentine; the dentinal tubuli were there, but seem to have followed no definite course, presenting a most turbulent appearance. The cementum had been small in quantity in the specimens, and presented no features for special notice. The extraordinary absence of pulp cavity in many teeth was worthy of remark: in all but two cases the pulp was wanting, and in those it was very fragmentary. In conclusion it would be a waste of time to describe irregularities which were not constant.

DISCUSSION.

Mr. ARTHUR UNDERWOOD had come with a very open mind, but still he thought it would be unfair to so able and carefully prepared a paper to allow it to pass without at least some kind of attempted comment. In the first place it would be generally recognized that Mr. Bland Sutton and Mr. Charters White had thrown a great deal of fresh light upon their subject, and he was of opinion that their paper would form a classic. Recently he came upon a case published in a Boston paper, it was a careful description of teeth lodged in two bones which resembled the parietal bones separated from each other by a suture. The teeth were called plainly molars and bicuspids, but they did not seem to Mr. Underwood to be anything of this plain description. He would be happy to give Mr. Bland Sutton the reference to the case if he desired. His next point was in connection with Mr. Sutton's remark that he did not believe there was any recorded instance of ovarian teeth with more than one fang; well, it was a dangerous thing to suggest that Mr. Sutton was possibly in error, but it seemed to Mr. Underwood that the specimen No. 994, which Mr. Sutton had passed round, had 2 fangs at the top; possibly if the bone were chipped away it might prove not to be so. Another point was a reference to epithelial pearls, possibly Mr. Bland Sutton was not aware of some interesting researches from the pen of a Frenchman who discussed these formations at great length, and endeavoured to prove that at times they were abnormal teeth, and at other times they were tumours. That reference he would also be pleased to give Mr. Sutton. With regard to the disorder of the tissues, it was obviously present, and he thought such disorder was always present in an abortive attempt to form a tooth. It was present when the pulp forgets to do its natural work and endeavours to form secondary dentine. When there were secondary teeth made they were always of a disordered kind. Of course Mr. Bland Sutton was careful to cut the particular section illustrated through the centre of the tooth, though it looked from the drawing as if it might be a little off the pulp. He would be glad if Mr. Sutton would put them in the way of obtaining such specimens as were exhibited. He (Mr. Underwood) would for his part promise to cut them, examine them, and report upon them. In conclusion he thought the society would be able to do greater justice to the paper later on.

Mr. Charters White said he had been careful to cut the specimen as near the median line as possible with a diamond disc and a dental engine. He must say that he very much regretted that he was unable to get more than two sections out of one tooth, therefore he cut each tooth into two sections, and he ground that down pretty flat and polished it so that he thought that they had obtained one side of the median line. He added, at present transverse sections had not been obtained.

Mr. Storer Bennett thought the society was to be congratulated upon the extremely able paper to which they had listened. And as this was the first occasion that Mr. Bland Sutton had been out after a severe illness, they would take it as a very great compliment that he had come down to deliver the paper himself. Mr. Bennett was exceedingly interested in hearing Mr. Sutton's remarks as to enamel being deficient on the crowns of teeth reminding them of the fissures that were to be seen in molars and bicuspids. Mr. Sutton said that at the bottom of these fissures there was fibrous tissue. Now on the authority of Charles Tomes it was known that they had Nasmyth's membrane, and it was very remarkable, as Mr. Sutton had pointed out, that cementum was either not present or was exceedingly thin; that instead of cementum on the Nasmyth's membrane there should be fibrous tissue, Mr. Bennett wished to ask whether he was correct in inferring that Mr. Sutton had found no trace of the membrane passing across the teeth.

Mr. George Cunningham (Cambridge) simply rose for the purpose of asking a question, viz., whether any caries had been found in these cysts. His reason for asking the question was, that at Buda Pesth he saw a cyst of the same nature containing carious teeth. His impression, from noticing Mr. Bland Sutton's specimen, was that caries was present in the various kinds of teeth.

Mr. Charters White, a casual observer might very often mistake some of the foramina for caries. They were brown and corroded, no polish at all on the surface, and they seemed to be eaten into by holes, more like worm holes than anything else, but with perfectly defined borders.

Mr. W. A. Maggs asked for information as to the condition of the multilocular cysts. And with regard to the multicuspidate teeth that seemed altogether exceptional, could Mr. Sutton give any more facts about them?

Mr. F. J. Bennett said that Mr. Bland Sutton's paper induced speculation in the absence of any apparent rational cause for certain departures from the usual course. With reference to calcification, Mr. Sutton had told them that there was no pulp cavity in the teeth from which the section was taken. If they looked at the secondary calcification nodules, which took place in the pulp chambers in old teeth, it seemed to begin in the middle and extend outwards. Might not these teeth, which were so eccentric in many ways, develop calcification in a precisely opposite manner? *i.e.*, commencing outwards and working towards the centre. It seemed quite possible, indeed more probable, as Mr. Sutton had said that in many of the teeth there was no cementum, or only very rudimentary indeed. Mr. Bennett remarked that in Richard Owen's "Odontology," published many years ago, there was a fine litho of an ovarian tooth, and in it there was no pulp cavity.

Mr. Bland Sutton replying said, he was extremely indebted to Mr. Arthur Underwood, and should be glad to be favoured with the references to the papers he mentioned. He might say, as to the tooth having a bifid fang, that upon looking at it again he thought Mr. Underwood was probably right. He (Mr. Sutton) had examined many hundreds of these teeth from bifurcated roots without finding them, that at last he supposed he must have got careless. But it was a point that he would take the earliest opportunity of putting beyond dispute. Should Mr. Underwood's view be correct, it would only modify the paper to the extent of stating that bifurcated roots were "of the greatest rarity," instead of that "they were unknown." Now with reference to caries, although he had intentionally excluded the subject in delivering the paper, it had in reality been included in the paper which had been prepared by Mr. Charters White and himself; that caries occurred in ovarian teeth was an assertion which would not hold water for a moment. These ravines in teeth always contained fibrous tissue. Caries in the teeth contained in ovarian dermoids in the sense employed for mouth teeth had yet to be demonstrated. With reference to Mr. F. J. Bennett's remarks, it was a curious thing that both Coleman and Salter had noticed that dentine radiates from the line rather than the pulp chamber. However, it showed the value of bringing a question of that sort before a society instead of writing the subject up in one's study, and packing it off to a journal. In thrashing a subject out before a society many valuable suggestions were often made in the course of discussion. With reference to Mr. Maggs' question, he would say that any number of teeth over twenty or fifty in these cysts was most rare. The dermoid before them was most exceptional. There was nothing peculiar about the teeth, but it would not be wise to draw any conclusion from them In conclusion, he wished to say that the discussion had been a most profitable one to him.

The President said it afforded him a great deal of pleasure to offer the thanks of the Society to Mr. Bland Sutton and Mr.

Charters White for their most interesting, able, and suggestive paper. They were all greatly rejoiced to see Mr. Sutton restored to health again, for had the illness been fatal it would have been a loss, not only to their society, but to the whole scientific world. The next meeting would be on the 14th April, when they would have a contribution from Mr. Henry Sewill on some points in the etiology and pathology of dental caries, illustrated by photo-micrographs of the tissues shown upon a screen by Mr. Andrew Pringle. There would also be a casual communication from Mr. Scott Thomson on splicing engine cords.

The meeting then separated.

EXTRACTS.

FALLACIES OF SOME OF THE OLD THEORIES OF IRREGULARITIES OF THE TEETH WITH SOME REMARKS ON DIAGNOSIS AND TREATMENT.*

By Dr EUGENE S. TALBOT, CHICAGO.

During the past few years new theories regarding the causes of irregularities have been advanced without eliciting much comment or discussion. At the same time men of ability continue to adhere to and advocate the old theories without giving reasons for the faith that is within them. This unsettled state of opinion is my excuse for reviewing them and calling your attention to their weak points. As long as the objections that can be raised against a theory are stronger than the arguments in its favour, there is an excuse for a new theory. Men of science cannot submit to either passively, but must prove all things before rejecting or adopting them.

A High Contracted Vault results from Thumb-sucking.

1. A high vault may be found in connection with thumb-sucking ; but this is not the case in many instances, and most individuals that have high vaults have never sucked their thumbs. If a mere coincidence cannot be taken for a cause, no reasonable conclusion can be drawn when this coincidence is limited to a small number of cases.

2. When the thumb is passively inserted into the mouth, no impression is made on the vault itself, though the parts between which it is inserted may be arrested in their development. A pressure necessary to produce a modification of the hard palate could not be

*Read before the First District Dental Society, State of New York.

borne; at least the child would find the comfort derived from thumb-sucking insufficient compensation for the distress endured. As soon as the lower teeth strike against the thumb with sufficient force to produce a pressure against the roof of the mouth, the uneasiness prevents the child from persevering in this position.

3. Thumb-sucking is begun very early in life, often as early as the first or second week. If an irregularity of the upper jaw would result, it would naturally appear before the permanent teeth are erupted, but the deciduous teeth are rarely found to be modified.

4. That a high and narrow vault cannot result from thumb-sucking alone, is shown by its extent. The deformity must appear where pressure is applied and confined to this area. That it should extend farther back is not reasonable.

In a recent work on irregularities we find the following statement regarding thumb-sucking: "In each case the jaws are held temporarily apart so that there could be no occlusion of teeth even though they occluded normally when the jaws were closed. This leaves the side teeth free to change their position if any influence is exerted to produce that result. In the act of sucking the cheeks are drawn in, and the strong pressure thus brought to bear upon the bicuspids and (occasionally) the first molars causes them to be bent inward. In this malposition they are frequently confirmed by the opportunity thus given to the other molar teeth to move forward, of which they are not slow to take advantage. The result is the deformity known as the 'saddle-shaped' jaw."

Since the child begins to suck its thumb at birth, or soon after, and ceases to do so about the sixth year in a majority of cases, and as irregularities of the temporary teeth are never observed in this region, this theory falls flat.

This summer I examined the mouths of five thumb-suckers at the sea shore. Two boys, twins, twelve years old, and a girl of nine, belonged to the same family. The boys had sucked their thumbs from birth, discontinuing at seven, probably from shame. The mother informed me that in each case the thumb of the right hand was inserted into the mouth with the palmar surface toward the tongue, producing pressure upon the teeth. These boys were strong and active, their jaws well developed, the vaults of medium height, the dental arches normal. The girl was gradually discontinuing the habit. She had also sucked her thumb from birth and held it in the same way. Another child, a girl of five, showed a slight forward movement of the right temporary central incisor, which could only be noticed on close inspection. The last case was that of a boy four years of age, who was sucking his thumb most of the time. He directed the palmar side of his thumb toward the upper alveolar arch. The pressure thus produced resulted in a slight absorption of the alveolar process, while the contour of the arch and the position of the teeth were perfectly normal. In none of the cases cited were the permanent teeth irregular.

That Irregularities are Produced bv a Force originating in the Sphenoid Bone and acting upon the Intermaxillary Bones.

In page 86 of his work, Coles makes the following statement: "The deformity known as the intermaxillary prognathism is the result of a force operating on the intermaxillary bone, such force originating in the body of the sphenoid and being transmitted by the intervening nasal septum."

It is observed in cases of idiocy, etc., that from inflammation of membranes in *utero* bones and sutures ossify early in life; on the other hand, it is observed in some cases that the same bones and sutures do not ossify till the thirty-fifth year. It stands to reason, with such difference in time of ossification there must be a marked difference in the size of the cranium: the more retarded the ossification, the more likely the cranium is to be large. Those pathologists that make a speciality of idiocy regard this premature or tardy ossification as an important means of differentiating different pathological conditions. Such differences must necessarily affect the base of the skull, for in this plane we find the greatest number of sutures. Coles had this in mind when he advanced his theory. The tardy development of the nose, which often does not assume the family type until late in life, corroborates this fact, for the face is in a direct line with the force exerted by the development of the bones at the base of the cranium, with which it develops simultaneously. But these conditions cannot affect the maxillary bones, for they are situated a considerable distance below the plane of the occiput.

If force could be communicated at all, it would have to be exerted nearly at right angles with its line of origin, which would lessen it materially. In this case the force would not only be exerted upon the intermaxillary bones, but also upon the maxillary, palate, turbinated, lachrymal, nasal, and malar bones as well, in other words, all the bones of the face would be acted upon, giving an apish appearance to the face, rather than producing prognathism. The fact that the sphenoid bone articulates with all the bones of the skull at the base of the brain probably led Coles to conclude that it must affect the intermaxillary bones, but the force exerted by the sphenoid bone is not in the line of the hard palate, but a considerable distance above it, diverging from it. The only way in which it would affect the intermaxillary bones is through the medium of the palate-bone and the palate; but the palate-bone is frail and contains a number of sinuses, so that all force would be lessened by these media, and the palate would be more apt to be bent out of shape than to communicate force to the maxillary bone.

2. The superior maxillary bone develops earlier, hence would exert more force on the intermaxillary bones than the sphenoid bone, for it must grow in every direction. Because of this priority of development it would be more apt to modify the sphenoid bone than be modified by it. To show that the maxillary bone is of far more potency in irregularities than the sphenoid is reserved for a discussion which is not the province of this paper.

Irregularities are Inherited and Congenital.

Just as a child may resemble a parent in form and features, so he may have an upper ar lower maxilla similar to that of one of his parents, but what is termed an irregularity of two or more teeth in one or both jaws cannot be inherited for the following reasons:

1. The size and form of one maxilla may be inherited from one parent while the teeth do not resemble those of the same parent; and even if the teeth are apparently of the same size, relation, and character, the denture as a whole shows marked differences when compared with another.

2. The character of two dentures depends largely on the character of occlusion and movement. In order that two upper jaws may be alike, it is not only necessary that the jaws and teeth shall have originally the same characteristics, but that the lower jaws must also be alike and articulate in the same manner and degree with the upper. If there is a difference of degree of development, differences in direction and occlusion must follow.

3. Irregularities often arise from premature or tardy extraction of a tooth. It would be difficult to find two cases in which the

above conditions are found, and the same teeth are extracted at the same time and under the same circumstances.

The usual cause of premature extraction being caries, the nutrition of parent and child, their environments, state of health, education, and occupation would have to be the same in order to produce the similarity of conditions that manifests itself in likeness of caries. The mode of life of the present generation differs from that of the past,—a fact easily explained. Climate is undergoing gradual changes; habits change with a difference of food and affluence or poverty; the occupations of parent and child are not often the same; permanence of habitation is not the rule; malaria and fevers are prolific causes of caries, and their prevalence differs with localities and periods of time.

A parent having been reared in a new portion of the country, leading an active life, living on food requiring thorough mastication, exposed to changes of weather, is likely to have a denture different from that of his son, who may have inherited the same form of jaw and similar teeth, but whose environments differ from those to which his father was subjected. Then there are the differences of the nervous system due to peculiarities of education and social conditions. The process of training and the surroundings during this period are rarely if ever the same in both parent and child.

I think I am correct in saying that jaws are growing smaller and caries appears earlier, though the size of the teeth remains the same. It may be objected that although in our generation these varied conditions are not likely to produce the same form of irregularity, in halcyon days of old this was otherwise. To this we reply that never in the history of mankind has there been such simplicity of life as to produce two dentures exactly alike, whether normal or irregular. Diversity of form is the law of organic bodies. It holds good in both the animal and vegetable kingdoms, extending probably even to cells. With all apparent similarity there is a great diversity of detail.

Instead of saying that two cases of irregularity are alike, it would be better if the dental profession would adopt the expression "Two cases of irregularity are similar." By doing so they would get nearer the truth and make room for individual peculiarities the observation of which is worthy of scientific consideration.

From the foregoing it will be seen that local conditions that cannot be the same in two individuals modify the arrangement of teeth.

Regarding the theory held by some that irregularities are congenital, it is only necessary to call attention to the fact that children are not born with teeth, certainly not with permanent teeth, which of course shuts out irregularities.

The Theory of Mouth-Breathing.

Contracted arches have hitherto been attributed to the pressure of the buccinator muscle on the alveoli in sleeping with the mouth open. This theory seems to be held generally for the reason that some cause of the contracted alveolar arch must be found, and in absence of any other that of pressure of the buccinator seemed plausible. This kind of reasoning does not appeal with much force to the mind, and includes important elements of error. It amounts to this : A contracted arch is found in some cases of sleeping with the mouth open. Pressure is the usual cause of dental irregularity. The contraction appears in the region of the bicuspids. No source of pressure being apparent, it is assumed that the buccinator exerts it. This is simply an opinion of possibility, not probability, much less inductive reasoning. It is based on the erroneous deductions (1) That some cases of mouth-breathing are representative of all cases ; (2) That pressure must necessarily be the cause of all irregularity ; (3) That the buccinator muscle exerts the pressure, as no other source of pressure is apparent. The human mind being restive under an acknowledgment of its ignorance, an opinion of possibility is hastily accepted as a theory.

In view of facts that every dentist must acknowledge, this argument cannot stand for the following reasoning :

1. It is inconsistent with our knowledge of the influences exerted by muscular structures in other parts of the body. Some of the muscles of the chest in respiration exert quite as much pressure as the buccinator during sleep, yet no one would expect to find the ribs modified by this process. The function of the buccinator is to keep the food under the molars in mastication. The pressure exerted by it on the crowns of the molars is not sufficient to affect the alveoli through the roots of the teeth ; but even if it could modify these spongy structures, its force would stop there and would not extend to the osseous vault, bending it out of shape. When one opens his mouth, he is conscious of a tension of the orbicularis oris, but not of a pressure of the buccinator. A study of the origin and insertion of this penniform muscle shows that its fibres are inserted along the edges of the jaw

and that they extend forward in a plane parallel to these processes. To produce a contraction of the arches by a muscular structure, the fibres would have to run at right angles to these uniting the two halves of the arches.

2. Muscles do not contract to a degree sufficient to produce the necessary pressure. It is true, as is generally asserted, that the tongue and lips are instrumental in changing the position of a tooth or teeth, but the action in these cases differs from that of the buccinator. The action of both tongue and lips is more or less voluntary, and in both cases what influence is exerted is due to repeated muscular *impulses* rather than a long-continued quiet *pressure*, such as that of any layer of muscles upon a portion of the osseous system.

In the former case we have force proper in the latter simply weight ; the first is active, the second passive. In sleep the voluntary muscles are at rest, except in those semi-conscious states we call dreams. It is therefore out of the question to speak of muscular contractions in connection with a voluntary muscle in sleep. When the mouth is open during sleep, due to some obstruction in the air-passages, it is the result of reflex nervous action, not direct volition.

3. But suppose for a moment that the direction of the fibres of this muscle were such as to permit of a contraction of the vault laterally, we should expect to find the modification of the osseous structure uniform. This would shut out semi-V and semi-saddle-shaped arches entirely, and a majority of other irregularities of the teeth in which there is bilateral asymmetry, for however much one would incline to the prevalent theory, no one would assert that the muscle will act on one side of the mouth while that on the opposite remains passive.

4. Partial V and partial saddle-shaped arches make it still less plausible. In these we met with sudden bends inward, where only one or two teeth may be involved, which could only be produced by a centralization of force on one given point, a peculiarity of function that has never yet been ascribed to muscles.

5. Lastly, if the buccinator acts as all muscles uniformly throughout its extent of contraction, below its median line it is just as efficient in producing a narrow contracted arch as in its upper portion, and we should expect to find the lower maxilla contracted whenever the upper one is, which is contrary to facts.

To recapitulate, the theory that the pressure of the buccinator muscle in sleeping with the mouth open is the cause of contracted arches is incorrect—(1) Because it is inconsistent with our knowledge of the influence exerted by muscular structures on the osseous system in other parts of the body; (2) Because muscles do not contract sufficiently to produce the necessary pressure; (3) Because by such pressure exerted on both sides of the arches semi-V and semi-saddle-shaped, partial V and partial saddle-shaped arches would be out of the question, and for the lower maxilla would be modified as much as the upper.

On Making a Diagnosis of a Case of Irregularity.

Irregularities have been divided into constitutional and local: the former affecting the body of the bone, the latter being accidental, affecting the teeth and alveolar process.

Frequently when a case of irregularity is presented we can tell by the general contour and profile of the face whether the case is one of the constitutional or local type, the external proportions being affected by a decided V-shaped arch, excessively developed alveoli, or underhung jaw. One of the first things a dentist has to learn is to observe carefully. In determining the correctness or incorrectness of the outline of the mouth and jaw, he instinctively takes it in as a whole, on the same principle that when we look at the picture of a friend we decide at once whether it is a good likeness or not, reserving our judgment on particular points until later.

Observe each jaw. See whether it has a normal outline or whether it belongs to the V-shaped or saddle-shaped variety; this will help you to decide about the appliance to be used.

Now comes an important feature of a correct diagnosis. Examine the occlusion, letting the patient open and close his mouth slowly. No detail must go unnoticed. The beginner should familiarize himself with the individuality of each class of teeth both as to outline and occlusion. For this purpose he is advised to study the very excellent article by Dr. E. T. Starr and F. L. Hise, in the August number of the *Dental Cosmos*, vol. xxxi.

When there is an asymmetry of the upper and lower jaws, one being larger than the other, the occlusion from the cuspid back is usually wrong. In such cases it generally strikes in front of the lower cuspid instead of between it and the bicuspid, disarranging the articulation of every tooth back of it. We cannot stop here to speak of the different forms of malocclusion; the dentist who never ceases to be a student will see these for himself.

The difficulty in local irregularities is usually easily detected, for it is found either in the alveolar arch or in the malposition of individual teeth.

Before giving your opinion inquire into the family history. Dr. Kingsley justly remarks that it is useless to try to correct an irregularity peculiar to a family type: nature reverts to her original design notwithstanding long-continued efforts. For this reason it is usually well to wait until the patient is of an age when it can be be determined what permanent form the jaw will assume.

When the arch is overcrowded and cannot be spread, or when it protrudes and the extraction of one or more teeth appears advisable for the purpose of obtaining space, care should be exercised in deciding upon the right ones. Examine to see which teeth are carious or diseased. Do not extract a first molar if it can be preserved with comfort to the patient. The cuspid is the most important tooth in determining the outline of the wing of the nose and upper lip and giving character to the face : for this reason never remove it when avoidable.

Eighteen years of experience in the correction of irregularities of the teeth and a practical knowledge of the laws of mechanics have taught me not to rely on any particular appliance. Frequently, though a certain appliance has worked well in one case it may not be efficient in another case of a similar nature, and not unfrequently two or three of the different forces are tried before one shows itself effective, this being due to the unknown factor of resistance which can be determined only by experience.—*Reported in Dental Cosoms.*

ABOUT PLATINUM.

Charles Wood, an assayer, in 1741 found in Jamaica some platina which had been brought from Carthagena and which he forwarded to London for inspection as a curiosity.

The first to mention platina by its present name, however, which means "little silver," was Don Antonio Ulloa, a Spanish mathematician, who, in 1735, accompanied the French academicians who were sent to Peru by their sovereign to measure a degree of the meridian in order to determine the figure of the earth.

After his return he published at Madrid, in 1748, a history of his voyage, and mentioned the abandonment of the gold mines in the territory of Choco on account of the presence of platina, which, being too hard to easily break or calcine, the gold could not be extracted without much expense and great difficulty.

It is reported in the *Chemical Annals* for July, 1792, that the miners of Choco, discovering platina was a metal, began to use it in adulterating gold, in consequence of which the Court of Spain, fearing disastrous results therefrom, attempted not only to prevent its export, but to conceal the discovery of the metal from the world.

To effect this all gold brought from Choco to be coined at the two mints of Santa Fè was carefully inspected, and all platina separated and given to the king's specially appointed officers, and when a sufficient quantity had accumulated, it was taken to the river Bogota, about two leagues from Santa Fè, or to the river Cauca, about one league from Papayan, and in the presence of witnesses thrown into the river.

From the great specific gravity of this metal, it being the heaviest known, together with its malleability and ductility, and the fact of its great resistance to the action of acids, alkalies and sulphurs, it has become known as the "metal of the chemists."

Some of the most important discoveries of modern chemistry would have been impossible without the aid of platina. It is so soft it may be readily cut with the scissors, and when formed into a mirror, reflects but one image.

Platina has been found in various parts of the world—Peru, New Granada, Brazil, St. Domingo, and in the gold washings of California, Australia and Borneo—but the principal source of supply is in the Ural Mountains of Russia and the auriferous sand of Kuschwa, in the Auralian Mountains of Siberia.

Platina is rarely found in pieces larger than a few grains in weight.

The chief uses of platina are for the various apparatus used in chemical laboratories, such as crucibles (first crucible was produced in 1784), spoons, blow-pipe points, tongs, forceps, and boilers or stills for concentrating sulphuric acid. A still of this kind, valued at 95,000 francs, was exhibited at Vienna in 1873, capacity 20,000 pounds of sulphuric acid daily.

An ingot valued at £4,000 was exhibited at the London Exhibition in 1862.

On account of the high degree of heat requisite to fuse or melt platina—melting point 1,460° to 1,480°—it is the only metal used for making the pins of porcelain teeth, and on account of its value and lack of any known substitute, has become the greatest item of expense in their manufacture.

It is also utilized for making fine jewellery, and a great and growing demand has been but recently created by the development of electricity.

The Russian Government began coining platina for general circulation in 1826 and continued until 1845, when by an imperial ukase the coinage was discontinued and the £500,000 issued called in because of the great fluctuation in the price of the metal.

The average production of platina metal from 1828 to 1845 amounted to 2,623.8 kilos or 5,784.48 lbs. per annum; from 1875 to 1884 inclusive, the average yield of the Russian mines was 3,483.3 lbs. per annum, showing a decrease since 1882, the maximum year of 45 per cent. in the yield. The Russian mines yield 80 per cent. of the total product of the world.

The price of platina, which has always ruled very high in consequence of the continually increasing demand, the limited source of supply, without any new discoveries of moment sufficient to relieve the market, is constantly advancing, so rapidly indeed as to cause serious apprehension for the future.

Those industries whose manufacturers depend largely on platina as their chief element of cost (and with no known substitute in sight), such as stills, crucibles, porcelain teeth, electrical and chemical apparatus, etc., are suffering more or less seriously from this increase in price, and for self-protection it would seem will be obliged to advance prices proportionately—*Electrical Review.*

LIVERPOOL DENTAL HOSPITAL.

The number of patients treated during the month of February was 1,987—Males, 1,036; Females, 951. Gold Fillings, 42; Plastic Fillings, 155; Extractions, 1,905; Under Anæsthetics, 53; Miscellaneous Cases and Advice, 87; Total, 2,242.—H. Fielden Briggs, D.D.S. and C. B. Dopson, L.D.S., *House Surgeons.*

BIRMINGHAM DENTAL HOSPITAL.

The number of patients treated during the month of February, 1890, was 379—Males, 119; Females, 152; Children, 108. The operations were as follows: Extractions, 364; plastic fillings, 68; gold fillings, 28; miscellaneous and advice, 106; Anæsthetics were administered in 21 cases.—Fred. R. Howard, *House Surgeon.*

REVIEW.

Dental Chemistry and Metallurgy. By Clifford Mitchell, M.D. Second Edition. Published by W. T. Keener, Chicago.

The publication of a second edition of Dr. Mitchell's book calls for a word of appreciation and comment. There is no other work, so far as we know, which contains such a mass of chemical and metallurgical information relating to substances and processes more or less intimately connected with the practice of dentistry. Here we have, within the two covers of a not unwieldy volume, the chemistry of drugs used in dental surgery—as apart from their therapeutics and pharmacy,—the chemical and physical properties of the numerous metals, precious and base, employed for various purposes by the dentist,—tables giving the chemical constituents of teeth, saliva, and calculi,—analyses and directions for the manufacture of various filling materials, together with sections on fermentation, the chemistry of caries, and the deleterious action exerted by certain substances on the teeth.

A large amount of useful matter has been brought together, and to many practitioners the book must prove of great service. It cannot be said that many new facts are offered for the consideration of the reader, but it is a manifest convenience to possess in a collected form, a statement of facts and theories, which otherwise would have to be sought for in sundry works on chemistry, physics, materia medica, dental surgery, and dental mechanics.

As a book of reference therefore, and suggestion, for the busy practitioner, we think it will deservedly find a place on the "useful" shelf of many a library, but with regard to its value for students, we cannot speak so favourably. In the absence of any similarly comprehensive work, we feel ourselves unfortunate in being unable conscientiously to recommend the one before us as a hand-book for students, except in the case of those who have already laid a solid foundation of chemical knowledge by means of information obtained from other sources. Let it not be thought that our criticism is mere carping, if we say that we object to the volume as a manual to place in the hands of any one fresh to the study of chemistry, on the grounds that it is at once too condensed and too diffuse. For it will be found, on the one hand, repeatedly throughout the book, and especially in the first two chapters, that statements are made with such a bareness and brevity as must inevitably repel and dishearten any reader unprepared by previous chemical education; whilst on the other hand, there is, in many pages, such a diffuseness, not to say chaotic looseness of information, as must appal the beginner by its extent and diversity—especially as important and unimportant facts are mixed up inextricably,—little or no indication, as a rule, being given as to their comparative value. These serious defects are obvious when one first opens the book, and a careful perusal of it makes them only the more glaring; the more one reads, the more one feels distressed at so much that is valuable being rendered to a great degree ineffectual and obscure. Sense of proportion, and ability to present facts in a way useful to the average student mind,—these are, for the most part, conspicuous by their absence, which is made all the more noticeable by the confused and inconsistent manner in which different kinds of type are used, or rather, misused.

Unfortunate as he is in style and method of arrangement, Dr. Mitchell may be congratulated on producing a book which is, in the main, accurate in fact—a most important consideration in a scientific work. Sundry minor mistakes, such as must inevitably creep into any publication of the kind, we do not notice. Of important errors there are very few: the worst is to be found on p. 11, and repeated on p. 35, where the statement is made that it follows from Avogadro's law that "the molecules of all bodies in the gaseous state are of the same size." This is quite incorrect, as is also the sentence in definition 2, p. 34, which reads: "atoms cannot, in all probability, remain free and uncombined." The latter inaccuracy is demonstrated by the author himself on p. 38, where he says that mercury, cadmium, and zinc "have one atom in the molecule," which is equivalent to stating that the atoms of these metals *may* remain free and incombined. Barium, stated on p. 38 to be monatomic, is not so. A general statement is made on p. 40 to the effect, that "when a current of electricity of sufficient strength is passed through a chemical compound in a state of solution, the compound is broken up into its constituent elements;" this is only true of a very limited number of substances. Antipyrine is not (see p. 284), a derivative of quinoline, but of pyrazol. It is much to be regretted that so limited a space should have been devoted by Dr. Mitchell to the chemistry of caries, a fuller account of which might with great advantage have been given.

The question of specialized training and practice is a vexed one, and we do not intend to discuss it here; but it may be said that the volume we are discussing exemplifies in some degree, both in its contents and method, the disadvantages as well as the advantages of special study. One of the advantages of concentrating one's energies on a particular subject or group of subjects, is that it becomes possible to gather together, within a moderate compass, the facts and principles which underly and govern the same; whilst the conspicuous drawback to such concentration is, that by the very limitation of thought and study which it permits, and in a sense requires, one is apt to lose a proper appreciation of the relative proportion of things.

We have been reminded, in reading this book, of a certain dish which was once described as containing "a deal of fine confused eating." Of the mental dish supplied in the book before us, we feel that the same words would be not inappropriate. The quantity of intellectual nourishment served up is considerable, and much of it may be said to be decidedly "fine" in quality, whilst the incongruities of arrangement and type are frequently as disconcerting and distasteful as it would be to have one's plate piled at once with fish, flesh, fowl, and good red herring.

Dental News.

COMPLIMENTARY NOTICES OF DENTAL WORK.—At the Annual Meeting of the Folkestone General Hospital, Mr. A. J. Crane, the Dental Surgeon to the Institution, received a high compliment from his medical colleagues upon the success attending his treatment of a fracture of both maxillæ occurring in a child.

AT a meeting recently held in the Townhall, Dewsbury, a very interesting ceremony took place, the presentation to the medical staff of a number of valuable articles as a mark of the esteem felt for the services rendered by them to the Dewsbury and District General Infirmary. Mr. Taylor, the honorary dentist, received a marble clock and pair of mantel ornaments, and the President, in presenting them, remarked that Mr. Taylor had done good hard work and skilful work for the infirmary, and his services were very much appreciated.

THE DENTAL RECORD, LONDON: APRIL 1, 1890.

The Etiology of Irregularity of the Teeth.

DR. TALBOT, who has made his name more or less associated with this subject, has recently addressed to the First District Dental Society of the State of New York, a paper dealing with what he called the "Fallacies of the Old Theories Concerning the Production of Dental Irregularity." The subject is very large, but it is also very important, and although the discussion which followed the paper was not exhaustive, it was sufficiently so to permit us to reproduce as far as space will permit the most salient arguments which it ventilated. Dr. Talbot has presented to the museum of the Odontological Society of Great Britain models of cases which he believes support his contentions, and we can strongly urge upon all dentists interested in the subject—and who are not?—a careful examination. Insisting upon the all-important influence of heredity and intra-uterine causes of dental irregularity, deficiencies and malformation of the palate, Dr. Talbot deprecates thumb-sucking, mouth breathing, &c., as determining causes of such departures from the normal. Dr. Barrett found difficulty in establishing a normal standard or type. He pointed out that it is necessary to trace back types not only to immediate ancestors but through congeners (the quadrumana) and proposed to demonstrate the prominent aberrations in types through these animals. The Collared Peccary is taken as a possible archetype of mammalian dentition. The arrangement of the teeth in these creatures is not an arch but half a parallelogram; a similar dentition occurs in the Cayote. The incisors are arranged in a line, there is a drawing in of the arch of the teeth and of the maxillæ at about the region of the last premolar. In the male Gorilla, the molars and premolars are almost in a straight line, no arch, but a drawing in of the premolars, so that the line they form with the cuspids and true molars is concave rather than convex, and the incisors are arranged at a right angle to it. In the Chimpanzee the same obtains, the outside line is concave rather than convex. In the Semnopithecus there is a swelling out of the line of the teeth, there is a slight convexity. Following the guidance of the teachings of "Evolution," Dr. Barrett tell us the archetype is the arrangement of teeth in a half-parallelogram. This arrangement however becomes more or less modified by anatomical (osseous) re-adjustments. Thus drawing back of the maxilla (the prognathism of the Gorilla being lessened) expands the arch and modifies the half-parallelogram into a semi-circle. Dr. Barrett would further regard many of the so-called aberrations of the "normal" arch as reversion to an ancestral type. The saddle-shaped jaw for example is the "normal jaw of the lower animals." Of course allowance must be made for the artificially manufactured malformations arising through premature loss of the deciduous teeth. It is perhaps hardly necessary to go so far back as Dr. Barrett does to obtain a workable "archetype," but if we do go so far back, it becomes necessary to establish a more precise relation between the archetype and the ultimate development. That Dr. Talbot's arguments and models are interesting no one will gainsay, but it seems to us to be open to grave question whether they advance us much in the search after an explanation of the commoner irregularities of the jaws. He deals with theories which are not accepted by anything like a majority of scientific dentists, and then proceeds to substitute hypotheses which appear to us to need far more proof than has at present been advanced.

GOSSIP.

THE Editor will feel much obliged if all letters and MS. which correspondents desire to send to him, be addressed "The Editor" of the DENTAL RECORD, 82, Mortimer Street, W.

WE have been repeatedly asked by correspondents the cause of the delay in the production of the new edition of "Sewill's Dental Surgery." We hear that it is in consequence of the great time consumed in preparing a number of *fac-simile* reproductions of photo-micrographs of the dental tissues, under exceptionally high powers, showing healthy and morbid anatomy. The completed work is expected to be ready for publication some time in May.

Doctors and Dentists with American Diplomas.—"According to Dalziel's Berlin agency (says the *Pall Mall Gazette*) by direction of the Privy Council, a census is being secretly taken of the number of doctors possessing American college degrees practising medicine and dentistry in the Empire. It is the intention of the Government to interdict the carrying of an American doctor's degree, a title assumed here principally by dentists. In German colleges there is no such degree as 'Doctor of Dentistry,' consequently many German students matriculate at an American university, generally in Philadelphia, Baltimore, or New York. They graduate with the degree of D.D.S. (Doctor Dental Surgery), and returning to Germany place the prefix 'Dr.' on their door plates. This is no longer to be permitted, as it is regarded as misleading to patients: an American medical degree being considered as next to valueless in Germany. In Berlin at present there are twenty-six German dentists with American diplomas. Their licences will be taken from them unless they call themselves plain 'Mr.'" If one may judge from recent expressions of opinion from the leading London Dentists and from the action of the Odontological Society which systematically ignores the American degrees, we should say that there is as strong a feeling in London against the assumption by dentists of the title of Dr. as in Berlin.

The Dental Hospital of London.—The 32nd Annual Meeting of this Institution was lately held at the Hospital, Leicester Square, under the presidency of Thomas Underwood, Esq., one of the Vice-Presidents. In the report, which was unanimously adopted, the Managing Committee congratulated the Governors on the continued success and prosperity of the Institution ; also on the great benefits which the Hospital continues to afford to the suffering poor, 54,630 cases having been treated during the year 1889, a large number of them painlessly (under anæsthetics), being 3,224 in excess of those of the previous year, and 32,636 in excess of the number treated in 1874, when the Hospital was removed to its present site. The Committee had been unable to pay off any part of the mortgage debt during the year, and that, unfortunately, there was £2,500 remaining of this debt, and they urgently appealed for funds to enable them to rid themselves of this encumbrance, incurred for the extension of the Hospital, rendered indispensably necessary to meet the growing wants of the Charity. Help, by an increase in annual subscriptions, is also earnestly solicited. The Charity is unendowed, and additional funds would enable it to greatly extend its usefulness.

GUY'S HOSPITAL DENTAL SCHOOL.—A Lectureship on Operative Dental Surgery has been founded, and Mr. Harold Murray has been appointed to the chair. The lectures will be delivered yearly during the Summer Session. The course will include the methods of examining the mouth for dental lesions, the exclusion of saliva during operations, the preparation of typical cavities for the reception of gold and other fillings. The lectures will deal with the scientific principles involved in the various methods of inserting the fillings now in use, individually or in combination with one another. Special attention will be directed to the treatment of pulpless teeth, and exposed pulps. The operative treatment of "Riggs' disease," the preparation of roots for pivots, the inlaying of teeth with porcelain, and the application of splints to fractured jaws will be fully discussed.

THE INTERNATIONAL MEDICAL CONGRESS IN BERLIN.—Great preparations are being made and no effort spared to render the meeting a success. Dr. Von Gossler the Cultusminister who has always put himself in the forefront in matters tending to advance medical science is interesting himself largely in the Congress, and has induced the government to make a grant of £4,000 towards defraying expenses. The Emperor it is reported will himself receive members of the Congress at Friedricsshkron, the palace of San Soucie, with its relics of Frederick the Great, is to be thrown open and the famous fountains of Potsdam are to play, so that, much that is interesting as well as beautiful will be brought within the reach of members of the Congress. The City of Berlin has voted five thousand pounds towards entertainment expenses. A special feature of the Congress will be the presentation of literary *souvenirs.* Of these, a new edition of Virchow's celebrated "Cellular Pathologie" will take the first place. The City of Berlin will present a Festschrift. The arrangements for the work of the sections are as yet incomplete, but are being rapidly got into order. The familiar name of Professor Victor Horsley appears as opener of a discussion upon the surgery of the central nervous system. The dental section has not as yet issued any definite programme, but we hear it is likely to prove a very interesting one. Special efforts are being made to obtain a reduction of railway rates for foreigners journeying to and fro from the Congress, and the Hamburg-American Packet Company has reduced its fares, saloon fare from Southampton to Hamburg being charged £2 5s. single, and £4 return (available for fifty days, but not after November 1st). The steamers call at Southampton *en route* to Hamburg for New York usually on Thursday. The agents are Smith, Sundius & Co., 158, Leadenhall Street, E.C., and 22, Cockspur Street, S.W., from whom all particulars are procurable.

Abrasion and Dental Disease in Monkeys.—Dr. Barrett exhibited before a New York Dental Society specimens of teeth in the jaws of Cynocephalus and a female gorilla, those of Cynocephalus showed "spontaneous abrasion on the anterior face of the left lateral incisor." This condition is by some attributed to over zealous employment of the tooth brush, a fact which led Dr. Barrett to speculate as to the particular kind of tooth powder Cynocephalus affects. The teeth of the female gorilla evinced caries, showing distinct cavities on the approximal surfaces of the central incisors. The anterior root of the first superior molar (the sixth year old molar) was denuded, while the lower incisors were badly decayed. Opposite the root of the *right* inferior first molar, marks of an extensive alveolar abscess were present. Evidence of pyorrhœa alveolaris also existed. As these creatures had not been kept for any length of time in captivity, the conclusions seem to be just, that spontaneous abrasion does not necessarily mean excessive mechanical attrition from tooth brushing, and that improper modes of life and artificial preparation of food, are not the only, if they be at all, the determining cause of dental diseases.

Transmission of Disease by Dental Instruments.—Writing under this heading, Dr. J. P. Parker, of Kansas, cites the following cases:—August 17, 1888, Miss F. consulted me about an eye trouble, and she stated that her throat and gums had been very sore for some days. On examination I found that she had severe double iritis, glandular swelling, and a coppery papular eruption distributed over the face and body. Being a very intelligent young woman she observed that I was puzzled and began to talk more freely. She stated that a dentist extracted a tooth for her about three months before, which he cut around with a dull knife and the wound had never healed, although the dentist had treated it a number of times and she had applied ever so much tincture of myrrh, etc. I examined the gums and found a chancre where the cut had been made. The syphilitic virus had been carried into the wound either on the knife or forceps.

On September 11, 1888, a young gentleman aged about 22 years, consulted me about a sore on his lower lip, and stated that the family physician had prescribed lip salve and which had always cured the sores he had on his lips before, but did not appear to do this one any good, and he said he had been referred to me by Miss F., to whom he was engaged. It was evident that the chancre on his lip had been acquired by direct contact through the act of kissing.

Guy's Hospital Residential College for Students, supplying as it does a long and keenly felt want, the opening of the New Residential Student's College at Guy's marks a new era in the history of the old hospital. Fifty years ago the matter had been discussed, but beyond this no further progress—at that time—appears to have been made. Again, in 1877, the project appears to have been under the consideration of authorities, and although plans were then prepared for a college, the matter seems to have drifted into abeyance. In the winter of 1887, however, a committee appointed for the purpose of considering a scheme whereby it would be possible to increase the number of senior appointments, reported that both in the interests of the students and the patients, it was advisable that such a course should be adopted. But it was felt that to augment the appointments of residents (house physicians, house surgeons, &c.), implied additional accommodation, and this fact seemed to offer an efficient barrier to the fulfilment of the scheme. With the object, therefore, of surmounting these difficulties and of giving practical effect to their views, the committee recommended the erection of a suitable college—a recommendation which met with prompt consideration and approval at the hands of the governors and staff to whom it was submitted—without delay the college was commenced, the excavations being made in August, 1888, and the result is the handsome building formally opened a few days ago by the Right Hon. W. E. Gladstone, M.P. The structure built entirely of red brick is of revised Elizabethan style, and is in quadrangular form. It consists, in addition to the space allotted to the residents, of the student's club, a warden's house, and further room for 30 residential students. The club rooms comprise, a handsome dining hall, smoking and reading rooms, and a gymnasium. The inaugural ceremony took place in the dining hall, when Mr. Gladstone, who was supported by the Bishop of Rochester, Viscount Cobham, &c., declared the new building open. Replying to the toast "Success to Guy's Hospital," proposed by the President (Mr. Hucks Gibbs):

Mr. GLADSTONE, who was received with great cheering, said, that the chairman had with great tact hit upon the only title which could possibly be pleaded on his behalf for the honour he now enjoyed of having his name associated with Guy's Hospital and of representing it on that occasion. He came amongst them after an absence of years, and even decades of years. That absence might be called truancy were it not that some forty or fifty years ago he was a pretty constant attendant, and took his share in the discharge of the duties pertaining to the office. He was very glad indeed to have the opportunity at last of showing that his feeling of sympathy with this great institution which had been dormant for a time—quite long enough perhaps to excite suspicion—was not altogether dead. There were three professions called the great professions, administering to the primary wants of mankind—the law, the holy ministry, and the medical profession. If they travelled back a short distance in the course of time, they found the last named almost without a recognised existence. It had had its luminaries in distant time; here and there they stood out in history as objects of great interest, filling an important part in society, enjoying respect in a high degree, but recognised as a great member in the body politic, it could hardly be said to exist. He was not aware whether botany now formed a recognised branch of medical education. He could not help wishing it did, because not only was it itself a most beautiful study, exercising the mind without fatiguing it, and stimulating the imagination without leading it astray, but it led to a careful observation of nature and to a habit of noticing the qualities of plants which were so remarkable and so powerful in their healing capacity. Perhaps his hearers would think it almost ludicrous if he told a little anecdote of his own, which was so simple and so slight as almost to be contemptible—but still it illustrated what he meant. As was pretty well known, he had been given to the pursuit of wood-cutting. By pure accident he drew his finger one day along a tolerably sharp bit of the edge of his axe and cut his finger. On searching about him he found he had no pocket handkerchief available; he wanted to staunch his little wound and he got a leaf and applied it. He was bound to say that this was not the result of botanical knowledge, it was a strictly empirical proceeding; but the curious part was that the healing of this little breach of continuity occupied exactly half the time unassisted nature would have required. Let them look at the extraordinary change that had happened in the development of the medical profession; as regards social position and influence, the advent of Drs. Friend and Meade in the last century was almost the earliest instance to which they could point of medical men assuming influence and power and general recognition. Turning to the immediate object of the gathering, the speaker expressed a strong conviction that the college would prove of great benefit, not only to the students themselves, but also to the hospital as an institution. The student in former times had had great difficulties to contend with. He found himself as a young man often with very limited means, and in earlier days, of limited education, plunged into the great ocean of the London population, with all its temptations, without guidance, without check, without the advantages of domestic life. Now they would enjoy the advantages of collegiate education, so far as regarded their profession and of dwelling under one roof. As an old Chancellor of the Exchequer he was extremely struck with the financial skill, the happy nature of the idea which supplied, without any danger he believed to anybody, the solid basis of credit upon which they had, without difficulty, been able to raise the means for the erection of the college. He warmly commended the self-denial of the medical and surgical staff, who had appropriated their future fees as a basis for the financial portion of the scheme. He trusted that the sentiment, "Prosperity to Guy's Hospital," would be found to be no mere dream, even of benevolence and philanthropy, but a solid and well built calculation. Mr. Gladstone resumed his seat amid tumultuous cheering, after having spoken for over half-an-hour. Subsequently the right hon. gentleman, together with Mrs. Gladstone, were conducted over the college and the wards. A reception by the governors and staff was held during the afternoon, and a great many ladies and gentlemen availed themselves of the opportunity of seeing the wards, school buildings, museum and chapel, all of which were thrown open to the visitors from 3 to 6. A capital selection of music was performed during the afternoon in the hospital grounds by the band of the M. Division Metropolitan Police.

CORRESPONDENCE.

[We do not hold ourselves irresponsible in any way for the opinions expressed by our correspondents.]

CLINICS.

To the Editor of the DENTAL RECORD.

SIR,—There are two sides to every question—many sides to most; and on the question of the true value of clinics there is a great deal to be urged against the views put forth by a writer in the last number of the RECORD. But first I would remark that it seems strange no hint was given of the evils and abuses associated with the clinic system which have grown up in the United States. These evils and abuses were fully exposed some few months back by one of the leading dental professors of Harvard University, and his paper, in abstract, was published in the *British Medical Journal.* He showed that a great number of the so-called clinics in the States constitute simply thinly disguised advertisements, either for the operator or his goods. In this country for a practitioner in any branch of the medical profession, including dentistry, to take out a patent for apparatus, instruments, or appliances, is, for sufficient reasons, into which I need not now enter, considered disreputable and incompatible with professional position. But in the States, although among the higher ranks the unwritten code of conduct called professional etiquette is as strictly obeyed as in Europe, there is a large class, particularly among dentists, who are willing to make a profit out of any invention, however trivial, over which they can acquire patent rights. A clinic is thus often really nothing more than an exhibition of tradesmen's goods, perhaps also giving an opportunity to offer for sale a license to use some more or less useful device or material.

But apart from all this, I venture to express my deliberate opinion formed upon experience, that the value of clinics has been very much overestimated. For the student clinical teaching is of course indispensable, but I question very much whether any properly educated practitioner has on any occasion derived any real profit from a clinic, or gained knowledge which he might not have acquired without its assistance.

If the advance of practice were through revolution not evolution, the case might be different. If suddenly some inventions were brought out which should at one stroke entirely revolutionize all methods of practice, and at once call for the use of hitherto unknown instruments and employment of hitherto unpractised methods, no doubt we should all need to begin over again and acquire instruction from demonstrations. But on the contrary, real progress is slow, and there can be no difficulty in any competent man keeping pace with the times. To a man who has had no opportunities, or has neglected those offered, to properly educate himself in the first principles of his profession in youth, when it can alone be done, and to train his fingers to the necessary point of mechanical dexterity, no amount of clinical instruction can be of the least use until he has supplied the fundamental deficiencies in his professional acquirements. On the other hand, an educated skilled man will have slowly modified his practice with the evolution of improvement. Take gold filling for instance, I am old enough to have known the time before the introduction of the beautifully plastic preparations of cohesive gold which now-a-days it is the fashion to use. But has any fairly good gold stopper found the least difficulty in availing himself of the new material—not likely; for it required as much skill, and fingers as highly trained to use the older preparations. The same with other modern improvements, such as the rubber dam and saliva ejecting apparatus. Can it be supposed that any operator able to overcome the much greater difficulties of excluding saliva and putting in a gold plug without these comparatively recent inventions would find the least difficulty in gradually adopting them in his practice. Finally, may be instanced the evolution of so-called crown bar and bridge work—a name, by-the-way, which associated as it is with cruel and fraudulent quackery, stinks in the nostrils of every decent dentist. This kind of work has been slowly evolved during years. The antiseptic method has gradually brought root filling to high perfection, and has taught us to deal with great certainty with many conditions of disease formerly intractable.

Root filling slowly led to crowning all classes of teeth—an operation not many years ago restricted to incisors and canines. Again, I would ask whether any intelligent competent operator desiring to do so, could have found the least difficulty in widening in this direction the scope of his operative procedures, in advancing from root filling to pivoting, from pivoting to crowning, and from crowning to bar work—the attachment of a united series of crowns to remaining broken down teeth. Nor can there have been the least difficulty in understanding the fully published explanations of principles and descriptions of methods which have been brought out at societies or printed in text-books during the period of progress. To a practitioner who had kept himself abreast of the times, the occasional difficult view of an operator at a clinic carrying out some new procedure would scarcely be in the least degree helpful; whilst to the ignorant or incompetent—to those deficient in fundamental knowledge and in manual dexterity, attendance upon occasional clinical demonstrations could not, I repeat, possibly be of service; they need first theoretical knowledge, and then systematic general mechanical training before they can understand or derive benefit from such instruction. Among those to whom clinics are quite useless there must be included another class of practitioners (and in this category I must place myself), namely, practitioners who are so devoid of natural aptitude that no amount of theoretical knowledge of patient perseverence ever makes of them highly skilled handicraftsmen. They lack the gift of fingers, and no exposition of what others can do helps them to advance beyond the limitations within which their feeble endowments confine them.

I remain, your obedient Servant,

Wimpole Street, *March*, 1890. HENRY SEWILL.

To the Editor of the DENTAL RECORD.

SIR,—Though we are probably all agreed as to the desirability of holding more frequent clinical meetings, it would be difficult to lay down any general rule as to the precise way in which they should be brought about; for while at one place an existing society might be both able and willing to take up this work, at another it might be necessary, as you suggest, to form a special clinical society. In London, however, the conditions to be dealt with, are, in some important particulars different from those existing anywhere else and my object in writing is, to suggest that here the wants of practitioners would best be served by forming a branch of the British Dental Association. Such a branch need not clash or interfere in any way with the objects or meetings of the Odontological Society. It could take up the question of clinical evenings, which that society has felt, and I believe still feels, itself unable to do. It would offer a platform for the consideration and discussion of political and educational questions which the Odontological Society considers to be outside its sphere of action. With a subscription of say half-a-guinea it should command a large membership, and find abundant material for both interesting and profitable meetings, and would thus supplement and carry forward the work which the Odontological

Society has so worthily begun. It would also stimulate the activity of those members of the British Dental Association who reside in London, by placing association meetings within reach, in a way which has not hitherto been done, and would probably result in adding largely to the membership of the Association in this city. Lastly, it would be the means of giving London members of the association a true representation on the Representative Board.

At present there seems to be some little mystery attaching to the method by which the London representatives are appointed. It is believed that they are nominated in the first place by the Business Committee; then confirmed by the Representative Board along with representatives nominated by the different branches; and finally they are elected by the members of the Association at the annual general meeting. Virtually then, if this be so, the London members of the Board are merely the nominees of the Business Committee, and the curious spectacle is seen of London practitioners being represented on the executive body by men in whose selection they have practically no voice. This undesirable state of things would be ended by the formation of a London branch which would nominate its representatives in the same way as the other branches do now.

It seems then from a consideration of the points noticed, that whatever may be thought desirable elsewhere, in London at any rate more advantages would attend the formation of a branch of the British Dental Association than of a special clinical society, and this suggestion I would therefore commend for further discussion by your readers.

Yours faithfully

A MEMBER OF THE B.D.A.

To the Editor of the DENTAL RECORD.

SIR,—I feel sure that many of your readers will be grateful to Mr. Mitchell for his interesting and well-expressed article on "Clinics," and to you for your leader in last month's RECORD, inviting discussion as to which is the best means of supplying the want which has been so long felt. As I have seen a great deal of the working of the British Dental Association in various parts of the country, and the great good it has done, I should like to give expression to a few thoughts which suggested themselves to my mind when I read your article, and to urge the claims of this association upon the attention of your readers. That a branch of the British Dental Association would supply in the most simple and effectual way all that is required I think cannot be denied, but it would also do a great deal more than this; up to now there has been no inclination shown on the part of the great majority of the members of the association residing in London and neighbourhood to take any interest in dental politics; they have exerted no influence, and consequently all has been allowed to fall into the hands of a few members, who, being willing to do the work, are left to control everything as they think best. Although the bye-laws of the association are based upon the elective principle, and although this principle has been more or less respected by the branches, in the building up of the association, we find that through the apathy of London members the despotic form of government practically prevails. The more experience I gain, the more convinced I become that there is a small party in the Association who are desirous that this state of things should continue. Now a branch would give to the members residing in London and district the opportunity of discussing subjects bearing upon the welfare of the profession as well as means for mutual self-improvement, and would also give them the privilege of nominating delegates to the Representative Board, so that their views might be made known and their influence felt. All that is required is for twenty or more members of the British Dental Association to be brought together, and a branch can be formed at once without waiting for any invitation or for the approval of existing societies. A little self-reliance (I allow it may be bad to find at present) will do far more than any amount of patronage from those who have too much to do, and too many meetings to attend already in connection with dental hospitals, the Odontological Society, the central work of the Association &c., &c., and who therefore feel that a London branch would be rather a burden, besides having a tendency to weaken the despotic power which they now possess, and which they firmly believe to be necessary for the welfare of the profession, but which in reality is degrading and demoralizing both to the profession and the Association.

In case it is decided to form a London branch it would give great satisfaction to the members of the Association in all parts of the country and do much to unite the profession into one harmonious whole, and to dispel those selfish, narrow-minded ideas, so well described by Mr. Mitchell, which we all so much deplore.

Thanking you for your kind invitation, and trusting that I have not trespassed too much on your space in availing myself of the opportunity so kindly afforded me of expressing the conclusions I have arrived at after several years of close observation,

I remain, yours faithfully,

10, Museum Street, York. THOS. EDWARD KING.

GAS OPERATIONS.

To the Editor of the DENTAL RECORD.

SIR,—Mr. Seymour is just a little one-sided in his articles on Gas Operations. It is all very well to say, we ought to have an anæsthetist to administer gas to our patients, but where are they to come from? Most medical practitioners know nothing whatever about the administration of gas, and to carry out Mr. Seymour's idea properly, medical practitioners all over the country would require to be trained in the administration of gas, and therefore I say, we practitioners in full practice are far more likely to administer gas satisfactorily and safely than men who know little or nothing about it. Another point is, in cases of urgency, it might be impossible for some hours to obtain the services of a medical man, is the poor patient in the meanwhile to suffer for our incapacity or temerity? There is also the case of patients of limited means, who could not afford to pay both doctor and dentist. Mr. Seymour in some of his letters uses the words "dishonest" and "disgrace" in regard to those who administer gas without medical aid. I think the same terms might be aptly applied to those who inflict upon their patients a double fee, as will no doubt have to be done when an anæsthetist is employed. The idea is altogether unworkable, and perhaps not desirable, as N_2O if given intelligently and a proper look out kept by assistant and operator is the safest anæsthetic we possess. I say this in view of the recent so-called death from N_2O in Scotland, which might more properly be called a death from fright and tight lacing than anything else.

I am, yours, &c.,

J. S.

DENTAL HOSPITALS AND ARTIFICIAL DENTURES.

To the Editor of the DENTAL RECORD.

SIR,—As the announcement that the authorities of the Dental Hospital of London contemplate supplying the *bonâ fide* necessitous poor with artificial dentures for the instruction of the students will doubtless be received by some with feelings of apprehension and misgiving, may I ask for a small space in your valuable journal whereby to express some views on this most important subject?

To enter minutely upon every side issue, probability, advantage or disadvantage, would involve me in too lengthy a discourse and far beyond the scope of a letter, I will therefore endeavour to give the main points only, leaving their elaboration as a natural sequence of thought.

Four aspects of the question may be taken :—(*a*) The necessity for thorough instruction in dental mechanics—about to become a prominent feature in the examination at the College of Surgeons; (*b*) The security of the institution against being classed with cheap dental establishments; (*c*) The moral influence on conservative dentistry by supplying artificial teeth gratis, and (*d*) The *boná fides* of the deserving poor.

It cannot be denied that the necessity for college training in this department has come about from various causes, amongst which are: the poverty of laboratories in the houses of reputable practitioners; the inability of those men to give time to pupils, owing to the pressure of surgery work; the danger of a young man being associated with the advertising quack; and the demoralizing influence in not a few, allowing pipes and pots of beer to be enjoyed during the daily work.

It appears to me that to secure systematic teaching, a permanent officer should be appointed at a salary worthy of his ability, and as a safeguard against him trafficking the institution, at £150 to £200 per annum. A fee of fifty or a hundred guineas to be paid by the student to a special fund for this department, in lieu of the present premium of apprenticeship, and following this, the student may be required to enter upon this course one year before he commences his dental surgery studies, so that the three years' instruction required by the College of Surgeons' regulations for the L.D.S. diploma may be complied with. The precise method of instruction need not be discussed here. Next in order, we are justified in a boast, and not an exaggerated one, that England is the home of true charity, and its institutions examples of order and regularity, so that any fresh departure in organization or operation is viewed with jealous curiosity, lest by any overt act its good name may become jeopardised. It is well known that on the Continent and in America, artificial dentures are supplied; and in the experience of two men who are well acquainted with the practice, the opinion has been expressed by one, that the "professors make a good thing out of it," and the other, that "they become competitors with dentists." Thus, if the patients are to be charged anything for these dentures, our institutions will deserve some condemnation. The premium paid by the student should be sufficient to cover all cost of materials used by him, and if his efforts result in anything of service to his fellow creatures, let that use be made, so that deliberate waste may not take place. This would give a satisfactory solution to two of the problems, the patient would receive his much needed denture, and the institution maintain its position as a charity, and successfully refute any charge of being a commercial enterprise.

The interest of the young practitioner should also be respected; and where a profit can be made, that profit should find its way into his pocket, and not to be absorbed by any institution. The student must pay for his instruction, the opulent public appealed to for such appliances and accommodation as are beyond his means of providing, and the poor *only* the recipients of his skilful offices.

How far our efforts to persuade the community to preserve their teeth will lose its influence by the introduction of this new system will remain to be proved. I think our experience of the indifference it shows to the ordinary rules of decent cleanliness, apart from special attention to the teeth, will give the opportunity to evade the prolonged operations which their preservation often demands, in the belief that their loss will be supplied by more easy means. Some penalty should therefore attach itself by allowing the inconvenience they endure, to mark the neglect they have practised in the past. The *bonâ fides* of a deserving person will rest on good ground if the institution has to draw from its coffers for the supply, for in justice to common sense its officers will see that their individual charity is not abused.

From the plausible intention in the interests of dental education always displayed by the authorities of the Dental Hospital of London, I trust the measure will be received with confidence but from the scope it offers for abuse I venture to make these suggestions in the interests of all concerned.

Your obedient servant,

F. HENRI WEISS.

Dean of the Faculty,
National Dental Hospital and School.

ANSWERS TO CORRESPONDENTS.

Mr. W. Voit.—We regret we cannot specify any particular dentist, as it is against our rule. Any first-rate London practitioner would do the work you require, the particular "method" to which you refer has no particular mystery about it, and is familiar to all "progressive," *i.e.*, educated dentists.

Anxious Enquirer.—There is no royal road to success save doing good work and avoiding dishonesty. Treat your patients just as you would wish them to treat you. In the long run if you aim at being a useful and honorable member of your profession you will find advertising in the local papers will do you more harm than good.

Mr. Breadey (Halifax).—The information you require can be obtained by writing to F. G. Hallett, Esq., The Examination Hall, Victoria Embankment, London, S.W.

A. D. F.—The only registrable qualifications of American origin are the D.D.S. (Chic.), and the D.M.D.Harv., and these can only be registered by a "Foreign Dentist," that is, a person who is not a British subject; or one who has practised for more than ten years elsewhere than the United Kingdom, or one practising in the United Kingdom at the time of the passing of the Dentists' Act (1878), for not less than ten years either in the United Kingdom or elsewhere. The diplomas you name are absolutely valueless here, and no dentist holding them could recover fees upon the strength of their possession. They are neither useful nor ornamental appendages to the name. You will find the whole matter discussed in 41 & 42 Vic., cap. xxxiii., p. 9, *et. seq.*

Sine Curriculo.—The best books are Tomes' "Dental Surgery"; Underwood's "Dental Anatomy" also "Dental Surgery"; Holden's "Anatomy" (Bones of Head and Face); Huxley's "Physiology"; a little Metallurgy, any Manual.

Scrupulosity.—We do not know of any published "Code of Ethics" promulgated for the benefit of dentists. We would suggest that you make one for yourself, based upon the model of what you think an honorable gentleman would be likely to do.

Monthly Statement of operations performed at the two Dental Hospitals in London, and at the Dental Hospital, Manchester, from January 31st to February 28th, 1890:—

		London.	National	Victoria.
Number of Patients attended		—	1832	1055
Extractions	Children under 14 ...	393	320	732
	Adults	1117	424	
	Under Nitrous Oxide ...	751	681	118
Gold Stoppings		400	97	31
Other Stoppings...		1369	359	174
Irregularities of the Teeth		83	68	--
Artificial Crowns		17	—	—
Miscellaneous and Dressings		475	344	287
Total		4,605	2,293	1,342

THE DENTAL RECORD.

VOL. X. MAY 1st, 1890. No. 5.

Original Communications.

ON SEPARATING TEETH.

By J. F. COLYER, L.R.C.P., M.R.C.S., L.D.S.

Demonstrator to the Dental Hospital of London.

THE main objects in separating teeth are to give space for the free use of instruments, whether for filling or examination purposes, and to allow the restoration of the contour of the tooth in filling.

Separation can be effected by either removing a portion of the tooth or by wedging the teeth apart by various materials or instruments ; it is to the latter method I propose to direct the following few brief remarks.

In young subjects the separation of teeth can be accomplished with a certain degree of safety. In the old, such is not the case, the result of wedging sometimes tending to a diseased action in the sockets and premature loss of the teeth. One author relating a case where the inflammation of the alveolar dental membrane caused by the separator spread to the pulp, leading to its destruction.

One should, I think, always consider carefully before separating teeth in a patient over forty, and our judgment should be guided by the condition of the patient's teeth, especially any tendency to pyorrhœa alveolaris, and by the presence of any constitutional condition where repair is not easily accomplished.

When considering the methods of separating teeth one finds they may be roughly divided into gradual and immediate.

For the gradual method tape or rubber is generally used, commencing with narrow breadths and gradually increasing the number till the required space is obtained. It is useful when the space is obtained, to let one or two days elapse before operating, as this will allow the tenderness caused by the wedging to subside to a certain degree.

It is also useful when instructing our patient how to use the tape, to prescribe a little tincture of iodine and aconite, to be applied to the gum over the teeth being separated, as this will also assist in allaying the tenderness.

Of the above, tape and rubber, the former is, I think, in most cases preferable; the disadvantages of the rubber lies in the fact that it works too rapidly and causes a greater amount of inflammation. When, however, the teeth are very close together, it is sometimes impossible to get a strand of tape up, the rubber is then very useful for commencing the separation.

Wood for wedging can be used in exactly the same way as tape, viz., commencing with thin pieces and gradually increasing the thickness. The disadvantage of wood over tape and rubber is that nearly always the operator has to change the thicknesses of the wood, whereas with the tape the patient is himself able to do it.

In preference to the above there are many who prefer to wedge with cotton, asserting that its action is just as effective and occasions not the slightest inflammation. It is best used as follows :—

Take a tuft of cotton and pull it into pieces so that the fibres are parallel to one another. Next reduce one end to a thread by twisting it between the fingers and thumb, pass this between the teeth to be separated, and draw it forward with a pair of tweezers. This gradually separates the teeth with a power which has scarcely any limit, and must be exercised with discretion. The point at which to stop being when there is just a feeling of discomfort.

The ends of the cotton tuft are then cut off pretty close to the enamel, and the saliva moistening the cotton causes it to separate the teeth beyond one's expectation.

Another extremely useful way of separating teeth, especially back ones, is at the first sitting to prepare the cavity roughly and fill the space up with some guttapercha, bringing it against the side of the adjacent tooth. The saliva causes the guttapercha to swell, and so separates the teeth. The cheaper forms are the best, since there is a greater tendency for them to swell.

When several teeth have to be separated, Mr. Coffin sometimes employs one of his expansion plates.

After wedging by the gradual method, the teeth are often found very tender, when this is the case the operation of filling should not be undertaken but the space should be kept, until the tenderness has passed off, by filling it up with some soft guttapercha.

Of immediate methods for separating teeth that by means of

wooden wedges is very simple. It is accomplished by cutting two narrow wedges of very fine grained wood, such as orange or box-wood, and inserting them between the teeth, one at the neck and the other at the cutting edge. These are then alternately tapped with a mallet until enough separation is obtained. The wedge between the teeth at the cutting edge is then removed and the other left *in sitû*.

Another method of inserting wooden wedges is with special forceps made for the purpose, one blade conveying the wedge the other a pad of rubber to protect the enamel from injury during the operation of introducing the wedge.

Of the special instruments made for separating teeth Perry's and Parr's are probably the best known in this country. Quite recently, however, Mr. Blandy has introduced, through the Dental Manufacturing Company, Limited, a separator (shown in Fig. 1); Hallam has also made one (shown in Fig. 2); the latter is stamped from

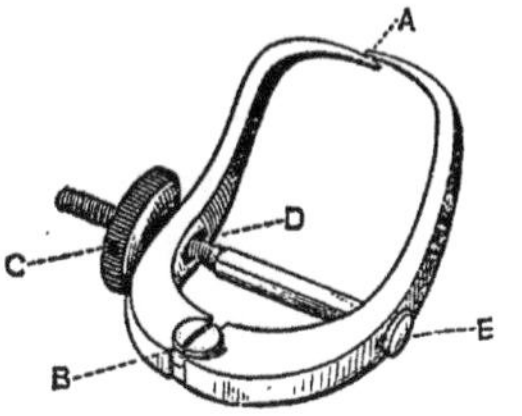

Fig. 1.

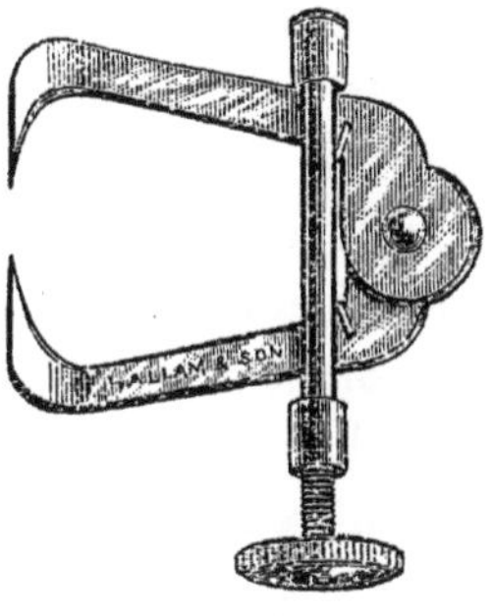
Fig. 2.

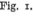

sheet steel, the former is wrought from solid cast steel; they each consist practically of a pair of wedges, one of which is placed between the teeth in front and the other behind, and the separation brought about by approximating them by means of a screw.

As to the practical utility of this class of instrument, in certain cases, there can be no doubt; a disadvantage of both the former is that they are to a certain extent a hinderance to the use of our filling instruments, this is not the case with the two latter, but in these the very act of application causes at times severe bruising of enamel.

Whenever applying these screw separators, the instrument should be kept firmly in position with the left hand, and the turns of the screw not made too quickly. A disadvantage one often meets with in Perry's is a tendency for the instrument to slip towards the gum;

this can easily be overcome by placing under the bows small pieces of either guttapercha, rubber or lead, just as turning the screws is commenced.

Parr's separator seems to be more universal in its use, but is certainly more clumsy. The two separators, illustrated, can be applied more quickly than either of the preceding, but their use is attended with far more discomfort.

In conclusion, it will, I think, be found best as a rule to commence separation by one of the gradual methods, completing with one of the immediate, and it should never be lost sight of that when filling after wedging, the main way to avoid pain is to keep the teeth perfectly steady.

A NOTE ON THE TREATMENT OF THE TEMPORARY TEETH.

By Nopac.

The indifference of the public to the welfare of children's temporary teeth is almost proverbial; but it may be questioned whether this is not to some extent encouraged by the unwillingness of dentists to undertake many operations for these little patients, owing to difficulties peculiar to the age of the patient, and to the different conditions met with in treating the temporary as distinguished from the permanent teeth. And yet a moment's consideration would make us realise more fully, than I fear we do in every day practice, the importance of these organs. They are the only means of mastication at the period of a child's most rapid growth, and at a time when surely every possible means should be employed of enabling it to lay the foundation of a good physique, which in these days of hurry and competition becomes every decade more necessary and perhaps more rare. It should then be the object of every dentist, not merely to pay careful attention to the temporary teeth of children, brought to him for advice or treatment, but also to impress on their parents the necessity of preserving them for mastication until the time comes for the eruption of their permanent successors. And yet it is hardly uncommon for parents to be told that they are too far gone to be filled, that they must be left as they are on the chance of their not giving much trouble, and that if they begin to ache badly, nothing remains but to get rid of them.

Something of the unwillingness of some dentists to do much for the temporary teeth, results, I think, from the failure of attempts to treat them on precisely the same lines as the permanent ones, when the conditions under which we work really justify and even require an altogether different procedure, and one which in the case of the permanent teeth would rightly be scouted as unscientific and reprehensible.

Crown cavities, when the pulp is not involved, are filled simply and effectively enough with amalgam; but interstitial cavities in the molars are difficult and unsatisfactory, partly from the relatively large size of the pulp chambers, which renders the pulp liable to exposure in cavities of even moderate size, and partly also from the impossibility of always excavating as thoroughly as desirable. If contoured amalgam fillings are attempted, the frailty of the teeth renders them very liable to break away, and if spaces are cut with a corundum disc, decay soon begins again at the cervical edge.

Some two or three years ago, Dr. Bonwill advocated treatment of interstitial caries of the temporary molars by filling up the space between the teeth as well as the cavities with guttapercha. Take the case of some slight decay between the two temporary molars involving both teeth. If the masticating surfaces are not materially weakened, he opens the cavities through the buccal walls with a pointed fissure bur, and having cleared them out, fills them and the space between the teeth with pink base-plate guttapercha packed into one solid mass. If the decay has involved the crown surfaces, he opens the cavities from above, excavates, and fills in the same way. Personally, I prefer, when as in the latter case the filling has to be bitten on, to use the hardest guttapercha procurable, and the kind I have found most suitable is Flagg's "high heat" guttapercha. Although more difficult to introduce, it has more than compensating advantages. It is very hard and wears comparatively little, absorbs little or no moisture, and does not seem to become "soppy" like some varieties; it is, also, possessed of little or no elasticity, and so does not tend to separate the teeth like the pink form, but simply keeps them in their places and prevents their being driven closer together, as they sometimes may be when extensively decayed, by the advance of the six year molars.

No doubt at first sight this method of filling will appear to many to be inartistic and unscientific, in practice, however, it will be found of much value. It keeps the mouth healthy by preventing the lodgment of food, &c., between the teeth, does not irritate the gums as might at first be expected, and is very comfortable for the little patient.

If the pulp of a tooth be exposed, it may be devitalized and thoroughly removed and rhizodontrophy performed, and the tooth filled in the same way, with a metal cap over the open pulp chamber.

TOTAL ABLATION OF THE BONES OF THE FACE.*

By M. PÉAN.

Surgeon to the Hospitals of Paris, Member of the Academy of Medicine.

MULTIPLE tumours of the bones of the face are relatively rare. An example of such was observed in a woman of 32, in whom the sphenoid, the three maxillaries, and the malars were invaded by osteo-fibromata consecutive to misplacement of teeth.

The first growth appeared at nine years. In 1884 one of M. Péan's colleagues resected the right upper maxillary which had been invaded. There was a recurrence and a short time after the left upper maxillary was in its turn attacked. The patient was seen for the first time by M. Péan in 1888. At this time the face was distorted, the left upper maxillary larger than the right, about the size of the head of a newly born infant; the lower jaw was swollen, the cheeks, the eye-lids, the nose were pushed out, the orbit, the buccal, and nasal cavities as well as the posterior nares were obstructed, the alveolar arch was thickened and the teeth movable and displaced without giving any appearance that two teeth among them were morbidly displaced by ectopia. The mastication, swallowing, speech and vision were impeded. Debilitated by suffering, and alarmed by the rapid progress of the tumours, the patient begged that some operation should be performed.

To make sure of thoroughly removing the growths it was necessary to take away the three maxillaries, the malars, and a portion of the sphenoid. Although no precedent existed for so extensive an operation and the sufferer appeared very weak to undergo it, it was agreed to operate, seeing that she would most likely succumb if something were not done.

---

* Communicated to the Academy of Medicine by M. Péan on the 14th of January, 1890 Translated for the DENTAL RECORD, by kind permission of M. Péan.

Accordingly at the first operation which took place on the 14th of December, 1888, M. Péan exposed the anterior surface of the maxillaries according to his usual method. The patient was placed

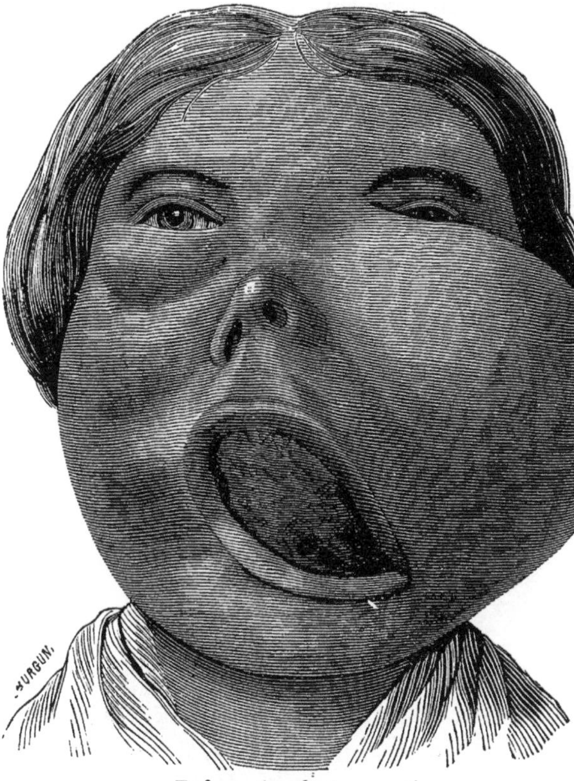

Before the first operation.

upon her back, with the trunk and neck raised, the pharyngeal *cul de sac* was plugged with sponges ; clips were put on the lips, cheeks, nose and septum. A median incision was then made through the upper lip and the tissues of the dorsum and root of the nose divided, the cheeks were dissected up with knife and scissors. As soon as the tumours were exposed, their exposed surfaces were cut away, a knife with a concave blade being employed. The other portions were cut away with cutting forceps. The superior maxillary bones, the malar bones, the pterygoid processes, the naso-orbital septum and the floor of the orbit were all removed. At this stage it was discovered that the upper lobe of the tumour occupied the lower part of the inferior plate of the sphenoid ; this was excised, and there was found a little molar hidden transversely in the spongy tissue. There can therefore be little doubt that this dental heterotopy had been the occasion of the neoplasm which was about to be removed. The existence of such an anomaly is perhaps without example in man, although with certain animals, notably the horse, heterotopic odontomes are frequent.

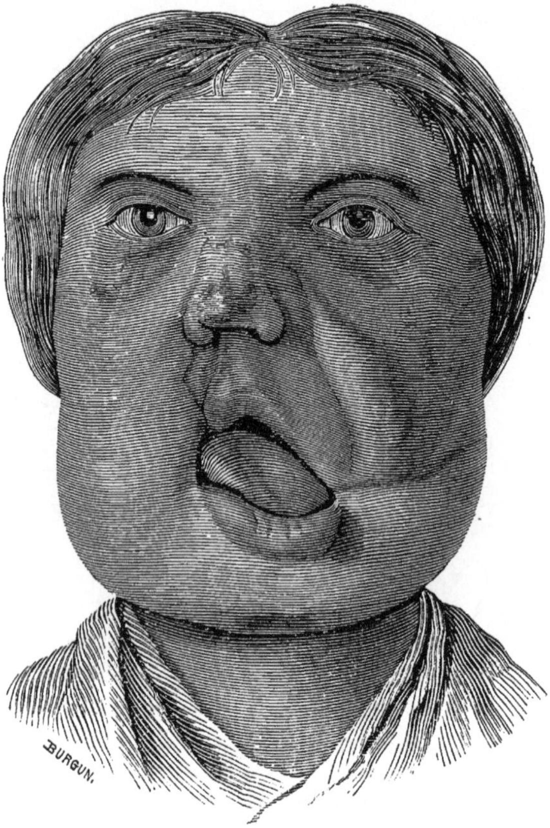

Before the second operation.

At the second operation which took place six weeks later, the lower maxillary was removed according to M. Péan's usual method; making a section of the soft parts from one angle of the jaw to the other along the lower border, and dissection of the periosteum and of the tumours on both sides of the bone, making a bilateral section of the ascending rami, removing the tumour in small pieces as it occupied the whole bone.

The operation was finished by detaching the muscles from the symphysis, and cutting across the middle line the periosteum which covered the lower border. At this point a permanent canine tooth was discovered hidden in a transverse position. This heterotopy surprised the more that the teeth of the lower maxilla were complete.

It is probable that this canine tooth had been the cause of the second tumour.

The result of the operation was favourable. Not only did the wounds unite by first intention, but no recurrence has as yet occurred (fourteen months after).

Besides, experience shows that these kinds of tumours when wholly removed do not often recur, although they contain, as in the case before us, some sarcomatous and myeloid elements disseminated in the midst of fibrous lamellæ and bony tissue in the layers which compose it. It remained to correct the malformation and to remedy the functional derangements following upon so extensive an ablation.

M. Michaels was requested to undertake the task of inventing some artificial substitute for the parts removed. (*See his description below*).

M. Péan summarises the following conclusions :—

(1) The total removal of the bony skeleton of the face can be performed with success.

(2) It is indicated in the case of osteo-fibromata following dental anomalies when these neoplasms occupy simultaneously the three maxillaries.

(3) In such a case it can be followed by a lasting cure.

(4) The mal-formation and functional derangements which it engenders can be corrected by prosthesis.

RESTORATION OF THE MAXILLARIES.*

By Professor MICHAELS.

M. MICHAELS describes his method of restoring the lost parts as follows :—The functional derangements in consequence of an operation so grave, the difficulty of nutrition, notably the abundant and constant loss of saliva, not to mention the deformity of the countenance, absolutely demanded some attempt at restoration whatever might be the issue.

The thing was far from being easy ; but a detailed description of

---

* Read before the Odontological Society of France, February 27th, 1890. Translated for the DENTAL RECORD, by kind permission of Professor Michaels.

the condition of the subject will enable you best to understand the complexity of the problem which had to be solved.

Upon examination I found a large and deep depression of the centre of the face, the cheeks were swollen, and sensitive to the

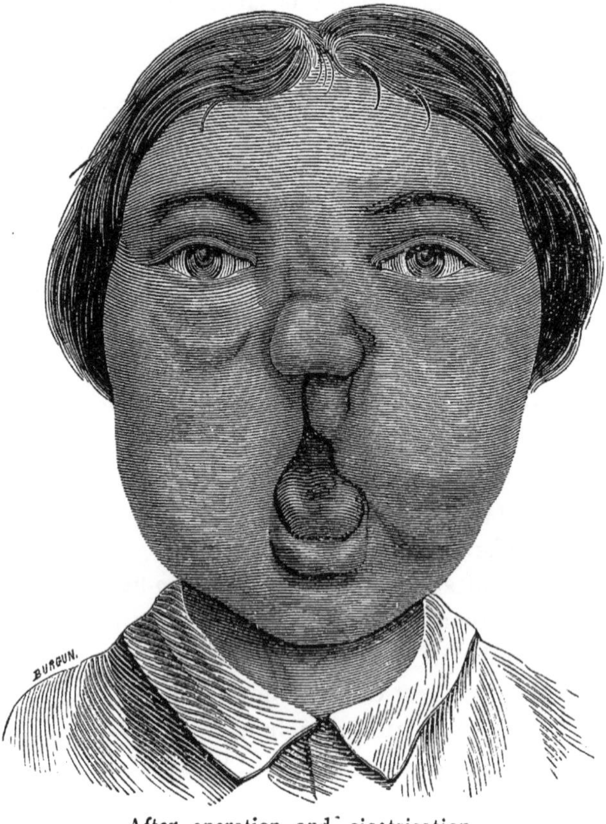

After operation and cicatrisation.

touch the nose reduced to the condition of a shapeless stump, the upper lip was like an exaggerated hare-lip with a cicatrix at the upper part of the section, its free sides directed into the mouth ; the lower lip was intact but drawn upwards and forwards at the angles by the contraction of the cicatrix in the upper lip, so that it appeared projecting and everted, the saliva flowing over it constantly and copiously.

The chin portion of the face had preserved its normal shape, but the cicatrix of the soft parts under the chin from one angle to the other along the inferior border of the maxillary was very different. This cicatrix on its inner side, considerably reduced the lower portion of the buccal cavity while the upper portion of this cavity had the form of a reversed funnel. This funnel was formed in front by the union of the internal face of the lip to the posterior face of the nostrils, and at the back by the soft palate, in height the opening corresponded with the cavity of the nasal fossæ which are so contracted that it was hardly possible to introduce the finger.

Let me add that there was a total absence of the middle meatus and of the inferior turbinate bones of the nose and total loss of the olfactory sense. The tongue was intact but paralysed, and performed its functions very imperfectly; it was disposed to project from the mouth, helping the outward flow of the saliva.

The sense of taste was preserved. The swallowing being defective and obstructed on account of the absence of the palatal arch the act caused the diffusion of liquids through the nasal fossæ. In repose the mouth was wide open allowing the tongue to project. The patient could with difficulty open and shut it, it was with the utmost exertion that she succeeded in making the smallest muscular contraction. Nutrition was painful and difficult; to feed herself the patient was compelled to make use of a long-necked bottle which she thrust into her mouth, the head well thrown back. To swallow the liquids she placed them in a vessel raised to the height of her arm. In the case of solids, after having conveyed the morsels to her mouth she pushed them as far as possible into the pharynx with her finger and then making an effort she swallowed. You mav judge that while food was taken into the stomach after this fashion without due mastication and insalivation, dyspepsia and gastric disorders were inevitable. Speech was so defective that it was almost impossible to understand her; conversation was carried on in writing. The lower eyelid of the right eye was deformed by the cicatricial contraction and the eye was constantly watering. In short, the patient in spite of the success of the operation was in a pitiable condition, condemned to a gradual decline by inanition and anæmia; one may question how long it would have been possible to have lived under such distressing conditions.

It was then important to correct as far as possible these malformations of the essential organs and to repair them. Were the ordinary resources of our art sufficient to cope with a case of such gravity? I was able to convince myself speedily that it was not in that direction that I should find the solution of the problem. How could I have devised the requisite means, if trusting to the traditions of the current prosthesis alone? The mobility of the soft parts yielding to the slightest pressure, the absence of anything solid to serve for a base which as you know is indispensable in this kind of work, made in this case all such attempts worthless.

All those who are familiar with the art of buccal restorations know that it is not an easy thing to take impressions of the soft parts of the mouth, and that the prosthetic pieces made under these conditions when put into place press upon and deform the soft parts with the result of producing painful irritations and excoriations.

Guided by these considerations, and strengthened besides by several fruitless attempts, made in this direction by skilful *confrères*, I set myself the task of devising the mechanism suitable for the proposed end in a different way. I succeeded at last in forming a solid base, on which I could manipulate when beginning this work.

We will describe the different experiments which I have made before arriving at the final result. It seemed natural to take the solid structure of the upper part of the head as a point of vantage of the system and a pair of spectacles would serve for the support of an artificial nose. But I determined not to have recourse to an artifice of this kind, and I resolved to make use of the fibrous cicatricial bridle of the upper lip, the only point of resistance of the upper buccal cavity, as the first and chief point of vantage for my operations. With this object I manufactured with the bowl of a coffee spoon a hook about 2½ centimetres in length, which by a turn of the hand I adapted on the curved part of the fibrous bridle ; its stem garnished with a mesh throughout its whole length descended thus obliquely and was continued outside the mouth. It remained to consolidate this axis by its free extremity. A compressor furnishing new points of support upon the face was indicated. The compressor was made of metal and of T shape. The lower extremity of the perpendicular branch of the T was furnished with a ring permitting the latter to slide the length of the axis of the hook. The horizontal branch, in the form of a cross, was adjusted externally on the lip surrounding the stump of the nose, adjusted exactly to the upper lip, thanks to a pad of gutta-percha which I took care to prepare. The hook put in place and the compresser brought by the sliding of its vertical arm into contact with the lip, I compressed the whole by the aid of a bolt, so as to have a resisting scaffold on which I could adapt the prosthetic pieces so-called. The upper artificial denture was made so as to attach itself to the branch of the great hook, kept in place behind as well as in front, and at once kept in place by a second spring bolt on the branch arm of the hook. The piece did not much resemble an ordinary denture ; its form was necessarily peculiar, owing to the abnormal conformation of the mouth. I was obliged to make an artificial velum applying it to the natural velum.

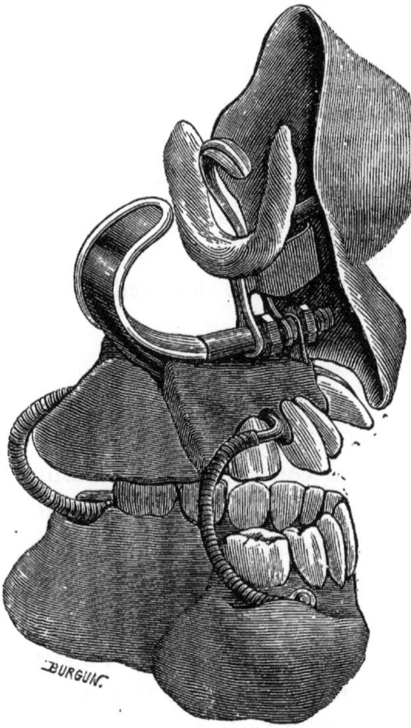

Apparatus devised by M. Michaels.

To protect the nasal cavity, the lower prosthetic piece, as every similar piece, was kept in position by the usual spiral springs used in dental prosthesis ; these springs were necessary in this case because without them the tongue would have constantly displaced the apparatus. After trial, the patient has found more support for the whole, thanks to this arrangement.

I was obliged to modify the system of the attachment of the springs with respect to the upper ; the springs attached to the lower artificial denture at a fixed point were re-united at their opposite extremity by a horizontal platina bar. Put in place this bar adapted itself to a groove designed on the buccal surface of the upper piece against which it rested.

In this way it became easy to manipulate the lower piece and to remove it from the mouth without displacing the upper arrangement.

The patient has derived benefit from this without suffering inconvenience. New difficulties presented themselves when it was necessary to make a nose and an upper lip. I wished, as I have already remarked, to avoid the use of the spectacles so disfiguring to a young subject. How then to avoid it? At length it was done; a small additional piece just permitted me to fix this on the artificial scaffolding represented by the compressor. A simple groove applied to the front of the perpendicular plate of the compressor was able to hold this adventitious portion; but so all important in an æsthetic sense. From the idea to the execution there was but one step. In other respects is was simple, an auxiliary branch whose enlarged extremity adjusted itself to the friction in the groove. The next step was to adapt a nose to the fixed part of the mechanism, and the nose itself.

I at first manipulated a nose in caoutchouc, which painted by a skilful artist appeared to me almost perfect, but I soon altered my opinion. It was simply frightful, and besides this, after having tried it I perceived that, in consequence of muscular movements of the face, it fell constantly forward, leaving a hideous void between the sides and the skin of the face. It was necessary to go over the work again, and I was compelled to take infinite pains in manipulating a suitable nose. At last, thanks to a happy inspiration, I succeeded in making a nose in celluloid, and I have effected without oil colours a tint for this factitious organ almost perfect, so that seen at a little distance it cannot be distinguished from the original organ. A last difficulty it was necessary to overcome; it was essential to find some means of preventing the nose from falling forward or becoming displaced.

The idea occurred to me to make a small hook with a tail, which was placed in the left nostril, that of the right being closed, and turned back astride on the fleshy part of the middle under partition of the stump of the nose. The tail of the hook terminated beneath in a small circle which was adapted to that of the principal hook; this arrangement kept the whole intact, and supported the artificial nose which was firmly fixed on the soft part of the face. Let us now survey rapidly the advantages which accrued, the æsthetic question apart, from the use of the prosthetic piece constructed with that object; I dare to affirm that the result has surpassed all expectation. After four months use, she has grown accustomed to the arrangement, placing and withdrawing it with facility; liquids no longer inundate the nasal cavity, she loses much less saliva, swallows with greater ease, opens and shuts the mouth naturally, takes nourishment without difficulty, speaks more easily, and there is

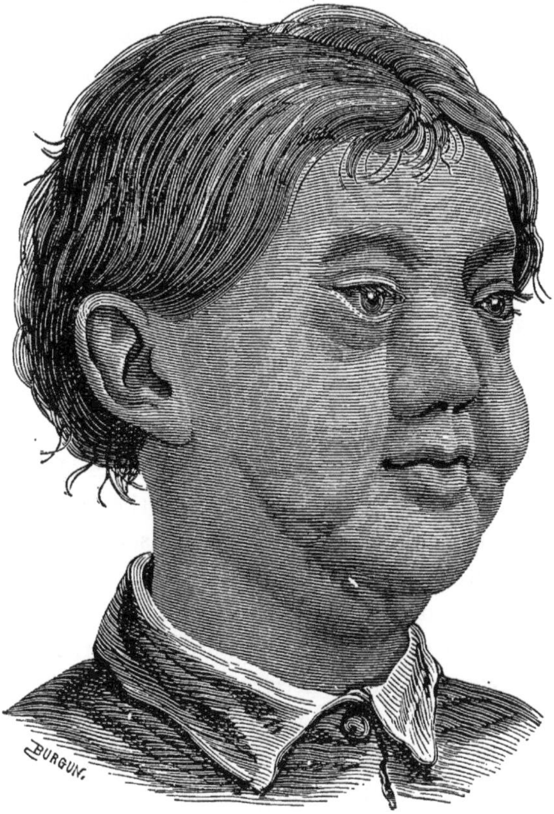

Restoration—the apparatus in place.

every hope that an improvement in the speech will follow as soon as use enables her to recover the flexibility of the tongue.

In conclusion, if I have described this experiment in all its details, it is not only on account of its interesting character or from the *amour propre* of an author satisfied with his work. It seems to me that useful instruction may be drawn from it. It is that we must never despair in most difficult cases when we are called upon for our good offices ; our art is fertile in resources, and we must seize every opportunity of realising, according to our ability, the improvement and the advance of which it is susceptible.

Reports.

THE ODONTOLOGICAL SOCIETY OF GREAT BRITAIN.

The ordinary monthly meeting of the above Society, was held at 40, Leicester Square, on the 14th ult. The President, Mr. FELIX WEISS, L.D.S.Eng., in the chair. There was a more than usually large attendance of members and visitors.

The LIBRARIAN (Mr. ASHLEY GIBBINGS) announced the receipt of the *Quarterly Journal of Microscopical Science*, *The Journal of Anatomy and Physiology*, and also an invitation to the 10th International Medical Congress to be held in August.

The CURATOR (Mr. STORER BENNETT) stated that by the kindness of Mr. Robbins he was able to bring to their notice two exceedingly interesting specimens, one Mr. Robbins had been good enough to give to the museum, the other had been lent by *The Field* newspaper. Both were similar, and were cases of over-growth of the lower incisors and deflected growth of the upper incisors in rabbits. Curiously enough the left upper incisor in both cases had taken $\frac{3}{4}$ of a circle and grown into the right side of the jaw. Mr. Robbins' specimen was also peculiar in the wearing of the molars owing to the irregular method in which the enamel was built up. The two very small incisors behind the ordinary incisors had become overgrown in a way Mr. Bennett had never seen before. They had received another specimen, presented by Mr. Redman, that of a supernumerary tooth occupying the position of a left upper incisor: it was a curiously shaped tooth, and looked as if it had been invaginated into the crown of the incisor itself. Mr. Henry Sewill had presented to the Society some photographs, taken by Mr. Andrew Pringle, illustrating some points in the etiology of caries and forming the basis of the slides to be shown in the course of his paper.

Mr. SCOTT THOMPSON showed an engine cord spliced by the method explained in the *International Dental Journal* of February and recommended the plan as a good one.

Mr. W. A. MAGGS read notes of a case of Defective Development of the Permanent Teeth, associated with Malformation of the Eyes and Anus, and showed models illustrating the patient's dentition.

The patient, a girl aged 18, was admitted to Guy's Hospital under the care of Mr. Brailey for chronic glaucoma of both eyes.

She was the eldest of six children. Her three brothers died in infancy from convulsions. Her two sisters, aged 17 and 13, were living, and in good health. The father was alive and well, aged about 41, the mother died of consumption aged 37. The patient was of medium height, dark complexion, fairly well developed head and face, dark abundant hair of fine texture. Some hair on the upper lip, eyebrows normal, but eyelashes scanty. Her anus was imperforate at birth, and had to be established by operation. With respect to the teeth, in the upper jaw she had a temporary and six permanent teeth; all the incisors and permanent molars were absent, but a temporary molar remained between the premolars on the right side. The palate was flat, and there was an absence of the alveolar process between the canines. In the lower jaw ten teeth were present. On the right side the incisors, second premolar and wisdom tooth were absent, but a caniniform supernumerary tooth was present between the canine and premolar. On the left side the canine second premolar and wisdom tooth were absent. The patient asserted that she had never had any teeth in the front of her mouth. The canine teeth were peculiarly peg-shaped, while the upper second premolars had two distinct cusps on the outer masticating surfaces. There was a tendency to dwarfing of the teeth, but all were well covered with enamel. The ophthalmic surgeon, Mr. Brailey, stated that both eyes were very deficient, the lenses were present, but there was all but a complete absence of irides. Each eye had thirteen dioptrics of myopia, which was not improved by spherical glasses. Mr. Brailey found nothing suggestive of specific disease. Mr. Maggs remarked that the chief interest centred in the fact that the teeth and eyes, which are mainly dermal organs, were malformed, the former being also deficient in number. The case was further interesting in that the nether portion of the alimentary canal, the anus, also of epiblastic origin, was imperforate; it was brought before the Society mainly as an association of congenital defects in organs derived from the same embryonic layer, viz., the epiblast.

Mr. ASHLEY BARRETT showed an electric lamp made by himself. The lamp, a Swan & Edison incandescent of 16 volts, having a concave reflector behind it and a convex ridge in front, was mounted on an arm with ball and socket joint giving freedom of movement in all directions. The construction was so arranged as to protect the operator from the glare and throw the light below the patient's eyes. Mr. Barrett also showed a device which he had been obliged to resort to in extracting a deeply buried stump of a lower third molar on the left side. He had unsuccessfully endeavoured with the aid of gas to get a grip of the stump with a pair of forceps, but they continually slipped off; he then tried with an elevator but could get no fulcrum. It occurred to him to make an artificial fulcrum in vulcanite, which he did with very satisfactory results.

Mr. LAWRENCE READ remarked that Mr. Barrett's lamp entirely excluded the light from the room, and asked what arrangement he had for finding his instruments?

Mr. ASHLEY BARRETT replied that he could so easily turn the ball and socket lamp in any direction that he constantly used it for finding anything he wanted, but at the same time a gas burner might be kept lighted and turned low.

Mr. HENRY SEWILL had spoken and written about dental caries perhaps more than most men in the Society. He was ashamed to say that it was only in recent times he had made thorough research with respect to the disease. He did not think that without the aid of Mr. Pound, of King's College, who as everyone knew was an expert of experts in bacteriology and staining organisms, he should now have undertaken it. Mr. Sewill had some sections more beautiful than had ever before been prepared, and this had been his inducement for bringing the subject upon which he had nothing new to tell them before the Society. Another inducement was, that he had been fortunate enough to interest Mr. Andrew Pringle, whose reputation as a physiologist and photomicrographist was well known. If he (Mr. Sewill) was to stop to express his obligations to every scientist to whom he had had recourse, his list would be a long one, but he would specially mention, Mr. Arthur Underwood, Mr. Charters White, and Mr. Charles Tomes.

SLIDES.

1. A section of developing teeth of a cat, taken from one of Mr. Charters White's sections, magnification 160 diameters on the slide, and 5,120 on the screen. This slide demonstrated that the natural blood supply of enamel came from the sac. The dentine commenced to be calcified before the enamel, and except externally there was no vascular supply besides that of the dental pulp which

was cut off by a mass of dentine. It was difficult to imagine the nutrition of the enamel pulp from the dentinal.

2. A section of developing dog's tooth prepared and stained by Mr. Arthur Underwood, magnification on the slide 240 diameters, on the screen 7,680. Dental sac, enamel cells, forming enamel, dentine, and odontoblasts were all clearly traceable.

3. Section of enamel organ, magnification 650 diameters on the slide, and 21,000 on the screen. Forming enamel, enamel pulp, external enamel cells and sac, all well defined.

4. A section of enamel by Mr. Arthur Underwood stained with chloride of gold. This was an exceedingly good section and a good photograph.

5. Section of dentine by Mr. Arthur Underwood, magnified 650 diameters on the slide, and 21,000 on the screen. Showing the point of junction with enamel.

All observers, though they differed in some small details, had come to the conclusion that caries was entirely due to external agents, and quite devoid of any pathological phenomena.

There was not the least doubt in Mr. Sewill's own mind that to imagine the presence in enamel of any physiological elements capable of pathological action was quite absurd. Protoplasm could not live isolated, it must be nourished. The physical character of enamel, and its absence of organic matter, precluded all idea of its performing any physiological action.

6. A transverse section of dentine unstained.

7. Showing structural defect in enamel from a section by Mr. Charters White, magnification 150 diameters on the slide and 7,800 on the screen. Granular enamel plainly seen, and a crack (part of it making an artificial section) being a flaw in the enamel.

8. A section of enamel and dentine. Mr. Sewill remarked that Gallippe and Hoppe Seyler had endeavoured to show that enamel undergoes changes and so becomes dense as years go on. The only way to prove whether teeth gained in density would be to cut sections from them at different periods of their existence, but even then the result would be very fallacious.

The photographs of sections of enamel and dentine largely explained the etiology of dental caries.

10. A typical section of the orifice of a cavity illustrating caries proper, magnified 80 diameters on slide, and 2,560 on screen.

Mr. Sewill remarked that Mr. Pound had in the course of the investigation cut and stained some eight dozen sections. Quite recently he (Mr. Sewill) had met with a lady having a re-inserted natural tooth. Mr. Pound had cut a considerable number of sections from that tooth and caries was shown to be absolutely the same in it as in a living tooth. Mr. Sewill further stated he had from Professor Miller of Berlin a series of slides illustrating caries artificially produced out of the mouth identical with that produced in the mouth. Several of the slides of artificial and natural caries had been mixed, and Mr. Arthur Underwood and Mr. Pound had endeavoured to separate them, but neither of them had been always successful, showing that in their essential appearance artificial and natural caries are identical. Of the bacteria which produce caries the micrococcus is the most frequent; they are found in groups, pairs, and chains. Dr. Miller says the pairs and chains are agents of lactic acid fermentation. Leptothrix is found in all cases especially on the surfaces. Bacteria proper are found everywhere. The torula, one of the true fermentation organisms was present, but not in great numbers.

11. A deeper section of the same tooth, magnified 160 diameters on the slide, and about 4,480 on the screen, showing the organisms penetrating along the tubes.

12. A finer section than No. 2, magnified 20,000 diameters on the screen. In this the microccoci could be seen forming pairs, groups, and strings.

13. A section of about the most advanced caries possible to cut a section of, magnified 950 diameters on the slide, and 21,000 on the screen.

14. A beautiful specimen of leptothrix. Why it so often happened that one organism was more abundant than another, it was difficult to say. This section was magnified 20,000 diameters on the screen.

15. A transverse section of carious dentine, magnification of photograph 650 diameters, 21,000 on screen. The tubes in this case were mainly loaded with leptothrix.

16. Photograph of scrapings of carious teeth, comma bacilli, a bundle of leptothrix, micrococci and various organisms.

17. Section of pipe stem appearance, caries just commencing, etching out of the tissue by acid. The so-called zone round the area of caries was once thought to indicate vital action of dentine, but

it was not possible, it was simply due to the softening of the dentine.

It was not necessary to multiply the specimens Mr. Pringle had been kind enough to take. Mr. Sewill had some six or eight dozen slides. But he did hope that a great many other individuals would go into the research of caries. It was really so simple that he did not see why students in every school should not go through the whole process.

There were a vast number of demonstrated facts; in the first place there was the anatomical facts indicating the pathology of enamel and dentine; there were the facts connected with predisposing causes; the fact that agents existing in the mouth can destroy dentine; the fact that caries is the same in pulpless teeth or teeth with living pulps. Then there was the fact that it occurs in teeth replaced in the mouth, dead teeth indicate changes absolutely identical with living teeth.

The President having eulogistically remarked upon the character of the photographic specimens, Mr. H. Sewill passed round some reproductions of the photographs by Messrs. Waterlow & Sons.

Mr. Charters White said that from the way in which Mr. Sewill's paper had been received it was evident that the Society thoroughly appreciated the work he had done, supplemented so ably by Mr. Andrew Pringle who was *facile princeps* in photo-micrography. In the early days of dental pathology Mr. White was inclined to adopt the physiological origin of caries. There were one or two points upon which his opinion was based at that time which convinced him that dental caries arose from within as well as from without, but in later years he had come to Mr. Sewill's conclusion that caries is due to external agencies in all cases, for if dental caries originated from within, it would very often if not always be found that a cavity existed in the dentine far removed from the external surfaces of the enamel, but it was not the case. Once he thought he had discovered a cavity below the enamel, but on careful examination he found it originated from a cavity in the enamel itself which he had overlooked. He thought that the conditions they had seen photographed on the screen, such as granular enamel, subjected the teeth to the attack of micro-organisms; once let such a condition be established on the enamel and the work proceeds by a sort of fermentation in the line of the tissues; the cavity becomes enlarged, micrococci multiply, and as yeast ferments, so they ferment until the dentine is exposed. These views were understood by everyone, so that he did not pretend to be stating anything original, but he had made these remarks rather for the purpose of supporting the opinions of Mr. Sewill with which he agreed.

Mr. F. J. Bennett thought that Mr. Sewill's delightful paper had been of the utmost service, not because it contained anything new, indeed the absence of anything new made discussion, if not impossible, at least unnecessary. But it was a great advantage for them to be able to see, by means of such pictures as Mr. Sewill had been able to obtain by the assistance of Mr. Pound and Mr. Pringle, the facts demonstrated upon which the opinions as to the etiology of dental caries rested. Mr. Sewill had so freely acknowledged the sources to which he was indebted in the course of his investigations that he felt sure that he (Mr. Sewill) would be glad to be reminded that the name of Mr. Arthur Underwood who had done so much, should always be associated with the name of Mr. Milles who had so ably worked in the same field. He felt sure that Mr. Underwood himself would be pained if his name were divorced from that of Mr. Milles.

ODONTO-CHIRURGICAL SOCIETY OF SCOTLAND.

The Annual Meeting of the above Society was held in March.

Mr. W. E. Satchell, L.D.S., Elizabeth Street, Hyde Park, Sydney, N.S.W., was, on the recommendation of the Council, nominated for membership.

THE EFFECTS OF BAGPIPE PLAYING ON THE TEETH.

Mr. Macleod said:—Recently one of the bandsmen of the Cameron Highlanders was having some teeth filled at the Dental Hospital. On overlooking the work being done, he observed a peculiarity in the teeth of the young man under treatment, and, on inquiry, found that the young man was a piper, and that the peculiarity noticed was caused by the mouth-piece of the pipe. Mr. Murray Thomson, the student under whose care the lad was, took two most excellent impressions, and he had now the pleasure of passing round the models obtained from these impressions, which would give a graphic idea of the peculiarity noted—viz., three crescentic-shaped apertures between the cutting edges of the six front teeth.

He had examined the teeth of various pipers since then, and all of them presented the same "wearing away" in a greater or lesser degree, varying with the density of the tooth structure and the time engaged in pipe playing. He found on enquiry that, on the average, it took about four years to make a well-marked impression, but that, once the enamel edge was worn through, the "wearing away" was more rapid. Every one was aware of the way in which the tobacco-pipe wore the teeth of the smoker, but this was not to be wondered at, the baked pipeclay being a hardish and gritty substance; but that a horn mouthpiece should have such an appreciable effect was, he thought, a matter of curious interest. He might mention, however, that the mouth-pieces suffered more than the teeth—the average life of a horn mouth-piece being from twelve to eighteen months, that of a bone or ivory one (a substance seldom used) being about two years. The peculiarity noticed was a crescent-shaped aperture  on the cutting edge of the front teeth in three localities—viz., between the central incisors, and between the lateral and canine on both sides.

Dr. Smith thought the case referred to by Mr. Macleod one which had never previously, so far as he knew, been noticed or described in any dental treatise or association. The different situations in which the wearing down of the teeth occurred, and which corresponded with the positions to which the mouth-piece was shifted while playing, showed that this was obviously the cause of the injury. The fact of a bone or horn mouth-piece producing this effect seemed more remarkable than the well-known similar consequences resulting from using a clay tobacco-pipe. But although the bone or horn was a much softer material, its action was possibly aided by the much harder bite capable of being sustained by it than could be borne by a clay pipe stem.

Mr. Leslie Fraser (Inverness) spoke of a case he came across in his practice. The patient was about twenty-five years of age, and had been playing the bagpipes for over seven years. The two central incisors were very much cut or worn towards the mesial line. They were also so very loose that he picked them out quite easily with a napkin between his forefinger and thumb. This patient always held the "chanter" between his two front teeth, and having rather a swinging gait, this probably caused a good deal of vibration between the mouth-piece and the teeth when he walked. The patient also suffered from Rigg's disease, more particularly in connection with the teeth in question. A plate of black rubber was inserted, and he finds he is able to grasp the mouth-piece quite as well now as formerly. How long these porcelain teeth will survive the strain is quite another question.

Mr. DURWARD exhibited a patient who had had the right half of the superior maxilla removed, along with a sarcoma. He had supplied the deficiency with a vulcanite denture, which restored the contour of the face, and also supplied the necessary masticating power—and invited the members to inspect the result. Of the improvement effected and the comfort imparted to the patient there could be but one opinion; and, in reply to a remark made by a member that such an arrangement could be but temporary, as there was always the liability of the growth to recur, Mr. Durward said that it was in any way an advantage to the patient that the remaining years of her life should be made as tolerable or comfortable as circumstances or rather art could permit.

Mr. MACLEOD showed models and described a case of artificial restoration of a large portion of the lower jaw. The loss of substance extended from the cuspid on the right to the second molar on the left. The loss was occasioned by the discharge of an army rifle beneath the chin.

Mr. MACLEOD exhibited an upper denture aluminium cast base, which had been worn with satisfaction and comfort. He also exhibited the Carrol Company's furnace flask and pneumatic crucible for working the material. He referred to the use of aluminium plates between twenty-five and thirty years ago—the drawback attending its use, and preventing its general adoption at that time, and explained that as many of these had now been removed, it might be worth while to place aluminium once more upon its trial, and determine its value as a dental base.

Dr. SMITH said he was somewhat interested in Mr. Macleod's communication on aluminium as a base for artificial dentures. He had himself about thirty years ago brought its use before the dental profession in Edinburgh, and had the honour of receiving the silver medal of the Royal Scottish Society of Arts for his mode of employing this substance in these cases. Mr. Macleod's method, in the very admirable piece of work handed round, was somewhat different from that adopted by Dr. Smith, inasmuch as Mr. Macleod's was a process of casting the metal so as to take the place, as it were, of the vulcanite in an ordinary vulcanite denture, whereas Dr. Smith's method consisted in striking a plate of aluminium and mounting the teeth upon it by means of vulcanite attached to the plate by a number of countersunk perforations. This obviated the necessity of contact with any other metal; as aluminium was peculiarly sensitive in this respect—the difficulty of soldering it or allowing any other metal to come in contact with it, such as even the platinum pins of the teeth, being that it corroded at the points of contact. Dr. Smith had exhibited to many of the dentists of the time sets made in this way, as well as some plates for the smaller lesions of the palate. One of these sets was worn by a well-known and respected old member of the profession for many years and was very little changed in the end. Its appearance was against the use of this metal, as it had a dull and leaden look about it. It was, however, very light and very cheap, and in most, though not in all cases, when properly handled, was fairly durable in the mouth. Purity of the metal was in all cases essential, and this he had found sometimes difficult to secure.

Mr. BROWNLIE had had no great personal experience with aluminium, as he did not look upon it as a metal that would ever be of much service to them, for reasons already quoted by Dr. Smith. A dentist in Glasgow—one of the advertising fraternity—had at one time taken up the matter rather warmly, and had gone the length of taking out a patent in the matter; but as he (Mr. Brownlie) had heard nothing of it of recent years from that source, he concluded that the dentist in question had discovered its defects, and abandoned its use.

Mr. WATSON mentioned that he had some experience in the making of aluminium plates while with his old master, Dr. Orphoot. They were made on the same principle as that described by Dr. Smith, but were found, especially when not kept clean, to corrode very rapidly, only lasting for a year or eighteen months.

Mr. BIGGS said that he had some considerable experience under Dr. Smith some twenty-eight years ago, and had assisted the doctor in constructing some of the plates for which he had received the medal of the Society of Arts. He could corroborate what Mr. Brownlie had said, that many years after this a patent was taken out for this very same process by a Glasgow dentist, who made a very great number of cases, but, latterly, even he had abandoned its use. It was interesting to see the apparatus and the cast denture in aluminium, but he could not say they had an attractive appearance. A set of teeth in gold would have a vastly higher apparent intrinsic value, and patients were not likely to appreciate a case approaching so much in general appearance to that of Britannia metal. He thanked Mr. Macleod for bringing the case before the Society.

Mr. WATSON handed round for inspection cultures of Miller's spirillum and Finkler's spirillum (or comma bacillus), and pointed out that the appearances of the two organisms under cultivation are exactly alike, and, by means of photo-micrographs showed that the microscopic appearances of both are analogous, although the one is found in the mouth and the other in the intestinal canal of cholera patients. They both grow up rapidly in culture media, and are undoubtedly distinct organisms.

Mr. J. A. BIGGS then read a paper upon the

TREATMENT OF IRREGULARITIES OF THE TEETH.

MR. CHAIRMAN AND GENTLEMAN,—At present I purpose not so much to enter into the etiology of the irregularities of the teeth, as to deal with the practical aspect of the subject, illustrated from models in various stages, and with the apparatus used from the beginning to the completion of each case.

Before commencing the subject proper I would like to remark the great diversity of opinion there seems to be as to the influence for good or evil in the early extraction of the deciduous teeth. On the one hand, it is advocated that the early removal of the deciduous teeth prevents crowding of the permanent ones. On the other, it is contended that such a procedure causes contraction of the jaws, and consequent over-crowding of the permanent set. My own experience is that infinitely more harm is done by too great haste in their removal, than by an error in the opposite direction. I certainly would not hesitate to remove a temporary tooth when I had sufficient evidence that it obstructed the permanent ones, and who has not seen even a tiny spicule suffice to divert a strong well-developed tooth from its normal position, as if it were there to dispute possession, and maintain the truth of the adage, that possession is nine points in the law. Yet I am not of opinion that extraction causes contraction of the jaws.

At an age when room for the permanent set might be deemed desirable, there are so many tooth germs, at all stages of development, hastening on to their destined goals, that I maintain there are sufficient factors present to promote the growth of the jaw, and that contraction is unlikely. I hold it more probable that extraction, for instance, at the age of from five to six, arrests the development of the alveolar process, until further demands stimulate it into new efforts. This is well exemplified in the case of a six-year-old molar if extracted at, say, eight years of age; at twelve there will be no trace of the patient ever having had a six-year-old molar removed. You will find nature has rather utilised the material already provided than exerted herself to produce it anew.

I pass round for your inspection the model of the superior maxilla of a young lady, aged 20. You will observe the bicuspids on one side almost touch those on the other; they are exactly five-sixteenths of an inch apart. With the model in your hands it is not difficult to define the reason for their displacement. The temporary molars were removed at so early a period, that the six-year-old molars were compelled to occupy their position. Consequently, when the bicuspids appeared, they were forced, for want of space, to occupy the position they now maintain. Of course if this case had come into my hands sufficiently soon, it would have been an easy matter to correct it. But the young lady lives at a considerable distance, her general health is not robust and she is inclined "rather to bear the ills she has than fly to others that she knows not of."

Her appearance is in no way impaired, she suffers no pain, and is not easily convinced that her general health may be impaired from the defective occlusion, as shown by her models, but rather looks forward to the time when she may rid herself of them all, and get others more beautiful, though less natural.

This is only one example of many similar cases where the symmetry of the mouth, and even the features, has been destroyed by this injudicious and premature extraction of the temporary teeth. So much then for the theory that early extraction of the deciduous is beneficial to the permanent teeth.

Again, I have heard it stated that the extraction of the six-year-old molar for a young person hinders the development of the sphenoid bone, stunts its growth, and thereby lessens the capacity of the brain case, and of course impairs functional activity of the brain. But I am of opinion that the sphenoid, the bodies of the maxillæ, and the adjacent bones, having independent developments, are capable of achieving normal dimensions, despite the existence of the teeth or the alveolar process, which may in a measure be considered an afterthought of nature, and not independent formations, like those just specified.

I will now, without further digression, proceed with my subject proper. I have here the model of a boy's superior maxilla. You will see a somewhat unusual form of irregularity. The right central has been thrown forward so much as to allow the lateral incisors to occupy its place in line with the opposite central. The model is accompanied by the appliance by which the irregularity was corrected. It is a vulcanite plate, filling the palate from molar to molar and forward to the incisors. You may observe the teeth are short, and poorly adapted for anchorage. I have, therefore, a wire round the molar on the left to make it fast there. On the right you see a long wire reach from the bicuspid round to and in front of the incisor. These wires are made of piano wire, and have a good reliable power. In front of the biscuspid there is a small ring of gold spring, to which a rubber band is attached. When in situation the band was stretched over the lateral, and the spring over the central. The lateral was drawn clear, and the central pushed back into position, a distance of over a quarter of an inch in the course of one month, much to the gratification of the boy and his parents.

The models I now place in your hands are those of the inferior and superior maxilla of a young lady, aged 12. I think it obvious that the abnormal condition here maintained is hereditary. This is a somewhat common type of irregularity, and one most difficult to correct. In the first place, you may observe that there is a defect in both jaws. The lower is small and receding, while the upper is prominent, causing a space between the lower and upper front teeth, when occluded, of fully half an inch, in addition to which the teeth in the upper are acutely V shaped and the canines stand forward in front of, and covering half the breadth of the laterals. The patient had quite a difficulty in closing her lips, and altogether an unsightly deformity was produced.

One of the great difficulties with this case was the shortness of the back teeth, the molar on the right side being only about a sixteenth of an inch above the surface of the gum, the first bicuspid about an eighth of an inch, and the second not erupted at all. The molar on the left is about an eighth, but the bicuspids fairly well developed. Such an arrangement you can readily see was not at all favourable for anchorage. However, a very accurately fitting plate was struck up for it, with a small loop of wire, soldered behind each central for the application of elastic bands, and a tube with a female screw, fitted and soldered behind each lateral, for male screws to push out the laterals. For the left bicuspids there were caps fitted to be cemented on, and square tubes were soldered to them, and for their accommodation there was a strong bar soldered to the side of the plate, on which they work backwards and forwards, the motor power being elastic bands fastened on cross-bars and to a ring at the back of the plate. On the right side the square tube was soldered to the plate, and the square bar made to slide in it for the retraction of the cuspid. By this device the teeth were brought fairly well into their positions. A retaining plate was then made, consisting of vulcanite, with a piano wire encircling the entire arch. This wire was divided in two, and a small jack screw fastened on one end, capable of revolving; the end of the other wire was screwed. When caught up by the jack screw it tightened the wire to any extent desired. Wooden wedges, placed judiciously against the lingual sides of the teeeh, enabled me to rotate the teeth as desired.

With the models exhibited and the difficulties to be overcome, you will, I think, see the utility of the appliances employed, in which, I trust, some originality can be discriminated. In the model of the completed case, so far as the upper is concerned, I think you will see that satisfactory results have been secured. I have had this case in hand for about nine months, yet the patient still wears the retaining plate at night, as it is possible the teeth might recede, although I think it improbable. The occlusion is no better than when I took the case in hand, but it is at least no worse, and the defect lies now in the lower, which, I hope, in course of time to take in hand, and when completed to exhibit the results to you. I might, perhaps, add that this patient lives at a distance of 30 miles, and after the first week I rarely saw her more than once a week, and often only once a fortnight.

The models of the next case I have the pleasure of bringing before you are somewhat similar, but even more complicated than the last. It came into my hands for treatment last October, and is evidently the outcome of heredity combined with lip or thumb-sucking. The patient is a female, aged 11, of good physique and a sanguine disposition. Her parents were much distressed at the deformity produced by the irregularity. It was with great reluctance I was persuaded to take the case in hand, and then I might, perhaps, mention, as being a practical point, not without firstly clearly establishing our financial relations, which were arranged to be independent of the result of my efforts.

From the models you will note there is not one single tooth, either in the upper or lower, that can be said to occupy a correct position—the two upper molars making the nearest approach to it. The occlusion is very defective, and the teeth honeycombed. The molars are also very defective, and in the lower jaw they and the bicuspids are barely above the level of the gums. They all seem to have been hurried into position, regardless of their condition of maturity, and show all sorts of imperfection in the enamel. To crown all, the two central incisors were poor, immature looking things, with, as before stated, defective enamel at their cutting edges and at the lingual aspect, and standing out so far that there was a space of five-eighths of an inch between them and the lower teeth. She had also fallen upon them, and the nerve in one of them was dead. A worse condition of affairs than this is hardly conceivable.

I first made a silver plate for the lowers, with a bar soldered round the front. To this bar was fastened a number of elastic rings to fit round the four front teeth, which brought them forward rapidly (that is in about three weeks' time) the distance of a quarter of an inch. I had then to make a small retaining plate until they became firm in their sockets. Meantime, I extracted the two centrals in the upper and made a plate, with a somewhat novel device, by which the laterals were drawn into position to act as their substitutes. Before the introduction of this plate, the laterals were three-quarters of an inch apart; they are now about one quarter apart. The canines have also been drawn in a little. This case is not completed; she is merely wearing retaining plates, as there is a danger in using too great haste.

The main aim here is, as far as possible, to correct the projection in the upper and the recession in the lower, so as to restore the features and expression, as her teeth are so poor that they are unworthy of consideration, but with the prospect of being able to give her substitutes, which afterwards will make her more presentable and prove more useful. Her mother and aunt both exhibited the same unfortunate peculiarities—the former having, previous to marriage, been under my treatment in respect to them.

I have here the models of a very similar case which came into my hands some years ago, and which I showed at the West of Scotland Branch of the B. D. A. The uppers protruded beyond the lowers to an unsightly extent, so that when the back teeth were closed, the lower incisors did not meet the upper by a distance of five-eighths of an inch. The lady was present at the meeting, and shown with and without the apparatus I am about to describe. The patient was young, but, unfortunately, too old to have the defect rectified by regulating devices. Yet she had such a fine face and expression that I deemed it desirable that something should be done for her. I therefore struck up a sort of glove for the lower teeth in (platinum), on which I mounted a set of six teeth, bringing them up to meet the uppers. They were finished with continuous gum work, and were a very considerable improvement to her. She does not wear them constantly, but reserves them for occasions, and kindly lent them for this meeting.

At our meeting of 1882, I brought before your notice a case of a child, about six months old, who fell and drove her two central incisors (upper) out of sight up into the alveolar process. The family physician (called in immediately) stated that as they were knocked out the mouth would soon heal up, but the swelling became alarming and I was consulted about it. I operated under chloroform and removed them. Not having seen a case similar at so early an age, I was doubtful whether the permanent teeth would suffer in consequence. Thinking it might interest you, I have secured models of the mouth after a lapse of eight years, which I now place before you. The centrals are now in position, and are in no way impaired. They are inclined to be irregular, but will probably right themselves as the other teeth come into position. Any displacement shown could not in any case be said to be the result of the accident.

The next case is that of a female, aged 11, in which the six front teeth have taken abnormal positions. The labial aspect of the right lateral is behind the lingual surface of the right central, the said central standing out too far. The left central has its lingual surface turned towards the mesial side of the right central, and its distal edge is standing in behind the left lateral. The canines stand forward right in front of the laterals; that, at least, is the position they indicate, as the mere points of them are all that are yet showing. I have been rather unfortunate in this case, as, after having almost succeeded in correcting them, and the patient was wearing a retaining plate, she had an attack of scarlet fever, during which the plate was removed, and unhappily the teeth again resumed, to a great extent, their former positions. You may see, from the models I hand round, the breadth gained at this stage.

I also show a couple of cases that have just come to hand—one in which the upper left canine is crowded out of the arch, and all the other teeth in situation ; the other where the two centrals are locked in behind the lower incisors, and which I have just begun to regulate, but possessing no particular points of interest ; and with them I conclude my paper.

Mr. Brownlie considered that much thought and discretion should be exercised before commencing regulating cases, as he had seen so much injury done to the teeth in the way of predisposing them to caries, resulting from the necessary pressure brought to bear upon them in pushing them into the required positions, and from the lengthened contact with the regulating frame. This he had had brought before him in a recent case, where, before treatment, the teeth were absolutely free from caries, but subsequently several had required to be stopped, and which he attributed to the result of the regulating process.

Mr. Dall suggested that a retaining-plate was liable to do injury to the teeth, as it had often to be worn for a considerable period. He had frequently adopted the plan of making what he might term a retaining-cage of gold wire, which consisted of two somewhat thick lengths of wire, the one fitted to the labial and the other to the lingual sides of the teeth, the two being connected by thin pieces of wire, passed between the intervals of the teeth where possible, and also over them, where the bite permitted, in such a position as to secure them in the positions in which they had been pushed by the regulating frame, and, where desirable, sometimes passing thin pieces of flat gold between the front teeth and soldering them to the main strand. In this way, he was of the opinion that greater cleanliness could be ensured and less consequent injury to the teeth.

Mr. Watson thanked Mr. Biggs for his interesting paper on irregularities, and expressed his admiration of some of the ingenious plates, &c., which Mr. Biggs had used in the treatment of cases. He was in the habit of discouraging as much as possible such cases, owing to the fact that they seldom paid for the time and trouble expended on them. Such cases required great discrimination and thought before attempting anything, and often proved extremely troublesome, while the results attained were not always very satisfactory. Mr. Brownlie's remark that often great harm is done in the treatment of irregularities, was, he thought a very true one, as there is not the slightest doubt that more harm than good is frequently done in interfering with the mal-arrangement of teeth, especially in congenital cases, besides the impress that may be produced on the teeth themselves while under treatment, in giving them a greater tendency to caries.

Mr. BIGGS said that he forgot who was the originator of the method Mr. Dall described (Dr. Guelfard's), but it was an easy matter to show the fallacy of Mr. Dall's deductions. In the first place, in answer to a remark by Mr. Watson, he stated that although it could not be removed for cleansing purposes by the patient, yet the wires were thin and the brush could get between it and the teeth, and so remove any *débris*. Mr. Biggs said that in his opinion the smallness of the wire was an element of weakness, as any friction, even though slight, had a greater tendency to cut the teeth ; and if the bristles of the brush were capable of getting between it and the teeth, it could not possibly be of any use in retaining the regulated teeth. Moreover, Mr. Dall spoke of having a piece of flat plate running between the centrals to steady the plate or cage, but he was of opinion that more injury would be done by such a contrivance in the course of three months than by such an arrangement as he had shown and described in three years. The teeth at that age being delicate and immature, it was necessary that as much facility for removing any cleansing as possible be provided, especially as retaining-plates had often to be kept in use for a whole year. Mr. Biggs thanked the various speakers for the kindly criticisms they had passed upon his paper, and was gratified that so many had concurred in his method of treatment. Several of the plates, they said, were novel, and he could assure them they were original.

THE PRESIDENT announced that the next meeting would be Thursday, the 13th November, and wished to all a pleasant summer ; and trusted they would come up next session stored with fresh and interesting facts and observations gathered during the long interval.

In the evening the members of the Odonto-Chirurgical Society dined in the Balmoral Hotel—Dr. Smith in the chair, and Mr. A. A. De Lessert acting as croupier. There were thirty-three present.

EXTRACTS.

THE PRIMITIVE TYPES OF MAMMALIAN MOLARS.

So much light has recently been thrown on the origin and mutual relations of the Mammalia by the labours of the Transatlantic palæontologists, that in the case of the limbs we have long since been able to trace the evolution of the specialized foot of the horse from that of the five-toed *Phenacodus* (see *Nature*, vol. xl. p. 57). Till quite lately, however, we have been unable to follow the mode of evolution of the more complicated forms of molar teeth from a common generalized type, although Professor Cope, by his description of the so-called 'trituhercular" type of molar structure, paved the way for the true history of this line of research.

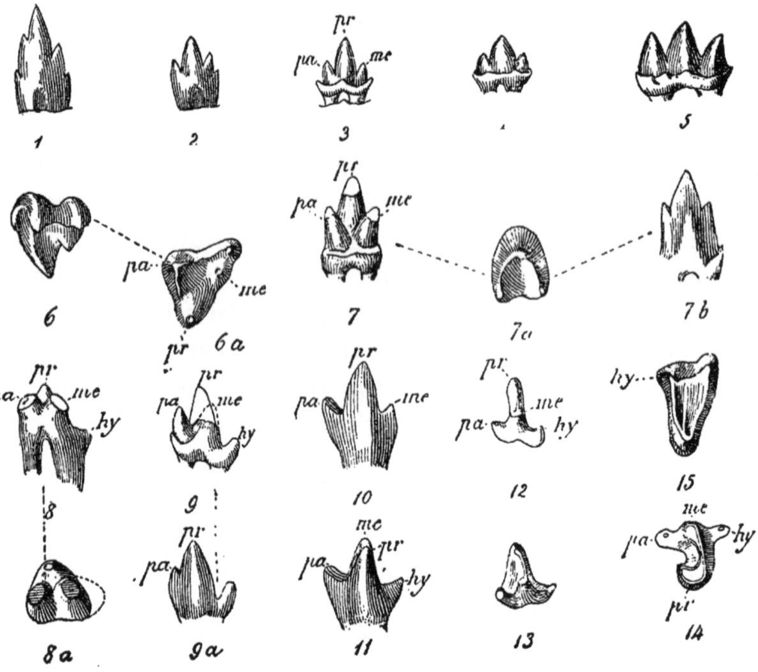

FIG. A.

FIG. A.—Types of Molar Teeth of Mesozoic Mammals. 1—5, Triconodont Type (1, *Dromatherium* ; 2, *Microconodon* ; 3, *Amphilestes* ; 4, *Phascolotherium* ; 5, *Triconodon*). 6, 7, 10, Tritubercular Type (6, *Peralestes* ; 7, *Spalacotherium* ; 10, *Asthenodon*). 8—9, 11—15, Tuberculo-Sectorial Type (8, *Amphitherium* ; 9, *Peramus* ; 11, *Dryolestes* ; 12, 13, *Amblotherium* ; 14, *Achyrodon* ; 15, *Kurtodon*. 6 and 15 are upper, and the remainder lower molars. *pa*, paraconid ; *pr*, protoconid ; *me*, metaconid ; *hy*, hypoconid. In the upper teeth the termination ends in cone.

The common occurrence of this tritubercular type of dentition among the mammals of the Lower Eocene at once suggests that we have to do with a very generalized form of tooth-structure ; and by a long series of observations Professor H. F. Osborn, of Princeton, New Jersey, has succeeded, to a great extent, in showing how the more complicated modifications of molars may have been evolved from this generalized type. These observations are of so much importance towards a right understanding of the phylogenetic relationships of the Mammalia that a short summary cannot fail to be interesting to all students of this branch of zoology.

The tritubercular molar (Fig. A, 6), consists of three cusps, cones, or tubercles, arranged in a triangle, and so disposed that those of the upper jaw alternate with those of the lower. Thus, in the upper teeth (Fig. A, 7), there are two cusps on the outer side, and one cusp on the inner side of the crown ; while in the lower teeth (Fig. A, 8, 8*a*) we have one outer and two inner cusps. This type, when attained, appears to have formed a starting-point from which the greater number of the more specialized types have been evolved. The Monotremes, the Edentates, perhaps the Cetaceans, and the extinct group of Multituberculata (*Plagiaulax* and its allies), must, however, be expected from the groups whose teeth have a tritubercular origin.

It appears probable, indeed, that "trituberculism," as this type of tooth-structure may be conveniently termed, was developed from a simple cone-like tooth during the Mesozoic period, and that in the Jurassic period it had developed into what is termed the primitive sectorial type (Fig. A, 9). The stages of the development of "trituberculism" may, according to Professor Osborn, be characterized as follows :—

(1) The *Haplodont* type.—This is a hypothetical type at present undiscovered, in which the crown of the tooth forms a simple cone, while the root is probably in most cases single, and not differentiated from the crown.

(*a*) The *Protodont* sub-type.—This sub-type is a slight advance on the preceding, and is represented by the American Triassic genus *Dromatherium*. The crown of the tooth (Fig. A, 1) has one main cone, with fore-and-aft accessory cusps, and the root is grooved.

(2) The *Triconodont* type.—In this Jurassic type the crown (Fig. A, 4, 5) is elongated, with one central cone, and a smaller

Q 2

anterior and posterior cone situated in the same line ; the roots being differentiated into double fangs. *Triconodon*, of the English Purbeck, is the typical example.

(3) The *Tritubercular* type.—In this modification the crown is triangular (Fig. A, 7), and carries three main cusps or cones, of which the central one is placed internally in the upper teeth (Fig. A, 6), and externally in the lower molars (Fig. A, 7). The teeth of the Jurassic *Spalacotherium* are typical examples. In the first and second types the molars are alike in both the upper and lower jaws ; but in the third or tritubercular type, the pattern is the same in the teeth of both jaws, but with the arrangement of the homologous cusps reversed. These features are exhibited in Fig. B.

These three types are regarded as primitive, but in the following sub-types we have additional cusps grafted on to the primitive tritubercular triangle, as it is convenient to term the three original cusps.

(a) Tuberculo-sectorial sub type.—This modification of the tritubercular type is found in the lower molars, like those of *Didelphys*. Typically the primitive tritubercular triangle is elevated, and the three cusps are connected by cross ridges, while a low posterior talon or heel is added (Fig. A, 9). This modification embraces a quinquetubercular form, in which the talon carries an inner and an outer cusp ; while by the suppression of one of the primitive cusps we arrive at the quadritubercular tooth, bunodont tooth (Fig. C), like that of the pigs. In the upper molars the primitive triangle in what is termed the secodont series may remain purely tricuspid. But by the development of intermediate tubercles in both the secodont and bunodont series a quinquetubercular form is reached ; while the addition of a postero-internal cusp in the bunodont series gives us the sextubercular molar.

There is no doubt as to the homology of the three primary cusps in the upper and lower molars ; and Professor Osborn proposes the following series of terms for all the cusps above mentioned. The first secondary cusps (hypocone and hypoconid) respectively added to the upper and lower molars are also evidently homologous, and modify the crown from a triangular to a quadrangular form ; but there is no homology between the additional secondary cusps of the upper molars termed protoconule and metaconule with the one termed ectoconid in the lower molars.

Terms applied to the cusps of molars :—

UPPER MOLARS.

Antero-internal cusp	= Protocone	—pr.
Postero- ,, ,, or 6th cusp	= Hypocone	—hy.
Antero-external ,, ...	= Paracone	—pa.
Postero- ,, ,, ...	= Metacone	—me.
Anterior intermediate cusp ...	= Protoconule*	—ml.
Posterior ,, ,, ...	= Metaconule	—pl.

LOWER MOLARS.

Antero-external cusp	= Protoconid	—$pr^{d.}$
Postero- ,, ,, ...	= Hypoconid	—$hy^{d.}$
Antero-internal or 5th cusp ...	= Paraconid	—$pa^{d.}$
Intermediate, or antero-internal cusp (in quadritubercular molars)	= Metaconid	—$me^{d.}$
Postero-internal cusp	= Entoconid	—$en^{d.}$

Having thus worked out the homology and relations of the tooth cusps, Professor Osborn gives some interesting observations on the principles governing the development of these cusps. It is considered that in the earliest Mammalian, or sub-mammalian, type of dentition (Haplodont), the simple cones of the upper and lower

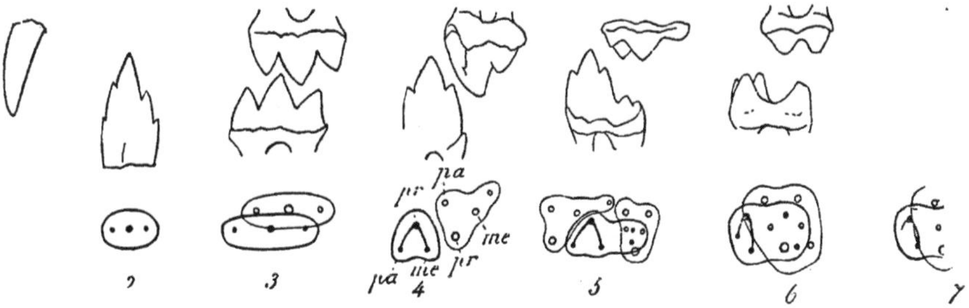

FIG B.

FIG. B.—Upper and Lower Molars in mutual apposition. 1, *Delphinus;* 2, *Dromatherium;* 3, *Triconodon;* 4, *Peralestes* and *Spalacotherium:* 5, *Didymictis;* 6, *Mioclænus;* 7, *Hyopsodus.* Letters as in preceding figure.

jaws interlocked with one another, as in the modern Dolphins (Fig. B, 1). The first additions to the primitive protoconid appeared upon its anterior and posterior borders, and the growth of the para- and metaconids involved the necessity of the upper teeth biting on the outer side of the lower (Fig. B, 2), this condition being termed anisognathism, in contrast to the isognathism of the

* The symbols *ml.* and *pl.* should properly apply respectively to the metaconule and protoconule, but since they bear the opposite signification in Fig. C, they are placed as above.

simple inter-locking cones. In the typical tritubercular type (Fig. A, 7) it has been suggested that the para- and metaconids were rotated inwards from the anterior and posterior borders of the triconodont type; but it is quite possible that they may have been

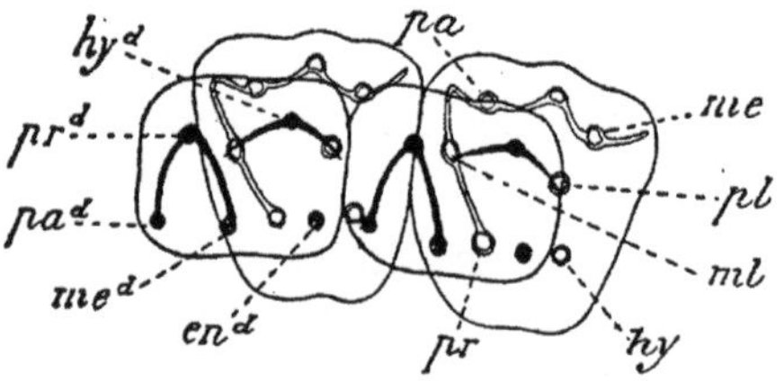

FIG C.

FIG. C.—Diagram of two upper and lower quadritubercular molars in apposition. The cusps and ridges of the upper molars are in double lines, and those of the lower ones in black. The letters refer to the table given above. The lower molars are looked at from below, as if transparent.

originally developed in their present position. By the alternation of the primitive triangle in the upper and lower jaws of the tritubercular type, the retention of an isognathous arrangement is permitted, the upper and lower teeth biting directly against one another.

Finally, Fig. C shows the mutual relations of the upper and lower teeth of the complicated quadritubercular molars, with the positions held by the primitive tritubercular triangles.—*Nature.*

DEMONSTRATION OF HYPNOTISM AS AN ANÆSTHETIC DURING THE PERFORMANCE OF DENTAL AND SURGICAL OPERATIONS.

A number of the leading medical men and dentists of Leeds and district were brought together on March 28th through the kind invitation issued by Messrs. Carter Brothers and Turner, dental surgeons, of Park-square, Leeds, to witness a series of surgical and dental operations performed in their rooms under the hypnotic influence induced by Dr. Milne Bramwell, of Goole, Yorkshire. Great interest was evinced in the meeting, as it is well known that Dr. Bramwell is quite a master of the art of hypnotism as applied to medicine and surgery, and is shortly to publish a work of considerable importance on the subject. Upwards of sixty medical men and dental surgeons accepted the invitation. Amongst the gentlemen present were the following:—Mr. Thomas Scattergood, Professor Wardrop Griffith, Mr. Pridgin Teale, Professor Eddison, Dr. Jacob, Dr. Churton, Mr. Mayo Robson, Mr. H. Bendelack Hewetson, Mr. Henderson Nicol, Mr. Moynihan, Mr. Littlewood, Mr. Henry Gott, Mr. Churton, Mr. Edmund Robinson,

Mr. William Hall, Dr. Braithwaite, Mr. Best, Mr. Wood, Dr. Light, Dr. Trevellyan, Dr. Caddy, Professor McGill, Dr. Turner (Menston Asylum), Dr. Hartley, Dr. Hellier, Mr. W. H. Brown, Dr. Bruce, (Goole), Mr. Dennison, Mr. Edward Ward, Mr. H. Robson, Mr. King, Mr. Glaisby, Mr. Sherburn, and Mr. Wayles. A letter expressing regret at his inability to be present was read from Dr. Clifford Allbutt, in which he reminded the meeting that he remembered the time—thirty-five years ago—when Lister performed several serious operations, using hypnotism as the anæsthetic, at the hands of a scientific lay friend in Lincolnshire. Mr. Jessop was also prevented at the last moment from being present. The object of the meeting was to show the power of hypnotism to produce absolute anæsthesia in very painful and severe operations.

The first case brought into the room was a woman of twenty-five. She was hypnotised at a word by Dr. Bramwell, and told she was to submit to three teeth being extracted without pain at the hands of Mr. T. Carter, and further that she was to do anything that Mr. Carter asked her to do (such as to open her mouth and spit out, and the like) as he required her. This was perfectly successful. There was no expression of pain in the face, no cry, and when told to awake she said she had not the least pain in the gums, nor had she felt the operation. Dr. Bramwell then hypnotised her, and ordered her to leave the room and go upstairs to the waiting room. This she did as a complete somnambulist.

The next case was that of a servant girl, aged nineteen, on whom, under the hypnotic influence induced by Dr. Bramwell, a large lacrimal abscess extending into the cheek had a fortnight previously been opened and scraped freely, without knowledge or pain. Furthermore, the dressing had been daily performed and the cavity freely syringed out under hypnotic anæsthesia, the "Healing Suggestions" being daily given to the patient, to which Dr. Bramwell in a great measure attributes the very rapid healing, which took place in ten days—a remarkably short space of time in a girl affected by inherited syphilis, and in a by no means good state of health. She was put to sleep by the following letter from Dr. Bramwell addressed to Mr. Turner, the operating dentist in the case.

[COPY]

"Burlington-crescent, Goole. Yorks.

"Dear Mr. Turner,—I send you a patient with enclosed order. When you give it her, she will fall asleep at once and obey your commands.

"(Signed) "J. MILNE BRAMWELL."

[COPY]

"Go to sleep by order of Dr. Bramwell, and obey Mr. Turner's command.

" J. MILNE BRAMWELL."

This experiment answered perfectly. Sleep was induced at once by reading the note, and was so profound that at the end of a lengthy operation, in which sixteen stumps were removed, she awoke smiling, and insisted that she had felt no pain ; and, what was remarkable, there was no pain in her mouth. She was found after some time, when unobserved, reading the *Graphic* in the waiting-room as if nothing had happened. During the whole time she did everything which Mr. Turner suggested, but it was observed that there was a diminished flow of saliva, and that the corneal reflexes were absent ; the breathing was more noisy than ordinary, and the pulse slower. Dr. Bramwell took occasion to explain that the next case, a boy of eight, was a severe test, and would not probably succeed ; partly because the patient was so young, and chiefly because he had not attempted to produce hypnotic anæsthesia earlier than two days before. He also explained that patients require training in this form of anæsthesia, the time of training or preparation varying with each individual. However, he was so far hypnotised that he allowed Mr. Mayo Robson to operate on the great toe, removing a bony growth and part of the first phalanx with no more than a few cries towards the close of the operation, and with the result that when questioned afterwards he appeared to know very little of what had been done. It was necessary in his case for Dr. Bramwell to repeat the hypnotic suggestions. Dr. Bramwell remarked that he wished to show a case that was less likely to be perfectly successful than the others, so as to enable those present to see the difficult as well as the apparently easy, straightforward cases.

The next case was a girl of 15, highly sensitive, requiring the removal of enlarged tonsils. At the request of Dr. Bramwell, Mr. Bendelack Hewetson was enabled, whilst the patient was in the hypnotic state, to extract each tonsil with ease, the girl, by suggestion of the hypnotiser, obeying every request of the operator, though in a state of perfect anæsthesia. In the same way Mr. Hewetson removed a cyst of the size of a horse-bean from the side of the nose of a young woman who was perfectly anæsthetic, breathing deeply, and who, on coming round by order, protested "that the operation had not been commenced."

Mr. Turner then extracted two large molar teeth from a man

with equal success, after which Dr. Bramwell explained how his patient had been completely cured of drunkenness by hypnotic suggestion. To prove this to those present, and to show the interesting psychological results, the man was hypnotised, and in that state he was shown a glass of water, which he was told by Dr. Bramwell was "bad beer." He was then told to awake, and the glass of water (so-called bad beer) was offered him by Dr. Bramwell. He put it to his lips, and at once spat out the "offensive liquid." Other interesting phenomena were illustrated and explained by means of this patient, who was a hale, strong working man.

Mr. Tom Carter next extracted a very difficult impacted stump from a railway navvy as successfully as the previous case. Dr. Bramwell described how this man had been completely cured of very obstinate facial neuralgia by hypnotism. The malady had been produced by working in a wet cutting, and had previously defied all medical treatment. On the third day of hypnotism the neuralgia had entirely disappeared (weeks ago,) and had not returned. The man had obtained, also, refreshing hypnotic sleep at night, being put to sleep by his daughter through a note from Dr. Bramwell, and on one occasion by a telegram, both methods succeeding perfectly.

At the conclusion of this most interesting and successful series of hypnotic experiments a vote of thanks to Dr. Bramwell for his kindness in giving the demonstration was proposed by Mr. Scattergood, Dean of the Yorkshire College, and seconded by Mr. Pridgin Teale, F.R.S., who remarked "that the experiments were deeply interesting, and had been marvellously successful," and said, "I feel sure that the time has now come when we shall have to recognise hypnotism as a necessary part of our study." The vote was carried by loud acclamations.

Messrs. Carter Brothers & Turner were cordially thanked for the great scientific treat which they had so kindly prepared for the many to whom hypnotism had been first introduced that day, and for the further opportunity afforded to the few who had seen Dr. Bramwell's work previously of studying its application as an anæsthetic. Mr. Henry Carter replied for the firm, and the meeting closed, the patients looking as little like patients as persons well could, giving neither by their manners or expression the slightest suggestion (except when external dressings were visible) that they had suffered or were suffering from, in some instances, extensive surgical interference.—*The Lancet.*

THE DENTAL RECORD, LONDON: MAY 1, 1890.

The Hypnotic State as a Workable Anæsthesia.

WE publish in another column some very interesting experiments performed in the house of Mr. Carter, of Leeds. Dr. Bramwell proposed to hypnotise several patients, and Mr. Carter tested the accuracy of the statement that the hypnotised were quite "anæsthetic" by extracting divers and sundry teeth. The suggestion is of course by no means new. Friedrich Anton Mesmer, who died in 1815, established a hospital in Vienna soon after the publication of his famous "Letter to a Foreign Physican on Magnetism," hypnotised for major as well as minor operations both in Vienna and subsequently in Paris. Esdaile, on April 4th, 1845, commenced in India a long series of operations, employing hypnotism as a means of destroying pain. Braid, of Manchester, and Elliotson, of London, had even before this asserted vigorously that although Mesmer was an unprincipled charlatan, and his so-called "secret" was all fudge, yet "mesmerism," or as Braid preferred to call it, "hypnotism," was a reality, and its powers for good far more widespreading than had been supposed. Within the last fifty years an enormous amount of evidence has been accumulated respecting hypnotism and the treatment of disease by suggestion, the result of which has been to dethrone the impostor's claim of a special magnetic power, and to bring these kindred subjects within the pale of scientific research and applicability. But it would be misleading to assert that that portion of the physiology of the brain which includes hypnotism, suggestion curing, auto-suggestion, and so on, is at present made light, or is explicable by any known principles. We understand some of the points which were dark, and recognise as fraud and chicane much which our forefathers accepted as diablerie, but when we come to explanations of the why and the wherefore, we must admit ignorance. Braid, as is well known, failed to perceive "unconscious suggestion." We now know that a posture, a word, will suggest to a "subject" actions which the hypnotiser desires him to execute. Braid taught phreno-hypnotism, asserting that pressure over the phrenologists "bump" of theft would produce mendacity in the subject, who would straightway acquire his neighbour's silver snuff-box. Pressure, we may be permitted almost to say, *counter pressure*, upon the bump of conscientiousness would, taught Braid, impel the penitent subject to return his neighbour's property and unveil his illicit appropriativeness. Coming into vogue in the "forties" hypnotism was soon distanced in the race for popular favour as an anæsthetic by ether (1846), and chloroform (1847), and nitrous oxide, which although introduced twenty years before, did not gain credence in London until 1868. None of the many workers in the field of neurypnology have doubted the feasibility of obtaining anæthesia by hypnotism or "suggestion," but most have been strongly impressed by the undesirability of its employment. The terrible power which may be exerted on those who can be made "subjects," and the almost absolute control which the hypnotiser, willy nilly, acquires over his patients, place both the hypnotiser and the hypnotised in positions the very reverse of healthy. Unconscious suggestion like auto-suggestion, will in some cases become dangerous as well as inconvenient. A well-known experimenter accustomed himself to auto-suggestion, *i.e.*, he used to render himself in a condition of hypnotism by fixation of his attention upon some object. However, after a time, he found that the smallest effort of attention, such as inditing a letter or signing his name, sent him off with his suggestion to sleep—a state of things subversive to his using his wits for the every day duties of life. In Esdaile's patients three weeks of preparation before the operation were often necessary before sufficient control could be exerted over the subjects, and as a rule many efforts at hypnotism have to be undertaken before an assured result can be predicted. These two drawbacks have kept hypnotism in the background as an anæsthetic, and there is little doubt that its use is attended with no slight moral danger.

PRESENTATION TO MR. FELIX WEISS, PRESIDENT OF THE ODONTOLOGICAL SOCIETY OF GREAT BRITAIN.—On Tuesday, the 22nd of April, at the residence of Mr. C. V. Cotterell, a presentation took place of a massive Silver Inkstand, bearing the following inscription:—

> "Presented to Felix Weiss, Esq., as a token of esteem and regard by past and present pupils on his being elected President of the Odontological Society, 1890."

All those who are numbered within the wide circle of Mr. Weiss's friends and admirers, will sympathise with the wish of his past pupils, to seize the present fitting occasion for giving honour where honour is due.

PRE-VICTORIAN SOVEREIGNS.—The time honoured custom of wrapping up the "filthy lucre" in a neat piece of paper before placing it in the receptive palm of the dentist or doctor, has we understand received quite a fillip since the banks have charged 6d. for exchanging pre-Victorian sovereigns. Those who never wrapped fees in paper, now do so invariably and do not scruple to use old coins. The moral of which is examine your fee before your patient departs, if, that is, you think you have the courage to refuse the coin.

OWING to pressure upon our space, we are compelled to postpone a number of letters and some Society proceedings until our next issue (June 1st.)

OBITUARY.

Mr. ALFRED HILL, L.D.S.Eng.

It is with sincere regret that we have to announce the death of Mr. Alfred Hill, of Henrietta Street, Cavendish Square, who although only in his 63rd year was fairly considered one of the veteran practitioners of Dental Surgery in London, he having been actively engaged in professional work for nearly 40 years. His name is intimately associated with the great Dental Reform movement as far back as the year 1856.

Until within a week of his death, Mr. Hill had been able to attend to his practice, but symptoms of an alarming character suddenly manifested themselves, indicating intestinal obstruction. The highest medical advice was obtained, but in spite of all care and treatment he succumbed on the 18th of April, after much suffering, at his residence at Ealing.

In the early days of the Reform movement Mr. Hill held an official position in the College of Dentists, indeed, at the famous meeting of Dental Practitioners, held in London in the autumn of 1856, he was elected in conjunction with Mr. Rymer, Honorary Secretary, and worked strenuously on behalf of that institution until its ultimate amalgamation with the Odontological Society. Here, again, his energies were called into requisition, and after the formation of the Dental Hospital of London, he for many years discharged the onerous duties of Honorary Secretary, both to the Managing and Medical Committees of that Institution. As Dental Surgeon to the Hospital, and as a teacher, Mr. Hill was deservedly popular. For 25 years his connection with the Hospital remained unbroken, and when his retirement from the staff took place it was amidst the universal regrets both of his colleagues and the students.

In 1877 appeared his book entitled "The History of the Reform Movement of the Dental Profession in Great Britain," a treatise of infinite value, as an authentic record of the early work and workers in the cause of Dental progress. This volume is too well known and appreciated to need further comment at this time.

Mr. Hill possessed many talents, notably among these were his great facility with pen and pencil, the former he used ungrudgingly in the cause of the advancement of the profession.

A man of marked rectitude and geniality he gained for himself many friends, and his life of uprightness and untiring industry affords an example not easily paralleled in the annals of the profession of which he was so distinguished and honored a member.

GOSSIP.

NATIONAL DENTAL HOSPITAL.—The last Smoking Concert of the season took place on Thursday, March 27th, at the Portman Rooms, Baker Street, W., under the genial chairmanship of the Dean of the School. About 160 were present, amongst whom were Drs. Hill and Waller of St. Mary's, Mr. W. H. Ash, and nearly every member of the Staff.

The programme, which included nearly every variety of entertainment, was received with hearty applause, particularly the contributions of Messrs. Genet (recitation), A. and H. Kelvey (banjoists), McLean (musical sketch), Pearce (legerdemain), Prager (impersonation), Bluff, Joyner, May, and Alfred Smith. The chairman took the opportunity to announce the generous offer of Messrs. Ash & Son to award an annual money prize of £3 3s. to the Students of the College for a paper on Dental Surgery, the competition to take place during the Winter Session.

INTERNATIONAL MEDICAL CONGRESS, 1890.—A short time since, in compliance with a request by the officers of the Berlin Congress, a committee was formed in London for the purpose of making known as widely as possible in England the object and arrangements of the Congress. On this Committee the following gentlemen have consented to act:—Sir James Paget, President of the London Congress; Sir Andrew Clark, President of the Royal College of Physicians; Mr. Jonathan Hutchinson, President of the Royal College of Surgeons; Mr. Bryant, Vice-President of the Royal College of Surgeons; Sir Edward Sieveking, late President of the Royal Medical and Chirurgical Society; Dr. Dickinson, President of the Pathological Society; Dr. Theodore Williams, late President of the Medical Society; Dr. Wade, President-Elect of the British Medical Association; Sir Joseph Lister, Dr. F. Semon, Sir William MacCormac, and Mr. Makins, under secretary to the London Congress. The committee met at the house of Sir James Paget and agreed to, as far as possible, further the success of the meeting by diffusing information regarding the business to be transacted. Mr. Makins (2, Queen Street, Mayfair, W.) was appointed secretary, and he will furnish on the part of the committee such details as may be arranged, to any members of the profession who may apply for them. It may interest intending visitors to Berlin in August to know that Messrs. Thomas Cook of Ludgate-circus, have very kindly undertaken to give every possible information and assistance. The most convenient routes are *viâ* Queenborough and Flushing, by which Berlin is reached under twenty-four hours.

	1st Class, single.	1st Class, return.	2nd Class, single.	2nd Class, return.
At a cost of	£5 2 11 ...	£7 14 6 ...	£3 14 11 ...	£5 12 4
Dover and Calais	£5 19 6 ...	£9 14 0 ...	£4 8 0 ...	£7 6 0
Ostend	£5 8 0 ...	£8 13 3 ...	£3 19 6 ...	£2 6 9

Viâ Dover and Calais takes 33½ hours.

For those who like a longer sea voyage and shorter rail, Berlin may be reached *viâ* Southampton and Bremen or Hamburg in one of the Great North American liners. From Hamburg to Berlin is five hours' railway journey, and to Hamburg *viâ* Southampton about twenty-four hours. The steamship *Augusta Victoria*, 8,000 tons and 12,500 horse-power, will probably leave Southampton for Hamburg on Thursday, July 31st. She is a fine new steamer in the Transatlantic service between Hamburg and New York.

DEATH AFTER THE INHALATION OF BROMIDE OF ETHYL.—A somewhat important case (says the *Lancet*) is now before the Berlin courts, in which a dentist is charged with having caused the death of a patient by means of an anæsthetic. The patient was a lady, and the dentist entrusted his pupil, whose age was under seventeen, with the administration of bromide of ethyl. Of this about an ounce was administered, together with four or five drops of chloroform. The patient is stated to have recovered completely from the effects of the anæsthetic, and to have felt quite well during the remainder of the day. The next day, however, she died, and a commission of medical experts has been directed to report upon the matter.

A USEFUL HINT.—*To mix Vaseline and Water.*—Vaseline and water may be mixed by the addition of two drops of castor oil to each gramme of the liquid. By this means iodide of potassium may be introduced into an unguent without danger of decomposition.

NOTICE TO CORRESPONDENTS.

Correction.—By an oversight in the Answers to Correspondents in our last issue, we are made to say that the American degrees, which under certain circumstances are registrable here, are D.M.D. Harvard and D.D S. Chicago, it should read, "D.M.D. Harvard and D.D.S. Michigan." The Chicago degree is not registrable here.

ANSWERS TO CORRESPONDENTS.

Mr. J. Gillespie.—A student proposing to take the L.D.S. receives no special examination in the subjects you mention. He is liable to be asked questions on them. The certificate of a competent teacher in Chemistry, and from a medical man or pharmaceutical chemist in pharmacy and *materia medica*, is all which is required. If he proposes taking the conjoint Board's diplomas he will be examined specially in these subjects.

LIVERPOOL DENTAL HOSPITAL.

The number of patients treated during the month of March was 2,245—Males, 1,109; Females, 1,136. Gold Fillings, 41; Plastic Fillings, 106; Extractions, 1,922; Under Anæsthetics, 80; Miscellaneous Cases and Advice, 152; Total, 2,301.—H. Fielden Briggs, D.D.S. and C. B. Dopson, L.D.S., *House Surgeons.*

Monthly Statement of operations performed at the two Dental Hospitals in London, and at the Dental Hospital, Manchester, from February 28th to March 31st, 1890:—

	London.	National	Victoria.
Number of Patients attended	——	2864	1092
Extractions: Children under 14 ...	451	367	660 (Children and Adults)
Extractions: Adults	959	609	
Extractions: Under Nitrous Oxide ...	776	601	133
Gold Stoppings	444	112	34
Other Stoppings...	1689	684	257
Irregularities of the Teeth	102	195	—
Artificial Crowns	38	—	—
Miscellaneous and Dressings	333	516	322
Total	4,792	3,084	1,406

THE DENTAL RECORD.

VOL. X. JUNE 2ND, 1890. No. 6.

Original Communications.

A VERY LARGE ODONTOME FROM THE HUMAN SUBJECT.

By J. BLAND SUTTON, F.R.C.S.

Assistant-Surgeon Middlesex Hospital.

IN this Journal (January, 1889) I drew attention to two large tumours which had been removed from the antrum, one in India the other in France, and described as exostoses. From a critical examination of the records and figures illustrating the microscopical characters of these supposed exostoses, I had no difficulty in coming to the conclusion that they were odontomes and the two largest examples of this form of tumour known to have occurred in the human subject. Further inquiry in this direction has induced me to bring under notice an additional specimen which has been previously known as an exostosis, but in reality it is an odontome and by far the largest example ever known to have grown in the human antrum; it has moreover an extraordinary clinical history.

The details of the case are recorded in *Guy's Hospital Reports*, vol. 1, 1836, by Hilton. The patient, a man aged 36 years, had a large osseous tumour occupying the antrum. The pressure of this tumour had caused the front wall of the antrum with the integument and soft tissues covering it to slough. The trouble was first noticed thirteen years before; as the cheek enlarged the eyeball became displaced and finally burst. For a long time the surface of the tumour was exposed, the suppuration being copious, and occasionally pieces of bone irregular in shape came away: at last to the man's astonishment the bony mass dropped out leaving an enormous hole in his face. The general appearance of this tumour may be inferred from the accompanying sketch in which it is shown of natural size. It weighed nearly fifteen ounces and measures eleven inches in its greatest circumference. The tumour which is remarkably hard, presents on section an ivory-like surface and on close scrutiny a number of closely arranged concentric laminæ. Sections ground thin and examined under the microscope show large numbers of lacunæ and canaliculi arranged in a very regular

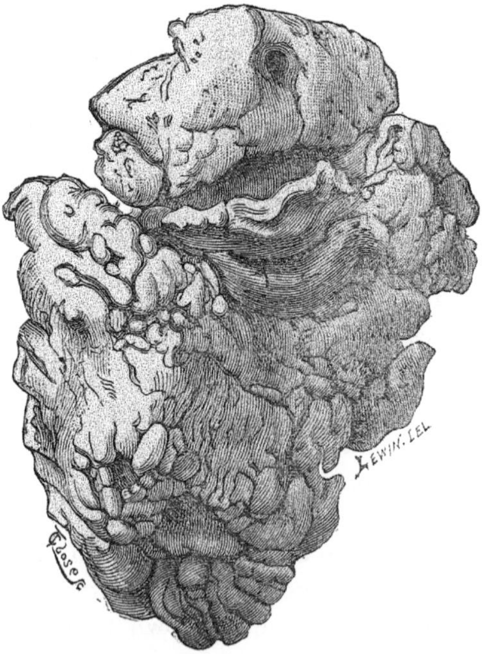

FIG. 1. A large odontome which was spontaneously shed from the antrum; weight nearly 15 ounces—Hilton's case. (From the Museum of Guy's Hospital.)

manner. I could not detect dentine and it is impossible without mutilating the specimen to be sure that no teeth are embedded in it.

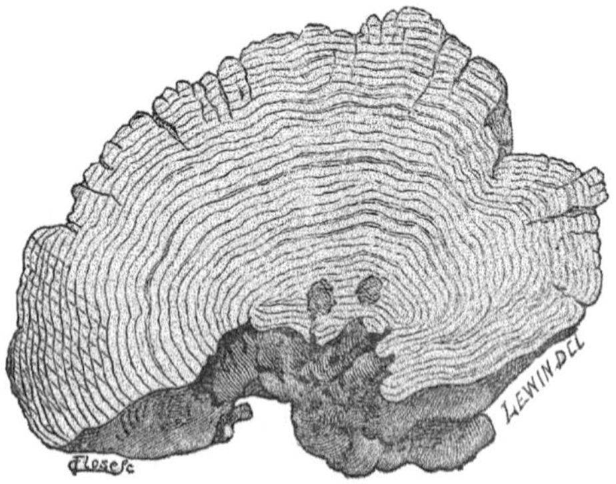

FIG. 2 A section of the tumour represented in Fig. 1 to show the concentric lamination.

As this tumour had no bony connections, occupied the antrum, and in the structure of its peripheral parts is so closely identical with odontomes which occur in horses, I have no hesitation in declaring that this particular tumour originated in one or more enlarged tooth-follicles, and is in fact an odontome. The chief reasons for this opinion are the following:—

On several occasions I have described in the *Transactions of the Odontological Society*, tumours in the maxillæ and mandible of goats, monkeys, marsupials, rickety lions and bears, composed of wavy lamellæ of fibrous tissue and bone, enclosing one or more teeth or denticles. In structure these soft tumours are identical with the follicle of a normal tooth, and as they arise from the

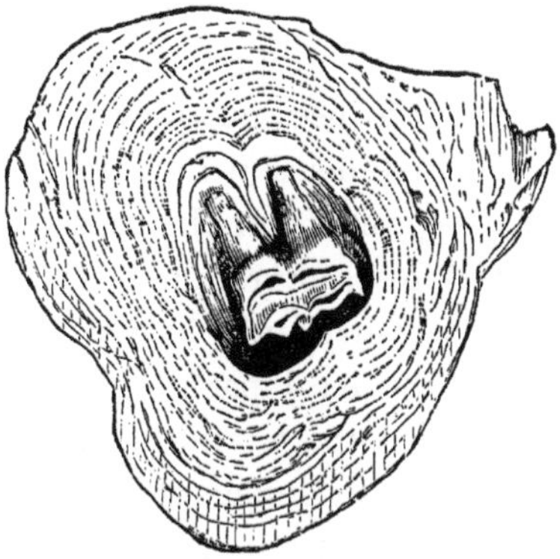

FIG. 3. A fibrous odontome from the antrum of a goat.

overgrowth of a tooth-follicle, I have ventured to call them fibrous odontomes, Fig 3. Similar tumours occur in the human jaws, and

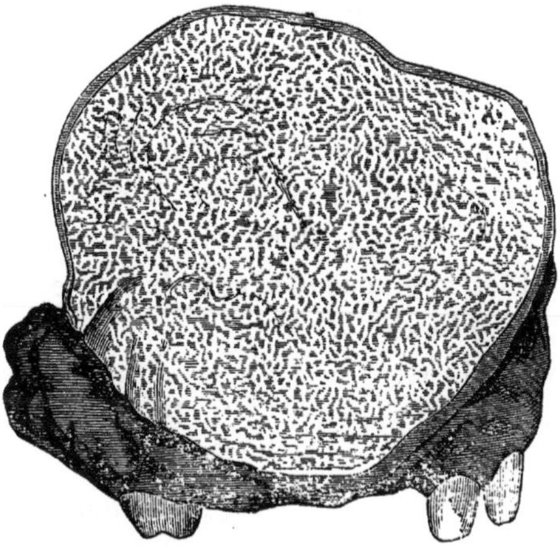

FIG 4. A fibrous odontome removed from the antrum of a boy aged 17 years. (Museum of St. Thomas's Hospital.)

they have been variously described as fibromata, osteo-fibromata and even myeloid sarcomata. For instance the Museum of St. Thomas's

Hospital contains a tumour of the upper jaw removed by Solly from a lad 17 years of age. It is described as an osteo-fibrous tumour. It is of rounded form, has a smooth external surface, and is attached to the roots of the first molar, canine and bicuspid teeth. Microscopically the tumour is composed of wavy fibrous tissue with tracts of calcareous matter interposed. The tumour was surrounded by a thin shell of true bone, Fig. 4. In some instances these fibrous masses ossify and the tooth or denticle becomes embedded in a mass of extremely hard bone. Ossification may commence at an early date and be continued by the periodontomal membrane depositing the bone in successive layers until a large mass is formed. This I believe to have happened in Hilton's case, and we may interpret the facts in this way:—A tooth retained and the follicle became thickened and subsequently ossified ; as the mass increased in size it invaded the antrum, growth continuing by successive deposits from the capsule. In time as the tumour invaded the nasal fossa, ulceration of the capsule and suppuration, as a consequence of irritation to which it would be liable would induce necrosis of the hard parts of the tumour as in the analogous case of eruption of a tooth, and finally lead to its eviction.

A study of this and similar specimens shows how unphilosophical it is to apply to all forms of hard tumours removed from the antrum the term exostosis.

It is significant that Virchow, in his classical work on "Tumours" mentioning this and similar cases, in discussing osteomata of the maxillæ, distinctly points out that they merit a new and more attentive examination.

A curious error has crept into text-books of Surgery and Surgical Pathology in consequence of the erroneous opinion held regarding the nature of some of these hard tumours from the antrum, to the effect that odontomes in man are limited to the lower jaw, I have therefore appended a table of the more important specimens, numbering in all

Lower Jaw.		Upper Jaw.	
Fergusson's	case	Hare's	case
Maisonneuve's	,,	Hilton's	,,
Salter's		Michon's	,,
Forget's		Duka's	,,
Heath's		Jordan Lloyd's	,,
Windle's	,		
Rushton Parker's	,,		

For a summary and figures of the above cases, compiled from several papers published in the *Transactions of the Odontological Society of Great Britain*, see *The Journal of Comp. Med. and Veterinary Archives* of New York, January 1890.

AN INAUGURAL ADDRESS.

By George Brunton.

President of the Midlands Branch of the British Dental Association.

Although dentistry as an art dated far back in the ages, as evidenced by the remains found in Egyptian and Etruscan tombs, dentistry as a science and art has only attained a recognised position in modern times. Dental literature proper dates from about 1536. A quarto volume was published at Frankfurt on "Zahnarzeney," without an author's name. In 1557, one De Castrillo, issued a book "Dentitione" at Valadolid. In Venice, one Bartholomaii Eustachius, published in 1563, a volume "Libellus de Dentibus," Monanvius, at Basle, in Switzerland, in 1578, Hamard Urbain at Lyons, France, in 1582, and Heurnius at Leyden, Holland, in 1605, also published works on Dentistry. The first Dental Pharmacopœia was published by Bunon of Paris in 1746, in the same year (also at Paris) "A Desertation on Artificial Teeth" by M. Mouton. John Hunter's great work, "Natural History of the Teeth," came out in 1771, and in 1778, his "Diseases of the Teeth." In the same year, at Edinburgh, S. H. Jackson published his "Physiology and Pathology of the Eruption of the Teeth"; in 1797, an 8vo volume was published by Dr. Chamant, in London, on "Artificial Teeth, Mineral Paste Teeth." J. R. Duval, a Frenchman, published in 1802, a volume "On the Accidents which happen during the Extraction of Teeth." Not, however, till 1820 do we find any work published on the mechanical art of dentistry. The first I find any mention of is "De l'art mechanique du Dentiste," in 2 vols., by C. T. De Labarre, Paris, I suppose, but am not quite sure where published. The first work published in England on the teeth bears the date 1687, but no author's name; it is a 4to volume entitled "Curious Observations on that part of Chirurgery Relating to the Teeth." The first work published in America "On the Human Teeth," by J. L. Skinner, New York, in 1801. About the same date an article was published in the *Medical Repository.*

Vol. I., No. 4, by Foot, "Why Defects of the Teeth are so frequent in America." Dentistry even formed the theme for a poet. We find Solyman Brown publishing a poem on "Dentologia" in 1833. Periodical dental literature however was first started in America by the publication of the *American Journal of Dental Science*, a monthly; England followed in 1843 with the *Quarterly Journal of Dental Science*, published in London, Germany in 1855, France in 1857, Italy in 1866, Spain in 1872, Denmark in 1873. But we have gone on too rapidly, let us hark back to the great English classical works, Hunter's "Natural History of the Teeth," 1771, and "Diseases of the Teeth," 1778. That worthy Scotchman, John Hunter, Surgeon-extraordinary to the king, and Fellow of the Royal Society, in whose works, still worthy of perusal, we find a clear statement of the knowledge of dental science and art in those days. If, as Mr. Gladstone said the other day, "Surgery began with John Hunter" they might, he (the President) thought, justly claim that dental surgery also began with him. The knowledge of the dentist was small in those days. His operations were limited to filling cavities in teeth without having first removed the decay, and they found the quack of to-day had got no further than that, with lead or gold foil. No attempt was made to shape the cavity, or even to dry it. If the filling would remain in the cavity, well and good; if not, the tooth was allowed to go on decaying, and was lost. The only effort recorded by Hunter to retain a filling by mechanical means was to be found in his "Treatise on the Diseases of the Teeth." In Hunter's day it seemed the ultimate skill of the dentist was in drilling a hole and putting a peg through the tooth and filling to keep the the two together. Extractions were mostly done with the key or the elevator. Examples of both instruments in all their hideous forms might be seen in their museums, and contemplating them they might try to realise the torture which patients in those days had to endure. Hunter said about extraction, "It generally happens in drawing a tooth that the alveolar process is broken, that they (the teeth) are naturally so fast as to require instruments and the most cautious and dexterous hand. It would be best of all to attempt the abstraction of a tooth by drawing it in the direction of its axis, but not being practicable by the instruments at present in use, which pull laterally, it is the next best to draw a tooth to that side where the alveolar process is the weakest, which is the inside in the two last grinders on each side of the lower jaw, and the outside in all the others." Was it any wonder that Duval found enough to fill a volume on the accidents which happen during the extraction of the teeth? or any wonder that a horror still lingered round the thought of submitting to "the most cautious and dexterous hand" for the extraction of a tooth? He need not tell those present that, instead of a fracture of the alveolar process generally happening, it was of rare occurrence with the well-trained dentist. Thanks to Sir John Tomes, Jean Evrard, and others, they had now instruments which enabled them to "pull a tooth in the direction of its axis," instruments which were adapted to fit each tooth so accurately, anatomically, that fracture of the alveolus was more the fault of the user than the consequence of the operation. In speaking of the decay of the teeth, Hunter said, "We have not, as yet, found any means of preventing this disease or of curing it." What wonderful progress had been made since Hunter's time! Through the microscope they had become acquainted with the minute anatomy of the teeth and associate parts; by their advance in mechanical skill, and the high development of the use of "the most cautious and dexterous hand," they were now able to cure the disease, not, however, in the way that surgeons cured disease, by removing the diseased portion, and allowing nature to do the rest, but by cutting out the diseased portion and substituting a foreign body, such as gold, amalgam, cement, gutta percha, &c., and restoring the form and functions of the tooth. The most cautious and dexterous hand had, along with education, been one of the most important means of raising dentistry to the high position which it had to-day attained. No machinery could be produced which will supersede, although it might help, the hand, in operative dentistry. Yes, they could cure the diseases of the teeth, and they had found out the causes which produced the diseases, but they were yet unable to prevent the diseases. True, some twenty years ago a clever American dentist thought he could do so, and claimed to prevent decay by anticipating it. His method was to file away the tooth so as to leave a space between them, but this method instead of preventing decay induced it, for the enamel (Nature's covering) being filed away, the fermentation of food, the acid secretions from the gums, and other causes, soon produced decay in the exposed dentine. Many practitioners in America, and some in other countries adopted this pernicious practice, the result of which led to much repentance. The pendulum had now swung over to the other side, and the conturist who followed Nature's teaching produced fillings which knuckle up to the adjoining tooth. Even cantilever fillings have been done (fanciful vagaries which bridge the space between the teeth). The science and art of dentistry had drawn so much from the collateral arts and sciences that a competent dentist might be expected to be well informed and somewhat practised in surgery and medicine, chemistry, physics, metallurgy, mechanics, electricity, &c. He was not infrequently called in by the physician or the surgeon, to find the cause for symptoms which puzzled him, and which symptoms he suspected to be in some way connected with the teeth. Affections of the palate, congenital and acquired, of the eye, nose, ear, tongue, throat, stomach, fractures of maxillæ, and many other troubles were often amenable to the treatment of the skilful dentist. The most perfect artificial restorations of parts of the face, lost by disease or operation, had been done, not by the instrument maker or the mechanician, but by the dexterous hand of the dentist. Their position, then, as useful members, of a profession depended not alone on a thorough knowledge of the subjects taught at school or college, but also on the thorough training and high development of touch of the cautious and dexterous hand. The training of the hand could never begin too soon. Boys who were educated with the intention of entering the medical or dental professions should have special attention paid to the training of the hand, but the training of one hand was not enough. Both hands should be well trained. How few operators there were who could extract teeth with the left hand as well as with the right, yet most practitioners would allow, the two-handed operator had the advantage. Having spoken of the importance of paying periodic attention to children's teeth, the president added that manual dexterity was first learnt by the dentist in the work-room, except in the case of those who had a natural gift. If a pupil was not after trial clever with his fingers, no matter how clever he might be with his head, he had better seek some calling which required more headwork than handwork. The dentist did a great variety of work with his hands, a larger range of work, perhaps, than any other craftsman or artist. Some startling facts were brought out when they went into statistics regarding the amount of precious metals used in connection with dental work. It was estimated, for instance, that at least 30,000 ounces of gold were used in filling teeth. They must add to that the gold used in constructing artificial dentures, the platina, paladium, silver, and other metals, the metallic oxides used in colouring teeth and gums. Miners, smelters, and goldbeaters were kept at work preparing metal for their use. In the United States alone there were 15,000 dentists in practice, this year 636 graduates received their diplomas, and 1,676 students matriculated. Germany and France had now their dental departments connected with their universities. In Berlin the Dental Institute was opened five years ago with five students. It had now 200. England, Scotland, Ireland, Russia, and Canada were all preparing students, and soon they would have to add Australia to the list. The dental profession in America, established originally as an independent profession, was now being affiliated with the medical profession, the standard of education was being raised, and a longer term of years was required at college. There was, however, a new trouble springing up in America. They have too many patents. Not only were instruments and tools patented, methods and processes were patented, companies were formed to work the patents, and the practitioner found himself hampered and taxed on all hands. The granting of patents had been a hindrance to the profession instead of a help, had introduced the trade spirit which sought to benefit itself at the expense of the other members of the profession, while on the other hand the professional spirit, like love, "seeketh not her own, is not puffed up, freely gives, because she has freely received." Dentistry should be just what the members of the profession choose to make it. If the trade spirit was allowed to predominate, it would become a mere money-making handicraft. What was the British Dental Association, and for what did it exist? The Diploma Committee after securing the granting of a diploma in dentistry by the Royal College of Surgeons, formed a large portion of the nucleus which grew into the British Dental Association in 1879. The objects of the association were first the administration of the Dental Act. There could be no question about its desire to do so. From the first hour of its existence it had had had that end in view, and had endeavoured to carry out the spirit of the Act, and to administer the letter of the law in such a way as to raise the status of the profession socially and politically, not only in the great metropolis, but in every town and village. It had more than once been a terror to evildoers, and would continue to be such as long as there were quacks who infringed the Act. The association held meetings for the reading and discussion of papers the discussion of subjects of interest to its members, the cultivation of a liberal spirit, and the dissemination of knowledge and information which might be of value to the practitioner. It published a monthly journal. The British Dental Associaton was at once conservative and liberal—conservative in the true sense, by protecting the public and the profession, as far as its means allowed, from the impositions of charlatanism. To the furtherance of this end, he would appeal to every registered practitioner to join their ranks, and by his consistent and liberal support to enable the association to put the machinery of the law in action against those who continued to degrade the profession by lying advertisements, show cases, patented processes, dental institutes, and other traps, to catch the unwary. It was liberal also in the true sense, by encouraging an interchange of knowledge and experience, by the reading and discussion of papers, the exhibition of modes of practice, the imprcvements or invention of instruments and tools, and the encouragement of that spirit of brotherhood which was the true bond of union. Looking back through the ten years of their existence they could not but come to the conclusion that the British Dental Association had to a large extent fulfilled the objects for which it was promoted, viz., the education not only of its members but also of the public.

SIMPLIFIED ORTHODONTIA BY ZIGZAG, SPRING, AND SHIELD, WITH SPECIAL REFERENCE TO ITS APPLICATION IN RECTIFYING THE FŒTAL ANGLE, V-SHAPED ARCH, AND CONTRACTED ALVEOLAR OR PALATINE PROCESSES OF THE MAXILLÆ.

By Frederick Sleep, L.D.S.

"Simplicity is a cardinal virtue in all matters of construction, and through lack of it about 75 per cent. of the patents granted in this country (U.S.A.) prove unprofitable."—Professor Guildford (*Orthodontia*).

Since Dr. Coffin introduced his simple method for expanding the alveolar arches, no department in dental science has received more attention from the thoughtful part of the profession than oral and dental deformity.

Yet, invaluable as the aforesaid method was in its application as contrasted with former treatment, its failure has been most significant in those very cases of malformation which have been perhaps a greater cause of perplexity than any other. I mean in the attempted

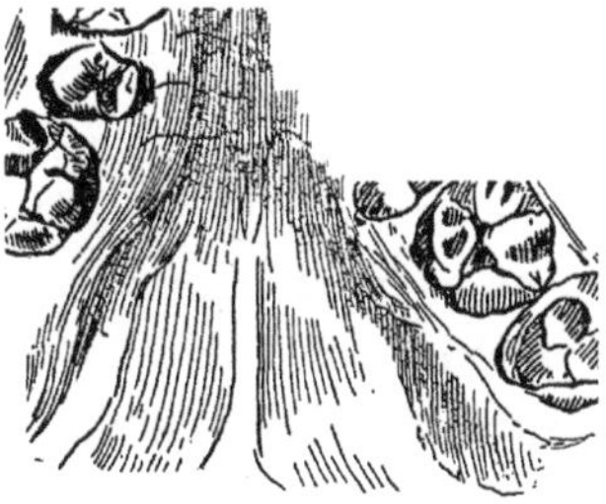

BEFORE TREATMENT.

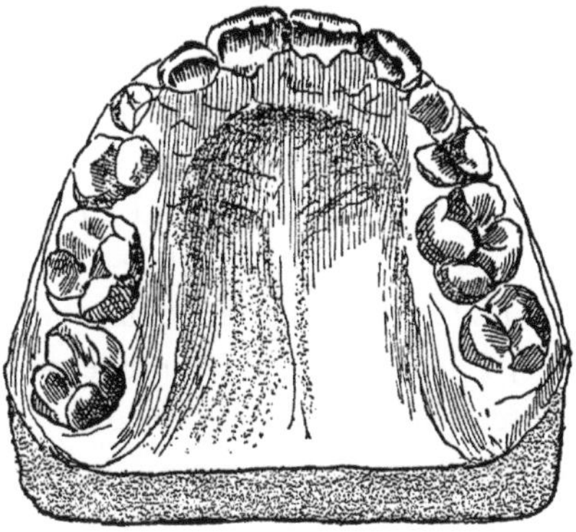

AFTER TREATMENT.

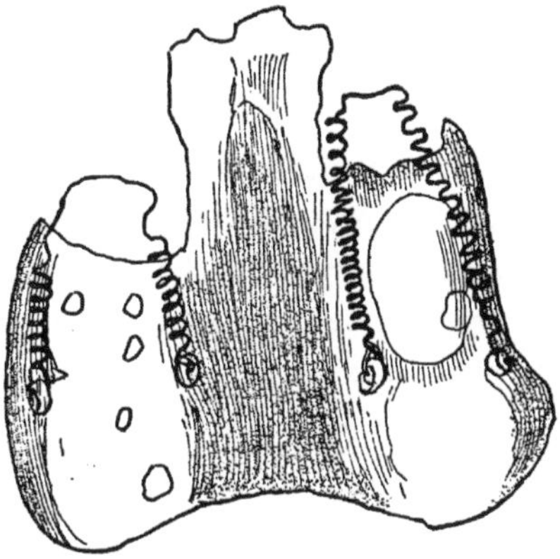

Nº 1.

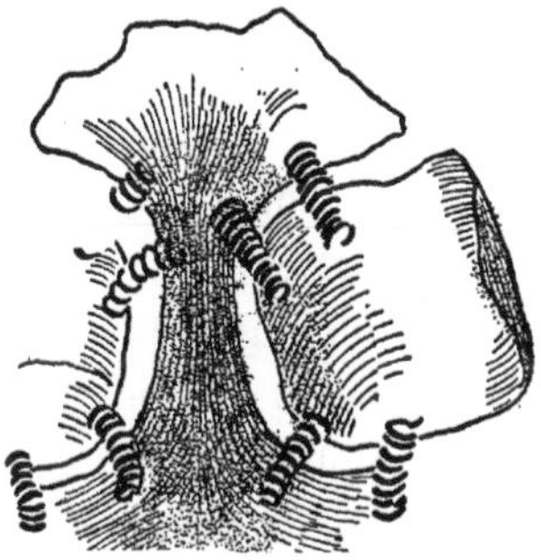

Nº 2.

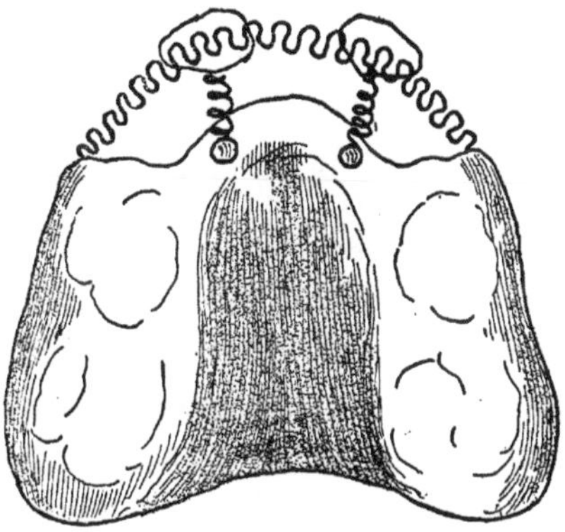

Nº 3.

obliteration of that abnormal angle which is found at the juncture of the added alveoli, which contain the true permanent molars, and that which terminates the position of the bicuspids and their antecedents, the milk grinders.

The theoretical ground that overlies the cause of this deformity has been and is the battle-field for our shrewdest intellects; but as the matter I am about to lay before the reader is a purely practical one, I leave theory, seductive and valuable as its pursuit proves, to those whose facilities for extensive observation make them better qualified for that obscure branch of the subject. We are all so much indebted to those who have paved the way to our successes, that I feel some qualms in indicating imperfection in their devices.

A liberal profession, however, is not supposed to be regulated by the laws of Media and of Persia, which allow neither criticism nor progress. To get a wider view, therefore, of the horizon, we must climb on the ample shoulders of our worthy predecessors and hope for and expect similar treatment ourselves.

Those whose practice has presented the special cases alluded to for treatment, must have observed to their mortification, that in expanding the central split plates of Coffin, we do but push apart bilaterally the angular abnormality we would obliterate, and often exert pressure on other parts already on the verge. Again, that by the tendency of the two parts of the plates to slide up the steep declivities of the sides on being pulled apart, there is an encouragement for the teeth and alveolar border to become "tipped" and so preclude further operation.

Moreover, the palate and teeth cannot be *modelled* by such an approach to the normal as we carry in our mind's eye. The split plates of Dr. Kingsley offer somewhat modified but similar objections, and the jack-screw traversing the palatine vault would inevitably rise the inborn impatience of the average British patient.

Dr. Talbot's spring, also, which is illustrated on page 129 of his recent work, is from its inclination to draw forward the posterior cornua in expanding to push outwards the last molar tooth already far enough on the border, and to decrease the room which may be otherwise gained between the bicuspids and antecedent teeth.

The case I shall take the liberty to illustrate in full, *ego*, without the usual "noster and nos," came under my notice about two years ago. The patient, a young lady, aged 14, daughter of a well-known merchant of the port of Plymouth. The case was undertaken somewhat languidly, for beside the aggravated deformity which precluded even my little finger touching the median line of the palate (*vide* plate 1), the young lady was eminently neurasthenic and like Niobe, all tears.

It was agreed it would be wisdom to precede and conjoin medical treatment with the transaction.

When, therefore, the patient reported herself fit and willing, Dr. Elliot Square, surgeon, called on me, and after a consultation, examination of the models and conversation on the prospects, the case was commenced.

Being at the moment too occupied for philosophic rumination, to gain time, I began routine practice with Dr. Coffin's plate, but seeing early the aforementioned defects, came to the conclusion that the case must be treated on other lines, or abandoned with less benefit than was desirable.

The superior maxilla, as the model indicates, protruded, making wide separation between the upper and lower incisors. So widely, indeed, that the lower lip was thrust habitually into the opening.

I determined therefore to extract the second bicuspids, to draw all the forward teeth back by the space gained, and to concentrate my energies on the fœtal angle. Dr. Square again attending, we administered gas and extracted the desired teeth.

The first bicuspids and canines were readily brought back in a manner, which for simplicity, ease of adaption, economy of time and substance, easy removability and replacement, may not readily be surpassed.

The base-plates and regulating attachments for this, and indeed for all, could each be made ready within thirty minutes for the flask, and I should forbear digressing to relate a manner of base making which ought, through the kindly zeal of Mr. Balkwill, to be more widely known, were it not for the fact that the old wearisome and damaging system of waxing up and pressing Coffin plates is described in Professor Guildford's valuable treatise, although the MSS. were criticised (as he tells us in preface) by twenty-five teachers of American Dental Colleges.

This then : the model having been lightly painted with a thick solution of rubber, a piece of rubber (I have found "horn" to lie steadier than most sorts) previously cut to lead pattern and previously softened on a hot-plate, is quickly adapted with wetted fingers from palate to teeth and over labial borders, pressing whilst still warm into every sinuosity.

The rubber overlapping all teeth in front of the first molars was now cut off with a hot knife, and the flattened ends of two compo swivel eyes were warmed and pushed into the rubber, one on lingual other on labial side, and parallel to one another, the same being done to both right and left sides of the plate (*vide* plate 3) and carefully vulcanized (being held at 260° twenty minutes before rising).

A piece of compo spring having now been pulled and partly stretched, a small portion midway between the extremities was strained and rubbed straight out over the extremity of a fine beck iron. This straight part of wire was adapted to hitch or yoke over the front of the forward tooth, and the spring being bowed was bound at ends in the parallel eye-holes (a provision against breakage). As the teeth closed up it was tightened again by removing plate and merely pushing the opened spring closer together and then replaced by patient or self.

In this way by acting on one side at a time for fear of moving back teeth forward, the bicuspids and canines were rapidly brought back.

The laterals and fronts were retracted in like manner by a single piece of opened spring looped over teeth and attached to the head of a swivel bolt. To economise space, for explanation the method is illustrated on plate 5. It will be found suited to draw back, push out, or even to turn a tooth on its axis, to replace the Lee Bennet screw, and to be easily inserted and removed by the patient. This last method, however, better suited for manipulating one tooth at a time, had better have been replaced by the zigzag method to be shortly described and to have been put in practice later on. The obnoxious angle now demanded attention. It was desirable to move the converging teeth and alveoli outward in their vertical positions, and to enlarge the palatine circle at the same time. Its accomplishment was alike a surprise and delight from the ready response of the parts to the simple device employed.

The palate being covered, and teeth capped with rubber in the manner before intimated, two pieces of spring previously stufied with wool and planished down to point at ends, were inserted and built over at extremities with rubber manipulated with hot knife (*vide* plate 4), and shields were cut as figured down palate, between affected teeth and through the external labial border with a heated blade.

When vulcanized, the shields were cut clean through the mark with a spring saw, and were then free on expansion to work in any direction, directly outward, semi-circularly, from front, backward, or in any other direction not required in present case. By manipulation out of the mouth, the distance of shields to plate daily widened and result (*vide* plate 2) quickly brought about.

After leaving case a week or two to secure implantation, the front teeth which had been left partly retracted and retained by T piece retainers for further treatment when greater expansion was secured, once more claimed notice. And, again, what was to me another novelty suggested itself.

Another plate being formed, a very fine gold wire (Ash's finest) was bent into convolutions about or more than $\frac{2}{3}$ length of the crowns of the teeth, and the terminal points of this zigzag (as I am pleased to call it) inserted in the labial flanges of the rubber at the median line of the external position of the bicuspids (*vide* plate 5).

This was tightened daily by being drawn together in or out of mouth with a fine pliers grooved near tips with a file.

All the inclined planes quickly marched inward and to the perpendicular.

Any tooth lagging or out of circle was quickly hurried by bending one of the toes of zigzag standing opposite the prominence, thus was any tooth turned or forced in any direction desired.

When finished the young lady wore the same plate as a retainer.

A word on regulating materials. I must declare my preference for gold before all others. It may by proper alloying be made more tenacious than steel, be more frequently bent without breaking, is better appreciated by patient, is not affected by the sulphur liberated in vulcanization, and is of the same value when returned as before, minus trouble of remelting and drawing out. Appliances containing caoutchouc and wood should be relegated to the cases of museums, both are unsanitary and liable to swelling and rottenness, whilst moreover elastic, instead of working by stages, allow no rest nor reparation. I have known the temporary application of a semi-vulcanized rubber wedge produce in a healthy subject a coated tongue, feverish symptoms and disgust; what then can we expect from its application over a much larger area in the mouth of a "strumous dyspeptic," which class I am convinced is largely represented by such dentures as the subject of illustration?

The lower maxilla being drawn back and pinched at same angle, the exposed nerves of the badly decayed first molars were respectively capped and destroyed and built up to shape so as to avoid further contraction.

The principle of regulating lower dentures being conveyed to any practical mind by the illustration appended, it is needless to engrave the lower plate, it being manufactured on the same lines with the exception that it is necessary to imbed a thick tinned knitting needle around the lower lingual border of the vulcanite, which should be somewhat thickened to allow strength for expansion of the independent wings or shields, and likewise, I may add, a piece of spring may, if desirous of extra strength, be put at each side of labial border of shield on either upper or lower plate in same manner as on lingual side, and would allow same range of movement. I enclose models of the lower before and after treatment for editorial inspection, the improvement being just as marked as the upper and all that could be desired.

I have hesitated several months before presenting this simple system, fearing I may be treading on antediluvian or pre-adamite ground, and have a rap on my knuckles for plagiarism and assurance.

So many of our best dentists are, unfortunately, so scrupulously hesitative and conscientiously reticent, that it is only too possible I am "bringing coal to Newcastle."

The nearest approach to the *shield* principle, however, that I can find, is illustrated in the work of Dr. Guildford just published; it is an independent splint, the invention of Professor Goddard, a modification of the Coffin plate being placed in apposition to the lingual faces of the incisors for their protrusion.

A friendly critic has again directed my attention to a very ingenious method of pivoted levers, and what I may term screw shields, the invention of Dr. Shaw, of Boston, for expanding the angle, illustrated in the *Cosmos* for 1888. A comparison, however, of his appliance may convince that though free from many faults adverted to in other devices, it will be found more complicated to manufacture and regulate, and to be less fitted for removal and replacement by the patient.

Lastly, another point of difference that should not be overlooked between this system of spring shields, illustrated, and the others I have been hardy enough to criticise will be found in this, that power is not wasted to act diffusedly against the unsupported halves of the maxillæ, but is economised by being applied just where required, whilst at the same time the posterior bridge of vulcanite holds and binds together the articulated palatal processes. Danger therefore of separating the median union of the suture is scarcely possible, neither to my mind is there the contingent possibility of causing disturbance to the foundation crest of the maxillary and palate bones on which the vomer and perpendicular process of the ethmoid rest, subject to the advancing forward pressure derived from the sphenoid.

Consequently, depression or obliquity of the septum of the nose and its accompaniment, disfigurement of the face, is avoided.

The applications of the zigzag, spring and shield, are of so varied a nature and range, that on conning the pages of the aforementioned works of Drs. Guildford and Talbot, there is scarcely a case illustrated I would not undertake in preference, to regulate by their simple or modified adjustment than by the varied methods taught, and I should feel a pleasure in indicating by diagrams simple applications of the same, but that I fear the aforementioned works not being in the hands of a tithe of our English readers, the references to plates they cannot refer to, will be wearisome, and an appropriation of space.

THE PHYSIOLOGY AND TREATMENT OF SENSITIVE DENTINE.

A Paper read before the Students' Society, National Dental Hospital.

By George M. Keevil.

Mr. President and Gentlemen,—Having been asked on several occasions to read a paper before this Society, I have always been obliged to decline on the ground of not being able to find a sufficiently novel subject for it, and although I cannot claim much novelty or originality for the title and matter of to-night's paper, yet it is a subject which is always being brought vividly and practically home to the mind of the dental practitioner, and for that reason I venture to hope that it may be sufficiently interesting to tempt you to sit it out.

In order to treat of this subject, it is necessary to briefly refer to the structure of dentine, well-known though it may be to most of you. This tissue is usually defined as consisting of a hard calcified matrix, permeated by a system of channels, which contain a process or elongation of the odontoblast layer of cells, this layer being in connection with those immediately beneath them, thus establishing an intimate connection between the pulp and dentine. This is alone sufficient to warrant a theory that the sensibility of dentine is dependent upon the pulp, but the fact that Boëdecker has demonstrated the presence of a minute plexus throughout the whole structure of dentine, derived from the ultimate branches of the fibrils, is an additional support to such a theory, dentine thus presenting an appearance of a nervous supply analogous to that of the other tissues of the body.

Salter believed that dentine has a nervous connection both with the pulp and periosteum, and in support of this he mentions instances of dentine retaining an intense sensibility after direct communication with the pulp had been cut off by the lesion of intervening tissue. As he observes, however, it does not necessarily follow that the connection between the pulp and dentine should be by a direct radiation in the course of the dentinal tubes, it may be circuitous, and thus an outlying mass of dentine retain its sentient connection with the pulp; and if we remember Boëdecker's demonstration just mentioned, this latter view would appear very probable, and more so because we can only admit that any connection between the pulp and periosteum could only occur in that portion of the tooth which is enveloped in that membrane. It is interesting, historically, to note that John Hunter did not consider dentine to be a tissue capable of transmitting sensation; he says that "teeth are occasionally worked upon by operators in the living body without pain," but he evidently had not had much experience in the matter. It has never yet been determined how the nerves of the pulp terminate. Tomes states that they terminate in a rich plexus beneath the odontoblast layer. Boll, however, in investigating this point, found that on treating a pulp with dilute chromic acid solution, an immense number of medullated nerve fibres could be traced onward into non-medullated ones, the ultimate destination of which however was uncertain, but he has seen them passing between the odontoblasts and taking a direction parallel to that of the dentinal fibrils in such numbers that he infers that they have been pulled out of the tubes, still, however, he has not seen a nerve fibre definitely to pass into a canal. His observations have been controverted by Magitot, who recently stated that he had fully satisfied himself that the nerves of the pulp become continuous with the stellate layer of cells, and through the medium of these with the odontoblasts. If this latter view be correct, the sensitiveness of dentine would be accounted for, without the necessity that nerves should actually enter it, for the dentinal fibrils would then be prolongations, so to speak, of the nerves, and as Tomes says, it is not necessary to assume that the dentinal fibrils should actually be nerve fibres, for many animals of a low organization are capable of sensation, although they have no demonstrable nervous system.

The foregoing facts plainly point to the conclusion that a certain degree of sensibility in dentine is normal; on histological grounds, there is also the following fact that dentine loses all sensibility on destruction of the pulp. Whether this degree of sensibility varies or not at different ages is uncertain. I have been unable to find statistics bearing on this point or upon another interesting point, and that is, what relation, if any, the sensitiveness of dentine bears to the state of the rest of the nervous system at the time of observation. With regard to the latter question, Dr. White in an article in the *Dental Review* mentions two or three cases in which a highly nervo-sanguineous temperament was accompanied by an exquisitely sensitive state of the dentine, and in one of them in which the children inheriting the parent's temperament were also affected with a like condition; more statistics, however, are required to show whether this was merely a coincidence or not. It is also said that the teeth of young persons, especially those just arriving at the age of puberty, are exceedingly sensitive, and to be more particularly marked in girls. It was formerly supposed that in aged, or senile dentine, the fibrils atrophied or became calcified, and that in consequence sensation was gradually lost, but Wedl proved that they were still there, and also retained their property of imbibition, it is only fair therefore to suppose that they still retained their sensibility. Regarding the uses of the sensations in dentine nothing definite is known. Mr. Coleman is inclined to accord them a special function, probably tactile, by which we are enabled to judge of the nature of substances which come under their action, and also to judge of the requisite amount of mastication, for it is an undoubted fact that persons with artificial teeth find at first considerable difficulty in ascertaining when their food has been sufficiently masticated; but it appears to me that this function, which is entirely dependent upon pressure, is more probably performed by the periosteum. It is suggested that the most likely use of the sensation is to give warning of the encroachings of caries, and to be intimately connected with the throwing out of secondary dentine. Being pretty well agreed, therefore, that a certain degree of sensation in dentine is normal, we must regard any exalted state of such sensibility as a pathological condition, but to what this hyperæsthesia is due is a matter which has been very violently discussed, without any definite conclusions being arrived at, the most usual thing to do in order to get out of the difficulty is to put it down to inflammation. The only thing which can be said against it is that the dentinal tubes are too small to admit blood corpuscles, but even this is a false objection, as there are countless numbers of immature corpuscles, the so-called "microcytes," which are capable of being exuded into the tubes. Thomas Bell, in endeavouring to establish the inflammatory theory says, that in many cases after breaking open a tooth, immediately after extraction, where the pain and inflammation had been severe, he found distinct red patches in the very substance of the dentine. He also states that on the examination of teeth of persons killed by drowning or hanging, he found the whole of the osseous part of the teeth, with the exception of the enamel, tinged a deep red. He places this against the objection of John Hunter and others, that the teeth have never been satisfactorily injected, and he especially mentions the case of a patient who died from jaundice, in which the dentine was found to be of a bright yellow colour. Amongst modern authorities who are in favour of the inflammatory theory may be mentioned Drs. Harris and Taft, but the worst of it is that no treatment based scientifically on this theory produces any satisfactory results.

Another and more plausible suggestion is, that the pulp itself is really the seat of the exalted sensibility, and the fibrils are merely the agents through which external impressions are conveyed to this central organ. Rational treatment based on this hypothesis would be the administration of such drugs, as acting on the nervous or circulatory systems, or both, should lower this exalted. Experiments involving the use of nervous and arterial sedatives have not tended to confirm this theory, although morphia is said to be of use in such cases as those which I have before mentioned in which great sensitiveness of dentine was a peculiarity of a nervous temperament, but in these cases, however, the hyperæsthesia cannot be considered to be a pathological state.

Another suggestion to account for this peculiar condition is, that it is caused by the crowding into the dentinal tubes, of bacteria, when disturbed by an exciting cause, and so causing pressure on the fibrils. Dr. Willmot's opinion is, that hypersensitive dentine as a pathological condition is analogous to that condition known as "teeth on edge," and is produced by the same general cause, the irritation of an acid. He says, that in these cases of "teeth on edge" from eating sour fruit, &c., the acid is concentrated and abundant, passing through pores and cracks in the enamel, acts on the peripheral extremities of the fibrils, and causes such irritability in the dentine that the slightest impact or change of temperature causes pain. He goes on to say that in the hyperæsthesia generally observed in general pratice, associated with caries, the irritating acid is very dilute, so that the effect is produced slowly, requiring for its manifestation greater changes of temperature or some chemical or mechanical injury, as the cut of an excavator, the difference of the two conditions being in degree only; in the former the irritant being in action for a short time only, and so soon becoming diluted with saliva, that an exalted sensibility rapidly subsides; in the latter the irritation due to an acid condition of saliva, is persistent, and the hyperæsthesia soon becomes chronic.

I have now tō pass to a more practical point, namely, treatment. The internal use of morphia has already been alluded to, the conclusion being that it is only of use in cases of systemic nervousness, and being a dangerous drug to play with should be excluded as much as possible from use by the dental practitioner, the risks not being counterbalanced by satisfactory results. In cases in which the sensibility is referable to an acid state of the secretions, a removal of the cause will at once suggest itself, cases such as these, and which occur so frequently in children, are easily corrected by the use of alkaline remedies, such as bicarbonate of soda or potash.

In such cases as are not included in the above, a lot may be gaining the confidence of the patient, by tact of manner and touch, and by proper use of sharp instruments, but it is in those cases, such as erosion cavities, in which the dentine is so hard as to require the determined use of the dental engine, which gives so much trouble, and to find a remedy for this class of case the whole *Materia Medica* has been ransacked from one end to the other, with very indifferent success. Dehydration by means of absolute alcohol, followed by warm air is one of the first things which should be tried, its apparent action being the subtraction of water from the organic material in the dentinal tubes, causing its contraction.

The next most primitive method of treatment is the application of creasote or carbolic acid, the latter by preference. Carbolic acid is a drug in which the relative dryness of the cavity and maintenance of the strength of the application produce proportionately satisfactory results, but it requires to remain for two or three hours to do any good. Dr. Flagg considers this drug to act in a two-fold way, both by forming insoluble phenates with the organic constituents of the dentine, and by anæsthetizing to a slight degree the pulp, rendering that organ less susceptible to irritation.

The next on the list of this class of remedies is a very favourite one, chloride of zinc; in using this drug it is absolutely essential that the cavity be as dry as possible, as success depends upon its being diluted, and in order to secure this, it has been recommended to place small pieces of it in the cavity and allow them to deliquesce of their own accord; fifteen minutes is usually sufficient time for this drug to produce its effects, unfortunately, however, its application is usually attented with intense pain, and I am not aware that any means have yet been found for avoiding this. Occasionally, in deep seated cavities, the application of chloride of zinc produces pain of a beating kind; it is an indication that the pulp is being affected, and this should be at once controlled by washing the cavity out with warm water and introducing a little oil of cloves.

Side by side with chloride of zinc may be placed nitrate of silver, which is said to affect the dentine to a greater depth and to be less painful, but the unfortunate discoloration which it produces is an effectual bar to its use, at any rate in front teeth.

The last of this series of drugs is arsenic; but although this substance is undoubtedly the best obtunder at present known, its use is almost unanimously condemned on account of its deleterious effect upon the pulp. If, however, its use is resorted to as a last resource, Dr. Harris recommends $\frac{1}{40}$th grain to be applied and allowed to remain for about an hour. It is doubtful, though, whether its employment is justifiable for the purpose of simply obtunding dentine.

Among other remedies may be mentioned tannin in alcoholic

solution, in creasote or in glycerine, sulphuric acid and cocaine, oxide of calcium, and the frequent administration of small quantities of nitrous oxide gas, has been said to be efficacious in some cases. These have all been used with more or less success, but their action appears to be very uncertain.

With regard to electricity as applied for the purpose of treating sensitive dentine, Dr. Harris mentions the galvanic cautery as being useful.

Dr. Flagg states that in many cases he has found galvanic electricity of great use in obtunding, but that it does not always bring about the result. He uses it by placing one pole of a large bichromate battery on the gum over the root of the affected tooth, the other being placed in the cavity, each pole for better connection being tipped with sponge ; it probably acts by producing a retraction of the organic material in the dentinal tubes, in the same way that electricity is known to cause the contraction of protoplasm, when applied to it as a stimulant.

In concluding my short paper, gentlemen, I trust that you will attribute its brevity to lack of material, not to want of painstaking in trying to get it together.

Reports.

THE ODONTOLOGICAL SOCIETY OF GREAT BRITAIN.

THE usual monthly meeting of the above Society was held on the 5th ult., at 40, Leicester Square.

The President, Mr. FELIX WEISS, L.D.S.Eng., occupied the chair, and there was a very full attendance of members.

The minutes having been read and confirmed, Messrs. J. O. Butcher, Jas. F. Colyer, Jno. Greenfield, Chas. F. Rylot, and R. Wynn Rouw were balloted for, and duly elected members of the Society.

The LIBRARIAN (Mr. Ashley Gibbings) announced the receipt of various books and publications ; among them being an Italian work, the English title of which was "The Pathology, Therapeutics, and Hygiene of the Cavities of the Mouth," the Year Book of th Scientific Societies, and a new Journal from Turin.

The CURATOR (Mr. Storer Bennett) had no report to make.

Mr. T. G. READ made a communication on "A method of making an all-gold crown, illustrating a convenient way of making and using a model." He said that a model was most useful when crowning bicuspids and molars, and in some cases incisors and canines. The metal band of the crown is roughly adapted to the stump, and feather-edged previous to fitting in the mouth, the portion passing under the gum is the same relative distance beneath it around the stump, and a very perfect occluding surface is obtained. When crowning a stump, the rubber dam should, if possible, be first adjusted, and the pulp canals filled. The broken-down crown should then be reduced in height to allow for restoration of the occluding surface, the stump being left standing as high as possible above the gum. Should it be necessary to cut away much tooth tissue, a long file cut fissure bur with a chisel point would be found useful for the purpose; drill two holes with the point for the labial to the lingual surface, one at the mesial, the other at the distal part of the crown. The tooth substance between these holes having been cut away, one blade of a pair of excising forceps is placed in the labial, and the other in the lingual opening, and the handles pressed together when the crown comes away. Small pieces of upstanding tooth substance close against another tooth may be readily removed with a wheel bur such as Dr. Meriam's, these projections can be cut from the inside without wounding the gum, and the unpleasantness of running a corundum wheel is avoided. The sides of the stump as far as the band is to extend should be made quite parallel, so that the crown may fit the stump quite closely and tightly. Previous to paring the stump, cocaine in crystals should be rubbed on the gums with the finger, then the enamel and overhanging or projecting tissue may be stripped off with suitable enamel chisels. The sides of the stump having been pared quite parallel, should be finished smooth by carefully passing a safety point shouldered fine file cut fissure bur around it. Then take a strip of thin metal—such as telephone plate—trim and bend this to the stump, when roughly fitted, press a small piece of softened composition to the band of stump, the patient then closes the mouth, and bites into the composition. As soon as it is hard, remove the impression of little band from the mouth. Cast a lower and upper model from this with the little band *in situ*, over this band make the metal band of the crown in coin gold, size 5, to fit it and correspond to the gum edge; the join should be at the lingual surface. Having fitted the band to the model, soften the end of a stick of composition and press the band on with the edge to go under the gum uppermost, this is feather-edged with a fine round file. Coin gold of the same substance of the band should be used for the cusps which should be struck up in White's die plate. Try the cusps to the occluding model and see if the bite will ride. Mark where it will, place the cusps on the male die of soft metal used to strike them up and with blunt punches knock down those places marked. The articulating surface is thus made perfect. Fill up some solder and mix it with a little Parr's flux, fill the interior of the cusps rather full and flow the solder over a Bunsen flame. The band should then be fine, fitted in the patient's mouth ; when this has been done, solder it edge to edge over a Bunsen flame using binding wire as a clamp. Contour the band with contouring pliers. If the canals have not been filled, twist a piece of binding wire with a bead or two upon it round the contoured band, place this on the stump and use it to hold the rubber dam. Soften the end of a stick of composition and press the band upon it, with the occluding edge uppermost, with a fine flat file. Cut the surface flat, remove the band from the composition, and try it and the cusps in the mouth, removing and replacing it upon the stick to cut away until the cusps are let in and the occlusion is perfect. Place the cusps on a soldering gridiron, borax the edge of the band, and adjust it in position on the cusps, so that when the shoulder which is on the cusps is cut away, the buccal and anterior surfaces will be perfect. Hold the work over a bunsen flame, and the solder in the cusps will melt and unite with the band. When soldered, if the lingual and posterior surfaces are not perfect, build them up with coin gold, scraps, and solder filings ; run the solder with a blow-pipe. Boil in acid, trim with a fine corundum wheel, and polish, holding the crown on a stick of composition. Horizontally groove the pulp chamber, dry it out and fill it and the anterior of the crown with oxy-phosphates of a creamy consistency, press the crown on the stump with a notched tooth-brush handle, strike the toothbrush handle once or twice with a lead mallet to expel any surplus cement. When the setting is hard trim away any excess of cement with a broken-back chisel. The mallet should be only used in the final stage, for, if properly made, the band may be pressed on the stump with the finger.

Mr. WALTER H. COFFIN remarked that in hearing a communication read with the rapidity that the one they had just listened to had been given to the meeting, it was quite possible to overlook some points. The only new point which he had been able to see was the fitting a base metal immediately, and adapting around that the permanent gold crown which would of course be too large, and then have to be closed up in the mouth and soldered. It seemed to Mr. Coffin that the filling of the permanent gold crown on the stump could be accomplished in the first instance as easily as in any other metal; he imagined, however, that Mr. Read found it more convenient to handle some other metal in the initial stage.

Mr. READ said the telephone plate band was not fitted to a nicety but only roughly; it could be done in about three minutes. Then the band was cast, or an impression taken, and an assistant could get the gum edge right. One advantage was that an assistant could do the work which would otherwise have to be done by the principal himself. Then the point was to get the gum edge right, in the specimen he had passed round, it was very shallow on one edge and deep on the other, it would be very difficult to make it in any other way.

Mr. H. BALDWIN narrated a case of chronic enlargement of the upper jawbone which had been under his observation for about eight years. The patient was an unmarried woman aged 39, and on first coming to him the enlargement was very marked, chiefly on the left under side of the molar region. For about six years after he first saw her it underwent very little change, but in the seventh year the enlargement grew considerably and the mucous membrane became pencilled over with blue veins, suggesting that the circulation was getting more free, indicating the necessity for operation. The growth was hard and bony to the touch. He had called it a case of hyperostosis, for want of a better definition, as it had many of the characteristics of that disease. The case was operated upon in the latter part of last year by Mr. Pearce Gould of Middlesex Hospital, the gum was deflected away from the growth, and the bone removed with bone-cutting forceps. It was found very easy to remove, and not of the ivory description which he had anticipated. The peculiarity of the case was, that wherever the partial plate, which the patient was wearing, touched the mouth, there the growth was much less marked; for several years everywhere where the plate touched was perfectly healthy, it was only in places where there was no contact with the plate that the growth developed. The plate seemed to have operated in preventing the occurrence of the growth and in no way to have irritated it. The model, which he showed, had been taken since the operation, and as that was performed only in December last, sufficient time had not elapsed to say whether a complete cure had been effected, but at present there were no signs of recurrence of the growth. One peculiarity of the patient was that the nasal processes of the maxillary bones were more prominent than is normal, and the question was whether this was a first instalment of a general enlargement or whether the nasal prominence were merely accidental, which would be cured by operation. There were sections of the growth under the microscope; it seemed to consist of a cancellous bony structure and the spaces were lined with fibrous membrane. Portions of the growth contained small cysts visible to the naked eye, about the size of a very small pea, lined with glistening membrane.

Mr. Howard Mummery then read a paper entitled—

NOTES ON THE PREPARATION OF MICROSCOPICAL SECTIONS OF TEETH AND BONE.

The paper was accompanied by an exhibit of photomicrographs thrown upon a screen by a lantern. Having referred in some detail to the disadvantages of the "decalcification method," Mr. Mummery said that his interest in the process he was about to describe was first awakened by a remark of Mr. C. S. Tomes, who told him some two years ago that Professor Moseley, of Oxford, had mentioned a plan of hardening sections of teeth with gradually increasing strengths of alcohol. No details, however, of the process were given by him. But these particulars were supplied by Dr. L. A. Weil, in a German Microscopical Journal, and were reproduced as an extract in the English Royal Microscopical Society's Journal, December 1888, p. 1042.

Mr. Mummery prepared some sections according to those directions, and was so pleased with the results that he had since cut nearly 200 specimens in the same way. By this method no decalcification is required, and the cells and connective tissue of the pulp, and also of the peridental membrane, are retained in their natural relations to the hard tissue.

The extract in the Microscopical Society's Journal stated that:— "Dr. L. A. Weil takes only fresh or nearly fresh teeth, and in order to allow reagents and stains to penetrate into the pulp cavity, divides the tooth immediately after extraction with a sharp fret saw below the neck into two or three pieces, allowing water to trickle over it the while." Mr. Mummery said that to procure longitudinal sections it was advisable to cut them a little to one side of the pulp cavity, just opening this enough to enable stains to penetrate. Continuing the quotation, "The pieces are then laid in concentrated sublimate solution to fix the soft parts. The sections are then washed in running water for about an hour and placed in 30 per cent. spirit for twelve hours, and for a corresponding period in 50 per cent. and in 70 per cent. spirit. To remove the black sublimate precipitate the teeth are then laid for twelve hours in 90 per cent. spirit, to which 1·5 to 2·0 per cent. of tincture of iodine has been added. The iodine is removed by immersion in absolute alcohol until the teeth become white. They are now ready for staining, and the stain which Dr. Weil recommends is borax carmine (alcoholic or aqueous solutions). After being washed for fifteen to thirty minutes in running water, they are left in the stain for two or three days; they are then transferred to acidulated 70 per cent. spirit, in which they remain, the watery-stained ones at least twelve, the alcoholic-stained ones twenty-four to thirty-six hours. They are then immersed for 15 minutes in 90 per cent. spirit, and then for half-an-hour in absolute alcohol, after which they are transferred to some etherial oil for twelve hours or more. The etherial oil is quickly washed off with pure zylot, and they are placed for twenty-four hours in pure chloroform; after this they are passed into a solution of balsam in chloroform. This balsam is prepared by drying in a water bath, heated gradually up to 90 degrees C. for 8 hours or more, until when cold the balsam will crack like glass on being punctured. The sections are allowed to lie for twenty-four hours in a thin solution of this dried balsam in chloroform, and then as much balsam is added as the chloroform will take up. The sections covered with the balsam solution are then placed in a suitable receptacle over a water bath kept at 90 degrees C. and this cooking is kept up until the mass of balsam, with the the teeth in, cracks like glass when cold. This requires two or three days. Thin pieces are then cut from them with a sharp fret saw, and they are then ground down in the usual manner"—first on a corundum wheel, afterwards on stone. Mr. Mummery said that the advantage of the sublimate appeared to be due to its coagulating the albumen of the tissues—it certainly seemed to be very efficacious in preventing shrinkage. His most successful sections had been ground down on a Washita stone, using a piece of cork, or the finger, and plenty of water. The *débris* could be very conveniently washed off the completed sections with a fine spray of water, blown through an ether spray apparatus. The section could then be mounted in chloroform balsam.

The process as detailed no doubt appeared very tedious and complicated, and was almost enough to deter anyone, who had but little leisure, from undertaking it; but when a number of sections were being prepared in different stages the passing on from one solution to another did not occupy much time. Wolrab's gold bottles in a rack formed excellent receptacles for the sections, a note being made on a label on the bottle of the stage they had reached. With this as with most other processes, there were of course a good many failures, some being caused by insufficient cooking, resulting in the pulp not being hardened enough, others by too prolonged cooking, which produced brittleness. The cutting down was certainly very tedious, and should be done on a slow-cutting stone. Again, without great care in grinding very thin sections, the pulp might break away at the last moment—only by practice could one learn to avoid this annoying accident. Borax carmine penetrated well and stained the nuclei very strongly, but did not give so much detail in the pulp as some other stains. Very good results might be obtained with aniline blue-black, which stained the nerve fibres as well as the nuclei and connective tissue. Mr. Mummery had not been very successful with hæmatoxylin, but had been told that Erlich's hæmatoxylin, which does not precipitate, would probably be the best stain to use in this process. The teeth he had made use of had been chiefly young bicuspids, some with the apex of the root still incomplete. He had also made sections of older teeth for comparison, and of some carious teeth and abscesses. In these latter he thought the process might prove very useful, enabling one to study the early stages of abscess formation.

Mr. Mummery, having expressed his indebtedness to Mr. Theodore Harris for the great help he had given him in preparing the sections, devoted the remainder of the time to pointing out the characteristics of the very beautiful specimens photographed on the screen. No description of these specimens will convey any adequate idea of their appearance, but a reference to one or two will serve to demonstrate the importance of the process.

A transverse section of the pulp of bicuspid tooth exhibited the pulp with its relation to the walls of the pulp cavity undisturbed.

The odontoblast layer was seen very distinctly differentiated from the rest of the pulp, lying in immediate contact with the semi-calcified portion of the dentine, the tissue, "on the border-land of calcification," that part of the matrix which had evidently undergone some change, being in advance of the line of complete calcification. The blood vessels were seen in transverse section, and also the slightly denser condition of the central part of the pulp, noticeable in many of the specimens.

The next slide from a similar pulp was interesting as showing in the large blood vessels in the centre what very delicate tissue could be retained in position by the hardened balsam during the process of grinding.

Another slide, taken from a tooth which was extracted before the apex of the root was completed, showed the odontoblast cells, which, together with their nuclei, had taken the stain deeply, not to be lying in close contact but to have distinct spaces between them. Mr. Mummery did not think this was due to shrinking in preparation, as he had found it in all the open ended bicuspid teeth which he had examined ; and other specimens prepared by this process seemed to indicate that there is no appreciable shrinkage of the odontoblast cell. Mr. Hopewell Smith, in a paper published in the DENTAL RECORD for August, 1889, speaking of the dentine after the commencement of calcification said : "Between some of the cells of the membrana eboris there are wide visible spaces, filled with homogeneous substance and small round and angular cells." Mr. Mummery remarked that Mr. Tomes also appeared to be a little shaken in his views on this point, for whereas in the earlier editions of his "Dental Anatomy," he said (p. 159, second edition) : "The odontoblasts are fitted closely together, and there is no room for any other tissue between them" ; in the third edition (p. 69) he says : "There is not much room."

Deposits of secondary dentine in the pulp are well exhibited by this method of preparation. The specimen shown was taken from a molar tooth, to all appearance sound, which caused intense neuralgia, rendering it necessary to extract it. The pulp was densely packed with secondary deposits, encroaching in every direction upon the nerves and blood-vessels. This deposit exhibits some curious concentric and radiating masses. The next slide was from a similar pulp, showing some very large deposits.

Another showed a tooth extracted from an old person, in which the whole of the pulp appears to be converted into a semi-calcified material, apparently of cartilaginous consistency, with islands of calcified tubular dentine. Mr. Mummery had been struck with the fact pointed out by Mr. Salter in his "Dental Pathology"—that many young and apparently healthy pulps show numerous deposits of secondary dentine. Mr. Salter, in the work referred to (p. 139), says this change is to a great extent reparative, and the result of trivial causes, though Mr. Mummery believes it never occurs unless the tooth has been in some way the subject of injury or irritation.

The specimens in which it was seen were certainly untouched by caries; but they may have been subjected to some form of irritation conveyed to the pulp from the great pressure caused by overcrowding.

Interglobular spaces in dentine are very well stained in the balsam process.

Caries in a fissure in the enamel.—This slide was prepared to show that the process, while keeping the relations of the carious portion to the calcified tissue, retains also in position tissue that has undergone a very considerable amount of disintegration.

A great number of slides were shown; and in conclusion Mr. Mummery expressed the hope that some of the points he had simply touched upon might suggest lines of investigation to those engaged in microscopical work.

THE PRESIDENT said they were greatly indebted to Mr. Howard Mummery for his very lucid and able paper, and for the beautiful illustrations, and he invited comments upon the paper.

Mr. F. NEWLAND-PEDLEY said he was able to confirm from his own experience the value of the process which Mr. Mummery had described, but like many other things, it was of some antiquity, having been known for the last fifteen years. Some five or six years ago one of his colleagues at Guy's wished to investigate the development of rider's bone, and it was necessary to show hard and soft structures at the same time: he (Mr. Newland-Pedley) cut sections by Mr. Mummery's method, and they were shown at the Pathological Society.

Mr. H. BALDWIN wished to ask Mr. Mummery whether the transparent portion which intervened between the dark layers was not chiefly formed of the unstained portion of the odontoblast cell, and whether the dark layer did not consist of the nuclei only of the odontoblast. Also whether the so-called spaces were not unstained portions of the cells? Again, as to the small groups of cells which were found in the periosteum, and which were said by some to be epithelial pearls, whether there were not some stain which would show whether they were of an epithelial nature or not?

Mr. ARTHUR UNDERWOOD said if it would not be taking a liberty to relieve Mr. Mummery of the trouble, he would take upon himself to answer two of the questions. If the parts were stained with gold the whole cell becomes perfectly stained, and the interspaces are quite marked, and that without confusion of substances, still more the transparent layer that lies between the cells is marked out quite plainly, being in no kind of sense a part of the cell, there could be no kind of confusion, there was no doubt that an interval does exist. Mr. Underwood thought that they ought really to feel very much indebted to Mr. Mummery for his epoch-making paper in dental microscopy. Though Mr. Newland-Pedley seemed to have been so happy as to have hit upon the same process a long time ago, still it had remained for Mr. Mummery to make it public property. All dental microscopists would feel under a great debt of gratitude for having solved the difficult problem how to cut hard and soft tissues together leaving them undisturbed by the influences either of the knife or the fluids. Mr. Underwood knew from experience how ready critics were to assert that the appearances were due to decalcifying fluids. He thought a tablet should be raised to Mr. Mummery for having delivered them from these tiresome critics.

Mr. CHARLES S. TOMES wished, in endorsing Mr. Underwood's remarks, to emphasize the fact that Mr. Mummery had been the first to produce preparations which would go very far towards necessitating a revision of much that had been written on the question of the development of dentine. The points in question Mr. Mummery had hardly touched upon, because until he had thoroughly worked the subject out he very rightly did not wish to say anything he might have to recede from. Mr. Tomes would not have said anything about it had not Mr. Mummery confined himself very much to the exhibition of the process, and had not Mr. Newland-Pedley said that the process was not very new, thereby implying that it was not worth while demonstrating what the process could do. This much he would assure Mr. Newland-Pedley that Mr. Mummery's demonstrations were entirely novel to him (Mr. Tomes); they showed things which he had never seen approached, and he felt sure they would give some results which would necessitate a great deal of re-writing.

Mr. GEORGE CUNNINGHAM desired to call attention to the fact that the photographs were all the work of Mr. Mummery himself, so that he was not only an able microscopist but also a photomicrographist who might vie with Mr. Andrew Pringle who had been described as *facile princeps*.

Mr. CHARTERS WHITE felt that he ought to add his testimony in favour of Mr. Mummery's very able paper. He (Mr. White) had been reading for the last thirty years on the subject of microscopy and photomicrography, and had made the subject a special study, but he was bound to say that he had never been so fortunate as to reach the process before. Decalcification of the bony tissues resulted in the destruction of the shape of the cells, and the presence of acid in the pulp made them very difficult to stain. Mr. White felt that Mr. Mummery had given the death knell to the decalcification of the tissues, and he would, for one, adopt the process new to him, because he felt it was capable of giving details which decalcification had never yet afforded. He would like to ask Mr. Mummery if the sections could be rubbed down in his process in the same manner which he (Mr. White) had always described for dry sections, because in that way it would be possible to get photographs much clearer and sharper.

Mr. WILLIAM HERN wished to ask Mr. Mummery if he could explain how it was that after a process of prolonged and powerful heating, soft tissue, which was known to contain a large per centage of water, seemed to occupy the same space as before the process.

Mr. CHARTERS WHITE said, if he might be allowed to reply, he thought the use of the corrosive sublimate as a fixing agent, and then afterwards the hardening in absolute alcohol prevented, any further change, for the soft tissue being saturated with Canada balsam could not possibly have its real histological elements altered.

Mr. HOWARD MUMMERY said, in reply to Mr. Newland-Pedley, that he was not aware that the process had been really well known before, although of course there had been hints of it, but he thought to Dr. Weil belonged the credit of bringing it out properly, and giving those minute details which were so necessary to practical working. With regard to Mr. Baldwin's questions, Mr. Arthur Underwood had so ably answered them that he did not think it was necessary for him to add anything. He (Mr. Mummery) quite agreed with Mr. Underwood that the spaces between the odontoblast layer and the fully calcified dentine are crossed by the tubes, and the spaces between the cells are not part of the cells. If Mr. Baldwin would look at the specimens under the microscope he would see that this was so. Mr. Mummery wished to thank Mr. Tomes for his very kind remarks. He quite agreed with Mr. White as to the evil effects of decalcification, and thought that the specimens might be cut down by his (Mr. White's) method, but at present he was only feeling his way, and had not adopted it ; the difficulty would be to be able to see if the pulp were sufficiently rubbed down. With regard to Mr. Hern's remarks, the water in the tissue is gradually taken out by the spirit, the shrinkage is avoided by slightly increasing the alcohol, and the balsam takes the place of the spirit. The value of the corrosive sublimate is very great, as it fixes the specimen and prevents the shrinkage which often takes place.

The usual votes of thanks having been passed, the proceedings terminated with the announcements for next meeting.

STUDENTS' SOCIETY OF THE NATIONAL DENTAL HOSPITAL.

THE ordinary monthly meeting of this Society was held on Friday, March 7th, at 8 p.m. P. W. GREETHAM, Esq., President in the chair.

The minutes of the previous meeting were read by the Secretary, and confirmed.

The Misses Brierly and Mr. Schilling were present as visitors, and received the usual form of welcome from the President.

Casual Communications.—Mr. E. G. CARTER showed the model of a mouth having a supernumerary tooth in the position of the left upper central, which was however in range though pushed very much on one side. Mr. Carter also showed some trays for crown work.

Mr. CLEMENTS exhibited a lower canine having two roots.

Mr. PERKS showed a malformed second upper molar, also the model of a patient's mouth illustrating arrested eruption. The patient who is 45 years of age has only quite recently erupted her left upper canine.

Mr. RUSHTON read a communication from Mr. Lankester relative to the system of teaching Dental Surgery in Philadelphia.

The PRESIDENT then called on Mr. KEEVIL for his paper (see page 257).

A discussion followed in which Messrs. ALLNUTT, HUMBY, PERLES, RITSON, RUSHTON, and the PRESIDENT took part, after which a hearty vote of thanks was accorded Mr. Keevil for his very able paper, and the meeting adjourned until Wednesday, April 2nd.

THE ordinary monthly meeting of this Society was held on Wednesday, April 2nd, at 8 p.m. P. W. GREETHAM, Esq., President in the chair.

The minutes of the previous meeting were read by the Secretary, and confirmed.

Miss Brierly was elected a member of the Society.

Casual Communications.—Mr. E. G. CARTER showed a case of erosion in a right upper canine.

Mr. ALLNUTT mentioned a case of hæmorrhage following extraction. The bleeding ceased within half-an-hour after the extraction, and came on profusely five days afterwards. The tooth removed was a first left upper bicuspid.

Mr. SPOKES mentioned the case of a family all of whom had teeth of a dark brown colour. This peculiarity was also demonstrated in the teeth of the grandparents and great-grandparents.

The gentleman who was to have read a paper, asked leave to be excused, owing to the work for the forthcoming examination in May leaving him insufficient time for its preparation. The President therefore adjourned the meeting until the second Friday in May, when Mr. Hill, Esq., M.D., B.Sc.Lond., will read a paper the subject of which will be duly announced.

EXAMINATION PAPERS FOR DIPLOMA IN DENTAL SURGERY.

ROYAL COLLEGE OF SURGEONS OF ENGLAND.

ANATOMY AND PHYSIOLOGY.

1. Describe the Hyoid Bone. Enumerate the muscles attached to it, and give the nervous supply of each.

2. Explain the terms Syncope, Apnœa, Dyspnœa, and Asphyxia. How is death produced by Asphyxia?

SURGERY AND PATHOLOGY.

3. Describe the principal affections of the Tonsil, with the appropriate treatment of each.

4. Describe the symptoms and treatment of Rheumatoid Arthritis of the Temporo-maxillary articulation.

DENTAL ANATOMY AND PHYSIOLOGY.

1. Which of the Dental Tissues are the more constant? Describe teeth in which one or more of the tissues are absent.

2. Give an account of Enamel-organs, from their first appearance to the completion of their functions. What are the chief modifications of Enamel?

3. What is the special importance of Mastication for the digestion of the several classes of food? Illustrate your remarks by reference to the Herbivora and Carnivora.

DENTAL SURGERY AND PATHOLOGY.

1. State, giving your reasons, the ages at which you would treat—

(i) Underhung "bite."

(ii) Undue protusion of upper front teeth.

(iii) Overcrowding of the teeth:—(*a*) By extraction of the 1st molar; (*b*) of the bicuspids; (*c*) cf the lower incisor.

2. Describe the operation of crowning Molars and Bicuspids. Under what circumstances is it advisable?

3. What is the general composition of red, black, and velum rubbers, dental alloy, celluloid, plate-gold, band-gold, gold solder?

ROYAL COLLEGE OF SURGEONS IN IRELAND.

PASS LIST.

THE following gentlemen, having passed the necessary examination, have been admitted Licentiates in Dental Surgery of the College:—Mr. S. A. T. Coxon, Wisbech; Mr. A. L. Harrington, Rochford; Mr. H. Hudson, Birmingham; Mr. T. Nottingham, Hull, and Mr. G. A. Story, Canterbury. The next examination will be held on Monday, July 21st.

ROYAL COLLEGE OF SURGEONS OF EDINBURGH.

PASS LIST.

AT the April sittings of the Examiners, the following gentlemen passed the First Professional Dental Examination:—John Charles Holland, Huddersfield; Henry Alexander Matheson, Edinburgh; Robert Nasmyth Hannah, Edinburgh; Murray Thomson, Edinburgh; David Wilson, Edinburgh; and Joseph Douglas Stewart

Shepherd, Edinburgh; and the following gentlemen passed the Final Professional Examination and were admitted Licentiates in Dental Surgery:—John William Daniels, Tyldesley, near Manchester; John Wesley Lloyd, Liverpool; and Alexander Wilson, Glasgow.

GOSSIP.

THE GUY'S HOSPITAL DENTAL SCHOOL.—A correspondent has favoured us with the following account of the work done at this school during the past year.

The Dental School has now completed its first year of existence, and its development has been very satisfactory. The alteration in the hours of attendance at first reduced the number of patients to zero, and there was a doubt expressed whether out-patients would be sufficiently alive to the advantages of conservative dental surgery to submit themselves to remedial treatment, which always entails sacrifice of time and is not always devoid of pain. The experience of the last twelve months has shown a steadily increasing number of applicants for treatment, and in February there were 255 extractions done under nitrous oxide gas, more than 50 gold fillings, and 124 other fillings, in addition to the usual work of a dental department. This does not represent the number of patients who presented themselves, but the amount of skilled assistance available to attend to them. Although the dental student has always completed a two or three years' course of dental mechanics before entering Hospital, it is perhaps months before he can be trusted to fill a tooth for a patient, and the time expended on his first fillings will average several hours each. At the end of a year each well trained student becomes a valuable assistant. The method of teaching adopted is that the Assistant Dental Surgeon for the day gives a clinical demonstration on one of the operations of dental surgery and supervises the work of the department, aided by students holding appointments. A chart is kept of every patient's mouth, on which is recorded the operations performed and the treatment adopted.

In the anæsthetic department the daily exhibition of nitrous oxide gas has met with great appreciation, and the number of gas cases is rapidly increasing. In order to avoid abuse of the charity no patient can obtain any operation, save an ordinary extraction, without the recommendation of one of the teachers.

The dental laboratory is now in use, and is rapidly being fitted up with all the requirements for the construction of artificial dentures, correction plates, and dental splints. There is room for twelve students to work at the time, and they are allowed to take models of patients' mouths and to construct dentures for them, carrying the work through all its processes from commencement to finish. The lack of adequate instruction on dental mechanics had long been felt by the London schools, but the difficulties of affording the necessary training had been deemed insurmountable. No attempt is made to supply the necessitous poor with artificial teeth, for such an undertaking would be quite beyond the province of a General Hospital, and the difficulties of administering such a form of charity will readily suggest themselves. Cases suitable for treatment are found within the Hospital, and the work done for them is absolutely free of charge.

The special lectures have been well attended, and additional courses of instruction have been organized, which more than meet the present requirements of the examining boards.

A course of lectures is delivered each summer on Operative Dental Surgery, dealing with the science of dental operations. There is also a summer course on Dental Microscopy, in which students prepare for themselves and mount specimens of teeth and surrounding tissues, human and comparative.

The department is now in thorough working order, and it may be confidently asserted that the coming year will bear favourable comparison with the past.

Dental Microscopy.—The impetus which has recently been given to the study of the microscopy of the dental tissues both in health and disease, gave an especial interest to the exhibits under the microscopes shown at the Odontological Society, when Mr. Sewill and then Mr. Howard Mummery read their valuable papers. We are informed that arrangements have been made by the Dental Manufacturing Company to supply slides identical with those prepared by Mr. Pound. We have carefully examined specimens of these which have been submitted to us, and find them excellent and most valuable for teaching purposes.

THE DENTAL RECORD, LONDON: JUNE 2, 1890.

Professional Ethics.

UNDER this title a graduate of Harvard addresses the Odontological Society of that place. Were the subject matter merely germane to our fellow practitioners across the Atlantic we might well afford to pass it by, perhaps with a sigh, but still, as of no business of ours. Dr. Boardman,* however, takes up a position which some of us over here have assumed, and speaks with so much assurance, from the purely commercial point of view, that it may be as well to point out that there is more than mere mid-summer madness in the view we have consistently advocated that dentistry is not a trade, a dentist is, or should not be, a glorified dealer in teeth and patent nostrums. The labourer is indeed worthy of his hire, but the hire need not be the end and aim of the labourer. If it be so, we contend he, the labourer, has fallen short of the ideal possibility of his calling, and has voluntarily assumed the "iron mask" of mediocrity of life-aim and dwarfed ambition. Nor is this mere "tall talking." We submit, and many will readily endorse our statement, that the truly happy life is the one over which the "dollars" do not rule supreme. It is a centuries-old saying, which experience has not disproved, that thieves may break through and steal our earthly gains, but no man can rob us of our self respect or of that subtle fragrance which belongs to a professional life well spent and honestly worked. Our greatest men, Carlyle's "heroes," Emerson's "representative men," Longfellow's "great men," whose lives remind us

> We can make our lives sublime,
> And departing leave behind us
> Footprints on the sands of time,

have not been millionaires, nor even worshippers at the shrine of mammon. Dr. Boardman insists that the

---

* See *Archives of Dentistry*, May, 1890.

higher ethics are talked but not practised. He seems a better man of business than logician, for if we read aright, his main contention rests upon this assumption:—Lawyers, doctors and other professional persons, save and except parsons (although why they should have more reason for living cleanly and self-denyingly than any honest worker for the good we fail to see), do not really accept higher ethics, therefore dentists should not do so. It seems to us that, at all events, in England the dental profession is numerous enough and influential enough to select its own line of conduct without copying traits, either good or bad, from other professions. Advertising or non-advertising, from an ethical point of view, resolves itself into this, does it by its results tend to raise or lower the individual? Dr. Boardman contends that advertising takes many forms, and seems to regard them as one and the same for "trade purposes." Whether, for example, "Mr. and Mrs. Blank" are stated to have returned to town in a footnote of the *Post*, or whether Mr. Blank draws attention in the advertisement columns to the special advantages of consulting him at his address. We have here nothing, however, to say about advertisements, save and except, that in so far as they react upon the individual we believe they are a mistake. The general culture, the mental grasp of the individual, indeed determine his life and his happiness, and the more highly cultured the man the less will he care to see his name associated with practices which those of the aristocracy of thought deem derogatory. So far from calling into operation penal clauses, we would invite every man to choose for himself, believing that the individual would from a wider vantage ground of observation prefer to adopt lines of procedure which in England, at least, are regarded as involved in the practice of professional ethics.

OBITUARY.

Dr. JULIUS POLLOCK.

It is with regret that we have to record the death of Dr. Julius Pollock, Physician to Charing Cross Hospital, which took place from pleuro-pneumonia on Sunday, May 11th. One of the younger sons of the late Right Hon. Sir Frederick Pollock, Bart., Chief Baron of the Court of Exchequer, Dr. Pollock pursued his medical studies at King's College Hospital, taking his M.R C.S. in 1859 and his M.D. (St. Andrew's) in 1861. Five years later he was appointed assistant-physician to Charing Cross Hospital, and in 1870 was promoted to be full physician and received his fellowship of the Royal College of Physicians. In only four years he was senior physician and lecturer on medicine, having in the meanwhile held the chairs consecutively of pathology and forensic medicine Dr. Pollock was for five years Dean of the Faculty, a post he resigned in 1874, and he then assumed the duties of Treasurer to the Institution.

GEORGE T. PARKINSON, L.D.S.Eng., OF BATH.

With great regret we have to announce the death of Mr. George Parkinson, late of Princes Buildings, Bath, in which city he had practised his profession over 40 years. He was a few years since elected as President of the Western Branch of the British Dental Association, and in the West of England he was widely known and greatly respected.

On retiring from active work about three years since, he elected to reside at Hampstead for the remainder of his days. About three months since he was unfortunately overtaken with a painful malady, to which he succumbed on the 28th of April, ult. He had just entered his 74th year.

His professional career commenced in Raquet Court, Fleet Street, where his grandfather, father and brother, formerly practised.

Mr. Parkinson's name has long been associated with the dental profession, his grandfather being in practice in Raquet Court as far back as the year 1770. He was second son of Mr. George H. Parkinson, of Raquet Court, and younger brother of Mr. James Parkinson, of Sackville Street, London, who was many years treasurer to the Odontological Society of Great Britain.

W. R. WOOD, L.D.S.Ireland.

The death of Colonel William Robert Wood occurred at his residence, 53, Norfolk Square, Brighton, on Wednesday, April 30th. Colonel Wood was born in London in 1842. His father, Mr. John Wood, for many years practised in Brighton as a dental surgeon. He died, when his sons were young children, and Colonel Wood became articled to his uncle, Mr. Councillor William Robert Wood, of Carlisle House, Pavilion Buildings. He was a student of the Metropolitan School of Dental Surgery, and took the medal for Mechanical Dentistry. He was elected in 1878 a Licentiate Dental Surgeon of the Royal College of Surgeons, Ireland ; at a later period he was appointed Consulting Dental Surgeon to the Brighton Dental Hospital. Colonel Wood may be regarded as essentially a public man ; and by his useful and indefatigable labours in connection with the Brighton Artillery Volunteers he will be chiefly remembered.

W. A. TURNER, L.D.S.

We regret to announce the death of Mr. W. A. Turner, whose name was recently associated with some interesting experiments on hypnotism, and which were reported in our last issue. Mr. Turner was only 32 years of age ; he died at the Grand Hotel, Paris, from pneumonia, resulting from a chill taken in crossing the Channel. Mr. Turner was a Licentiate in Dental Surgery of the English College and much respected among his friends and patients.

C. H. BROMLEY, M.R.C.S., L.D.S.

On Sunday, the 4th of May, at 1, Portland Terrace, Southampton, Charles Henry Bromley, M.R.C.S., L.D.S.Eng., honorary dental surgeon to the Royal South Hants Infirmary, aged fifty-one.

GEORGE SLEEP, L.D.S.Ireland.

We regret to announce the death of this gentleman at the early age of 32. Besides being a skilful dentist, Mr. Sleep was a keen lover of nature, and an enthusiastic student of psychology. He had paid much attention to mesmerism and possessed considerale power as a medium. Mr. Sleep was also a successful landscape painter and took much interest in leading Art classes. His useful life was terminated from bronchitis ; he died at his residence, 40, Keppel Street, Russell Square.

BURTON LLEWELLYN HARDING, L.D.S

All those who knew Mr. B. L. Harding of Harrogate, and later of Guernsey, will regret to hear of his early death in Tasmania at the age of 34, after a painful illness from phthisis. He was a man of considerable promise, holding the English Licentiate, and being a prizeman of his year at the Dental Hospital of London.

CORRESPONDENCE.

[We do not hold ourselves responsible in any way for the opinions expressed by our correspondents.]

GAS OPERATIONS.

To the Editor of the Dental Record.

Sir,—In reply to your correspondent "J. S.," I trust you will allow me a word or two, although I think your space might be taken up by a worthier pen than mine.

He says "It is all very well to say we ought to have an anæsthetist to administer gas to our patients, but where are they to come from?"

I think as a rule that any town which has a sufficient population to support a dentist, is generally favoured with one if not more medical men. In fact, I think there are many who say the medical profession is overcrowded, and that they cannot find a town to practise in which does not already possess more medical practitioners than they desire.

Then I did not say that the medical men should necessarily administer the gas themselves. I advocated the presence of a medical man when gas was given (*see* my letter in December, 1889).

I did not say the medical men should give it. I left that an open question; but allow me to say all medical men are not destitute of intelligence, and if "J. S." would allow them to see him give gas a few times, and if necessary explain to them what he wishes them to do, they would be quite as capable of giving it as himself.

Permit me to point out that it is greatly to the advantage of the dentist to have both hands free, especially when he has a difficult case in hand, such as an impacted lower wisdom.

It saves time to have the elevator or forceps ready in hand and not being lumbered up with a bag and face-piece, he can go to work immediately the face-piece is removed, and when operating under gas time is *very* precious.

The left hand, if free, is ready immediately the face-piece is removed, to hold aside the lip, cheek, or tongue, and act as a support to the jaw (especially in the lower) while the right slips in the forceps or elevator. Then, whilst operating, the dentist is perfectly free to give his whole attention to the work in hand, and is not troubled either with the pulse or respiration, that being left entirely to the medical man; he is responsible for the patient's life, the dentist for his operation.

Should anything go wrong the much desired assistance is at at hand; it is useless to send for a medical man when life is extinct.

N^2O may be the safest anæsthetic we possess; but no anæsthetic is totally free from danger, and it is only right and just that we should minimise that danger as much as possible, and as I have mentioned before, Dr. Dudley Buxton says (Anæsthetics) "It cannot be doubted that to give any individual an anæsthetic subjecting him to a minimum of danger is all one person can do."

As to not being able to secure the services of a medical man for several hours. If a dentist is unable to secure the services of one medical man, he may be able to obtain those of another; but even supposing a medical man cannot be secured for several hours, is it not better for the patient either to put up with the pain of the operation without gas (if it be so very urgent) or else to wait, rather than run the risk?

As to patients with limited means who cannot afford to pay the double fee. If the patients be poor, they generally attend a medical man who charges them low fees, and who will be quite as willing to trust them with his services at a gas case, as he would with a bottle of medicine.

The question of fees can generally be arranged, and medical men are not by any means a stony-hearted set of people.

"J. S." says the idea is altogether unworkable. I cannot quite agree with him in that; if I am not mistaken the leaders of our profession in London and other towns, find it workable.

Finally, your correspondent speaks of "temerity." There is a difference between "temerity" and "prudence"—the former word means "rashness" or "unreasonable contempt for danger" the latter means "caution." I am Sir, yours &c.,

103, Sandgate Road, Folkestone. GEORGE SEYMOUR.

CLINICS.

To the Editor of the DENTAL RECORD.

SIR,—In the April number of the DENTAL RECORD a communication appears attempting a reply to my paper upon "Clinics." That "most subjects possess two sides" never should be in debate; being an axiom. Because the observer of the reverse side of this subject possesses a limited range of vision, it does not necessarily follow that its horizon is limited to the confines of his curtailed capacity for observation and appreciation. A man in a well would necessarily view the universe at a disadvantage, and due allowance would be made for any opinion he might advance respecting it. I quite understand how clinics might possibly be taken advantage of by schemers to further their own base ends, and how the best of ideas may be perverted by those who never had, and never will have, anything but the gratification of their own sordid ends in view. I have no doubt but a few choice specimens of this class exist in England as in the United States. I should be sorry to believe that the rank and file of the profession in both countries were unable to combat successfully these parasites whenever manifest.

Your correspondent must possess—with many others I am sorry to say—a peculiar reasoning capacity that would debar another a privilege he himself would enjoy, viz., that of protecting an invention which might conduce to the benefit of both patient and operator by promoting results hitherto imperfectly attained, even if attained at all; while he without any compunction of conscience would copyright a literary production, which is according a dignity to many productions, the authors of which must experience as great a sensation of pleasurable surprise as the purchaser does of unmitigated disgust and disappointment, they proving an *exposé* of the "reblocked and ironed" ideas of some one else, instead of what they purport to be.

In the case of the literature study, thought, and possibly research may have been bestowed upon the work, what about the inventor? Thought, study, and a correct appreciation of the underlying principles, coupled with a far more valuable quality than that possessed by the literary man pure and simple, especially when considered in connection with our profession—the capacity for *doing* a thing, instead of *talking* about it. I think the solution of the protection problem should be left to the individuals immediately interested, instead of to a self-constituted board of censors, who complacently roll their eyes and "thank God they are not as other men," instead of, during a lucid interval, thinking how much progress would be evidenced in their vicinity if they were. I cannot for one moment agree with your correspondent when he "questions very much whether any properly educated practitioner has on any occasion derived any real benefit from a clinic, or gained knowledge which he might not have acquired without it." If "clinical instruction is indispensable to the student," why is it any the less so to the active practitioner?

Any man if left to himself and his own—frequently narrow surroundings, will soon find himself in a rut so deep that he soon sinks out of sight of not only his professional brethren but also of the public whom he imagined he had been serving with benefit. If any man should be a perpetual student, and preserve an open and receptive mind it is a dentist.

To attempt to argue that the published proceedings of societies, and the description of methods can take the place of their demonstrations, at a time when medical, dental and technical schools of all kinds are shortening their lectures, by devoting more time to the practical application of their precepts, is at once suggestive that possibly another Rip Van Winkle has developed. Your correspondent, I imagine, will hardly be prepared to deny the Royal Society being a thorough representative institution; what are the methods pursued by it in its continued presentation of scientific, artistic, and abstruse subjects? Wherever apparati, experimentation, or tangible evidence can be introduced to illustrate a subject it is done. The fact that it is done, is evidence sufficient that the best minds of our most able instructors thoroughly appreciate the value of practical illustration. Wherever dentistry is recognised as a profession, it has been the practical go-ahead men—men who could practice as well as preach, and had the courage of their convictions to demonstrate successfully that which many times the mere theorist had proved impossible. Such men as the former are those to whom the profession must revert with pleasure, and thank for the present enviable position it occupies, they are the men who have gone hand-in-hand with their literary co-labourers, demonstrating the value or fallacy of the different lines of practice, and making possible the grandest combination of science and art the world has ever been compelled to acknowledge.

Dentistry is peculiar in the fact that frequently theory and practice are at variance, therefore, *all* avenues of knowledge should be entered, explored, and their treasures developed to the greatest possible extent. I am sorry to note the admission that a profession had been followed—the practical development and application of which should constitute its greatest charm to its advocate, thereby proving a blessing to those who would avail themselves of its possibilities—by one, who instead of enjoying to the full a life well rounded out by an assurance of work well accomplished, at last realizes he was by nature ill adapted to play the part successfully he had hoped for when entering upon his career, I can understand how crushed hopes has resulted in metaphorical "dead sea fruit," and would cover with the mantle of charity the evidences of an unrealized ambition.

"By their works ye shall know them" is a saying well worth considering by the members of our profession; thorough earnest men, and plenty of them, is what we need, both in theory and practice, let their theories be based upon tangibilities, not upon a gauzy foundation which causes their builders to tremble lest the breath of practical enquiry should cause them to fall in ruins at the first test they may be subjected to.

There is evidently a void that the present work of existing metropolitan societies does not fill, as evidenced by other communications to your valuable journal. The profession is awaking from the somnolent condition it has too long been in.

The spirit that tabooed the idea of women doctors and women dentists, has a more bitter tonic in store for it than that evolution proved to be. In conclusion I would say, let us have a full and free discussion upon this subject, let it be intelligent and worthy of our profession, then I do not fear the verdict of our dental brethren upon such a vital subject as "clinics."

Yours truly,
W. MITCHELL.

Upper Brook Street, W.

FLAGG'S PLASTICS AND PLASTIC FILLING.

To the Editor of the DENTAL RECORD.

DEAR SIR,—The third edition of this book appears again with an extraordinary statement. On page 56 two assays of alloys are stated to be made by me, but which in no respect, and in no proportion of any metal bear the slightest resemblance to any alloy ever made by me, nor would alloys, made according to the published assay, have any properties like any alloy I make. In one assay *two* important metals in the alloy are not even mentioned. Dr. Bogue is aware that the assays are not correct, and no doubt Dr. Flagg is also aware of the fact.

Dr. Flagg also expends much eloquence on the properties of gold and platinum in alloys. It is evident that *the* use of gold in an amalgam has never entered into his mind, and he remains unaware that gold is used in amalgam in this country, at all events solely for the purpose of making it clean and pleasant in working, and that its other properties are comparatively unimportant, and in many respects similar to those of tin. It is very well known that the setting time of any silver-tin alloy can be ruled by the proportion of platinum added. Why Dr. Flagg should take so very much trouble to inform his readers that he does not know this, is not easy to explain.

THOS. FLETCHER.

Warrington.

MONTHLY STATEMENT of operations performed at the two Dental Hospitals in London, and at the Dental Hospital, Manchester, from April 1st to April 30th, 1890 :—

		London.	National	Victoria.
Number of Patients attended		—	1806	1015
Extractions	Children under 14 ...	497	347	578
	Adults	994	510	
	Under Nitrous Oxide ...	794	571	113
Gold Stoppings		257	104	36
Other Stoppings...		741	321	202
Irregularities of the Teeth		60	134	37
Artificial Crowns		28	5	9
Miscellaneous and Dressings		533	191	422
Total		3,904	2,183	1,397

THE DENTAL RECORD.

VOL. X. JULY 1ST, 1890. No. 7.

Original Communications.

CALCIFICATION.

By SIDNEY SPOKES, M.R.C.S., L.D.S.

WHEN the Dental Student has made himself acquainted with the arrangement of the soft tissues which constitute the formative organs of the future tooth, he has next to consider the process by which these soft structures become changed into the hard organs known as teeth.

In addition to other observations bearing upon this subject, a paper on the "Secretion of Lime by Animals" has recently appeared in the Report issued from the Laboratory of the Royal College of Physicians of Edinburgh. Mr. Irvine and Dr. Sims Woodhead point out that the carbonate of lime present in sea-water is only one tenth of the whole lime salts present, whereas in the coral, shells and calcareous plants formed from the sea by animal and vegetable life the whole lime is practically in the form of carbonate. On the other hand, sulphate of lime is largely present in sea-water, and these observers thought that this salt might be assimilated and then elaborated as carbonate. They experimented upon laying hens, the only lime supplied to the birds being the pure hydrated sulphate. It was calculated that during six weeks 954 grains of carbonate were elaborated in the form of egg-shell from the sulphate of lime supplied. On examining the oviduct it was found to be secreting lime, the epithelial cells containing lime in minute granules which, incorporated with the organic matter, appear to form the egg-shell. "It is interesting to note in this connection that the epithelial cells are evidently in a state of great functional activity, as a consequence of which the nucleus is considerably obscured, and that along with the lime there is secreted some other substance (probably the organic material in which the lime is eventually embedded)." Having pointed out how the sulphate of lime may become changed into the carbonate these observers again refer to the special function of the epithelial cells in secreting the lime brought to them by the blood and lymph. "This lime evidently accumulates in the epithelial cells and is then thrown out on the free surface, just as urate, oxalates of lime, soda, &c., are secreted by the renal epithelium." As a result of the tissue waste by the activity of the cells, carbonic acid is present to combine with the lime secreted, and an analogy is drawn to what occurs in the formation of bone where, it is said, the organic basis is laid down by cells which, at the same time, actually secrete the salts of lime derived from the blood and lymph. "The osteoblasts are the secreting cells." This statement may perplex some students who, perhaps, are taught that bone is formed by the ossification of the osteoblasts themselves; and perhaps some exception may be taken to the analogy being true. Another exception is pointed out by the authors—that in the formation of bone, where the amount of phosphoric acid salts in the blood and lymph is large and there is no special development of carbonic acid gas, the phosphates predominates. Whilst it is admitted that the above processes are "merely suggested," those interested in the subject will be glad to know that further investigations are promised; the great difficulty, it is said, being the ignorance at present existing as to the changes effected by protoplasm upon the constitution of inorganic salts. With regard to the conversion of lime salts, and secretion of carbonates, the authors say "that the process is the result of a combination of two forms of activity, the purely chemical and what we must call vital, must be taken for granted; and it is this vital part of the process which appears to eke out the possibilities of chemical reactions taking place." While it may be strictly true that secretion can only take place in a living medium, it may perhaps be asked whether it is possible to regard the conversion of soft organised material into a more or less hard mass as necessarily a vital process; for it has been done in the laboratory. Leaving on one side for the moment the consideration as to whether the cells concerned are themselves the receptacles for deposition of lime salts or whether they secrete something which afterwards becomes impregnated, the larger question presents itself—what is the relation, chemical or vital, between the inorganic salt and the organised material? In connection with this, every well-regulated student bears in mind the names of Rainie, Ord, and Harting, and it may be useful to present, although in a necessarily condensed form, some account of their observations, if only to save reference to distinct papers.

Rainie, in 1858, published a book "On the mode of Formation of Shells of Animals, of Bone, and of several other structures by a process of Molecular Coalescence, demonstrable by certain artificially formed products." Amongst other things he claimed to have discovered a process by which carbonate of lime can be made to assume a globular form, and he explained "molecular coalescence," the process by which that globular form is produced. He also came to the conclusion that the rounded forms of organised animal bodies depended upon physical and not on vital agencies. In a broad-mouthed bottle a solution of gum arabic saturated with carbonate of potash was allowed to stand until the carbonate of lime set free from the gum and the triple phosphate set free by the alkali were settled at the bottom. Two clean microscope glass slides, inclined against each other, were inserted, and the bottle filled up carefully with a filtered solution of gum arabic in common water. It was then covered up and kept perfectly still for three weeks or a month. The soluble salts of lime to be decomposed by the carbonate of potash are contained in the gum (in combination with the malic acid) and also in the common water; triple phosphate is also contained in the gum and set free by the alkali. The deposit formed upon the slides in the gum is of a globular form instead of the crystalline found in ordinary solutions.

Dr. Ord, 1870, found by experiment that where uric acid was deposited in the presence of albumen it took the form of either small crystals with rounded angles, or of dumb-bells, or of sub-spherical bodies or even spheres. Glass tubes with a plug of isinglass jelly at the lower end were placed in a weak solution of chloride of calcium and then filled up with a slightly alkaline solution of potassium oxalate. After three months the plug was opaque with earthy deposit and stratified, forming a layer of greatest density near the calcium solution. The forms varied on the oxalate side from those on the calcium, and a series of gradations led from one to the other; the coalescence forms were characteristic of the calcic end, the crystalline of the oxalic end of the plug. Very many other experiments were made. When gelatin was used and magnetised, the general result was an extraordinary increase in the size of all the forms, crystalline and non-crystalline, but no new forms nor a greater tendency to sphericity. The effects of light and heat were tried ; no decisive results were gained in the former, but in the latter a kitchen specimen gave coalescence forms three or four times as numerous as the crystalline, whilst in a garden specimen this condition was more than reversed. Albumen was coagulated in tubes at a temperature not exceeding 200°, and oxalate of calcium deposited in these plugs at a temperature of from 50° to 60° took almost entirely the coalescence forms. Albumen was evidently much more active than gelatin in controlling crystallizing force. When phosphates and carbonate were arranged in proper proportions, it was found that the phosphate of lime was evenly distributed through the albumen in definite strata, not forming crystals or spheres, but cementing the albumen to great hardness, particularly at the line of greatest density. Carbonate of lime always formed spheres at the higher temperatures, but at lower temperatures showed attempts at crystallization by the formation of spines sticking out from the spheres. In the bone-salts experiments the carbonate of lime was subdued, so to speak, by the phosphate, and an even sub-crystalline but continuous deposit was produced. The use of a phosphate as a cement and manipulator of the less tractable carbonate, is well indicated in these experiments ; the strength of the carbonate seems necessary in all hard tissues that have to be tough. But the carbonate alone does not seem fitted to form tissue, tissue destined to be the seat of active interstitial change, therefore in the bird's high temperature and great vital activity we see associated a great predominance of phosphate. In the tortoise, with its low temperature and sluggish processes, a great decrease of phosphate and increase of carbonate ; and in the shells of Invertebrata, where interstitial change does not prevail, the carbonate alone or with but little phosphate suffices. In cases where this does not seem to hold good the explanation may be found in the nature of the animal matter with which the salts are associated.

Professor Harting published "Researches in Synthetical Morphology on the Artificial Production of Some Organic Calcareous Formations." He caused calcium carbonate and phosphate to combine, *in the nascent state*, with organic substances by using salts which by their double decomposition produce insoluble salts of calcium. After several weeks a considerable number of forms are developed which are mostly found in nature. The most frequently occurring form affected by calcium carbonate, in combination with albumen, gelatin, or the other organic substances used, he called *Calcospherites*. When these are formed in the midst of the liquid and the surrounding parts are perfectly tranquil, they are quite spherical; they become larger in proportion as their formation takes place with greater tranquility and slowness. They often contain a nucleus, and all those which attain a certain size are seen to be formed of concentric layers and very fine radiating fibres. Similar calcospherites, of spheroidal shape, are met with in nature in the form of different concretions in the bile, urine, and the saliva of certain animals; pearls are calcospherites, which in the course of time have attained remarkable dimensions. When the fluid is not kept quiet other forms occur, modifications of the calcospherite; one very remarkable is called *conostat*, characterized by a cup-shaped enlargement which becomes filled with air, and floats. The most remarkable of all the conditions, which assist in determining the shape of the calcospherites, consists in the fact of their mutual adhesion when they are developed in the neighbourhood of one another. Calcospherites consist of a combination of calcium carbonate with organic matter, which is the sole residue when the calcareous salt is removed by treating with an acid. If the development has taken place in albumen, or a liquid containing albumen, the fundamental substance is no longer albumen. The albumen is transformed into a substance, the chemical relations of which are those of conchyoline, and resemble those of chitin. This Harting calls *calcoglobulin*. It is not necessary however to cause albumen to combine with calcium carbonate and then to decompose the resulting compound in order to obtain calcoglobulin It can be obained by placing a fragment of chloride of calcium in albumen. After some days the albumen dissolves the calcareous salt and is transformed into calcoglobulin, which presents also, in part, a fibrillar structure, and, having been washed, gives all the reactions of that substance.

If calcium phosphate is liberated by the double decomposition of calcium chloride and a neutral phosphate in albumen or gelatin no combination takes place. But if calcium carbonate is present there is a combination of the organic matter with the two calcareous salts.

From the above quotations it will be seen that it is not difficult for any student to make calcospherites for examination, and thus prepare the way for understanding better the relationship of the cell and the lime salt in the living body.

With regard to the question as to the conversion of the odontoblast in the formation of dentine, there is a passage in the paper communicated by Mr. C. S. Tomes to the Royal Society, "On the structure and development of Vascular Dentine," which seems to have escaped the text-books. In describing the capillaries clothed with odontoblasts, it is pointed out that when the latter calcify the capillary becomes solidly embedded in dentine. "And this is a strong argument in favour of what is known as the "conversion theory," of the development of dentine; supposing these odontoblasts to be calcified and themselves converted into dentine, there is no difficulty in seeing how the capillary comes to be enclosed in a tube of dentine, having the same calibre as itself. But if the odontoblast cells secrete the dentine, as maintained by Hertz and others, how is the process to be completed when there is no longer room for an entire odontoblast or the half of an odontoblast between the rigid wall of already formed dentine and the capillary? One can hardly conceive a secreting cell going on shedding out from its end its secretion when it has been reduced to, say, one tenth of its length; and unless one is prepared to accept such a conception, this observation of the structure of a Hake's tooth-pulp becomes fatal to any "secretion" hypothesis of the formation of dentine."

THE FIRST PERMANENT MOLAR.

By J. F. Colyer, M.R.C.S., L.R.C.P., L.D.S.

Probably no tooth in the whole dental arch has given rise to more discussion as to its treatment than that of the first permanent molar, and in the following remarks no new idea has been advanced, but the question of treatment has been briefly reviewed. The six-year old molar is of special interest to us from more than one point of view.

Physiologically it is the most useful tooth in the whole arch, since it presents the largest area of crown surface, is situate in a position where mastication is greatest, and is admirably adapted to bear the strain thus put upon it, inserted as it is into the malar process, the thickest portion of the maxillary bone.

Pathologically, the first permanent molar is of interest, since it is more liable to caries than any other tooth, caused probably by its structure being weakened in its development at a period when nutrition in the child is often at fault.

The six-year olds are also of great importance in preserving the integrity of the arch, since should they be lost prior to the eruption of the second permanent molars, irregularity may frequently be caused in the other teeth ; or if later than this period, the second bicuspid and second molar will constantly tilt towards each other, and thus lose their use in mastication to some extent, or cause disarrangement of the bite.

From these facts it is evident that our decision on a course of treatment in these cases will at times be a matter of the utmost difficulty.

In the six-year old then, we have these two great characteristics, the one militating against the other, *idem est* :—its physiological utility in mastication and its pathological tendency to decay. Presuming these to be set off against each other, our treatment will almost inevitably turn upon the question of irregularity.

Probably the best method of treating the subject will be to assume the various cases that most frequently come before our notice and discuss them separately.

(i.) *Given an overcrowded mouth and moderately sound six-year olds.*—There can be no question of our treatment in these cases, the bicuspids should be removed, and the molar, a tooth of far greater importance in mastication, should be saved. The same treatment will apply when a slight cavity may exist in the six-year old molars.

Some practitioners always make it a rule to remove the six-year olds rather than the bicuspids on account of the greater liability to decay in the former. We would ask them to remember that the molar has withstood the secretions of the mouth for a much longer period than the bicuspid, and hence there is no reason why it should be a weaker tooth. We may even lay it down as a rule, that a six-year old molar remaining healthy until the age of twelve is far less prone to approximal decay than the bicuspid.

(ii.) *Given an overcrowded mouth and carious six-year olds.*—There can be no doubt that in these cases we should adopt radical treatment and not only should we extract such molars as are carious but we strenuously advise the removal of all four six-year olds. Nature will usually speedily overcome any crowding, and the gaps left will be gradually filled by the twelve-year old molars and second bicuspids. The travelling backwards of the bicuspids is brought about in the following manner: each aspect of the crown surface of these teeth presents practically an inclined plane. Now these antagonistic planes will naturally act upon one another in the direction of least resistance, and should the four six-year olds have been extracted as suggested, we get the bicuspids moving backwards to at least partially occupy the spaces left.

Should only one first permanent molar be extracted, the opposing teeth in the other jaw will be locked, we shall fail to get any natural backward action, and shall have to resort to artificial means in order to pull back the bicuspids. I need scarcely mention here that mechanical contrivances should always be avoided if possible. Again, should only one six-year old be extracted, the corresponding tooth in the other jaw is to all intents and purposes useless in mastication.

Hence with an overcrowded mouth and carious six-year olds, we strongly advise the extraction of all four.

(iii.) *Given a case with practically no overcrowding and carious six-year olds.*—The amount of decay that has taken place, and the number of six-year olds attacked by caries, must be taken into account. It is very unusual to find one of the six-year olds carious and the other three sound, but should this be the case we should be inclined to adopt conservative treatment and endeavour to save the tooth.

Now since six-year olds are so pathologically liable to decay, we shall find it at all times an exceedingly difficult matter to put a permanent filling into these teeth. We should bear this fact prominently in mind when considering our treatment. Should our filling fail shortly after insertion, we shall be worse off than ever.

Hence we should undoubtedly advise extraction of all four six-year olds should approximal decay have attacked them, and should we not feel absolutely certain of introducing a permanent filling.

As a rule the wisdom teeth, from the fact that they are placed so far back in the dental arch, are of practically little or no use in mastication. Should, however, the treatment of extraction have been adopted, they will come forward together with the second molars and take up to a large extent their normal functional use in the trituration of food. In no case, however, will they be as serviceable as the six-year olds, should the latter have been preserved.

We have yet to briefly discuss our general treatment of the six-year old and the time at which it should be extracted, presuming this course of treatment has been chosen.

Only in exceptional circumstances should we extract the first permanent molars before our patient is from eleven and a-half to twelve years old, and should they be carious, we must patch them up or treat them in the ordinary way, in order that they may last until the age specified. For stopping purposes, Sullivan's amalgam certainly stands *facile princeps*, as it appears to exert a hardening influence in the dentine. Should the pulp have to be drilled, great care must be taken with our drills, as the apical foramina are necessarily large.

Presuming then our patient has arrived at the age of twelve, the question arises, should we extract the six-year olds just as the second permanent molars are appearing through the gum, or should we wait until the latter are fully erupted? I think the time should depend on circumstances. Should our extraction be performed on account of the unhealthiness of the six-year olds, it should be proceeded with just before the eruption of the second molars, so that the latter may come well forward. Should there be much irregularity, however, and a good space is required, we must defer our operation until the second molars are fully erupted.

A PRACTICAL METHOD OF ELECTRO-GILDING GOLD DENTURES, BRIDGE-WORK, AND COLLAR CROWNS.

By H. Fielden Briggs, D.D.S.Mich., L.D.S.Glas.

First prepare in the following manner a stock solution of gilding fluid. (1) Take of pure gold 30 grains and digest in aqua regia ($H N O_3 + 3 H Cl.$); (2) evaporate *almost* but not quite to dryness; (3) dissolve this in twenty ounces of water; (4) then add half ounce of cyanide of potassium. This fluid will last a long while, and should be kept in a bottle ready for future use at any time.

To Gild: Heat gilding solution in jar in saucepan of water to about 150° Fah. While this is heating, polish the denture with whiting, wash well with plenty of soap, and place it into a basin of clean water; then avoid handling or exposing it to the air.

Attach to the positive electrode a thin sheet of fine gold, which should be not less in area than the piece to be gilded.

To the negative electrode attach the denture. When the gilding solution is heated, place the positive and negative electrodes with their attachments into it.

In a few minutes a dull brownish yellow deposit will be found on the denture. Polishing on the lathe with whiting will produce a rich deep gold appearance, giving the plate uniformity of colour, obscuring the distinctness between it and the solder, and giving a perfectly finished aspect which lasts for many years.

By using a battery of six (1 quart) Leclanché cells and keeping the sheet of gold always attached to the positive electrode, a piece can be gilded at any time in a very few minutes.

Reports.

GENERAL MEDICAL COUNCIL.

DENTAL BUSINESS.

Dr. MACNAMARA said he had been asked to bring forward a matter of some importance with reference to gentlemen whose names appeared in the Dental Register. Many of these gentlemen were anxious to get higher qualifications with the object of getting them introduced into the Dental Register, the question that he wished to ask was:

(*a*) "That whilst recognizing the fact that such are not registrable in the *Medical Register*, he will ask the PRESIDENT whether titles conferred by the several Medical Authorities subsequent to the passing of the *Medical Act* (1886), but not conferred in accordance with the provisions contained therein, said titles being conferred on Registered Dentists only after *bonâ fide* examination, are or are not registrable in the *Dentists' Register* as 'additional qualification' under the provisions of Clause 6 of Section 11 of the *Dentists' Act* (1878) which runs as follows:—

> 'The GENERAL COUNCIL may, if they think fit, from time to time make, and when made, revoke and vary orders for the registration in (on payment of the fixed fee by the orders) and the removal from the *Dentists' Register* of any additional diplomas, memberships, degrees, licences, or letters held by a person registered therein, which appear to the COUNCIL to be granted after examination by any of the Medical Authorities in respect

of a higher degree of knowledge than is required to obtain a certificate of fitness under this Act.'

(*b*) "That he will ask, through the PRESIDENT, whether it is, or is not, the opinion of this COUNCIL that, with the object of raising the status of Registered Dentists, facilities should be afforded them of obtaining such additional titles after sufficient examination."

The question resolved itself into this. They knew well enough that if anyone chose to be examined not in accordance with the requirements of the Medical Act (1886) that title would not be entitled to registration in the Medical Register inasmuch as it would not be a qualifying examination in medicine, surgery and midwifery. The first question that cropped up was as to what was meant by a higher title and he insisted on the fact that by higher qualifications was not meant a higher title in dentistry. He could refer members to several instances in the Dental Register in support of his contention. He pointed to the entry of one gentlemen who was registered as licentiate in dental surgery of the Royal College of Surgeons in Ireland, and in addition to that were appended the titles of M.D., M.Ch., of the Dublin University. He would have no difficulty in finding others, but that single example was sufficient for his purpose, viz., to show that the higher title was now necessarily one in dentistry. If these titles were given now they would not entitle the holder to registration in the Medical Register, but they would entitle him to put them in the Dental Register as additional qualifications. He urged that the very lively ambition to have a special qualification in surgery or medicine was one to be encouraged. They would not give the holders the right to practice but would appear as a feather in the cap and in fact as a higher qualification.

With reference to his next question he said he would ask whether it was or not the opinion of the Council that, with the object of raising the status of registered dentists, facilities should be afforded for enabling them to obtain additional titles after special examinations. He pointed out that no matter how high or how severe the examination might be which they might have passed it would give them no right to demand registration in the Medical Register, and therefore could be no title to practice since it would at the best only entitle them to insert it as an additional qualification in the Dental Register. If this could be legally conceded he thought that the desire was a laudable one and one to be encouraged.

The PRESIDENT said the question was a complicated one, but fortunately they had precedents to guide them. There had always been a conflict between the legal opinions obtained as to the right of the Council to act in this matter. The strict legal opinion was that the Dental Register was for Dentists only; but on the other hand, and without going into further argument he might say that it had been decided by the Council that additional qualifications might be capable of being put upon the Dental Register: they might be thereby going contrary to the opinion of their legal advisers, still the Council in the exercise of its discretion and in virtue of its powers, had ordered additional qualifications to be put upon the Dental Register. He had again taken legal opinion and again he might state that if the Council had put such qualifications on the Register they had done so solely by reason of their power. Not only had this course been taken with regard to surgical qualifications which might be thought to be more or less allied to the department of surgical dentistry, but it had been done also in respect of medical qualifications in respect of which the connection was less obvious.

Dr. MACNAMARA was anxious to know whether after an Act of Parliament had been passed which provided that no qualification should be admitted to registration in the Medical Register, unless it was a complete qualification, whether they would admit them as additional qualifications in the Dental Register. He recalled that there was nothing in the Medical Act (1886) which took away the power of the various bodies to grant diplomas, except that one of putting a single diploma upon the Medical Register. For instance, they could not prevent the College of Surgeons of England issuing their single diploma if they thought fit, although it would, of course, be valueless in so far as registration was concerned; but it could be granted nevertheless. It remained then to be seen whether that power should be continued and whether the Registrar should be allowed to put such single diplomas as additional qualifications on the Dental Register. He said that they had already exceeded their legal powers, and it remained to be settled where they would draw the line. His own opinion was that the Medical Council having exceeded its powers by putting on the Dental Register qualifications which would confer no status in regard to the Medical Register, they must ask themselves whether this power should be extended so as to include special titles by authorising the Registrar to continue to register additional qualifications on the Dental Register. He then asked the Registrar to read a report which he had drawn up on the subject.

The REGISTRAR read the report which was as follows :—" (*a*) Acting on the powers conferred by the cited Section of the Dentists' Act (1878), the General Council, on April 28th, 1881 (Minutes, vol. xviii., p. 82), resolved that every registered dentist holding any of the surgical qualifications set forth on Schedule A. of the Medical Act (1858) should have such qualification or qualifications recorded in the Dentists' Register as evidence of the possession of a higher degree of knowledge. Moreover, on July 8th, 1882 (vol. xix. p. 119), this right was extended by the Council to any or all of the qualifications named in Schedule A. of the Medical Act.

" Seeing, therefore, that the entry of such qualifications in the Dentists' Register confers no right to practise medicine or surgery, but merely records the possession of a higher degree of knowledge, the provisions of the Medical Act (1886) do not restrain the Council from registering in the Dentists' Register the titles specified in this question.

" (*b*) As to this question, that is put, through the President, to the Council itself."

The PRESIDENT said that with regard to Dr. Macnamara's second question it must be dealt with by a special motion. It was not for him, as President, to elicit the opinion of the Council on the point which he had raised.

Dr. MACNAMARA said he thought it would be more respectful if he put the question through the President.

Sir JOHN SIMON said it had been resolved that qualifications under Schedule A., possessed by dentists, should be inserted in the Dental Register, they being then qualifications to practise, but now that they had ceased to be qualifications to practise he was very doubtful whether this was at all desirable, unless it was a qualification under the Medical Act (1886). He said that if fragmentary diplomas were to be entered upon the Dental Register, it would produce great confusion in the minds of the public. He thought that it was undesirable to go on perpetuating fragmentary diplomas in any form, and that it would be much better to enact that no diplomas except under the new law were to be admitted to registration even as additional qualifications in the Dental Register.

Dr. MACNAMARA gave notice that he would bring forward a motion on the subject on the following day.

The standing orders were suspended to admit of the completion of the business in hand.

Dr. GLOVER said that in the absence of Mr. Banks he had been requested to ask a question of the President in reference to the alleged frequent admissions to the Dental Register under Clause 37 of the Dentists' Act. He pointed out that there were two ways in which a person might obtain entrance to the Dentists' Register, one by giving evidence of having passed the qualifying examination for a dentist, and the other under Clause 37 of the Dentists' Act. He contended that it was time that this method of obtaining entrance to the Dental Register should be discontinued. It was provided that registration on the ground of apprenticeship should not be continued after 1880 unless in exceptional cases, but he wished to call the attention of the Council to the fact that the registrations under Clause 37 in favour of persons who had no dental education in the present sense of the word were still continuing in considerable numbers, and if his information were correct, with considerable, he would not say carelessness, but at any rate kindness on the part of the persons responsible for this, though he did not know who really was responsibie. He called attention to the fact that the number of persons registered under Clause 37 since 1880 was larger than of regular licentiates, there being only 248 of the latter as compared with 312 of the former. He said that this condition of things excited serious dissatisfaction in the minds of those who had gone through a regular course of training when they saw others admitted to the Register without having gone through any sort of education. Mr. Banks had received letters on the subject from the President of the Irish Branch of the British Dental Association, the President of the Scottish Branch, the Central Counties Branch, the West of Scotland Branch, the Midland Branch, &c., and he himself had received several communications on the same subject. He read an extract from a letter addressed to him by the Secretary of the Midland Branch, in which it was urged that there had been ample time for all *bonâ fide* practitioners under the Act of 1878 to register.

The PRESIDENT said that Dr. Glover was to ask a question and he was waiting to hear what it was.

Dr. LEISHMAN said that he had given notice of his intention to bring forward a motion on the subject.

The PRESIDENT asked what was the question.

Dr. GLOVER said it was to ask by what authority these registrations were made, and after what kind of investigation?

The PRESIDENT requested the Registrar to read the statement that had been prepared on the subject.

The REGISTRAR read the following statement:—"Every application for registration under Section 37 of the Dentists' Act (1878) is carefully investigated, and the process of investigation sometimes occupies several months. The applicant is required to furnish, besides other particulars, a Statutory Declaration, taken before a Commissioner of Oaths, embodying all the necessary details of the case; and in this Declaration his master is required to join. A certificate of birth has, moreover, at the suggestion of the British Dental Association, been of late demanded.

"Each such application is considered by the President, and additional information, if deemed necessary, is sought for from the applicant.

"Furthermore, whenever a doubt arises in regard to any legal points in connection with such application, the case is always referred by the President to the Council's legal advisers, and is sometimes also remitted specially to the Executive Committee. An example of this may be seen on page 223 of last year's volume (xxvi.) of the Council's minutes, where it is recorded that, on November 25th, 1889, the Executive Committee directed two such apprentices to be registered.

"Applications under Clause 37 of the Dentists' Act are not unfrequently accompanied by recommendations from well-known persons, either registered dental practitioners, or registered persons, medical practitioners, or even by Members of this Council itself, as for example, one sent in on the 7th of April last, which is still under investigation.

"Vague complaints are sometimes made in regard to these special registrations, and these now and then proceed from a dental practitioner who, having himself been registered in the same way, states that the person complained of, knows nothing whatever of dentistry, and goes on to request to be furnished with full particulars in regard to the application of such person. In consequence of the vagueness of such complaints, the President on December 6th, 1889, found it necessary for the conduct of the business of the office to direct the Registrar to state that if application were made in writing by a secretary or other authorised person on behalf of the British Dental Association an answer would be sent in each particular case, giving the information desired.

"Accordingly, on February 14th, 1890, in reply to such a request from the Secretary of the British Dental Association, the Registrar, with the President's authorization, furnished—in regard to what was considered as a typical case—the fullest information, including even the name of the Commissioner of Oaths, before whom the Statutory Declaration was made; but, hitherto, nothing further has been heard about the case.

"Thus, all possible care is taken in regard to applications under the said Section of the Dentists' Act, though, in consequence of the framers of the Act having placed no limit of time to such form of registration, such applicants cannot legally be rejected, as, in fact, has been intimated by solicitors acting for certain applicants. For dentists who were in practice before July 22nd, 1878, a distinct limit of time was set forth in the Act; but in regard to these applications under Section 37, no limit whatever is prescribed in the Act.

"Of necessity, by lapse of time these applications are diminished in number. For five months past there have been received no more than ten of any kind; of these four have been summarily rejected, four have been acceded to, and two are still under investigation."

Thursday, June 5th.

Mr. MARSHALL, President, in the chair.

On the motion of Dr. HERON WATSON, seconded by Dr. PETTIGREW, it was agreed, "That the Dental Committee appointed under Clause 15 of the Dentists' Act, for the purpose of erasure from, and restoration to the Dentists' Register, consist of the following members:—The President (chairman), Sir William Turner, Sir Dyce Duckworth, Dr. Macnamara, Dr. Quain."

Dr. MACNAMARA moved: That it is the opinion of this Council that, with the object of raising the status of Registered Dentists, facilities should be afforded them of obtaining such additional titles, after sufficient examination, as are mentioned in Sub-section 6, Section 11, of the Dentists' Act (1878). He said it was desirable to get in the minds of dentists a wish to obtain higher qualifications than those which entitled them to be put on the Dentists' Register. They should be encouraged to raise themselves from the mere mechanical to the more surgical aspect of disease. He did not think much argument was necessary to enforce the view that the Council would look with pleasure on anything that would improve the status of the dental practitioner. Several Irish practitioners had got themselves as it were, out of the ruck. It was a very praiseworthy, laudable ambition to get a qualification entitling him to be on the Medical Register as well as on the Dentists' Register, and the Council should encourage that as much as possible.

Mr. CARTER seconded the motion.

Sir WILLIAM TURNER asked Dr. Macnamara how he proposed that the facilities should be afforded for obtaining such additional titles. He thought that the motion should read that facilities should be afforded by the authorities conferring qualifications.

Dr. MACNAMARA was quite willing to add those words.

Sir WILLIAM TURNER: Does Dr. Macnamara mean dental qualifications or medical qualifications?

Mr. MILLER: It must be medical, because the whole thing refers to what has been registered as additional qualifications hitherto, namely, surgical and medical qualifications.

Sir WILLIAM TURNER: Then kindly insert "facilities should be afforded them by the medical authorities."

Sir JOHN SIMON asked if there was any reason to suppose that the Bodies did not afford facilities.

The PRESIDENT said the College of Surgeons would very likely ask the question whether they could really hold such an examination now, but if the Council declared their opinion it would lead the way to their affording such facilities.

The resolution was thereupon agreed to in the following form:— "That it is the opinion of this Council that with the object of raising the status of Registered Dentists, facilities should be afforded them by the medical authorities for obtaining such additional titles after sufficient examination as are mentioned in Sub-section 6, Section 11 of the Dentists' Act, (1878.")

Notice of motion had been given by Dr. LEISHMAN, "That the attention of the Dental Committee be called to the frequency with which the names of certain persons are still entered on the Dentists' Register under Section 37 of the Dentists' Act, 1878.

The PRESIDENT said he wished to explain that the purposes for which the Dental Committee were appointed did not include this function. They were appointed for a special purpose, and they could not undertake other duties.

Mr. MILLER said they were appointed for a special purpose, which was set forth very clearly in the Dentists' Act.

Dr. GLOVER hoped that the consideration of the matter would be deferred until the next day.

Dr. LEISHMAN: Do I understand that this is incompetent as a motion?

The PRESIDENT: I think so. That is my impression.

Dr. LEISHMAN: Is it competent to move that a certain question relating to dentists may be remitted to the Dental Committee for consideration?

Mr. MILLER: The Committee is appointed for a special purpose in respect to the erasure of names from the Dental Register.

Dr. LEISHMAN: Then alter it to the Executive Committee, and I give notice of that for to-morrow.

Friday, June 6th.

Mr. MARSHALL, President, in the chair.

Dr. LEISHMAN, in moving "That the attention of the Executive Committee be called to the frequency with which the names of certain persons are still entered on the Dentists' Register under Section 37 of the Dentists' Act (1878)," said that this subject had been brought under his notice by several members who occupied a high position in the dental profession, and who were all gentlemen who had gone through a curriculum, and passed an examination and who had become somewhat impatient that the operation of certain clauses of the Dentists' Act should cease. He was quite aware that the Council had no power to say that this action was to cease, and he would not now bring it under the notice of the Council if he had not what he believed was clear evidence that there had been a great amount of fraud and wilful misrepresentation. Men's names under Clause 37 had been put on the Dentists' Register on false evidence and false affidavits. The curious thing was that this was a clause by which it was made possible under the Dentists' Act, which said: "Any person who has been articled as a pupil and has paid a premium to a dental practitioner entitled to be registered under this Act, in consideration of receiving from such practitioner a complete dental education shall, if his articles expire before the first day of January, 1880, be entitled to be registered under this Act." His indentures, therefore, ought to have terminated on January 1st, 1880. One would think that ten or twelve years after the passing of the Act the number of these men would be dwindling away, more especially as the longest term of apprenticeship in such a case that he ever heard of was seven years. Twelve years had passed, but he was told that last year there was a considerable increase in the number of men who presented themselves for registration under the clause. He knew himself of several cases of men who could not by any possibility be described under the terms of the first paragraph of the clause—men who were simply workmen, but who, somehow or other, managed to get themselves interpreted as apprentices. One case was very striking. He had the real initials, and from the date he could identify the individual on the Register. He would call him A. B. He was admitted to the Register in 1888 under Clause 37 of the Dentists' Act of 1878. He was apprenticed in a town in an eastern county after the passing of the Act. Then the first step towards registration was that he applied for it and was refused, but on what ground he (Dr. Leishman) was not informed. Then on further application by a solicitor, the Dental Committee decided to consider the matter on an affidavit by the man to whom A. B. was apprenticed. He declined to make the affidavit, having already dated back the indentures, and regretted it, and he was afraid of getting into trouble if he made an affidavit. Finally A. B. was accepted upon an affidavit that his master would not make an affidavit. He (Dr. Leishman) knew something of the class of men who had gone on the Register under this clause, and it was strange that the numbers were so large after twelve years. Gentlemen who had got to the position of dentists on the higher level were very much annoyed, and looked to the Council, with some show of reason, for some sympathy. They would be pleased to know that the Council would turn attention in this direction, and do something to prevent the evil. He believed they had a most substantial grievance.

Dr. Glover seconded the motion. The President was kind enough to give an answer to his question, and to say that by lapse of time these applications were diminishing in number. Last year there were twenty-nine, the year before twenty-four, the year before only nine. In the last three years there had been sixty-two; in the previous three years fifty-seven, so that the process of diminution was not going on so fast as could be wished. The President also said that every application was most carefully investigated. That, he was sure, was the intention, but the cases showed that the amount of attention was insufficient to detect serious defects. Following Dr. Leishman's example he would not mention names, but he would give a second example. The man and the master had both sworn to the facts. The facility with which certain facts were sworn to was very painful. It was even possible to get man and master to swear to things that did not bear investigation. Then it might be said that additional information was got from the applicant, but the applicant was an interested party, and if he had made up his mind to it he went on giving information. Then it was said if there was any doubt the Committee applied to the legal adviser of the Council. On page 228 of the volume for 1889, it was said, "Read application from two apprentices, with opinions from the Council's legal advisers to the effect that, although it is doubtful whether these applicants have a right to claim registration, the Executive Committee has in such cases power to make direction for registration." There the legal advisers were evidently against the registration, but the Executive Committee were of very kindly mind, and seemed to be generally inclined to yield. One sentence, there was that much dissatisfaction arose from rival practitioners. He thought that was an unhappy phrase. One case was that of a man who at the time of his application was a joiner, and still was a joiner. When he applied for registration he was fifty years of age, while the master when he assumed that position was of the ripe age of eighteen years. He had now slipped off the Register, and was in the occupation of a driver of a tram-car, no doubt being engaged in a business for which he was better fitted. Mr. Miller had addressed several letters to him, but happily he was too busy to answer him. He (Dr. Glover) was informed that the President was warned of these facts before registration was effected.

The President: Will you give the date of that case?

Dr. Glover said the man was registered in 1889, but he did not wish to give particulars, as his object was not personal. He did not know that he need say more, having, he thought, said enough to show that this state of matters must be remedied. Dr. Leishman's notice seemed slightly inadequate—just enough to direct the attention of the Executive Committee to the serious nature of some of their admissions to the Register, but he would not ask for any addition to the motion at present. He suggested that the members of the Council should have time to make enquiries before the registration was actually granted.

Sir W. FOSTER said the Council generally erred on the side of good nature. Some time ago he wrote to the Registrar about a case of this kind, and in the future he should be very careful about recommending anybody for the Dental Register who had not gone through the curriculum. No doubt they all had confidence in the carefulness of the Committee, who, while careful in the past, would be still more so in the future.

The PRESIDENT said he had not the smallest objection to passing the resolution; on the contrary, he should be exceedingly pleased. Of all the unpleasant duties he had to perform these were the most unpleasant. He could give no answer with regard to the cases that had been mentioned, because he had not investigated them. He had, however, investigated each individual case as it came before him, and had obtained the information which the rules required him to. What more could he do? Was he to constitute himself as a kind of detective policeman? Was he to send round and ascertain whether this man or that was actually declaring a falsehood? There was a remedy. If the British Dental Association showed clearly that some false statement was made, of course action could be taken. As to the proposal that these things should be submitted to individual members of the Council, he was quite sure that without a great deal of trouble they do not get better information than they received now. They must take documents as they appeared on the face of them. If a man declared he was able to be a master at the age of eighteen that was his fault. The advantage the British Dental Association had over the Committee was that they searched the record and tried to find out something after the man was let in. Theirs was an *ex post facto* examination. The Committee were entrusted with certain powers, and they faithfully carried them out, but if the Council wished anything more to be done he did not object. There was nothing like negligence on the part of the Committee, and sometimes they took legal advice as to their actual position. If they were cheated there was a mode by which punishment could be secured, but if the Executive Committee were expected to examine into all these cases the Council must be prepared for a sitting of the Executive Committee to last four days or a week. He could see no objection except on the score of expense.

Dr. LEISHMAN said his object was simply to get the matter looked at by the Executive Committee, in order to ascertain if there was any better way of managing these things. If the gentlemen who had dental qualifications were aware that the Council took some interest in their affairs it would help them considerably.

Dr. HERON WATSON said that in some cases, at all events, the British Dental Association had proved that certain persons had given false affidavits. The best thing for them to do was to bring a few prosecutions, which would do a great deal of good. It was impossible for the President or any member of the Executive Committee to do it.

The motion was agreed to.

DENTAL BOARD OF VICTORIA.

THE ordinary meeting was held on 28th March, at 8 p.m. Present—Dr. L. A. CARTER, D.D.S. (in the chair), Messrs. KERNOT, and POTTS.

The minutes of the second annual meeting were read, and were found to be correct.

The minutes of the previous meeting were duly read and confirmed.

The UNDER-SECRETARY (Mr. T. R. Wilson) wrote, by direction of Mr. Deakin, to acknowledge the receipt of the Board's letter of the 14th of March submitting a report of the proceedings of the Dental Board of Victoria during the year ending 28th February, together with a statement of the receipts and expenditure for the same period.

The CHIEF COMMISSIONER OF POLICE wrote to advise the Board of the name of the dentist who was recently alleged in the Press to have been guilty of indecent behaviour towards a female patient. The police were unable to obtain such evidence as would justify a criminal charge against the person in question.

CHARLES BRANDT, of Wandong, wrote to inquire if he could practise as a dentist in Victoria. From the facts stated in the letter it appeared that the applicant had a certificate of competency, and had passed the examinations required in Stockholm, Sweden.

The Board decided to request the applicant to forward full particulars of his career—number of years in practice, &c.—for its information, and his certificates, for inspection.

George N. Heyward, an applicant for registration as a dentist, protested against being called upon to pay the full fee for registration, and gave a number of reasons why this should not be insisted upon. The Board had already decided that the full fee demanded by law must be charged. Applicant to be advised that the Board saw no reason to alter its previous decision.

Mr. Alfred Boot (of Dunedin, N. Z.), wrote to make inquiries as to the particulars of the "modified examination" which one Charles William Hay had passed, as Hay was an applicant for registration in New Zealand. The Board decided to furnish the writer with a copy of the regulations under which the examination was held, and to advise him that the examination was a very elementary one, consisting of *viva voce* questions before the whole Board, and that it had been held to remedy the grievance caused by the fact that the candidates had been unable, owing to unforeseen circumstances, to make application for registration by the time prescribed by the statute.

Mr. George Thomson, L.D.S., wrote to say that he had been advised that an unregistered man was practising as a dentist at Dr. Singleton's dispensary, Collingwood. According to section 17 of the Act, No. 960, no person shall hold any appointment as a dentist or dental practitioner or dental surgeon in any hospital, infirmary, dispensary, or lying-in-hospital, unless he is registered under the Act as a dentist or is a legally qualified medical practitioner. The Board decided to draw Dr. Singleton's attention to this section of the Act, and to inquire if there was a dentist in the institution referred to, and if so, to ask for his name.

Clement Haddon, a registered dental student, wrote to inquire whether four years' professional education would be insisted upon for candidates for the "modified examination;" his indentures were for three years only. The Board decided to advise the writer that it considered that upon completion of his indentures he was entitled to present himself for the "modified examination."

Edmund E. Howarth, a registered dental student, wrote to inquire what text-books would be necessary for the "modified examination." Applicant to be advised that the information would be forwarded as soon as possible.

The editor of the *Australasian Journal of Pharmacy* wrote to say that he would be pleased to publish monthly the report of the minutes of the meetings of the Dental Board.

W. D. MACGREGOR furnished the necessary explanation with regard to a discrepancy in his articles of indenture. The applicant was accordingly registered as a dental student entitled to go up for the "modified examination."

JOSEPH ABRAHAM and ARTHUR H. BELL applied to be registered under the third schedule, and forwarded their articles of registration for inspection. The Board decided to register both applicants as dentists.

The sub-committee appointed to arrange the text-books for the "modified examination" were requested to meet during the month.

Mr. POTTS and the SECRETARY were appointed a sub-committee to obtain a seal for the Board.

Ordinary accounts were passed for payment, and the Board adjourned.

DENTAL ASSOCIATION OF VICTORIA.

THE Council of the Dental Association met on Thursday evening, the 20th March. The president, Dr. SPRINGTHORPE, occupied the chair. There were also present—Messrs. Iliffe, Carter, Clarke, George, Kernot, M'Gregor, Reeve, Stevens, and Thomson. The secretary reported that he had had an interview with Mr. Lynch, the deputy sheriff, and pointed out that registered dentists were now, by law, exempt from attendance on juries. It was decided to furnish the sheriff with the list of registered dentists, so that their names might be omitted from the jury roll. Mr. Alfred H. Lewes, of Branxton, New South Wales, and Mr. R. Shackell, of Coburg, were unanimously elected members of the Association. The sub-committee furnished their report with regard to the immediate establishment of a dental college and hospital in Melbourne. The report was received and discussed, and its further consideration was adjourned.

THE STUDENTS' SOCIETY OF THE VICTORIA DENTAL HOSPITAL OF MANCHESTER.

THE fifth annual meeting of the above Society was held May 22nd. Mr. DAVID HEADRIDGE in the chair.

The minutes being read and confirmed, Messrs. F. L. Tanner, and G. Kershaw were admitted members.

Mr. J. C. LINGFORD presented a model of a lower jaw showing a supplemental canine.

Mr. P. R. SIBSON exhibited a well-marked case of dilaceration.

The report of the Council giving a brief *resumé* of the work of the past session was received with much applause.

The Treasurer's report showed a balance to the credit of the Society of £18 9s.

The CURATOR's (Mr. D. Headridge) report of the library and museum showed an increase in both the number of books and specimens presented.

The following were elected officers for the ensuing session:—

President.—G. G. Campion, Esq.

Vice-Presidents.—H. C. Smale, Esq.; G. O. Whittaker, Esq.; P. A. Linnell, Esq.; C. H. Smale, Esq.

Secretaries.—Mr. P. R. Sibson (re-elected), Mr. J. C. Lingford.

Treasurer.—Mr. D. Headridge (re-elected).

Curator and Librarian.—Mr. J. C. Stokoe.

Councillors.—Messrs. Coogan, Fisher, Sherratt, Stokoe.

DENTAL HOSPITAL OF LONDON ATHLETIC CLUB.

THE Third Annual Dinner of the above Club was held on Saturday, May 31st, at the Holborn Restaurant, the chair being taken by J. SMITH-TURNER. Nearly one hundred were present, the evening proving as anticipated, very successful. The usual loyal toasts having been proposed and duly honoured, the Chairman in an appropriate speech proposed the "Dental Hospital of London Athletic Club," coupling with it the names of the two energetic secretaries, Messrs. FORSYTH and PREEDY; Mr. PREEDY, in replying, referred to the success of the club during the past year, stating that he thought it had now obtained a firm footing. The other toasts proposed were those of the "Hospital Staff" by Mr. C. S. TOMES, responded to by Mr. MORTON SMALE (Dean); the "Visitors" by Mr. WOODHOUSE, responded to by Mr. J. TURNER; and the "Chairman" by Mr. HEPBURN. The Musical Society contributed selections during the evening; Messrs. Hepburn, Barrett, and Wheatly also assisting with solos, the singing of "Auld Lang Syne" bringing a very pleasant evening to a close.

Dental News.

Clifford and Another *v.* Brown.—Mr. Justice Grantham, sitting without a jury, heard the above cause. This was an action brought to recover £111 arrears of weekly payments agreed to be paid by the defendant to the plaintiffs in respect of the practice of a dentist at Ealing. The facts were shortly as follows:—By an agreement dated June 23, 1886, between the plaintiffs and defendant, the plaintiffs agreed to take the defendant into their service for a term of one year as a general dental assistant. The plaintiffs were to pay the defendant £4 per week salary, and a further £5 for every £100 received by the defendant. The salary and commision were guaranteed to be not less than £5 per week. The defendant was to pay the plaintiffs £40 per annum for the house, Lyncombe Villa, Ealing, by weekly instalments, and the defendant was to devote the whole of his time to the practice. After the defendant had had three months' trial it was agreed that the defendant should keep all the fees of the practice and should pay the plaintiffs the weekly sum of £3 for twelve years from July 3rd, 1886; then the practice, furniture, instruments and house were to become the defendant's property. It was alleged on the part of the plaintiffs that the sum of £111 was due in respect of the said weekly payments. The defendant denied liability, and further contended that it was agreed that the practice of a dentist should continue to be carried on and advertised under the name and style of Clifford Eskell, but that the plaintiffs refused to carry on the practice under that name and style, and withdrew the advertisements of the said practice, whereby the defendant became discharged from his agreement, and he counter-claimed for damages in respect of the plaintiffs' refusal to carry on practice under the said name, and the withdrawal of the advertisements. Mr. Justice Grantham gave judgment for the plaintiffs for the amount claimed with costs. Mr. G. Candy, Q.C., and Mr. Rosenthal were for the plaintiffs; Mr. Channell, Q.C., and Mr. H. Lloyd for the defendant.

PARTRIDGE *v.* GENERAL COUNCIL OF MEDICAL EDUCATION AND REGISTRATION.

This was an appeal from the judgment of Mr. Baron Huddleston at the trial of the action. The action was brought for unlawfully and maliciously removing the plaintiff's name from the Dentists

Register kept by the defendants under the Dentists Act, 1878. It appeared that in 1868 the plaintiff commenced practising as a dentist in London, and under the Dentists Act, 1878, for the first time a register of dentists was required to be kept. The plaintiff was at this date engaged in practising dentistry, but he did not wish to be entered on the Register in respect of having so practised, and accordingly he passed an examination and obtained a diploma from the Royal College of Surgeons in Ireland as a licentiate in dental surgery, and was entered on the Dentists' Register in respect of this qualification. Every applicant for a diploma is required by the Royal College of Surgeons in Ireland to declare that if the diploma is granted he will not seek to attract business by advertising or by any practice considered by the College to be unbecoming, and that he agrees that the diploma shall be cancelled on its being proved to the satisfaction of the President and Council of the College that he has done so. The plaintiff entered into this undertaking. In 1883 the plaintiff became suddenly blind, and was unable to attend personally to his practice. He thereupon started a dental institution in South Kensington, and employed qualified assistants, whom he paid. He advertised this Institution. In July, 1885, the College of Surgeons in Ireland withdrew the plaintiff's diploma on the ground that he had advertised in connection with his profession and notified this fact to the General Council of Medical Education and Registration. This latter body, upon the ground that the plaintiff had lost his qualification, on June 2nd, 1886, ordered his name to be erased from the Dentists' Register. A *mandamus* was granted by the Court directing the Council to restore the plaintiff's name to the Register on the ground that they had not held any inquiry and had not acted under Sections 13 and 15 of the Dentists Act, 1878. The case is reported in 19 Q.B.D., 467. The plaintiff's name was accordingly restored to the Register on September 18, 1887, and the plaintiff brought this action to recover damages for the wrongful erasure of his name during this period. The General Medical Council subsequently held an inquiry under Section 15 of the Act, and on November 25th, 1887, ordered the plaintiff's name to be removed from the Register. The action was tried before Mr. Baron Huddleston without a jury, and he held that the action was not maintainable without evidence of malice, and gave judgment for the defendants. The plaintiff appealed.

Mr. Waddy, Q.C., and Mr. Lyon, for the plaintiff, contended that the defendants were acting not in a judicial capacity, but in a ministerial capacity, in removing the plaintiff's name from the Register, as they did not purport to act under Sections 13 and 15. Secondly, if the defendants were acting as a *quasi*-judicial body, the fact of their removal of the name without any inquiry was evidence of malice. The trial was begun with a jury, when the learned Judge said that he was prepared to nonsuit the plaintiff on the ground that there was no evidence of malice. To enable the plaintiff to appeal straight to the Court of Appeal, the jury were discharged by consent and the Judge gave judgment for the defendants. But it must be taken as if the Judge held that there was no evidence of malice to go to the jury, and if he was wrong in that there should be a new trial.

Mr. Reid, Q.C., and Mr. Muir Mackenzie, for the defendants, contended that, whether the defendants acted under Section 11, or under Section 13 in erasing the plaintiff's name, they were not acting in a merely ministerial capacity, but were acting judicially.

The Court dismissed the appeal.

The Master of the Rolls said that the case was being tried with a jury, when, for a reason which he could never understand, the case was left to be tried by the Judge without the jury. That was equivalent to treating the case as if the jury had never been there, and the question whether or not there was evidence of malice to go to the jury could not arise. The Judge must have found, and must be taken to have found, that there was no malice. No one could possibly suggest any malice. There was, therefore, no malice in fact. Then how did the defendants fulfil the duty imposed upon them by the statute? He would undertake to inform them how they ought to act when inquiring whether a name should be erased from the Register. They ought to make careful inquiry whether there was any ground for doing so, and they ought to communicate with the person against whom any accusation was made and ask for his explanations. He did not go so far as to say that they ought to hear the witnesses, if there were any, in the presence of the accused, but they ought to communicate the evidence to him and ask for his explanations upon it. They ought to do this before deciding erase a name. It was quite clear that the defendants had not done in this case what they ought to have done, and the Court had granted a *mandamus* to re-insert the plaintift's name in the register. But it was quite a different question whether an action would lie against the defendants for having acted wrongly. The duties were imposed upon them by the Dentists Act, 1878, and they were intending to act under the Act. Assuming that they were acting under Section 13, then, in his opinion they were acting in a judicial capacity. It was said that they intended to act under Section 11, and not under Section 13. In his opinion, if they intended to act under the Act, and erroneously acted under the wrong Section, they would not be liable if the act was not merely ministerial. But assuming that they acted under Section 11, was their act a merely ministerial act? He thought clearly not. In his opinion the giving an order to the Registrar under that Section was not a merely ministerial act, but depended upon the exercise of their discretion. This proposition seemed to him to be true—that where a public duty was imposed upon persons by statute, and that duty consisted in the exercise of a discretion, the act done in performance of that duty could not be said to be merely ministerial, but must for the purposes of protection be considered as judicial. The protection could only be got rid of by showing that the act was ministerial. The protection, therefore, existed in this case, there being no malice, and the appeal must be dismissed.

Lord Justice Fry agreed that where there was a public duty imposed by statute, and a discretion conferred in the exercise of that duty, the duty was a judicial and not a ministerial duty. The scheme of the Dentists Act, was that the Registrar should perform the ministerial acts, and the duties of the General Council with respect to the Registrar were of a judicial character. The General Council in this case seemed to have considered that the Register must automatically follow the qualification, and that they had power to make such corrections by giving an order to the Registrar to that effect. They were wrong, but they were exercising a discretion in giving the order to the Registrar which the statute conferred upon them. The General Council had no duties in connection with the Register which were not discretionary in their nature. In his opinion, for these reasons the General Council were acting in the exercise of a discretion imposed upon them, and were therefore acting judiciously. The action, therefore, would not lie without proof of malice.

Lord Justice Lopes concurred.

THE FIRST PROSECUTION UNDER THE NEW ZEALAND DENTISTS ACT.

THE first prosecution under the New Zealand Dentists Act for the unlawful assumption of the title of dentist marks an epoch in the colonial history of this branch of the medical profession. In Christchurch, on March 6th, J. D. Hellewell was charged before Mr. R. Beetham, R.M., on the information of Audley Edward Merewether, that, not being a legally qualified medical practitioner, and not being registered under "The Dentists Act, 1880," nor under any other legal enactment, he did unlawfully use the title of dentist. Evidence was taken, Mr. Joynt appearing for the informant, Mr. Widdowson for defendant. The Bench imposed a fine of £5, with costs. This conviction practically dispels the opinion that a "carriage and four" may be driven through the New Zealand Dentists Act with impunity, and will cause less surprise than the long delay in testing this question, and that initial proceedings should be left to the sole responsibility of a dental student. In June last, at a meeting of dental delegates held in Wellington, a New Zealand Dental Association was formed upon the bases of the British Dental Association, and which a few weeks ago held its first conference at Dunedin. One of the primary objects of this Association is to maintain the provisions and carry out the intention of the Dentists Act, in other words to prevent the use of the title of Dentist, or any equivalent thereof, and the practice of dentistry by any but legally qualified persons, that is by persons whose names appear upon the Dental Register of New Zealand, or upon that of the United Kingdom, or Imperial Register. At the recent conference several cases were cited of at least *primâ facie* gross violations of that Act, demanding prompt legal action. Was the Association prepared to institute proceedings? The Dentists Act, it was said though evident as to intention, was inexact and incomplete in its wording, and could be evaded; that, as it now stood, it would be impossible to obtain a conviction. Eminent legal opinion, it was believed, had confirmed this impression. It was decided to obtain further legal opinion. Accordingly, the question of the adequacy of the Act as now worded, and of the legal liability of the alleged cases of violation, was placed before Sir Robert Stout, who held that the Act as it now stood was quite adequate to deal with such cases, and that where the Act was as he deemed defective an amendment could be readily drafted and make "assurance doubly sure." Events, however, moved faster than the action of the Association. The Association, it was thought by some, was cautious to timidity. It was rightly felt by dental students, who, at great cost, were loyally complying with the conditions of the Act, and in some instances seeking higher qualifications than the Act demanded, to be a gross injustice that others who had not complied with those conditions, and who held no legal qualification whatever, should be allowed to practise as if duly registered and qualified. Better no law than a law any man sufficiently unscrupulous could evade with safety. It was simply the deep sense of this injustice, and probably a degree of impatience at the cautious step of the Association, that led Mr. Merewether, a dental student of Christchurch, to institute, solely on his own responsibility, the above prosecution. The premature and widespread decay and loss of the teeth in this and other Australasian colonies is on all hands acknowledged and deplored. How far this miserably defective dental condition affects the public health in these colonies it is impossible to tell—that it does so to a serious and depressing extent cannot be doubted. Yet the difficulty of preserving the teeth is great, and becomes greater every year. This is the vocation of the dentist, his most legitimate as it is his most beneficent task—how difficult and important, and how necessary and reasonable the public demand for the best possible skill and treatment, is shown by the fact that throughout Europe and America the standard of qualification has been raised higher and higher.—*New Zealand Herald.*

CLAIM FOR RENT.

Croydon Building Society v. Goodman.—This was a claim for £13 15s., for one quarter and a-half's rent for rooms at 92, North End. An agreement was put in showing that a person called Dr. J. Wilks, who represented himself as the manager of the Dental Supply Company, took the rooms on behalf of that Company at a rental of £50 a year. That company, it was stated, was composed of the defendant, Mr. Goodman, and two others whom they had difficulty in finding, and therefore they sued Mr. Goodman, treating Dr. J. Wilks as his agent.

Mr. Black said the defence was that the defendant, Mr. Goodman, was not a member of the Dental Supply Company, and gave no instructions for the taking of these rooms.

Various letters were put in on behalf of plaintiffs, including one from the defendant, dated the 3rd of December, in which he stated that Mr. Wilks was not in his employ, nor was he then a member of the Dental Supply Company at Croydon. Another letter from Mr. Wilks, dated 30th December, stated that he was sorry to say, from circumstances over which he had no control, that he was unable to begin business in Croydon as the Dental Supply Company, and enclosing the key of the premises, together with £5 for his liability. That, Mr. Bower (counsel for plaintiffs) said, of itself would show that Wilks was the tenant, but they had a clerk to show that the money was actually paid on behalf of the defendant Goodman, and that the ingenious trick was resorted to in order to evade the liability of the latter. Mr. Bower stated that in the rooms at North End were found some papers advertising a "revolution in dentistry."

His HONOUR: A blessed one, I hope.

Mr. BOWER: A bloodless one. Those advertisements were exactly the same as those issued by Mr. Goodman at Ludgate Hill, where he practised, the only difference being that Mr. Goodman's name was on those issued at Ludgate Hill, and that of the Dental Supply Association, Croydon, on those found on the premises at North End.

Mr. BLACK then stated the defence, that Wilks was not at the time he took the rooms in the employ of the Dental Supply Association, but that he intended to set up for himself, and adopted that title as he was not a registered dentist.

Evidence was called in support of the above statement, and his Honour then summed up. He said in this case the defendant was sued for certain rent due under an agreement which was made by a man of the name of Wilks, purporting to be carrying on business as "The Dental Supply Association," in premises at North End. Wilks did not remain there very long, in fact he levanted without paying the first quarter's rent. The defendant Goodman was sued in consequence for this rent, when he replied that Wilks had no authority from him to pledge his credit, and further that he was never a member of the firm of the Dental Supply Association at Croydon, although he knew Wilks. Mr. Goodman had been called, and he said that he had been carrying on business with his brother in St. Paul's Churchyard, under the name of the Dental Supply Association, but that the Association had been dissolved nearly two years ago, and that it never had anything to do with the Dental Supply Association at Croydon. It was a grave question as to how far Mr. Goodman was to be believed, and he (his Honour) regretted that he had come to the conclusion that Mr. Goodman was not a gentleman whose word could be accepted. In the first place, Mr. Goodman, according to his own confession, was asked whether he considered Mr. Wilks a fit and proper person to rent the premises, and he was bound to tell the simple truth. But what did he do? He knew that Wilks had been a failure at West Bromwich, and was in an impecunious state; but he sat down in a deliberate manner and gave Wilks a good character, stating that he would be found a good and reliable tenant. That was not the action of an honest man, but was most dishonourable and dishonest, and he believed it was written solely for the purpose of deceiving Mr. Auber. There was another point in the case, why did Goodman pay £5? It might have been a good thing to do, but probably it was a case of conscience, but he did not pay it like a man, and tell the plaintiff "Well, I'm very sorry, Wilks is gone, and the affair is a failure." No! He went to some solicitor and sent the money as coming from a friend. The whole thing savoured of trickery, and was not done in a straightforward manner, and he (his Honour) could not but come to the conclusion that for certain purposes Dr. Wilks and Mr. Goodman were one and the same. He gave judgment for the plaintiff for the whole amount.

A CHESHIRE FARMER AND HIS FALSE TEETH.

A CASE was heard at Crewe County Court on April 9th, before his Honour Judge Hughes, in which the plaintiff was Charles Edwards, farmer, of Nantwich, who sought to recover £20 from Albert Maurice, dentist, of Liverpool, for the detention of a set of teeth. The plaintiff's evidence was that several years ago he bought a set of teeth for £15. The teeth were plated with gold and encased in vulcanite. A few months ago he went to the defendant and requested him to make some alterations in the upper case so as to make the teeth more comfortable. The alterations were made, and afterwards, at plaintiff's suggestion, the lower set was repaired. Subsequently, while sitting in the defendant's room, the plaintiff suddenly jumped up and demanded an explanation, stating that he had not received back his right set of teeth—that while his teeth were set in a gold plate and cost £15, the set produced were largely vulcanite, and there was not a pound's worth of gold on the case. There was a scene in the defendant's office, and because the plaintiff declined to leave the defendant walked out. The plaintift's wife and daughter described the original set of teeth with the gold plate. The defendant said that the gold on the old case had been placed on the new, and while he could not swear it was the same piece of gold, he believed it was. A man named Rigby, who modelled the case, said it was the same piece of gold, and that none of it had been taken away. The judge said that the action suggested a serious accusation against the defendant, for which there was no ground. He gave judgment for the defendant with costs.

EXTRACTS.

A BOGUS UNIVERSITY.—THE SALE OF AMERICAN DIPLOMAS.

A MOST astounding account of the systematic way in which the business of selling the degree of M.D. has been conducted in some parts of America was recently published by the *Boston Sunday Herald*. According to the report before us, there are five of these "bogus diploma mills" in the United States (one each in New Jersey, New York, Ohio, Vermont, and New Hampshire), and one in Canada, at Montreal. The investigations of our contemporary were specially directed to the proceedings of an institution calling itself by a high-sounding title—"Universitas Trinitatis, Collegium Medicinæ et Chirurgiæ, Reipublicæ Vermontis." Its Dean lately forwarded to Mr. A. H. G. Hardwicke, described as a well-known hardware dealer of Buffalo, a beautiful Latin diploma which declared that the faculty admitted him to the rank of doctor of medicine, with "all rights, freedoms and honours belonging to that station." Now, it does not appear that Mr. Alan H. G. Hardwicke had proved anything of the kind, nor that the "examining instructors" had had, or indeed seriously sought, any opportunity of ascertaining that he was "well grounded in medicine and surgery." In fact Mr. Hardwicke knew nothing of medicine or surgery, being, as has been already said, a successful and respected dealer in hardware. For the purpose of investigating and, if possible, exposing the whole system, he applied to the person calling himself Dr. H. F. Bradbury, Dean of the Trinity University.

At first some small pretence was made of requiring some sort of examination. This is what "the Dean" says in his first letter :—

"We can get you a much better article than the Bellevue. We can get you an article from a college in Ohio for 150 dols., dated 1880, or one from a university in one of the New England States for 60 dols. This latter will be dated the coming May. Your brother has ordered one of the latter. I enclose circular. All business must be done with me, not sent to the university. I should like very much to see you. Wish you could come this way, and when here get your article. You should send thesis, and also pass some kind of examination, so you can swear in court of law it was granted after due examination. Send money by express." This was on the 13th of April, 1889. By the 22nd of April the Dean will be more easily satisfied as to his correspondent being able to show that he is well grounded in medicine and surgery. "If you write a good thesis," he tells him, "we will pass you on the examination." The *Herald* having made inquiries on the spot, it was finally determined that Mr. Hardwicke should attempt to obtain one of the diplomas. No great difficulty was encountered, and, after a little fencing, the Dean consented, on the 18th of August, "To send the goods c. o. d. This," he adds, "is something I never did, and it is not customary in this business. However, if you give me your word as a gentleman that you will take the article from the expressman just as soon as it gets to Buffalo, without any delay or exposure, I will send it." Accordingly, the following letter was, on the 27th of August, 1889, addressed to "Dear Mr. Hardwicke," whom the writer, so far as appears, had never seen, "We have shipped to you this a.m. goods, c.o.d. 60 dollars, per agreement. We sent by the name of E. L. Needham, as we did not wish to put our name on the express. Please take it as soon as arrived.—Yours faithfully, Dr. Bradbury." In it the recipent, "a well-known dealer in hardware," be it remembered, found his learning set forth in most official Latin :—"Quoniam inter omnia Academica Corpora, secundum leges institua [*sic*] mos antiquus et honestus factus est, magno honore donare, eos qui studium fideliter dederint Literis et Scientiæ et Artibus Utilibus, atque se interdum integriter portaverint, Igitur quum Alan H. G. Hardwicke" [hardware merchant, to wit !] "Nobis se Arti Medicinæ per tempus usitatum et secundum leges operam dedisse demonstrait" [*sic*], and so on.

Secundum leges, there is the rub. The articles of incorporation had been duly "recorded March 25th, A.D. 1889, at 8 o'clock a.m. by E. A. Booth, town clerk." So that it would seem that this university, founded, according to the modest claims of its parents, "for the purpose of education and charitable purposes," but confining its operations mainly, if report be true, to selling diplomas *doctoris medicinæ* to hardware dealers and others, is not an illegal body; neither is it, if the report in the *Herald* states the case correctly, the only institution of the kind in Vermont.—*Britsih Medical Journal.*

ACTION OF THE PEROXIDE OF HYDROGEN UPON THE TEETH.

By W. D. Miller, PH.D., D.D.S., Berlin.

W. H. Rollins,* after calling attention to the fact that the enamel of the teeth loses its polish under the action of peroxide of hydrogen, reports upon an experiment which at first appears to indicate that this agent, for some years extensively used in the human mouth, may have an effect upon the teeth far more injurious than any that has ever been ascribed to salicylic acid even by its most zealous opponents.

Rollins placed a freshly-extracted tooth in an ounce of peroxide of hydrogen (strength not given) obtained from a thoroughly reliable apothecary, and found that after four hours the enamel had completely lost its polish, and that in the remarkably short time of two days the whole tooth had become so soft that it could be bent between the fingers. He uses a solution of peroxide of hydrogen for decalcifying teeth of which he wishes to make cuts.

A decalcifying action as intense as that indicated by the above experiment would unfit any agent for use in the mouth. Unfortunately, in the account I have seen nothing is said of the reaction of the solution made use of, and I very strongly suspect that it was decidedly acid. There are here in use two different preparations of peroxide of hydrogen, the medicinal and the technical; the latter of these usually has a strong acid reaction. A sample which I recently examined contained 0·3 per cent. of hydrochloric acid.

It would naturally be well for every practitioner who makes use of the peroxide to demand a preparation free from acid, or one in which the acid reaction is so slight as to be of no consequence; or if the solution, on testing with litmus paper, is found to have an acid reaction, it should be neutralized and filtered before using.

In the following I wish to call attention to an action of the

---

* *Correspondenzblatt für Zahnärzte*, 1889, Heft 2 (from *British Journal of Dental Science*).

peroxide of hydrogen upon teeth out of the mouth, which is directly the reverse of that observed by Rollins. In a lecture on the peroxide of hydrogen delivered by Busch before the Odontological Society of Germany, the lecturer presented three glass vessels for inspection, the first of which contained a number of sound teeth, the second a cross-section of an elephant's tusk, the third a section of a walrus tooth, all in 10 per cent. solutions of the technical peroxide of hydrogen.

The reaction of the solutions was neutral or but slightly acid. The bottom of all the vessels was covered with a fine white powder, while the liquid was clouded by a precipitate of a more flocculent nature.

An examination of the teeth which had been lying in the solution for six weeks showed that the enamel had not been very seriously affected; it had lost its polish, and on drying was found at some points to have become superficially opaque and chalky.

The action upon the roots was much more pronounced. They were softened to a depth of about one-half millimeter (at the apices still more), and could be readily cut with a knife. The softening was not, however, of the nature of a decalcification; the roots were not cartilaginous, as when softened by acids, but rather chalky, cutting very much like soapstone, suggesting the thought that the organic constituents which hold together the lime-salts have heen destroyed.

The powder covering the bottom of the vessel was readily soluble in acids with a slight residue, and was found to consist of 14·7 per cent. organic matter and 85·3 per cent. inorganic matter (lime-salts). The flocculent precipitate above-mentioned consisted of glutin which had been dissolved and was subsequently pecipitated by the gradual change in the reaction of the solution.

The effect upon the section of ivory which had laid for six months in the solution was very remarkable. On attempting to remove it from the vessel it fell into "a thousand pieces," very much like a piece of charred paper. Small pieces of it placed in solutions of various acids, mineral and vegetable, were speedily dissolved, leaving a very delicate, fragile, and transparent residuum. The other pieces, on being dried, were rubbed up into a powder with the greatest ease.

The analysis gave 10·65 per cent. organic matter, instead of 38 per cent. which I found in normal ivory.

The solvent action of the peroxide of hydrogen upon the

basis substance of dentine may be further illustrated by the following experiment: A cross-section of the tooth of a whale (Catodon) after being decalcified was brought into 10.0 ccm. of a 10 per cent. solution of technical peroxide. In twenty days the greater part of the section had been dissolved; the solution gave a dense precipitate on addition of a drop of tannic acid.

The result seems to leave no room for doubt that neutral or nearly neutral solutions of peroxide of hydrogen act upon dentine by destroying or dissolving the organic matter by which the lime-salts are liberated or their bond of union destroyed. At all events the agent in question should be used with some caution, and when applied repeatedly, or when used as a mouth-wash, as suggested by Busch, the necks of the teeth should be particularly watched and the use discontinued in case the disintegration begins to show itself.

These observations have a certain interest from another point of view, inasmuch as they show us what we should have to expect in case decay of the teeth resulted from a destruction of the organic matter by bacteria, thus permitting the lime-salts to fall apart, as was formerly maintained by some authors. If such were the case, the decayed dentine would be reduced to a chalky, friable mass, which might be readily pulverized in a mortar, and not to the tough, cartilaginous mass which we actually find.

NOTE.—A still more intense action was produced upon teeth by keeping them for some weeks in a 5 to 10 per cent. solution of caustic potash. The ends of the roots could be crushed between the fingers and easily cut with a knife. They were not decalcified, but disintegrated. If decayed teeth are placed in the same solution, the decayed dentine will in the course of time be completely dissolved, a fact to which my attention was first called by Prof. Busch. The question arises in this connection whether there may not be other substances in the human mouth under certain conditions which, in the course of years, may in a similar manner dissolve out the organic basis-substance of the teeth, leaving the friable tissue to be worn away mechanically. Attempts to account for erosion by the action of decalcifying agents have thus far not led to a satisfactory solution of the question, and it might be well in future while searching for the cause of erosion to bear in mind that the teeth may be acted upon by agents which attack primarily the organic as well as by those which attack only the inorganic constituents.—*Dental Cosmos.*

DENTISTRY IN JAPAN.*

By ATSUHIKO KATAYAMA, D.D.S., YOKOHAMA, JAPAN.

BEFORE I describe dentistry in Japan, a brief sketch of the medical science of Japan is necessary.

Our ancient medical science was almost similar to that of China, but since the Hollanders opened a trade between Holland and Nagasaki (southern part of Japan), somewhere about two hundred years ago, the Dutch Medical Science has prevailed and made great progress. And again, since the first treaty between the United States and Japan was concluded by Commodore Perry in 1854, England, Germany, Russia, and other countries following suit, our medical science has made a sudden and successful progress. Notwithstanding, our Dental Science was very poor and scarcely practiced till 1873, yet as soon as Medical Science established her successful position, Dentistry began to follow. In 1873, our Government created a "Dental Board of Examiners," that examines twice yearly.

Since the law is formed in this manner, this Department has made a progress similar to the Medical Science. One of our ancestors in Dentistry was a famous professor of fencing, about five hundred years ago. He himself often felt very inconveniently the lack of a Dental Science. Frequently, while he was teaching, accidents would occur in which teeth were broken or loosened. Whenever an accident occurred to a person's teeth, the professor operated on them. For instance, if the crown were broken, he made a tooth with a piece of wood or wax temporarily; if it were a loosened tooth, he extracted it with his thumb; if a case of hæmorrhage, he stopped the bleeding by pressing his finger on the place until it ceased. At length, he succeeded in making artificial teeth, also in the extraction of teeth and the stoppage of hæmorrhage. Thence he called himself a dentist. Since he became a regular dentist, there have been many original native dentists practicing dentistry until the present time.

Their methods of practicing were entirely different, in every respect, from those who are practicing in civilized countries at the present time. They never filled cavities in teeth nor treated the teeth. They only knew how to extract the teeth and to make artificial plates.

* Thesis for the degree of Doctor of Dental Surgery, Ohio College of Dental Surgery, 1890.

When they had a patient who had a bad toothache, they either lanced the gum, or put a pellet of cotton saturated with oil of cloves or essence of peppermint into the cavity. If they could not relieve the pain they extracted the tooth, whether it could be saved or not.

Their general method of extracting, using full power, and placing a piece of paper on the tooth to resist the slipping.

This method succeeded almost every time, but sometimes when they met very difficult cases they used a hammer and a wooden stick, which they applied to the tooth and then knocked it out or in. However, this was very seldom done. They had a very peculiar method of extracting the deciduous teeth—so peculiar that we have never understood it. The child was given a piece of paper, which it was told to bite or hold firmly with the tooth that was to be extracted. The dentist, standing at a small distance from the child, would ask, "Are you ready?" and when the answer "Yes" came, he would clap his hands and go to the child and let him open his mouth; then the tooth would drop on the floor with the paper. Nobody has ever ascertained what was used on the paper, but some suppose that they put a very adhesive wax on the paper, or, according to others, a piece of sticky candy was used, because some of the children said the paper tasted sweet. We claim that it must have been a piece of extra adhesive wax, though it is uncertain. The method of making artificial plates was almost the same as that used in civilised countries to-day. They had neither metal nor rubber plates; only fine wooden plates were in use, and they had no porcelain artificial teeth.

They first took impressions with beeswax (without impression tray), and after it had hardened enough to handle, hard wax, or a kind of plaster of Paris, was pounded into the beeswax impression for a model. After getting this model, it was generally painted with some colouring matter, especially red. A carved imitation of the model was then produced (cherry-wood being considered the best wood) which was put over the painted model; the paint marked the protruding parts. It was then carved again and again, until the paint marked the whole inside of the wood carving. After this was finished, they were ready to set ivory, wood, bone or marble teeth in the carved wood. Holes were carved on the margin of the wooden plate in which the teeth were set. They did not set more than eight teeth, that is from the central incisors to the bicuspids silver or gold pins taking the place of the molars.

The teeth were retained in their place by small, strong threads. In a case of "partials" they never made a plate, something like bridge-work was used, tightening it in the mouth by the neighboring teeth or staying it by gold or silver clasps. They made two kinds of plates—white-teeth plate and black-teeth plate, the former being for men and unmarried women the latter was for married women only. It will not be out of place here to tell *why* our Japanese women blackened their teeth after marriage and *how* it was done. The substance with which the teeth are blackened is a solution made by dissolving a piece of iron in an acid. When they apply it to their teeth the substance is first rubbed on with a brush, then a little powdered tannic acid is applied with a brush, and this is repeated until the teeth are thoroughly black.

As we dentists know, the enamel of human teeth is very hard and smooth, so that it cannot retain any colouring matter on it long; consequently, if a woman has well-developed enamel, it is almost impossible for her to keep her teeth black, but on the contrary, badly-developed enamel retains the colouring matter for several days. The colouring matter adhering to the enamel is entirely dependent upon the good or bad development of the enamel; therefore, if a woman has well-developed enamel, she uses a diluted solution of acetic or sulphuric acid, which she applies with a brush. This she does first to roughen the surface, after which she proceeds to blacken her teeth; these operations are repeated until she succeeds.

We do not know exactly when the custom of blackening the teeth began, but we can suppose it had its origin in the sixteenth or seventeenth century, when the country was so much disturbed by her civil wars. At that time many of the feudal chiefs of the Emperor were scattered around the country living in obscurity or privacy, and as they were known to be both brave and patriotic, a feeling of dislike crept into the people's hearts against the inactive and *unsoldierly* literary men. The military art was exalted and flourished vigorously. The women, reflecting the men's opinions, selected the brave military men for husbands instead of the sedate literary men.

If once married, though the husband immediately lost his life on the battle-field, the bereaved wife never married again, and this should be remembered to the honour of our women's lives. Then began the practise of blackening the teeth after marriage; this was the sign that the wife's virtue was sacred to her husband, and also the oath that no future marriage would ever take place.

The reason given for blackening the teeth is quite poetical; it appears that teeth once blackened never resume their natural color, and that women once married are never unmarried.

This custom is almost entirely unseen at the present time, except among old women. Our Japanese married women's custom was bad but it appears to me that the cramped foot of the Chinese woman and the compressed waist of the European woman is fully as bad and much worse for general health. As custom becomes "second nature" all over the world, civilized or uncivilized, our country has distinguished herself by the most complete and rapid revolution of old customs and the adoption of European civilization. No country in the range of history, excepting our own, has in the short space of twenty-five years made such a complete change in *public sentiment*, *habits* and *government* without bloodshed.—*Dental Review.*

GOSSIP.

ODONTOLOGICAL SOCIETY.—We are obliged to keep back our report of this Society until our next issue, owing to the necessity of reporting fully the important meeting of the Medical Council.

GUY'S HOSPITAL DENTAL SCHOOL.—We learn there were five new entries in May for the L.D.S.Eng., viz., Messrs. F. J. Blewitt, P. Harrison, J. S. Sewill, H. B. Stoner, C. Read. There is a steady increase in the amount of work done; the present average of dental operations performed is 1,000 a month. Two of the new entries have already passed the second professional examination of the Conjoint Board.

CHARING CROSS HOSPITAL MEDICAL SCHOOL.—On June 18th the Rev. S. F. Cumberlege, rector of St. Paul's, Covent Garden, presided at the presentation of prizes awarded to the successful students of this school. The report of the executive, which was read by Mr. Stanley Boyd, the sub-dean, stated that the new school buildings had been progressing towards completion, and the number of students had increased. Seventy students had entered—33 general, 24 dental, and 13 occasional—the average number in daily attendance being

190; 30 had passed the first examination of the conjoint board, 26 the second, and 22 the final. Out of 65 vacancies in the Indian, home, and naval services, 32 of the successful candidates received a portion of their training in the Charing Cross School. The prizes were then distributed by the Chairman, the Llewellyn scholarship falling to Mr. H. S. Baker, the Golding scholarship to Mr. G. H. Hooper, the Governors clinical gold medal to Mr. J. B. Williams, and the Periera prize to Mr. J. Busfield, the last mentioned receiving also several other awards. The Chairman, in addressing the students, observed that the report held out good ground for relying upon the increasing reputation of the school. The expense that had been incurred in making the buildings more commodious and the teaching more perfect should act as a stimulus to increased study; and he was happy to say that there was universal testimony to the fact that the character and conduct of the Charing Cross Hospital students of to-day were very different indeed to what they were some years ago.—A hearty vote of thanks to the chairman was accorded, and the proceedings were brought to a close.

Among the prize winners the following "dentals" took a conspicuous place:—E. B. Jones (Anatomy, Physiology, Chemistry—prize); W. R. Barrett (Physiology); T. Coysh (Practical Chemistry, Dental Surgery, 2nd prize); C. J. Allin (Practical Chemistry); A. W. W. Hoffmann (Medicine, prize—Practical Medicine, prize); J. P. Oliver (Practical Medicine); C. Schelling (Dental Surgery); W. May (Dental Surgery—1st prize). All we can say is "Bravo Dentals!"

APPOINTMENTS.

Colyer, J. F., L.D.S., M.R.C.S., L.R.C.P., appointed Assistant Surgeon-Dentist to the Charing Cross Hospital.

Ellwood, Francis Henry, L.D.S.I., has been appointed Dentist to S. Joseph's Convent, Redhill, and Hon. Dentist to Hope Lodge Training Home, Redhill.

Morris, John, L.D.S.Eng., has been appointed House Surgeon to the Liverpool Dental Hospital.

Penfold, William, L.D.S.I., has been appointed Honorary Dentist to the London Homœopathic Hospital, Great Ormond Street, Bloomsbury.

THE DENTAL RECORD, LONDON: JULY 1, 1890.

"Raising the Status of Registered Dentists."

It is with mingled feelings that dentists will peruse the report of the recent proceedings of the General Medical Council which we publish on another page. All will admit the expediency of raising the social status of our profession, or indeed, any other profession, but how many will acquiesce in the measures which Dr. Rawdon McNamara proposes to adopt for that purpose is quite another question. As matters stand at present, we possess a distinctive and exclusively dental diploma, the L.D.S., and facilities are offered those whose ambition aims at further qualifications to acquire the diploma of the conjoint examining board and so blossom forth as M.R.C.S., L.R.C.P., L.D.S. Still, the distinctive feature is the L.D.S., and there is no doubt that at least the dental board in London have determined to make that qualification accessible only to those whose knowledge and manipulative skill are of a thorough nature. Improving (?) upon this scheme, Dr. McNamara suggests, and the Medical Council have ratified the suggestion, that it shall be competent for an L.D.S. to take the single diploma of M.R.C.S., or other single diploma, to add, as he gracefully puts it, "a feather in their caps." It would seem the status of our profession stands in sore need of being raised, if it be honestly deemed advisable to fling to us a tinsel diploma to adorn our head-pieces and so save us from Bottom's fate and they "write us down an ass."

The single diploma would carry us how far? It would neither entitle us to practice as a dentist nor as a doctor; it would give us no prestige among our medical friends, who would, according as they were loafers or workers, scream at us for thieves and robbers for having climbed into the fold by ways other than that accessible to them, or point the finger of scorn at those who, aiming at the rotundity of the ox, had at best achieved only the bloated distension of the frog.

Among our *confrères*, how should we stand? The L.D.S. men whose means, or time, or what not, had compelled them to take the dentist's diploma alone, would hardly regard as master masons those whose achievements had been tempered of their severity by the fostering hands of the Medical Council, while the zealots whose heads and hands seek not rest until the solid work of thorough all-round knowledge is gained would prefer a diploma which allows them to run neck to neck with the medical students of their general hospital, and not be content with a Bowdlerised edition—the medical curriculum with the hard words left out. The London students would certainly say, thank you for nothing were they to have the M.R.C.S. flounted before them, while for the Irish and Scotch colleges to grant a diploma whose *raître d'être* is merely of a *cosmetic* nature, would hardly promote union peace and concord, nor would it subserve any useful purpose.

In hospital appointments, the value of a single diploma in days when the medical profession has been taught to regard a dual diploma as a minimum, must be very questionable, and would certainly label a man as second-rate when competing against L.D.S. men only and L.D.S. men who have taken the dual diploma of the conjoint board, for the presumption now is that the L.D.S. man, if a first-rate dentist, was prevented from prosecuting his studies, whereas the gentleman with the feather in his cap advertises the fact that he had time and money to go for something beyond the bare L.D.S., but shied at the test imposed for the acquisition of the dual diploma. Except for the cosmetic attraction of wearing a cap adorned with a single feather, the scheme seems to us valueless, and further, the exception, makes it the more worthy of condemnation by an intelligent and independent profession.

ROYAL COLLEGE OF SURGEONS OF ENGLAND.

THE following gentlemen, having passed the necessary Examinations on the 12th, 13th, 14th and 15th of May, were at an ordinary meeting of the Council on the 12th instant admitted Licentiates in Dental Surgery :—

BARRETT, WALTER RUSSELL, Charing Cross and Dental Hospital, 25, York Place, Portman Square, W.

BOWTELL, HERBERT RICHMOND, Charing Cross and Dental Hospital, 146, Richmond Road, Hackney.

BRIAULT, ERNEST HENRY LEWIS, Charing Cross and Dental Hospital, 30, Richmond Crescent, Barnsbury, N.

CARDELL, ARTHUR JOHN, Charing Cross and Dental Hospital, 23, Victoria Road, Clapham Common, S.W.

CARTER, HENRY CHARLES, St. Mary's and National Dental Hospital, 181, Edgware Road, W.

COX, ARTHUR BROOKS, M.R.C.S.Eng., Middlesex and Dental Hospital, Middlesex Hospital.

DAVIDS, ERNEST CORNILS, Middlesex and Dental Hospital, 30, Monmouth Road, Bayswater.

DERWENT, ARTHUR HOLMES, Manchester Hospital, 10, Park Terrace, Bishop Street, Moss Side, Manchester.

HAYMAN, HOWARD LITTLE, Charing Cross, and Bristol and Dental Hospital, Clevedon, Somersetshire.

HERN, GEORGE, Middlesex and Dental Hospital, 12, Hamilton Road, Ealing, N.W.

HOFFMAN, AUGUSTUS WILLIAM WISTINGHAUSEN, Charing Cross and Dental Hospital, 16, Beauclerc Road, Hammersmith, W.

HORDERN, JOSEPH BROOKHOUSE, Charing Cross and Dental Hospital, Spencer Villa, Leamington Spa.

MOON, WILLIAM DRAPER, Middlesex and Dental Hospital, 85, Newman Street, W.

OLIVER, JOHN PERCY, Charing Cross and Dental Hospital, 121, Queen Street, Cardiff.

PREEDY, EDWARD JOHN, Charing Cross and Dental Hospital, 360, Camden Road, N.

READ, SIBLEY WALTER, London and Dental Hospital, 30, Finsbury Square, E.C.

READ, STANLEY, Charing Cross and Dental Hospital, 12, Old Steine, Brighton. Sixteen Candidates were referred.

CORRESPONDENCE.

[We do not hold ourselves responsible in any way for the opinions expressed by our correspondents.]

GAS OPERATIONS.

To the Editor of the DENTAL RECORD.

DEAR SIR,—The sensible and very temperate letter of your correspondent, "J. S.," which appeared in the April number of the RECORD, commends itself to my unqualified approval. The gas question has so frequently been presented to us from a medical stand-point that the opportunity of regarding it from the vantage ground of a dentist is refreshing. "J. S." truly remarks that, "Medical men know nothing whatever about gas operations." We possess, in abundance, their own evidence of this.

It cannot be too distinctly recognised that no amount of academical learning can supply the want of practical knowledge; nor is it the privilege of anyone to know everything about dentistry without learning anything. There can be no objection to the presence of medical men at gas operations. It would be unfair, alike to the patient and his medical attendant, for the dentist to raise any, should he, the patient, express a wish for such presence.

I do not agree with those writers who, arbitrarily, lay down the law, that no gas operations ought ever to be performed in the absence of a medical man; nor do I think it can be expected that any capable dentist, who is doubly qualified by practical training, being both an experienced anæsthetist and a skilful operator, will ever stultify himself by conducting his practice on principles to harmonize with the limited attainments of others.

The dentist who fully realizes his responsibilities, who respects himself and the lives of his patients, does not willingly delegate to another the duties of either administrator or operator. Some writers contend that the two duties ought always to be separated. I do not hold this view. There are many cases where advantages and better results may be obtained by a contrary method. This teaching has recently been combated by a leading London anæsthetist* who says, "He has never before met with anybody who has taken up this position," *i.e.*, the position taken up by myself. This remarkable assertion has been made in face of the fact that precisely the same position has been adopted by specialists who have had the greatest experience, and who now stand pre-eminently in the forefront of successful gas operators.

Dr. Guilford, who can show a record of tens of thousands of successful cases in his useful little manual on nitrous oxide, published three years ago, says, p. 53, "Some writers insist upon having the

* *Vide* "An Additional Note on Nitrous Oxide," by Dr. Dudley Buxton, *British Journal of Dental Science*, October 1st, 1889.

assistant administer the gas, so as to leave the operator entirely free. *We see no necessity for this; indeed, we prefer to be both administrator and operator.*" The italics are my own.

With the mere anæsthetists, who are not skilful operators, or *vice versâ*, there is no alternative: the duties must be divided or the gas left alone; and it becomes incumbent upon them to defend to the utmost their only position.

Yours faithfully,

Stramongate, Kendal. J. Otley Atkinson, L.D.S.

WHY NOT?

To the Editor of the Dental Record.

Sir,—In a recent paper before the Odontological Society the author inadvertently dubbed some of its members "Fellows," a title which has no existence; but why not? Has not the time arrived when the title might be made the blue riband of the profession? To be conferred only upon those, who, by their researches, widen the bounds of scientific knowledge; upon such men as Mr. C. S. Tomes, Dr. H. D. Miller. Bestowed with the care that the Royal Society and the Geographical Society observe, would it not be an incentive to research, and become a coveted honour?

Your obedient servant,

June 20th, 1890. Epsilon

ALUMINIUM AS A DENTAL BASE METAL.

Mr. James Wallace, of Glasgow, writes:—In your issue of May 1st, I read the discussion on "Aluminium as a Dental Base," by Mr. Macleod and others, with considerable interest. I may state what was the reason which led me to use aluminium, and subsequently to take out a patent for it. (I do not want to argue at present, however, who used the metal first, as that can be ascertained, as a matter of fact, by reference to dates).

About 30 years ago, when I was a student at the Andersonian University Glasgow, under Dr. Penny, Professor of Chemistry, he gave a lecture on aluminium, and said that it might do for dental purposes if a solder could be found for it. After the lecture we had a conversation. When I suggested that it might be used in combination with vulcanite the Professor became quite enthusiastic over the matter and requested me to make an upper set of teeth for him with the metal (he was wearing a gold plate at the time that was very unsatisfactory).

After the new denture was made, he wore it constantly for two years, when the metal was as pure and perfect as when it left the polishing brush. I then took out a patent for it. The Professor wore the aluminium till his lamented death; his wife wore one for thirteen years, and within the last month I made a new case of teeth for a patient who was still wearing an upper denture in aluminium that I made for her 26 years ago. No metal can be compared to it for dental purposes if it was always made pure, but, when I used it, it was shamefully manufactured, and irregular in character. Not infrequently, when the plate was being struck up, it would go into reeds and indicate the unprepared clayey matter. This was my principal reason for giving up the using of aluminium, for such impure material would get corroded in about five years.

THE DENTAL RECORD.

VOL. X. AUGUST 1ST, 1890. No. 8.

Original Communications.

A FEW REMARKS ON DENTAL REFLEXES.

By H. MACNAUGHTON JONES, M.D., Hon. M.A.O. M.Ch. F.R.C.S.I. & E.

(*Formerly University Professor Queen's University, and Examiner in the Royal University*).

THE part played by the teeth in originating reflex irritations is now well established. But this source of a distant neurosis is hardly kept in view as frequently as it ought to be in the daily practice, both of the practitioner and the dental surgeon. The latter, especially, must have frequent opportunity of recognising in carious or otherwise affected teeth, an explanation of some puzzling disorder which has baffled the therapeutic skill of the physician or the more specialised aid of the "Specialist," the attention of the latter being very naturally concentrated on that affection of nervous system, eye, ear, uterus, or other organs for which he is consulted. Since the fact has been recognised that the teeth and eyes are frequently the cause of severe headache, facial neuralgias, and more especially in the instance of errors of refraction, reflex gastric disturbances, such as nausea and sickness, dental and ocular affections, in their relation to these disorders, have had greater attention paid to them than was the practice some years since. I think that the sensitiveness of the teeth and the secondary consequences of dental disorders are more felt by women than men. This is not a matter for surprise when we remember the greater susceptibility of women to various neuroses, both visceral and peripheral, the physiological predisposition to which, the frequently recurring changes of female life bring about. No gynœcologist can any longer ignore the possibility of dental irritation being a superadded source of a headache, which he is inclined to look on as "neurotic" because he can find nothing abnormal in the pelvic viscera, or which persists after he has perchance rectified some such uterine cause of reflex disturbance as a flexion or version of the uterus, or some irregularity in the catamenial flow. It is quite possible that the amenorrhœa, which may be associated with anæmia predisposes to the general circulatory or nervous disturbance which promotes the susceptibility to reflex irritation started in the numerous peripheral terminations of the fifth nerve.

Cerebral or facial vaso-motor changes, due to pelvic disorders, are very common in the many ovarian and uterine affections of women. Various forms and degrees of headache accompany and aggravate such affections. Neuralgia is a frequent concurrent symptom. This neuralgia is constantly felt in the course of the fifth and facial branches. And if search be made beyond this local evidence of nervous disturbance we may find, in cardiac rhythm or systole, proof of general increase or diminution of vascular tension. Such deviation from the normal blood current, both in quality and quantity, must have an effect in starting a stimulus in nerves, already prone to irritation through chronic disease in the tissues they supply, perhaps, themselves also, chronically inflamed and vascular, or encroached on by enlargements and pressed on by morbid effusions. I have this day seen a patient with white and gold stoppings in the upper and lower left molar teeth, and overcrowded incisors: she suffers from periodical tinnitus aurium of the left ear, the hearing is nearly normal, there is nothing discernible save some slight catarrhal changes in the membrana tympani, yet there is violent neuralgic pain apparently starting in the ear and radiating in the course of the facial branches. This lady has been wearing a pessary for some time for retroversion of the womb, to which she ascribes all her ills. And many times I have known neuralgia of the ear, occurring without any inflammation or other abnormal conditions of the ear, unquestionably due to a carious tooth, and the pain has been immediately relieved by its removal. Such neuralgic attacks are as I shall show accompanied occasionally by tinnitus. Such a local symptom generally points either to an interference with the equilibration of the air in the tympanum or the fluid in the labyrinth, or at least, to sufficient irritation in the auditory nerve tract from nucleus to cortex, to start this symptom. The communications of the fifth with the facial and auditory nerves through the otic and spheno-palatine ganglia; the distinct supply of the tensor tympani by the fifth nerve, and of the stapedius by the facial—the two muscles which are most important in regulating the equilibration of the fluid in the labyrinth—offer the anatomical explanation of such a reflex aural irritation springing from a dental cause in the superior or inferior dental branches of the fifth nerve. This possible reflex disturbance of the fluid equilibrium in the labyrinth, through an irritation existing in the teeth demands additional attention in face of the fact stated by Foster that the "activity of the tensor tympani is regulated by reflex action." Nor in estimating the various reflex relationships of fifth nerve must the fact be overlooked that the origin of the sensory root of the fifth anastomose with all the motor nuclei of the nerves arising from the medulla with the exception of the abducens (6th) (Landois and Stirling). There are other anatomical points in regard to the connections and communications of the fifth nerve which are of interest to remember in discussing any of those reflexes which irritation of the dental branches may produce. It may be well in the first place briefly to tabulate these.

SOME ANATOMICAL POINTS BEARING ON DENTAL REFLEXES

1. Nuclei of origin of Fifth.	The connection of the motor nucleus with the cortical motor centre of the opposite side, and its connection with the descending root. The anastomosis of the sensory root with all the motor nuclei of the nerves, arising from the medulla save the sixth.—(LANDOIS and STIRLING)*.
2. Distribution to dura mater and arachnoid from fifth nerve	The supply of the dura mater from the fifth nerve through the recurrent branch from the Gasserian ganglion, superior maxillary, ophthalmic division of fifth, the communications between the branches of the carotid plexus of the sympathetic, going to the dura mater, with the Gasserian ganglion and Meckel's ganglion, through the vidian. Besides the facial and spinal accessory, the motor division of the inferior maxillary of fifth sends a branch to the arachnoid, while the fifth also participates in the supply of the pia mater.
3. Distribution to scalp and communications of Fifth.	Supra-trochlear, infra-orbital, from ophthalmic; temporal of orbital, from superior maxillary; auriculo-temporal, from inferio maxillary. *"All the cutaneous offsets of the fifth nerve, form communications with the adjacent ramification of the seventh nerve."*—(QUAIN.) The intercommunications between the great auricular, small and great occipital (from the second and third cervical nerves) and the posterior auricular of the facial, form a connecting link between the cutaneous branches of the second and third cervical, and the fifth nerves. This anatomical connection has an important bearing on the concurrence of cervical with dental neuralgia.

Landois and Stirling, "Text Book on Physiology," 1889.

Important communications of fifth with other cranial nerves.	With the facial through the Chorda tympani; temporo-facial and temporal; malar; infra-orbital; buccal; supra-maxillary.	
	With the Auditory.	The upper division of the auditory nerve communicates with the geniculate ganglion of facial, and so, by means of the large and small superficial petrosal nerves, with Meckel's and the otic ganglion, respectively.
	With the glossopharyngeal.	Jacobson's "tympanic branch" with the small superficial petrosal and otic ganglion-section of the fifth nerve is followed by inflammatory changes in the tympanum of the rabbit.—(BERTHOLD and GRÜNHAGEN.) Also, in relation to *ocular*, *auditory*, and *nasal* reflex irritation, these distributions of the fifth nerve have to be remembered.
Other Distributions.	Eye.	The origin of the long ciliary branches through the sensory root of the lenticular ganglion: the infra- and supra-trochlear branches to the eye and lachrymal apparatus, the supra-orbital cutaneous twigs to the scalp and frontal pericranium. Communications with the third, fourth, and sixth nerves through the ophthalmic of fifth.
	Ear.	The communication through the otic ganglion with the tympanic plexus. The muscular supply from the otic ganglion to the tensor tympani and the tensor palati.
	Nose.	The supply through the branches of Meckel's ganglion, and the naso-palatine nerve, to the hard palate and the middle and inferior meati, soft palate, tonsils, septum nasi, and ethmoidal cells.

I have ventured thus to remind the readers of this paper of the connections and distribution of the branches of the fifth nerve which are in themselves sufficient to explain some of the occasional reflex symptoms that may be traced to an irritation of the dental twigs. The connections of the fifth nerve with the sympathetic are of primary importance in so far as they bear on the vaso-motor effects of irritation of the dental twigs. These effects are manifested in allied conditions of blood pressure, increase or dimunition, in the ciliary circulation in the eye, in the vessels of the tympanum and labyrinth in the ear, and those of the septum and turbinate bones in the nose. The same observation applies to the scalp, frontal pericranium, and dura mater. Though the auditory nerve in common with the optic and olfactory has no connection directly with the sympathetic, yet there are the communications from the carotid plexus with Meckel's ganglion through the deep and great superficial petrosal (forming the vidian) and the filaments that proceed from the sympathetic around the middle meningeal to the otic ganglion. There are indirect connections also through the tympanic branch of the glosso-pharyngeal, and the communications with the facial nerve through its geniculate ganglion and its branch to the stylo-hyoid muscle.

The vaso-constrictor fibres (contracting blood vessels) pass from the anterior roots of the upper dorsal through the sympathetic cervical ganglia (Gaskell) to the carotid artery, and thence to the special arteries supplying the parts before named. The vaso-dilators arising from the entire spinal cord find their way in the same manner to the smaller vessels. The knowledge of the existence of these distinctly opposed vaso-motor nerves, one diminishing the blood supply and raising the blood pressure, the other increasing it and lowering the blood pressure, helps to explain some of the seemingly paradoxical effects following on stimulation of the fifth nerve, as for instance, an increase or diminution of the intra-ocular vascular tension from decayed teeth and supra- or infra-orbital nerve excitation. Still more seriously touching on this question is the knowledge that "pressor" nerve fibres exist in the trigeminus which excite the vaso-motor centre in the medulla and cause a rise* of blood pressure. The annexed diagram (Landois and Stirling) will serve to illustrate these brief observations on the connection and distribution of the fifth nerve.

Before referring to the particular case which prompted this communication, I desire to make a few remarks gleaned from my own experience of the effects of decayed teeth on the eye and ear. The communication of Mr. Henry Power to the Odontological Society of Great Britain (November 5th, 1883), dealt so fully with the literature of "the relation between dental lesions and diseases of the eye" that it would be waste of space to go into the question

* "Text Book on Physiology," by J. McKendrick, M.D., F.R.C.S., vol. ii., p. 294, 1889.

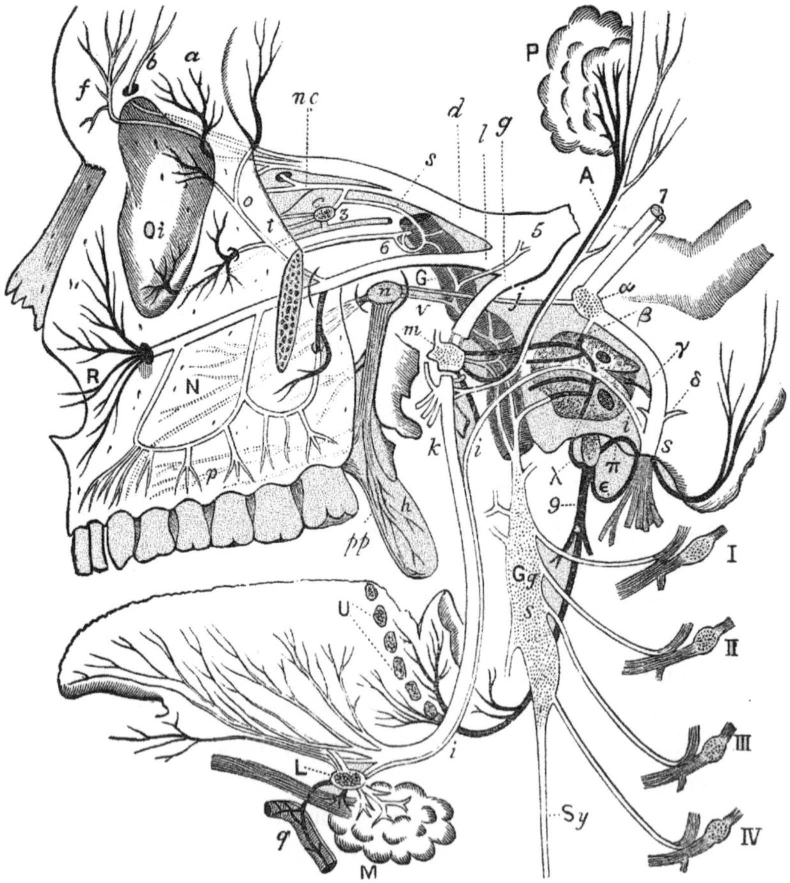

Semi-diagramatic representation (after Landois and Stirling) of the nerves of the eyeball, the connections of the trigeminus and its ganglia, together with the facial and glosso-pharyngeal nerves. 3. Branch to the inferior oblique muscle from the oculomotorius, with the thick short root to the ciliary ganglion (*c*), *t*, ciliary nerves, long root to the ganglion from the naso-ciliary (*nc*); *s*, sympathetic root from the sympathetic plexus surrounding the internal carotid (G); *d*, first or ophthalmic division of the trigeminus (5) with the naso-ciliary (*nc*) and the terminal branches of the lachrymal (*a*) supra orbital (*b*) and frontal (*f*), *l*, second or superior maxillary division of the trigeminus (R) infra-orbital, (*n*), spheno-palatine (Meckel's) ganglion with its roots, (*j*), from the facial, and *v*, from the sympathetic, N, the nasal branches, and *pp*, the palatine branches of the ganglion; *g*, third or inferior maxillary division of the trigeminus, *k*, lingual; *i*, *i*, chorda tympani, *m*, otic ganglion, with the roots from the tympanic plexus, the carotid plexus, and from the 3rd branch and with its branches to the auriculo-temporal (*a*) and to the chorda (*i i*), L, sub-maxillary ganglion with its roots from the tympanico-lingual, and the sympathetic plexus on the external artery (*q*). 7. Facial nerve, *j*, its great superficial petrosal branch, *a*, ang, geniculatum, β, branch to the tympanic plexus; γ, branch to the stapedius; δ, anastomatic twig to the auricular branch of the vagus; *i i*, chorda tympani; *S*, stylo-mastoid foramen. 9, Glosso pharyngeal; λ, its tympanic branch; π and ε, connections with the facial; U, terminations of the gustatory fibres of 9 in the circumvallate papillae, *Sy*, sympathetic with *G g*, *s*; the superior cervical ganglion, I., II., III. .IV., the four upper cervical nerves; P, parotid; *m*, submaxillary gland.

DIAGRAM OF THE THIRD DIVISION OF THE FIFTH NERVE, ITS CONNECTION AND BRANCHES.

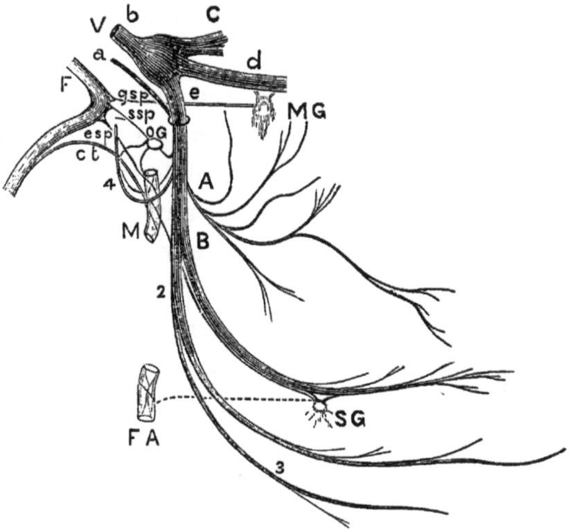

V—Fifth Nerve. b, large sensory root with the Gasserian ganglion; a, smaller motor root joining inferior maxillary nerve. A, anterior division of the inferior maxillary nerve with its branches to the muscles of mastication and buccal branch (mainly motor); B, posterior division; I, its lingual branch; 2, the inferior dental branch, with the twigs to the teeth, and the mental branch; 3, the mylo-hyoid branch; F, the facial nerve with its (c t), chorda tympani branch going to (S G) sub-maxillary ganglion as its motor root. O G, otic ganglion, g s p, great superficial petrosal connecting the facial nerve with (M G), Meckel's ganglion, s s p small superficial petrosal connecting the facial nerve with the otic ganglion; e s p, external superficial petrosal connecting the middle meningeal, (M), plexus with the facial nerve. (F A), facial artery, communication with sub-maxillary ganglion.—*From* "Herman's Physiology."

fully here. I regret that my old Eye-hospital notes are not now available, for I should have had a better opportunity of verifying by an analysis of cases the teaching of my hospital experience on some points of importance in regard to the relation between morbid dental conditions and certain ophthalmic affections. The various reflex affections arising during the dentition period in children are clearly recognised. Perhaps, two of the most frequently occurring are general convulsions and bronchial irritations. Many times I have seen the error fallen into of attacking with expectorants and counter irritants, a lung which would have been more easily relieved by bromide of potassium and belladonna. In the face of my own experience, I am not sure, as is now generally thought, that the depletion of the gums, produced by the old practice of scarification did not occasionally relieve such reflex irritation; not of course with the view of facilitating the eruption of the teeth, but of relieving the congestion of the gum. I have many times seen the immediate good effects of gingival depletion, in children suffering from the fever of dentition and from other reflex troubles arising from delayed eruption.

And this recalls to mind the old and pernicious system of the administration of calomel during dentition as a prophylactic against convulsions, and which led to the differential diagnosis by Mr. Hutchinson, between mercurial teeth and those of hereditary syphilis. Few children escape the traditional castor oil of infancy, the calomel course of dentition, and the vermifuges of a later period. "Teething" and "worms" accounted for most of the ills of the growing child. Nor can there be any doubt that normal as well as abnormal dentition have been credited with causing various troubles with which the physiological process of eruption has little or nothing to say. "Superstition and ignorance" says Henoch, "here lend a hand, especially in practice among the poor, which it is often very difficult to undo afterwards" (Lectures on Children's Diseases, New Syd. Soc., 1889). This author ascribes to rickets a much more important part in the production of convulsions in children than to dentition. "It is only rarely," he says, "that convulsions are observed in teething children who are not ricketty." It is widely known that gastric disturbances or indigestion start the nervous impulses that lead up to convulsions in young children, still my experience (a considerable one for many years) in the affections of children, has convinced me that, as a constantly occurring predisposing or collateral condition, the irritation of dentition exerts a powerful influence in causing convulsions

I have repeatedly known the occurrence of such convulsions preceded by the recent appearance of a tooth through the gum, and the effort of a second to escape; and the cessation of such convulsive seizures, after a period of dentition has passed, proves the part played by the teeth in their causation. "Also" says Henoch, "the indisputable fact that obstinate vomiting, diarrhœa, a spasmodic cough or eczema of the face which for days or weeks has defied all treatment, will all disappear as soon as one or a couple of teeth emerge from the alveolus, and this can only be explained by the reflex action from the dental branches of the fifth on the peristalsis and the vagus or the vaso-motor nerves." Mr. Power's reference to phlyctenular inflammation * in his paper before alluded to, is another instance of this correlation of the dentition period and a

* *Loc.-cit.*

common ocular affection of infancy and childhood, a correlation with which every ophthalmic surgeon is cognisant.

A leucophlegmatic condition of the child predisposes to this response of the vaso-motor nerves to the dental irritation of the sensory dental branches. The same remark applies to spasmodic and spurious croup. Dental irritation causes periodical and alternating strabismus, occurring quite independently of convulsions. In addition to the older ophthalmic writers referred to by Mr. Power, we find Wardrop (1808) under the head of "Squint from Teething," remarking "the squint in such cases is sometimes slight and goes away when the teething process is completed. In other instances the squint is to a greater extent, and is permanent." *

But this knowledge of the occasional source of strabismus in prolonged or severe dentition does not absolve the practitioner from the responsibility of attending to any optical defect in the eyes of children over two years of age, and meeting such by the aid of suitable lenses or operation. The fact that after the age of five, cases of anterior polio-myelitis (infantile paralysis) are rare (Charcot)† and that the great majority of cases occur between the ages of six months and three years makes the association of this disease with the dentition period something more than a mere coincidence (Barlow ‡). All the cases I have ever seen of infantile paralysis have occurred in children under three years of age. In none was there any direct relationship to be traced between the teeth and the acute stage or onset of the affection. In all the patients, where any cause could be ascribed it has been that of exposure to cold, causing dilatation of the vessels in that portion of the spinal cord to which this reflex excitation is transmitted. On two occasions I have known the serious mistake made of confounding this affection with acute morbus coxæ. I cannot see any difficulty in view of our knowledge of the relation and connections of the nuclei of the fifth nerve, and the researches of Gaskell proving the origin from the anterior *cornua* of the cord of the vaso-motor nerves, and the connections of these with the trigeminus, in conceiving, that an irritation of the dental nerves is capable, by reflex excitation of the sympathetic, of starting a myelitis in the anterior cornua of the cord, especially in the cervical region. Henoch points out, in reviewing the symptoms of a case in

* "The Morbid Anatomy of the Human Eye," by James Wardrop.

† Charcot "On Diseases of the Nervous System" (New Syd. Soc., 1881).

‡ Barlow "On Repressive Paralysis," 1878.

which facial paralysis accompanied the paralysis of the right upper extremity, that an encephalitis of a very limited nature must have occurred in the neighbourhood of the nucleus of the left facial nerve, and he remarks that it is not quite certain that analogous changes do not occur in the brain in some cases to those found in the spinal cord. Henoch says that he has not been able to make sure of teething as the cause of the paralysis in a single case. Ross* in commenting on the fact that dentition is the most frequently assigned cause of polio-myelitis, remarks that "it is probable that too much rather than too little importance has been attributed to this process in the production of the affection."

Dr. E. D. Mapother in one of his papers on dermatology,† incidentally gives the details of an interesting case of reflex tonic spasm producing closure of the jaws (trismus dentium), due to impaction of a wisdom tooth in the coronoid process of the jaw, a displacement accompanied by disease of the adjacent molar. The spasm disappeared under ether, and was cured permanently, though of eighteen months' duration, by the extraction of the teeth. So far back as 1778, John Hunter, as pointed out by Dr. Mapother, noticed that the half erupted condition of these teeth had a tendency to cause approximal caries, while aphonia and amaurosis have been attributed to the same cause or the malposition of the teeth. For months Dr. Mapother's patient had been fed with fluids sucked from the point of a teaspoon. A somewhat similar case in the person of a gentleman I had under my care a few years since. The patient was anæsthetised with ether, but the spasm which was associated with great rigidity of the maxillary muscles yielded with difficulty, though I used specula and clamp to effect separation.

Mr. Sewill's case, recorded before the Odontological Society, of permanent cure of severe spasm of the orbicularis palpebrarum and neuralgia, with attendant facial hyperæsthesia, by removal of the carious incisors and some molars, is an interesting one.‡

I may here note in connection with this case, that removal of the teeth is not always attended by rapid relief of the facial spasm. In June, 1870, a lady, aged fifty, consulted me for severe spasm of the muscles of the right side of the face, attended on the least excitement by closure of the eye, and dragging of the mouth. She had had

* "Diseases of the Nervous System," by James Ross, M.D., in 1883.

† "Papers on Dermatology," by E. D. Mapother, M.D., 1889.

‡ "Dental Surgery," by Henry Sewill, M.R.C.S., 1889.

carious teeth on that side, in the upper and lower jaws. All these had been extracted before consulting me. This had cured the dental pain, but not the spasm. There was acute pain in the head, especially over the occiput ; for this she had been repeatedly blistered. She had suffered, she said, from toothache, but not from neuralgia of the *face*. Under the use of galvanism, bromides, arseniate of iron, and quinine, with other tonics, she was greatly relieved, but not quite cured. In the following year the spasm recurred with severe pain in the head, which again, in a measure, yielded to remedies. She would consent to no operative interference. It may be doubtful in this case, if the neuralgia proceeded from the teeth ; but it is not the only instance of a severe facial neuralgia apparently dependent upon decayed teeth which I have known to persist despite the removal of the entire offending teeth.

The shifting nature of facial neuralgia, referred at different times to various localities, and the more intermittent character of the affection, with its periodical return at certain times of the day or night, are important features of the affection which enables us to differentiate it from ordinary toothache, while more active manifestations of associated disorders of other cerebral nerves help us to differentiate mere peripheral from central disorders.

In a record of neuralgia of the fifth and facial nerves associated with tinnitus aurium, I found that out of 260 cases of tinnitus seven were suffering from neuralgia of these nerves, and seven more complained of severe headache. Though I have no record of the condition of the teeth in these cases, still I am aware that in many the teeth were affected, and it is only reasonable, on physiological grounds, to infer that the decayed teeth may have had a share in causing the tinnitus, or in starting the morbid condition of the tympanum which accompanied it. Rarely, however, in aural cases is *deafness* attributed to the teeth. This is my experience. Some of these cases of facial neuralgia were associated with serious eye complications. I take the following case as an instance. A single lady, aged 60, consulted me for a sightless and painful glaucomatous eyeball ; the eye had been affected for eighteen months ; this onset of symptoms she stated had been attended with severe neuralgia of that side of the face and head, accompanied by attacks of conjunctivitis ; these attacks of neuralgia persisted side by side with the progress of the affection ; I enucleated the eye. This may arise from the patient and surgeon overlooking the teeth as a probable source of the ear mischief.

Neuralgic and radiating *pain* in the ear associated with dental pain is common. In the eruption of the wisdom teeth such pain is not unusual. Still, occasionally, the origin of deafness is ascribed to toothache. A lady, aged 34, consulted me in 1888 for deafness and tinnitus. She was positive the deafness at first appeared when she was suffering from severe toothache. There were carious teeth of the upper and lower jaws. She was quite healthy in every other respect. The membrana tympani of either ear was rigid; there was collapse of the Eustachian tube—she had the teeth attended to but the deafness and tinnitus continued. I cannot say that I regard disorders of the teeth as anything more than an occasional source, or coincidental one, of retinal trouble or glaucomatous states of the eye. I may have, from ignorance of the possible relationship, overlooked this cause of retinal irritation, increase or diminution of ocular tension, or other intraocular conditions. While I quite recognise the possibility of such dental sources of ocular mischief existing, I believe they occur but rarely. Once a lady consulted me for loss of vision in the left eye, which she asserted had commenced about six months previously, in consequence of a large maxillary abscess that had formed in the corresponding upper jaw from a decayed tooth. When I saw her the eye was typically glaucomatous. The following is a case in point.

Mr. D——, aged 47, sedentary occupation (writing), sight of right eye five months affected, began with neuralgia of the side of the face, and in the teeth; this caused a sense of tightness in the eye, now has a black shadow before his eye occasionally, $V=\frac{1}{5}$ of left eye, $V=\frac{1}{2}$ right; hypermetropic; health otherwise good; tension of right eye$= +3$; right optic papilla congested, retina hyperæmic. There were several decayed teeth on each side. At this time I saw this patient only once; the teeth I directed to be attended to. He returned after an interval of two years, improved considerably in vision but with a return of the neuralgic pains in the teeth, and complaining of tinnitus and abscess in the left meatus; I then had some teeth extracted. The ear symptoms disappeared on treatment.

Mr. Tomes, in his classical work on dental surgery*, in his chapter on secondary affections due to diseased teeth, quotes the case of Mr. Hutchinson's,† in which lagophthalmos and neuralgia of the left eye were ultimately cured by extraction of the five lower

* "System of Dental Surgery," by Sir John Tomes, F.R.S., &c. 3rd edition, by Charles Sismore Tomes, M.A., F.R.S., &c. † Odontological Soc., 1885.

molars, a minute pulp exposure in one of these being sufficient to sustain the lagophthalmos after the neuralgia had been cured by the removal of the others. Temporary injection of the conjunctival vessels and even temporary ciliary congestion occasionally occur after dental operations, or are associated with toothache and dental neuralgia. After the fracture of a tooth in extraction I have seen such ocular irritation maintained for days.

Long since Donders attributed to irritation of the secretory fibres in the trigeminus, the occurrence of glaucoma, and the experiments of Hippel and Grünhagen show, that irritation, in the trigeminus nucleus in the medulla oblongata, is followed by a considerable increase of the intra-ocular pressure; the same result follows the peripheral trigeminal irritation caused by introduction of nicotine into the eye*; such a theory, however, is only sufficient to explain the occurrence of glaucoma in a very limited number of cases and accounts for its presence on quite different pathological grounds from those which are generally accepted by ophthalmologists, both as regards the crystalline lens and the filtrating media. The fact before referred to of the presence of "pressor" or constrictive nerve fibres existing in the trigeminus has an important bearing on this association of trigeminal irritation with glaucoma.

The case which has prompted this contribution is an example of a reflex irritation from affection of the teeth, which has hardly received that consideration which the importance and frequency of the relationship demands. Dr. Lauder Brunton, in a paper which he contributed to St. Bartholomew's Reports,† drew special attention to those forms of headache which are dependent upon disorders of the eyes and teeth, as well as those which are due to disorders of indigestion. His attention was attracted to the relation of headache and carious teeth by his discovery of its occurrence in his own person, finding a commencing caries in the last molar tooth on the same side as the headache. "Not unfrequently," he says, "when I have pointed to a decayed molar as the origin of the headache, the patient has said, 'but I have no pain in the tooth,' and to this I usually answer, it is quite natural, you get the toothache in another part of your head." Dr. Lauder Brunton has noticed as the special seats of headache associated with teeth, the temporal and occipital regions; this location he attributes to an affection of the vaso-motor branches

* Ross on "Diseases of the Nervous System," (*loc.-cit.*, p. 510).

† "Disorders of Digestion," by Lauder Brunton, M.D., F.R.S., 1886.

of the temporal and those of the occipital artery through the sympathetic system, a vascular spasm causing the pain in the head. He has noticed a tenderness in the scalp over the affected regions and this I have myself several times verified. Dr. Lauder Brunton says that a decayed molar in the lower jaw usually gives a temporal or occipital headache, and a decayed molar in the upper jaw causes temporal headache, rather farther forward than that caused by the lower jaw. Caries of the incisors, or eye teeth, is more likely to cause frontal or vertical headache. There is one strong clinical feature which assists in the differentiation between ocular and dental headache, viz.: the frequent occurrence of megrim in the former and its absence in the latter. I, myself, have suffered for years from severe, periodical, ocular megrim, of late, unattended with headache, and though I have few unstopped teeth, have never had dental headache. I believe in this, as in kindred dental associations, there generally is a constitutional state or diathesis which tends to promote the reflex irritation.

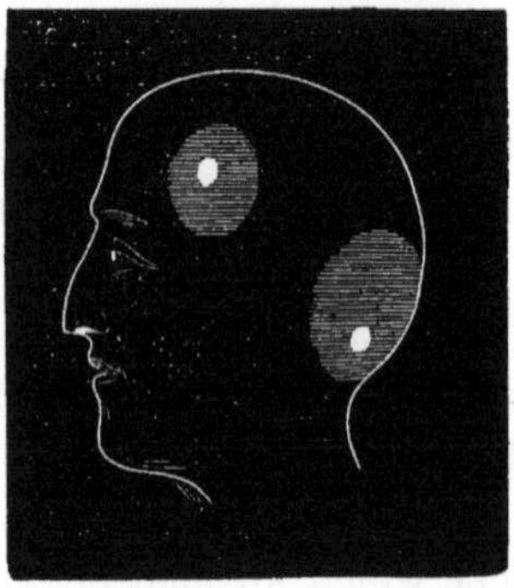

Dr. Lauder Brunton's painful regions in Dental Headache.

In June, 1885, I was consulted by a lady, aged 33, for severe and constant headache, mainly felt across the forehead, and the summit of the head. At times this pain, as she described it, "felt like a band fastened so tightly that it would be a relief to burst it open." When it reached its climax it was felt all over the head, but always worse at the left side, especially over the left orbit, the skin over which occasionally became red and swollen. She described a sensation "inside the head like cords cracking," she was by no means what one would term a "neurotic" subject; the headache commenced in 1882, during her pregnancy, and became more intense after her confinement; she tried various remedies, and consulted different medical men with a view of getting relief. She had change of air to different health resorts, and had exhausted the usual run of neuralgic remedies. Complaining of obstinate costiveness and pain in the back, I made an examination and found an enlarged and retroverted uterus. This I replaced, and having seen it permanently restored in its normal position, and placing her on a course of arseniate of iron with quinine, combined with the use of hydrobromic acid and bromide of zinc, she left London, and I hoped that the reflex disturbance had been due to the corrected uterine disorder. This was in June, 1885; she then assured me that her teeth had been recently overhauled, and gave her no distress whatever; there was no complaint of vision. In March, 1886, she returned as bad as ever. I then determined to have her teeth carefully inspected, which they were; some old stoppings being removed, some sensitive cavities were discovered and these were filled. There was no pain in the teeth. I also determined to carefully test the eyes for any anomaly of refraction. There was some apparent myopia (less than a dioptric in each eye, complicated with astigmatism) I atropinised the pupils, and then discovered that there was a low degree of a vertical hypermetropic astigmatism, which had produced an artificial myopia from spasm of accommodation. The astigmatism took some trouble in its correction, but was finally and completely met; the patient finding considerable relief to her eyes from use of glasses, which she still wears for near work. I now hoped that I had overcome another source of reflex irritation; however, this was not so, and during the latter part of 1886, the entire of 1887, and the greater part of 1888, the patient's sufferings rather increased than diminished, notwithstanding that I exhausted every conceivable remedy, including a long trial of the galvanic current applied over the painful points, and the use of Charcot's discs, which I obtained specially for her.

In October, 1888, she came to London in despair. I thought of placing her under a Weir-Mitchell course, including head and general massage, and with this view she went into a Medical Home. While there she complained of neuralgic pain in the teeth, at both sides of the upper jaw. Mr. Baly examined the teeth and found evidences of slight caries and periostitis in several.

Stoppings were applied in the right lower first molar, the right first and second lower bicuspids, the first left lower molar, the right upper first and second bicuspids; two painful and carious upper molar teeth were extracted. There were no wisdom teeth.

She remained in the home for some weeks subsequently to the

teeth being attended to. I found no relief was given to the head. She then went for a change of air to St. Leonards, and while there had an attack of inflammation and abscess beneath the first upper molar. She immediately came to London, and contrary to my wish, insisted on having all her remaining upper teeth, all of which had stoppings, removed. Accordingly, nine teeth were extracted in November, 1888, Dr. Dudley Buxton administering the anæsthetic. Suffice it to say that from the time of the extraction of the teeth, she gradually began to improve; within three months she had lost the pain in her head, and has been for the past year, completely restored to health, passing through a perfectly normal pregnancy and successful labour in 1889.

The following report from Mr. Badcock shows what the condition of the teeth was which were extracted:—

"On examining the teeth one is at once struck by the fact that *all* are carious, and exostosed, and moreover, that these conditions are distinctly proportional to one another, varying in amount from large mesial and distal cavities, with marked apical enlargement in the case of the lateral, to carious fissures and slightly thickened cementum in that of the molar.

"That the exostosis was the immediate cause of the neuralgia is pretty certain, and I am led to this conclusion by the consideration of the following facts. Firstly:—At no time while the case was under my observation were there any localised symptoms whatever.

"Secondly:—No relief followed treatment of any tooth or teeth other than extraction.

"Thirdly:—On section and microscopical examination of four of the teeth I find no evidence of intrinsic or extrinsic calcification of the pulp; but, on the contrary, the pulp cavities are normal in every respect.

"The thickening of the cementum is probably not sufficient to have given rise to symptoms had the general health been normal. That this was not so is shown by a carious condition of every tooth, at the points corresponding to the gingival margin, where, in some cases, fittings had been inserted, but these had failed to arrest the progress of decay.

"As to the cause of the exostosis, I am inclined to attribute it partly to extension to the dental periosteum of slight pulp irritation, due to caries; and partly to the fact that the teeth have for a long time been subjected to severe irritation as evidenced by large facets; these especially were marked on the lingual aspects of the incisors and canines."

In reference to this case, the following observations of Mr. Tomes are of importance: "There are cases, however, in which the presence of exostosis even of slight amount produces great misery. A certain tooth is pointed to by the patient as the cause; its removal brings relief, the complaint returns, another tooth is fixed upon and removed with a similar result. Another and another follow, and it is only after all the teeth in the upper or the lower jaw have been removed that the patient gains permanent immunity from pain."* Mr. Tomes gives some interesting cases as examples of this persistent pain until extraction of all the diseased teeth had been effected. Two cases occurred under his observation in which epilepsy appeared to be consequent upon diseased and exostosed teeth.

I regard the case as one of the greatest interest, not only to the dental practitioner, but also to the physician or surgeon; three causes were coincidently in operation, to any of which experience proves severe reflex headache might be attributed. When I had successfully relieved two of these, and thought that I had combatted the remaining one, by twice having the teeth carefully examined and treated, the hidden source of the mischief still remained until the radical cure of extraction was resorted to. The practical lesson from such a case is obvious.

In 1888, I was consulted by a patient, aged 60; he came complaining of violent neuralgia of the face and hemicrania. He had tried a variety of remedies without effect. On examining the teeth I found an old tooth plate, which had not been removed for four months, and which covered some carious stumps; there were also two highly inflamed and sensitive teeth, covered with tartar, and the gums generally were in a most unhealthly condition. I recommended, in addition to other remedies, attention to the teeth. I did not hear of the sequel of the case.

In 1885, a lady, aged 35, consulted me for persistent headache, attended occasionally with nausea and sickness; in this case there was extensive erosion of the os uteri. I hoped by curing this, and other general treatment to cure the head symptoms, but I was disappointed. Fortunately, I remembered the teeth as a source of irritation, and found that there were eight carious teeth in the upper jaw, all of which she had removed; this was followed up to the time I last

* *Loc.-cit.*

heard of her, by considerable though not entire, relief from the headache.

A young lady, aged 20, consulted me last year for a neuralgia of the head and face of two years' duration ; her health in every other respect was good. On examining her teeth I found that she had not a single sound tooth in the upper jaw ; my prescription was a reference to a dentist. I have not heard of her since, but I could by reference to past cases adduce many similar proofs of the correlation between carious teeth and severe headache. This paper has, however, quite exceeded my original intention in writing it, my only object being to add my testimony to that previously offered with regard to the importance of not overlooking the teeth as a source of obscure affections the causation of which has not been ascertained. The dentist and the physician should be more commonly in touch than they have been to secure this result.

THE VASCULARIZATION OF THE DENTAL TISSUES.

By A. Hopewell Smith, L.D.S.Eng., L.R.C.P.Lond.
Late Assistant Demonstrator of Histology at Charing Cross Hospital Medical School.

In determining the relationship which exists normally between the vascular supply of the dental tissues, and the tissues themselves, it is necessary to consider the origin of the blood-vessels, their arrangement and mode of distribution, and the areas governed by them. Where great development is taking place, there is free blood-supply ; and the more complex the organisation of a part, whether in anatomical structure or location, or in physiological function, the more abundant anastomosis of capillary blood-vessels is found. And this anastomosis is most important in governing the growth of the tissue, as on it depends the hypertrophy, and atrophy, or normal conditions of the part. For should the blood-stream be increased or accelerated, then overgrowth results, while, on the other hand, should it be diminished or occluded, it is followed by shrinkage, atrophy, degeneration and death.

Hence the blood supply of the hard and soft dental tissues is of vital importance : when normal, the tooth undergoes the changes consequent on development, and finally, is erupted in a perfect condition ; when abnormal, hypertrophies, and atrophies of the whole or parts of the tooth are produced, and irregularities of external configuration, defects in quality of the organic and inorganic substances, and other deviations from typical forms occur.

The most satisfactory subject for the purposes of the examination of capillary arrangement, is an injected section, in which the functional activity of development is most progressive, and most clearly observable—a section, whose genetic cells are most busily engaged in producing the various dental and peridental structures—a section, in short, which exhibits the birth of the life-history of a tooth. Here it is found that the tissues formed from each layer of the primitive blastoderm, are supplied by a separate set of vessels: there is an external or superficial, and an internal or deep network, the former being distributed to the tissues which are epiblastic in origin, including gum, and certain parts of the enamel organ; the latter to those arising from the mesoblast, including dentine organ, dental sac, and surrounding bone. Thus, the external set of vessels is distinctly separated from, and has no connection with the internal deeper set, except at one part, namely, the periosteal membrane, where they meet and anastomose freely with each other.

The external set supplies the enamel organ and gum. On examination of the enamel organ proper, it is found that its external part is absolutely free from any closely-meshed network of capillaries. The layer of cells forming the external epithelium, and the thin branching cells of the stellate reticulum have no blood-supply. One or two large non-branching vessels cross the space occupied by the reticulum, from the thick gum lying external to the enamel organ. These, having advanced as far as the stratum intermedium, suddenly break up into numbers of small capillaries, and form a beautiful plexus, which supplies the cells of this intermediate layer and the internal epithelium. But the capillaries are placed very closely together over the layer of ameloblasts—a fact explained by the activity and importance of these cells in the formation of enamel, and their consequent necessity for a large blood-supply. Little need be said of the vessels of the gum. The stratum corneum, lucidum, and granulosum, are non-vascularized; the rete malpighii and fibrous connective tissue of the dermis differing greatly by being provided abundantly with numerous long, straight vessels, which ramify in all directions. It is clear, therefore, that the nourishment of enamel organ and fibrous tissue of the gum emanates from the same source and is quite distinct from and different to that of the other dental structures.

The internal set supplies the dentine organ, dental sac, and surrounding bone.

In the dentine organ, the pulp has by far the largest and most important system of capillaries. Here, one large vessel enters at the apical foramen of the tooth, and occupying its axis proceeds sinuously outwards, to end near the newly-formed dentine. As it proceeds its calibre becomes somewhat diminished in size, and, in a thick plexus of vessels its branches terminate beneath the odontoblasts. There appears to be no regularity in the arrangement of the primary branches: they leave the large arterial trunk at a considerable angle—in some sections this approaches to and occasionally exceeds a right angle. The secondary and other branches have a similar arrangement. The greater number of the minor distal branches run parallel to the line of dentine under cover of the odontoblasts, between and around which their ultimate ramifications are distributed. These cells and the small round dentogenetic cells which lie closely to them have, therefore, an abundant supply of blood, brought about in a similar manner to that which obtains in the cells of the stratum

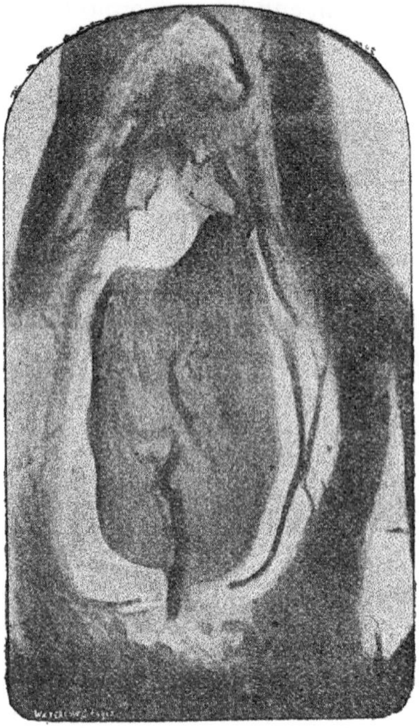

Transverse Section of Jaw of Fœtal Kitten. × = 70.
The detailed explanation of the micro-photograph will be found in the text.

intermedium and internal epithelium. The comparative size of these pulp vessels is much greater than that of the fine, closely set capillaries of striped muscle fibre: they bear a slight analogy to them, but none of the globules or spherical dilatations found in the walls of the latter are to be observed in the former. The advantages of this peculiar method of arrangement of vessels—the sinuous primary arterial trunk, the branches coming off at various angles, the minute anastomosis beneath the dentine—are manifest at once. It is evident that they are thus distributed, first, to give as large an area of blood-supply to the pulp tissues in as small a space as possible, and, second, to prevent shock or any other extraneous influence acting injuriously on its delicate elements. Thus a flow of blood to the part is maintained—constant and uniform—two necessary factors in the production of perfect development, growth, and nourishment.

The accompanying woodcut is taken from a micro-photograph of a transverse section of the lower jaw of a fœtal kitten, the capillaries of which are injected with Berlin blue. It shows the arrangement of the vessels in the pulp and enamel organ, alveolus and dental sac, and the non-vascularization of the oral epithelium and stellate reticulum.

Included under the term "dental sac" are cementum and periosteum.

It is difficult to determine absolutely whence cementum obtains its blood-supply. It would seem to come chiefly from the periosteal vessels. Microscopic appearances demonstrate this. That it is freely vascularized is an undoubted fact, and it is equally certain that the dentine is not the medium by which blood comes. Hence it is fair to presume that the same vessels which supply the alveolo-dental membrane, vascularize cementum also. Wedl * has pointed out that the periosteum has three sources for its blood-supply, viz., from the gum, from the pulp, and from the adjacent alveolus. In regard to the first, it has already been shown that the external and internal sets unite in this situation, the vessels of the gum running deeply inwards to anastomose with the internal set, which supply the dental sac. But also, loops of capillaries from the main arterial trunk of the pulp can be seen spreading outwards and joining the before-mentioned vessels. And in addition, numerous off-shoots from the capillaries of the alveolar bone run towards the cementum and form thick plexuses with the other two. Periosteum therefore is most richly vascularized, and forms, by its method of attachment, the vascular bridge, so to speak, between the living tissues of the jaw and the living tissues of the tooth.

The vascularization of the bone of the alveolus calls for no comment here, being identical with the blood-supply of bone elsewhere.

Briefly to summarise, it can be said that of the soft tissues, the pulp, as being the most important nutritive agent, has the

* *Pathologie der Zahne*, 1870.

greatest, and the gum the smallest system of capillaries; while in the enamel organ the reticulate cells and the external epithelium are destitute of any vessels whatsoever.

On blood-supply, nourishment and vitality depend. Of the three hard dental tissues, enamel is placed absolutely without the pale of nutrition: from the time of its calcification it has been non-nourished, only the ameloblasts, for the work of enamel formation, have been vascularized. Cementum by means of the circulation through its lacunæ and canaliculi is highly vitalized: a state of semi-nutrition or a degree intermediate between these two is found in dentine.

This is carried on in a peculiar and indeed unique manner. It may be said that the method of maintaining the vitality of this tissue has no analogue elsewhere. It is evident, *primâ facie*, that no capillaries can or do traverse the dentinal tubules—the anatomical conditions of the parts are against it. It is likewise impossible for the corpuscular elements of the blood to exude through the vessel walls and distribute themselves along the boundaries of the tubules. For then, dentine would undergo a deep pink pigmentation. One occasionally meets with stained dentine. This, however, is pathological, and follows on rupture of the pulp capillaries, and exudation of blood which by a form of capillary attraction has penetrated the dentine through its tubules, and imparted to it its colour. But it is quite compatible with modern scientific evidence to assume that from the vessels on the surface of the pulp an exudation of plasma, and the fluid constituents of the blood does take place, which entering the tubules, nourishes not only the dentinal matrix, but also the fibrils themselves. If a tooth, in a fresh condition, be fractured, and its pulp chamber opened, the surface of this cavity is seen to be bathed in a thin film of fluid which possesses the properties of protoplasm, and this comes from the blood-vessels: in other words there exists between the layer of odontoblasts and the fully-formed dentine, a thin stream of plasma whose function is to sustain the life of the dentine, and also the cells of the membrana eboris.

For these reasons, dentine is only semi-vitalized, and while enamel cannot withstand the ravages of disease and death, dentine but feebly resists their powers, the functions of the former being merely mechanical and protective, those of the latter only approaching a degree nearer to activity and life.

Reports.

THE ODONTOLOGICAL SOCIETY OF GREAT BRITAIN.

THE ordinary monthly meeting of the above Society was held on the 2nd of June. The President, Mr. FELIX WEISS, L.D.S.Eng., in the chair, and a full attendance of members and visitors.

The minutes having been read and confirmed, the LIBRARIAN (Mr. Ashley Gibbings) announced the receipt of "Black's Study of the Histology and Characteristics of Dental Membrane," together with several volumes and guides to the Natural History Department of the British Museum, for which they were indebted to the kindness of Professor Flower.

The PRESIDENT mentioned that a new list of the Bye-laws of the Odontological Society had just been printed, and copies might be had on application to the Secretary.

Mr. SIDNEY SPOKES read notes of a case of faulty development of enamel. The patient, aged 25, married, wished to know if anything could be done for her "brown teeth." A central incisor had been recently removed, owing to necrosis of the alveolar process. The four first permanent molars were also lost. All the remaining teeth were brown in color, the upper being darker than the lower. The approximal surfaces were affected by caries. As the patient was anxious that something should be done, the upper teeth were removed with the object of replacing them by artificial ones. In ordinary cases of defective enamel, it is usual to see transverse grooves across the teeth marking the period of interfered development of tissue, but in the present case the grooves are in the long axis of the teeth, showing that the process was interfered with during the whole period of calcification; in some places there was a total absence of enamel, the exposed dentine having apparently been sufficiently hard to survive, in spite of the absence of enamel. Elsewhere the enamel occurred in irregular masses. A transverse section through a bicuspid plainly showed the transverse striation of the enamel prisms, while spaces or channels existed in the long axis of the tooth, and these in places were connected with transverse branches mapping the tissue out into areæ. The family history revealed the fact that the "brown teeth" were hereditary, and had appeared through several generations. They were not so dark when first erupted, but became worse as they grew older, in some cases becoming almost black.

The PRESIDENT asked Mr. Spokes if he had seen any of the teeth he had referred to.

Mr. SPOKES replied that he had only seen those in the patient's mouth : he had been promised an opportunity of examining the teeth of the mother, but had not yet seen her.

The PRESIDENT desired to know whether Mr. Spokes had had an opportunity of judging of the colour of the enamel below the surface.

Mr. SPOKES answered affirmatively, and stated that he had made a section of the teeth, but there was nothing much to account for the colour ; it showed that the structure was bad ; a good deal of porosity existed, the teeth absorbed something, and they became browner.

Mr. WALTER H. COFFIN wished to know if he were correct in inferring from Mr. Spoke's remarks that in no case did brown teeth occur as a reversion through white.

Mr. SPOKES : Yes, that is so according to the chart.

Mr. ALFRED SMITH read notes of a "Case of Epulis." The patient was a girl aged 19, and was seen last August. On examining her mouth, Mr. Smith discovered an epulis arising from the left upper central and lateral incisors as large as a filbert. It commenced to grow in 1887, and was excised in the hospital in August, 1888. About five months later it recurred and the surgeon told the patient it would be necessary to remove the adjoining tooth. She expressed reluctance and left the hospital to think the matter over, allowing the epulis to grow untouched until August, 1889. The patient still objecting to lose a sound tooth, it was decided to remove the growth by Paquelin's benzine thermo-cautery, which was successfully accomplished. The wound healed up in a fortnight and there had been no recurrence of the growth since. Mr. Smith exhibited and demonstrated the action of the cautery used.

Mr. GEORGE BRUNTON remarked that he had just such a case to operate upon, and would be glad if the cautery referred to might be exhibited, which was accordingly done.

Mr. J. DENNANT (Brighton), exhibited a contrivance which, though very simple, he had found very useful. He called it an Iodine Dresser. Most practitioners had doubtless experienced the difficulty that patients had in applying iodine to their gums, they generally stain their lips, and practitioners also stained their fingers. This contrivance, which could be made at an extremely small cost, consisted of a stem of black vulcanite with a slot at the top end, into which a little wool is twisted, and perfectly avoided the staining alluded to.

Mr. George Brunton mentioned that tinctura iodi decolorata does not stain the gums.

Mr. C. Robbins stated that he used a still cheaper instrument which answered the purpose: he always instructed his patients to use a common match.

Other members also mentioned having used an ordinary match for many years.

M. W. H. Coffin thought that anything of that kind which the practitioner used himself was much more convenient if the end were bent at an angle.

Mr. Betts thought that the great advantage of the lucifer match was that it could and would be thrown away when used, and a new one used next time. He did not think that there was the same certainty of the vulcanite stems being thrown away, however cheap.

Mr. George Brunton felt that he owed some apology to the society for introducing such trifling matters to their notice as the following, but he would run through them as rapidly as possible. First, he wished to show some *bleached* rubber dam: it was easily done; soak it in cold water, and wrap it up. When dry it is white, and will remain so for a considerable time. Secondly, he used a little pad (shown) for applying an astringent to the mouth and stopping the flow of saliva. He used a strong astringent known as chloralum, which stopped the saliva for a couple of hours, enabling him to work without the rubber dam. He also exhibited a few cutters for running round crowns and trimming roots for pivots. Sometimes he found that in using the syringe one was apt to soil a patient's dress; to avoid this he used a piece of rounded glass with a hole in it, which he placed over the patient's mouth. Mr. Brunton also showed the kind of mouth mirror he used into which he was able to fit glasses himself by running a little cement on warm. He preferred the oval shape mirror, and used with it an attachment to keep down the mouth-piece of saliva ejector when working on the lower jaw. He also exhibited some Rouge Discs for finishing gold fillings; they were made of a French paper known as "rouge" paper, and when both sides of the discs were required to be used, they could be made by glueing the backs of the paper together with shellac.

Lastly, he had three models of cases taken from the mouth, which he would like to present to the society if they were thought worthy of a place in it. One was a model of a syphilitic case, showing "Hutchinson's notch." Another a remarkable spreading of molars in the upper jaw, the upper were quite outside, and overlapped the lower molars. The last case was one of six deciduous incisors in the upper jaw.

The PRESIDENT asked what cement Mr. Brunton used for repairing his mirrors?

Mr. G. BRUNTON: The same as supplied by the depôts for mending teeth.

Mr. WALTER COFFIN wished to know if that cement would stand immersion in hot water?

Mr. W. A. HUNT (Yeovil), said that he had himself found a difficulty with that very cement; it underwent rapid expansion or contraction with heat or cold, and therefore would not do for anyone accustomed to put their mirror in hot water.

Mr. G. BRUNTON remarked that he never put his mirror in hot water; any mirror would be rapidly destroyed in that way, whether that cement or any other had been used.

Mr. KIRBY (Bedford), said with reference to the very interesting model showing six deciduous temporary incisors, he would like to ask Mr. Brunton whether he had had an opportunity of seeing his patient later and knowing whether the corresponding teeth in the permanent set were abnormal.

Mr. G. BRUNTON hoped to see the patient shortly—it was not one of his own patients. If he could take a model of the permanent set he would certainly supply it to the society.

The PRESIDENT said the first paper on the agenda was one by Mr. Leonard Matheson, but with that nice consideration which he (the President) hoped would always distinguish their profession, Mr. Matheson had waived his claim to precedence in favour of Dr. Silk, who was a visitor; with the concurrence of the society he would therefore call upon Dr. Silk for his paper.

Dr. J. F. SILK then read a paper entitled:—

AN ANALYSIS OF A SERIES OF ONE THOUSAND NITROUS OXIDE ADMINISTRATIONS RECORDED SYSTEMATICALLY.

He stated the object of his paper to be two-fold; first, he wished to emphasize the importance of keeping systematic records of *all* gas administrations. Whether the individual cases presented features of special interest or not, he was of opinion that they should always be recorded, for by such means alone could satisfactory explanations of the many curious anomalies in practice be hoped for. In the second place, he wished to give an example of such systematic recórds, and for this purpose he had analysed the first thousand cases that he had recorded upon a definite plan. To thoroughly appreciate and correctly explain the action of a drug upon the human body, it was essential to compare the facts obtained by three distinct methods of investigation, viz., the physiological, the pathological, and the clinical. As far as nitrous oxide was concerned, the happy absence of *post mortem* records seriously limited the pathological element; and although there was probably still much to be learned as to the physiological action, the lesson on a recent commission must be borne in mind, and they must hesitate to dogmatise on the action or the method of administration of a drug when experience is obtained solely in the physiological laboratory, or at best corroborated the experience of the clinical observer.

Physiological investigations, such as those so ably carried out by Dr. Dudley Buxton, combined with the clinical observations of many, was the desideratum. Each one of them might endeavour to add to the common stock of knowledge by keeping clinical records of cases, though lack of time, opportunity or ability, excluded them from the laboratory. As to the way in which to keep notes so as to furnish the largest number and most uniform observations, it must be recollected:—(1) That the patient as a rule was a comparative stranger to the anæsthetist, who, for details as to past and family history, was obliged to depend upon such information as a third person was able and willing to afford; (2) That physical examination and undue cross questioning were frequently resented; (3) That the phenomena observed were purely objective, subjective sensations not being trustworthy; (4) That the whole duration of the process was very short, and much had to be done in the time; (5) That information as to after-effects were seldom obtainable.

These considerations determined Dr. Silk in the adoption of a *tabular* record. The form which he had used in recording nearly 3,000 cases he handed round, but thought perhaps it was rather too elaborate for general use, though with modifications it seemed capable of doing good service. Proceeding to the analysis of cases—

Table I. briefly summarised the various points arranged under three main divisions :—

TABLE I.

GENERAL SUMMARY.

Antecedent Conditions.	Phenomena.	After Effects.
Sex. Age. Physical State. Consecutive Administra- Gas used. [tors. Time. Methods.	Respiratory. Circulatory. Muscular. Nervous. Digestive. Genito-Urinary.	Immediate. Remote.

TABLE II.

DETAILS OF SEX AND AGE.

	7 years and under.	8-14.	15-49.	50-60.	61-70.	p	Totals.	Average Age.
Males	3	25	201	8	3		240	24·18
Females ...	4	50	681	15	4	6	760	24·32
	7	75	882	23	7	6	1,000	24·28

With reference to the physical and mental condition prior to administration, in the majority of the cases in which notes were made, the circumstances were trivial; in twenty-one neurotic, trouble was more or less marked, he did not include simple nervousness. In two cases there was a family history of insanity, and in both the administrations were troublesome, giving rise to much hysteria during recovery. There were but three cases of those who were subject to epileptic fits; one a healthy girl aged 18 who had gas twice. The first time there was nothing noteworthy; the second, after the removal of the face-piece, she struggled to get her hands up, and afterwards described her feelings as pain in the forehead where the epileptic aura commenced. In four cases of phthisis there was nothing out of the ordinary. In one case of valvular disease of the heart, that of a girl aged 16, who had previously had an attack of acute rheumatism, the patient had gas four times, the lividity following being more lasting than normal, and on one occasion a tendency to syncope ensued. Diabetes one case; the urine being examined no change was found. In nine cases of pregnant women, nothing had gone wrong, and he remarked that in seven he would have been the first to hear of it if there had; but in most there was a tendency to vomit. In the only case during lactation the patient had a bilious attack next day, and the infant seemed upset; this point Dr. Silk thought worthy of more attention than was generally given to it. Of consecutive administations of gas—*i.e.*, where the patient was allowed to regain consciousness and then after a few minutes submitted to the anæsthetic, he had sixty-five records: in 12 per cent. there was more or less retching; in two instances there were asphyxial symptoms necessitating pulling forward the tongue; in 9 per cent. there was marked hysteria with crying and screaming on recovery. In six out of nine recorded cases of remote effects, the records were unfavourable, but in 73 per cent. there was nothing to call for remark either as to immediate or remote effects. The average quantity of gas used was between four and five gallons, and the average time during which the face-piece was in position, was 67·5 seconds. The duration of the anæsthesia was very variable, as it was exceedingly difficult to know when sensibility was recovered; the absence of the conjunctival reflex or the presence of jactitations was no guide. In some 400 cases the duration had sufficed for that extraction, on the average, of 2·2 teeth per case, but of course this gave no idea of the actual duration of anæsthesia.

As to the method of administration, in 44 cases the gasometer was used; in 467 cases the gas was administered quite pure; and on 502 occasions the supplemental bag or its substitute was employed. The tabulated effects of the two methods were as follows:—

	Total Observations.	Effects.				
		Immediate.		Remote.		
		Nil.	Bad.	Observations.	Nil.	Bad.
Pure	467	81·16	18·84	28	39·28	60·72
Supplemental ...	502	75·9	24·10	33	48·48	51·52

He should mention that he had more than one remark in his note book to the effect that he was inclined to believe that the use of the supplemental bag tended to accelerate the onset of anæsthesia.

Passing to phenomena, with regard to the circulatory system, the diagram he handed round would be recognised as being taken from one of the many excellent tracings made by Dr. Dudley Buxton, by whose kind permission it was exhibited. Dr. Buxton's tracing was, if it might be so termed, a model of standard tracing, and was, if Dr. Silk understood rightly, taken under exceptionally favourable circumstances; such a tracing as Dr. Buxton's one could hardly hope to obtain in ordinary every day experience. At the same time it would be observed that there was a strong resemblance between his and Dr. Buxton's tracings, *i.e.*, general acceleration of pulse, loss of tidal wave, accentuation of the dicrotic curve, increase in heart force. With regard to the muscular system, rhythmic movements of arms or legs were frequent, and Dr. Silk was at a loss to explain them. Opisthotonos was most common in females, and was invariably accompanied with profound anæsthesia.

With reference to the condition of the pupils, on 797 occasions in this series of cases he had made notes, and in 64 a rough attempt at measurement, in the latter the average size of the pupil before administration was 3·64 mm.; at the height of the narcosis the average size was 5·5 mm.—an appreciable dilatation no doubt, but hardly what was understood as "a dilated pupil." Of unmeasured cases, the following notes were made: decided dilatation, 366; more or less dilatation, 96; little or no dilatation, 94; dilatation followed by contraction, 20; after dilatation, 15. Dr. Silk did not think that pupil dilatation could be solely relied upon as a test of the completion of narcosis.

Micturition occurred in ten cases, or one per cent.; all were females: in three of these there was opisthotonos, and in one much struggling. Erotic movements and sexual illusions were present in six cases—all females, five of whom were unmarried, and one married and in an early stage of pregnancy. There was great difficulty in getting records of after-effects, but probably more or less headache was the rule rather than the exception.

DISCUSSION.

The PRESIDENT having invited discussion on Dr. Silk's very interesting paper

Mr. W. A. HUNT (Yeovil), said that in order to save time he would at once take advantage of the President's invitation, and ask

Dr. Silk a question. Twenty years ago he (Mr. Hunt) gave up watching the pupils and also the cornea, nor had he watched patients as to dilatation, but he had observed sometimes that a tear would trickle down one side of the face only, showing clearly that the action of the sympathetic nerve was confined to that side only. Had Dr. Silk noticed any inequality in the dilatation?

Dr. Silk replied that in the recorded series he had not met with any inequality, but he had one case on his note book, which, however, he had not yet had an opportunity of examining very carefully.

Mr. Walter H. Coffin wished to ask Dr. Silk on the point of dilatation, whether he was accustomed to give instructions to his patients as to closing the eye. In many cases the patients close the eye before administration, in others the administrator told them to keep the eye open. He thought some difference in the size of the pupil might be accounted for in that way. He would also like to ask whether Dr. Silk advocated mptying the bladder before administration as a matter of routine.

Dr. Silk said, with regard to opening or shutting the eye before administration, he generally found that the patient was placed in the full glare of the window, and he did not know that any difference would be made by shutting the eye. His average was taken from a large number of cases, and any slight difference there might be would reduce itself; he should think that in the majority of cases the eye was open. With reference to urinating, he thought all administrators would endeavour to get the bladder empty, but it was not always possible—it was a good routine practice.

Mr. L. Matheson, interposing, desired to say that if any members were shrinking from discussing Dr. Silk's paper out of consideration for him, he should be quite willing to defer his paper to another meeting.

The President thanked Mr. Matheson and said that it would certainly seem desirable, with so good a meeting which included several eminent anæsthetists, that they should fully discuss Dr. Silk's valuable paper.

Mr. George Brunton thought that the opportunity of discussing the paper should not be lost, and wished to say that some of the principal points had not yet been touched upon, one of them, viz., the pulse tracings, he should personally like to know more about, as many of their men were not in the habit of taking them at all.

Mr. Woodhouse Braine did not know whether they ought to have anything to 'say about ether. There was one little point; during the last twenty years in which he had given it, he had had five or six cases in which the patients—boys chiefly, under the age of 16—on the following day were very drowsy and suffered from delusions; one person refused to take food, alledging that poison had been put into it. It was quite certain that the result of ether was to produce delusions. But it had been pointed out by one of the physicians to St. Luke's Hospital that this condition had degenerated into idiocy. With reference to epilepsy in the administration of gas, Mr. Braine was quite sure it might be given with perfect safety to epileptic patients, and he knew of cases where gas had been administered while patients were actually under an epileptic seizure. He was called in to give gas to an epileptic in Bloomsbury Square, and when he arrived the boy was in a state of epilepsy, Mr. Braine administered the gas notwithstanding, and when the boy recovered he did not have any of the after effects of long sleep to which he had previously been subject. In these patients he had always noticed that they came under the effects of anæsthesia very quickly. When the anæsthesia deepens after the removal of the face-piece, it was he thought generally in cases of extraction of lower teeth, and his explanation was that it was due to the tongue being forced back out of the way for the convenience of the dentist. Mr. Braine very rarely gave gas in private a second time, because the patients did not recover so well—it was quite a case of fees against comfort. With reference to rhythmic movements, he thought they very often began in a voluntary movement on the part of the patient to show that they were not insensible, because he had asked patients afterwards and they had replied, "Well, I thought if I did so you would know I was not insensible." He thought it a bad plan to allow them, because when commenced they often got exaggerated in the end, and the patient's hands would get in the way.

Mr. Bailey thought that the Society should give Dr. Silk a hearty vote of thanks for his paper and for having given them the tabulated records of cases. He thought there was no doubt that those who were in extensive practice would find some difficulty in the way of keeping a tabulated record; in private practice there would be diffidence on the part of patients in answering some questions. The question of sex would not present any difficulty, but age was a delicate matter about which to ask a lady. But in hospitals it could be done, and tabulated records should be kept. With regard to epilepsy, he quite agreed with Mr. Braine. In reference to after intensification of effects, Mr. Bailey said in taking out lower molars the patient would sometimes get cyanotic, and the operator would become alarmed, but if the tongue were got out of the way the patient recovered. Mr. Bailey had never advocated pulling the tongue forward, and he had never seen the necessity of it if the gag is taken out of the mouth and the chin put up. With reference to pupil dilatation, his opinion was that in profound anæsthesia it is always dilated. He was perfectly sure that in all his own cases the pupil was dilated. In one case of extreme dilatation the patient, a man, was delighted that he felt so comfortable after the administration, showing that the dilatation had no ill effect. There was a little difficulty when Dr. Silk talked about taking the face-piece off. Jactitation, which is the only known reliable symptom of complete anæsthesia, one got in five or six seconds. The mouth-piece is taken off, and he would say absolute anæsthesia continued for about twenty seconds; that seemed a short time, but a great deal could be done in it, one could extract a tooth in three seconds. Dr. Silk stated that he gave pure gas: Mr. Bailey was rather astonished at the quantity. Whether he (Mr. Bailey) was extravagant or not he did not know, but he usually marked off his 100 gallon bottles for fourteen inhalations, that would be about seven gallons for each patient. However, the best way to get at the actual quantity used would be to ask the house surgeon of the hospital, and this he would do. He thought even four gallons a small quantity: perhaps he did not give the gas in the way that Dr. Silk did. He (Mr. Bailey) gave it using a face-piece with an expiratory valve only, no inspiratory. He did not see his patients get blue. His Cattlin's bag was very small, only one-and-a-half gallons. Children were most liable to opisthotonos, women next, and men least. He (Mr. Bailey) could only remember a few cases of men having opisthotonos. One patient he had who fought a long time after the tooth was out—about half a minute; he was a very intellectual man, his fear was that he should go off again. Mr. Bailey was perfectly sure that gas might be given in almost any condition of heart disease. He had chiefly risen for the purpose of thanking Dr. Silk for his very interesting paper.

Dr. Dudley Buxton said that at that late hour of the evening it would be wholly impossible to attempt an adequate criticism upon Dr. Silk's paper. There were, however, some points upon which he would like to touch. In reference to the question of the advisability of administering nitrous oxide gas to epileptics and persons of unsound mind, Dr. Dudley Buxton proposed to offer the result of his experience, which had been pretty wide. It had been pointed out by Dr. Savage, of Bethlem Hospital, and by others, that attacks of acute mania had apparently been determined, in those predisposed, by the administration of laughing gas, chloroform and ether. It was a mistake, he thought, to suppose that true delusions followed such anæsthetics unless in the predisposed, and further, even in persons who had a bad family history, or had themselves been mentally affected, he believed from his experience that such recurrence of attacks was very rare. In instances in which he had given gas to lunatics, for extractions and for surgical operations, he had had no particular difficulties, and certainly none but what a little tact could overcome, and he had not met with exacerbation of the patient's condition. Subsequently, indeed, they had seemed cowed and more tractable after the anæsthetics. Epileptics and persons the subject of epileptiform convulsions, took laughing gas very well. Dr. Dudley Buxton did not think that taking that anæsthetic in any way increased the chance of their having a fit, but if a fit did come on he did not consider it any indication for discontinuing the anæsthetic. In a tolerably long series of brain cases with which he had assisted his friend and colleague, Mr. Victor Horsley, he had had to deal with many in whom slight causes originated epileptiform seizures, and in only one case had a fit occurred whilst gas was being given. Upon this occasion he went on with administration, and the patient became unconscious, while no complications occurred. Dr. Dudley Buxton asked whether Dr. Silk's cases were taken from records of hospital patients or of private patients, and he made the enquiry because he felt the statistics given must be allowed for in a different way, according as one or the other class was dealt with. Hospital patients were herded together in out-patients' waiting rooms and were, from reasons into which he need not enter, always very highly nervous and excitable, and not at all favourably placed for taking gas. It was a common remark for them to make as soon as they resumed consciousness, "Did I scream?" They went to sleep with the idea that they would scream, and as a result they awakened doing it. He thought to get the full value of the records of cases, that they should be divided into different classes, according as they were private or hospital patients. He did not quite agree with Mr. Bailey when he said it was impossible in private practice to elicit the required particulars. As a rule, the dentist knew the patient's family, and his (Dr. Buxton's) experience was, they were always most ready to help forward any investigation. He was quite sure that Mr. Bailey, with that suave manner which formed so conspicuous a trait of his bearing, could obtain particulars of his cases, and would by so doing, confer a benefit upon the profession. Turning to the question of heart disease, he would emphasize most strongly what Mr. Bailey had said. He was quite sure that valvular disease of the heart was *per se* no reason for refusing to administer gas, but rather a strong reason for giving it. The only cases that had in his hands given rise to unpleasant symptoms, were those of the functionally feeble heart, and the heart weakened by degeneracy of its muscular coats. He had no hesitation in saying that even in these cases the effects of the shock was far more likely to be detrimental to the well-being of the heart than could be those of nitrous oxide gas when properly given. There were many other points upon which he would have liked to have touched, were he not warned by the procession of time that all things must come to an end.

Dr. Silk felt that he had to thank the society very heartily and sincerely for the very kind manner in which they had received his remarks. He had no idea that he would be displacing anyone or leading to a transfer of business to another evening. He was very sorry that Mr. Matheson's paper should have been postponed, at the same time he was very much indebted to him for having allowed his paper to take precedence. There had been so many speakers who had raised questions of the greatest importance, that he could not hope to answer all of them at that late hour. Mr. Braine had raised the question of ether, and he (Dr. Silk) hoped Mr. Braine would not think he was being treated cavalierly, if he said with Mr. Bailey that he regarded it as rather outside the scope of the paper. With regard to epilepsy, he did not know of any reason why gas should not be given in such cases. With reference to rhythmic movements, the rhythmic movements as he meant them were distinctly not those which commence with the patient drawing attention to his condition; they were not the movements of lifting the warning finger, they were the movements of the knee. Mr. Bailey had said something about the after intensification of the anæsthesia. Dr. Silk was glad that Mr. Bailey agreed with him that there was an after intensification for about twenty seconds, that might account for the fact of the pupil being dilated. But what he wished to point out was that before the dilatation you get jactitation and so on. Some question had been raised by Mr. Bailey as to the quantity of gas; Dr. Silk did not regard the point as of much importance, but one could very readily see that with no inspiratory valve Mr. Bailey's average and Dr. Silk's were easily accounted for; he did not think there was any great discrepancy. Dr. Dudley Buxton had asked if the recorded cases were those of hospital or private patients: he (Dr. Silk) did not quite agree with him as to the difference between one class of patient and the other; it was rather a difference of degree than of kind, which education alone would account for.

The usual votes of thanks having been adopted, the society adjourned to November 3rd, when papers by Mr. L. Matheson and Mr. Storer Bennett will be read.

REVIEW.

Transactions of the American Dental Association, 1889, at the Twenty-ninth Annual Session. Philadelphia: The S. S White Dental Manufacturing Co. 1889.

It may seem somewhat late in the day to offer a review of this publication, recently to hand, but to those of our readers who are fond of comparing things dental, in the American and English schools, some account of the proceedings of the last meeting, held at Saratoga Springs, may be interesting. Moreover, although the American Association would seem to differ from the British Dental Association, both in its constitution and its methods, it may be of advantage, on the eve of the meeting to be held at Exeter, to take a short note of the work done "on the other side." The mode of proceeding seems to be as follows: After opening the Session with prayer, and calling over the roll, reports of the various committees are received and miscellaneous business transacted. The real work of the meeting is arranged by the formation of Sections, the largest of which appears to be the one dealing with Operative Dentistry, and there are morning, afternoon and evening sessions.

In addition to the President's Address the following papers were read :—"On the Growth of Enamel," by Dr. Frank Abbott. The author strongly supports the views of Heitzmann and Bödecker. The internal epithelium of the enamel organ is not directly converted into the hard tissue, but there is an intermediate process whereby the epithelial cell is replaced by "medullary corpuscles," the re-arrangement of which forms the true ameloblast, to be afterwards again split up into "medullary corpuscles," described as being finely granular, and then calcified as the enamel prism. An analogous process occurs in connection with odontoblasts in the formation of enamel. With regard to these statements, one can scarcely help recalling how Owen formerly described the nuclei of the cells of the pulp lengthening, and then dividing both longitudinally and transversely to develop secondary cells which continue included within the primary cells. As to the second disintegration in the complicated metamorphosis described by the American observers, may it not be asked whether the finely granular condition noticed in the "few perfect specimens in Bödecker's collection" is not to be ascribed simply to the impregnation of the ameloblasts with lime-salts in the form of calco-spherites? The paper further points out that the original enamel organ is not of sufficient size to suffice for the production of the whole enamel, although the ameloblasts are recruited from the *stratum intermedium*. "Both the last-named layer and the blood vessels in the myxomatous enamel-organ have been observed and depicted by John Tomes as early as 1848—an admirable instance of acute observation of lasting value."

"Dentistry in China and the East," by J. Ward Hall, of Shanghai. According to this paper there are nine Americans practicing on the coast, but the patients are drawn from the English, American and Continental residents, "so that the four hundred millions of Chinamen do not figure in the matter at all." The author's advice to the young dentist is to stop at home, and the paper closes with some not very consoling remarks as to the social status of dentists in England and India.

Dr. Harlan's report of Section V. dealt with the value of essential oils.

In Section VI. the report on "Implantation," by H. A. Smith, and the discussion which followed, contain references to the usual disputed points, such as the salvation of the pericementum, the age of the tooth, the perforation of the antrum, &c., but although words of warning, nay, of despair, were made use of, no one yet seems bold enough to condemn the operation. One case mentioned in the report may be here reproduced : In implanting a first bicuspid, the antrum was "accidentally" penetrated while the socket was prepared. "The severe hæmorrhage which followed evidently came from a wounded arteriole in the lining membrane of the cavity. While the tooth was in place the blood escaped through the natural opening of the autrum, dripping into the throat behind the soft palate. After a few days, serious complications arose, endangering the life of the patient, and not until five weeks after the operation was restoration complete."

In the same Section was a paper by Dr. Talbot, who has attempted to explain the causes of irregularities of the teeth and jaws, and has offered a system of classification. Numerous observations in asylums led the author to the conclusion that irregularities are commonly associated with idiocy ; and this agrees with the well-known opinion of Dr. Langdon Down, expressed in his paper to the Odontological Society. Another interesting matter discussed in Section VI. was the proposal for a systematic examination of all the pre-historic crania to be found in the museums of the United States, in order to get all the information bearing upon dental science. The association voted the sum of five hundred dollars towards the expenses necessary, and amongst others on the committee appointed to co-operate, is Dr. Barrett, who, some years ago, published the results of his examination of about two thousand pre-historic skulls. He came to the conclusion that the people then living suffered from caries very nearly to the same extent as those of to-day. Dr. Brophy read a paper dealing with some of the remote causes of trigeminal neuralgia, and narrated a case due to the pressure of a lower denture, necessitating somewhat heroic treatment. There was marked enlargement of the nerve at the mental foramen, and the author appears to think this condition occurs more often than is suspected. In an edentulous jaw, especially where the foramen is situated near the upper border, it will be well to relieve the plate and avoid pressure at this point.

Section II. was concerned with Dental Education, Literature, and Nomenclature. It was reported that the number of dental colleges had risen to thirty-one, and that seven hundred and ninety-six persons had graduated, making a total of 2,642 for the last four years ; whilst in England we may imagine that an increase in the schools may be productive of good, it may be doubted whether in the United States the increase has not already exceeded the limit which gives rise to healthy competition. One college in favour of the three-year system had decided to extend the college term to seven months in each year, but felt themselves obliged to arrange a two-years' graded course of instruction, and the report remarks: "It is painful to chronicle a backward step, although, undoubtedly the institution is justified in pursuing this course while 'the fences are down all around.'" It was decided to recommend that all the dental colleges should increase the course of study to a three-year graded system of not less than five months each; "while some dental colleges may not be conducted strictly for the best interests of the profession, there are now no bogus colleges in the United States." The papers read in this section were: "Some thoughts on Education," by Dr. Atkinson; "Oral Surgery and who should Perform it," by Dr. Tenison; and "The Necessity for Independent Dental Journalism," by Dr. Louis Jack.

The report of Section III. on Operative Dentistry alludes to the use of electricity, the treatment of exposed pulps, and immediate root-filling. With regard to the latter, it is said that "a number of reported cases of adverse results has induced caution, and the necessity for a more careful discrimination in the selection of cases for this operation is clearly indicated." Crown and bridge work is thought to be so important that it has been made a specialty, occupying an intermediate ground between operative and mechanical dentistry. A paper was read by Dr. Jackson on appliances for correcting irregularities, and one from Dr. Herbst on glass fillings. The discussion in this section turned upon root-filling, and afforded an opportunity for the expression of very various opinions. A paper had been read upon this subject, but the committee were instructed not to publish it, and therefore it does not appear in the *Transactions*. The points referred to by the speakers were principally with regard to the position and number of the foramina in the root, the direction of the canal and the advisability of enlarging it, the permeability and the contents of the dentinal tubuli, and the use of gutta-percha, hickory, and oxychloride. Altogether, this copy of the *Transactions* enables one to form some idea as to the work done and the method of doing it. There is certainly a wide range of subjects and a very free expression of opinion, but the general impression left on one's mind is that the individual expressions of opinion are too dogmatic, as who should say: "I know *my* experience is the only true one, I cannot account for the results you claim, and I am satisfied with my own." In other words, there would seem to be a tendency to forget that the scientist should cultivate an open mind.

DENTAL SURGERY FOR MEDICAL PRACTITIONERS AND STUDENTS OF MEDICINE. By A. W. BARRETT, M.B. (Lond.), M.R.C.S., L.D.S.E. London: H. K. Lewis.

To say that we cannot congratulate the author on this, the second edition of his work, is to express our opinion but feebly. The book is lamentably behind the times; it is, in more than one important statement, inaccurate; and as a text book it is quite inadequate, both by reason of most serious omissions, and because of the want of lucidity in such instructions as it does contain.

It must be freely admitted that it is no easy task to write a book on special surgery for the use of the general practitioner; one of the chief difficulties being to avoid, on the one hand, the Scylla of elaborate and detailed description which can only puzzle and confuse the average practitioner, untrained in special work and study, and on the other hand, the Charybdis of instructions so brief as to be practically useless, and calculated only to mislead the unwary reader into supposing that operations requiring the very greatest nicety and anxious care, may be undertaken with a light heart and fingers unaccustomed as a rule to work of any greater delicacy than the passing of a catheter, the opening of an abscess, or the setting of a broken bone. It has not been given to Mr. Barrett to steer the middle course of pithy brevity, either in his enumeration of symptoms, or his description of operations.

Again, it is no doubt desirable and necessary to keep down the size of a handbook, but in such a one as that now under discussion, it would have been quite possible to substitute for much that is practically useless to the general practitioner, some attempt at a respectable account of dental and dentigerous cysts,—of antral disease as connected with the teeth,—of alveolar abscess,—of neuralgia of the fifth nerve,—of the serious influence for good or evil which the condition of the first permanent molars may and often does exert on the general health of a young child,—of the part played in the production of decay and odontalgia by pregnancy and febrile diseases,—of the many forms of reflex nervous disturbance which may be set up by dental disease. These most important subjects, and others of scarcely less weight, are either entirely ignored, or touched upon in such a casual manner, as to render what is said concerning them of no practical value whatever.

To instance inaccuracies :—The account of dental caries is unscientific and misleading ; and the one reference to neuralgia of dental origin must leave a reader unacquainted with facts under the impression that the only form of dental disease which produces neuralgia of the fifth is chronic periostitis of old roots, as a matter of fact this being but one and not the most frequent of the dental causes of neuralgia. To speak of trismus and fistulous openings through the cheeks as the results of *chronic* disease, is to credit chronic with what is certainly in nine cases out of ten due to *acute* inflammatory action, whilst to leave the practitioner to suppose that after the application of arsenious acid there is no need to clear the pulp canals, is to sanction, and indeed teach, a method of practice both pernicious and discreditable.

With regard to immediate torsion we entirely disagree with the author, for it has been shown over and over again to be a most valuable and successful operation when performed with due discrimination. The use of nitrate of silver in the treatment of pyorrhœa alveolaris is to be severely deprecated, since quite as good results may be obtained by other drugs (aromatic sulphuric acid for example), without the unsightly discoloration produced by lunar caustic. That erosion (by the author quaintly termed "Hunter's Denuding Process") is produced always and solely by the friction of brushing, is a fiction long ago exploded.

Quite at variance with the opinion of most experienced anæsthetists is the statement boldly made, that "for anæsthetising hysterical patients of either sex"—for the extraction of teeth be it remembered—"chloroform is more serviceable than gas" ; and it is certainly news to us to hear that a patient "recovers consciousness less rapidly" after inhalation of ether than after that of chloroform.

In speaking of Mr. Barrett's book as being sadly behind the times, we do not, of course, desire or expect, in a work intended for general practitioners, a detailed exposition of all the latest and best methods of work ; but the general tone of the volume, and the character of the instructions given, are such as to present but a very poor picture of the capabilities of modern dentistry.

We are strongly of opinion that such a book is not only incomplete, but positively injurious, if it does not contain an emphatic introductory statement, pointing out, in the first place, the extreme delicacy and exquisite accuracy and finish necessary to the success of all but the most elementary dental operations ; and in the second place, insisting upon the folly of attempting anything more than such simple operations unless one has undergone the years of special education which can alone give a surgeon the requisite knowledge and ability for the practice of modern dental surgery.

Manual of Dental Surgery, including Special Anatomy and Pathology. By Henry Sewill, M.R.C.S , L.D.S. Third Edition. London: Balliere, Tyndall & Cox.

Books on professional subjects are written "for practice" or "from practice," the author has "something to say" or he wants to "say something," or, on the other hand, he may be a teacher at a hospital school, and may have had some special experience on the subject about which he writes, he may have conducted some original researches that are valuable to his profession. The readers of this manual must judge for themselves why this book has been written. The early editions were very poor indeed, when compared with this new one, which is very nicely arranged and profusely illustrated, but the claims made in the preface of original researches is nowhere borne out in the subsequent pages. There are plenty of records of original work, but it has invariably been undertaken and carried out by others. Mr. Pound, Mr. Pringle, Mr. Charters White, Mr. Arthur Underwood, are all mentioned as having done good original work for the author, and some of these names appear very often in connection with the series of very beautiful and valuable micro-photographs that are found in the book.

The grounds, therefore, upon which Mr. Sewill has constituted himself a teacher are a little difficult to find, more especially after an admission made in this journal a short time since as to the mediocrity of his operative powers.

The chapter on caries is decidedly the best in the book and is well worth perusing ; but the chapter on its treatment is not so good, the preparation of cavities might be better, there is far too much cutting away of tissue in interstitial cavities recommended, little or nothing about preserving as much as possible of the front wall of a cavity in the incisors, while grooves are advised to be made that it would be impossible to accurately fill with gold. That in these days anyone should deliberately advise the use of india-rubber wedges for the separation of teeth that have to be filled is strange indeed, while tape and separators are dismissed with a few words. Surely humanity demands that the relative positions of these processes should be reversed, even if the india-rubber is not omitted entirely.

The chapter on diseases of the pulp is good, but a Donaldson's bristle is not the best instrument with which to remove a dead pulp. Nor is cotton wool soaked in antiseptics by any means the best filling for root canals. Something non-absorbent, such as gutta-percha or even sealing wax is preferable. Something might with advantage to the reader have been said for or against immediate root filling, a practice that is rapidly gaining many advocates.

No new light is thrown upon the difficulties surrounding the diagnosis of exostosis or the treatment or cause of pyorrhœa alveolaris, or erosion, all subjects of great importance to the dental surgeon, and why, if it be right, as it certainly is, to fill eroded cavities it is wise to wait until the erosion is deep, as stated by Mr. Sewill, is difficult to follow.

In the description of pivoting no mention is even made of the most perfect manner of performing this operation by means of a tube and split pin, and the chapter on crown and bar work is quite too meagre in its dealing with the subject, for it is one that is of great importance to the dentist and it is to works on dental surgery that he would naturally turn for a description of how to proceed in such cases, equally as much as he would for pivoting "the mechanical processes which it includes" and which do come within the scope of a manual in dental surgery. All dentists have to do crowning, while very few will be called upon to diagnose or treat the varieties of odontomes that are met with.

The chapter on extraction is fairly good, except that it seems strange to see the ordinary old-fashioned straight forceps recommended for the extraction of lower bicuspid and molar teeth in preference to the hawk's bill.

It is in subjects that are on the borderland between surgery and dentistry that the book is, perhaps, weakest In such matters, for instance, as stomatitis and ranula ; in the first case very much more might be said on the subject, and certainly a few more varieties mentioned, while the second is quite wrong. Ranula is never an obstruction of the duct of a sublingual salivary gland, and never contains saliva, but has been proved many times to be caused by the enlargement of a sublingual mucous gland, and in nearly every case the duct of the salivary gland can be traced across the ranula, as in another particular. Epulis is poorly described and the dentists having to operate upon such a thing, and wishing to know how to proceed, would certainly receive rather a disappointment if he referred to this manual for any help.

If only for the plates and the chapter on dental caries wherein is epitomised the latest knowledge on that disease, the book should be on the shelves of every dentist's library. The "get up" of the book is excellent, its type clean, and the printing and production of the plates most commendable.

GOSSIP.

ALL communications for the Editor should be addressed to 82, Mortimer Street, London, W. Much confusion and loss of time will be avoided if readers will bear this in mind.

THE British Dental Association holds its Annual General Meeting at Exeter this year, under the presidency of Mr. Browne Mason, of that city. A strong programme is published.

A VERY successful entertainment was given on Wednesday, 23rd ult., at the Stanley Exhibition by the officials of the Dental Hospital and London School of Dental Surgery. Mr Thomas Underwood distributed the prizes.

MR. ASHLEY W. BARRETT, B.M.Lond., M.R.C.S., has been appointed examiner on the Dental Board of the Royal College of Surgeons of England *vice* Mr. Winterbottom. The present examiners are Messrs. C.S.Tomes, S.J. Hutchinson, Morton Smale, and A. Barrett.

WE hope shortly to publish the Articles of Association issued by the Victoria Dental Association, a society modelled upon that of the kindred British Dental Association. The founders of the Colonial Association will receive cordial sympathy and support from fellow-practitioners in the mother-country; they have a fine field of useful labour open to them.

IT is, we believe, pretty generally understood, that before long some important changes will take place in the executive of the British Dental Association, owing to the proposed resignation of some of the leading officials. Rumour mentions Mr. Smith Turner and Mr. Morton Smale as likely to retire from the presidency of the Representative Board and Secretaryship of the Association respectively. Mr. F. Canton is spoken of as a successor to Mr. Smith Turner, but the secretary's name has not as yet been divulged.

THE DENTAL RECORD, LONDON: AUG. 1, 1890.

Implantation at the National Dental Hospital.

Dr. Younger, of San Francisco, who was the first to perform the operation of Implantation, was asked to demonstrate his method during his recent stay in London. Accordingly, on the 18th ult., some twenty gentlemen were present, by invitation, at the National Dental Hospital. Dr. Younger first gave a short account of the operation, explaining by means of a diagram, the method of obtaining the necessary flaps of gum. He does not now think it necessary to have the scion tooth in a fresh state, but holds that the dried remains of the pericementum are important in securing an attachment in the new socket, and that there results a vital union. The patient, a young lady, then took her place in the chair to have a tooth implanted in the situation of the second left upper bicuspid, which had been lost some years. A local anæsthetic mixture containing cocaine was injected, the needle being pushed in deeply. The operator expressed his regret that the composition of this mixture is at present a trade secret, but spoke favourably of his experience with it. The new socket is made by instruments which combine the reamer and the trephine, and a sliding spring enables one to gauge the length of the root to be inserted, so that the socket shall not be made too deep. The scion tooth was "one without a history" with a not very long root, one side of which was bare, but the other was said to have pericementum upon it. The pulp canal had been cleared out and filled from the crown just before, and the tooth was laid in bichloride of mercury solution until required. It was tried in the new socket two or three times until the latter was the right size and length, and then pushed forcibly home, no ligature or splint being used. The operation was skilfully, neatly and quietly performed, and the patient on being asked afterwards as to pain said that "it did not hurt much," and that the boring for the socket was not as bad as having a tooth extracted. She apparently had some unpleasant sensations in the throat, which were thought to be due to some of the anæsthetic mixture having been swallowed. On presenting herself the following morning, the patient said she had been troubled with nausea during the night, but that her mouth was quite comfortable, and she would not know that anything had been done, except that the former space was filled up. The tooth appeared comfortable, the gum quiet, and after seeing that the bite was not raised, the patient was dismissed for a week.

Dr. Younger had just received from Berlin a favourable report from a patient upon whom he had operated last February. This is the most extensive case he has yet undertaken, and as it has not yet been published and is of an unusual character, it may be briefly mentioned. A young lady, aged twenty, with mal-development of the upper jaw and a well-marked underhung bite had associated with these conditions a deficiency of teeth. The two centrals were present in the upper jaw, but much separated; there were some teeth in the bicuspid region, but no molars. This patient had twelve teeth implanted altogether within six weeks, including two centrals in the lower. In the upper jaw a modification was practised. Instead of distinct sockets in the bone a series of deep grooves was made in the front, and the teeth were practically inserted between the jaw and the gum. In this way the "bite" was so rectified that it is now a normal one, and the patient's appearance is greatly improved. The case will be shown during the Congress in Berlin.

APPOINTMENTS.

Cumine, Rupert H., L.D.S.I., has been appointed Hon. Dental Surgeon to the West Ham, Stratford and South Essex Hospital.

Gregory, Thomas, L.D.S., has been appointed Assistant Dental Surgeon to the Edinburgh Dental Hospital, *vice* Wm. Wilson, M.B, C.M., L.D.S., deceased.

Repairing Gold Fillings.—It is claimed as a novelty in the method of repairing gold fillings building directly on the gold after it was annealed in the tooth. A separate flame and a chip blower to blow the flame on to the freshly filed surface of the gold was for some time used by Mr. S. S. Southruth, and from this has been evolved the present appliance.

CORRESPONDENCE.

[We do not hold ourselves responsible in any way for the opinions expressed by our correspondents.]

ENCOURAGEMENT TO DENTAL STUDENTS.

To the Editor of the DENTAL RECORD.

DEAR SIR,—There can be no doubt that the future of the profession depends on those who are now students, and every possible encouragement should be offered to keep them well up to the mark. At the Derby meeting of the British Dental Association Mr. Henry C. Quinby, of Liverpool, and myself, offered each the sum of £20 annually for five years, to be expended on prizes for proficiency in operating, and it has since been decided that Mr. Quinby's contribution shall be divided into two prizes, of £12 and £8 respectively, for the Liverpool Dental School, and that my own should be divided in a similar manner for the Manchester school.

It is desirable that similar prizes shall be at the disposal of all the Dental Schools in the United Kingdom, and we ask your careful consideration of the matter. Competition is the essence of success, and everything should be done to encourage the rising generation. These prizes, at both the Liverpool and Manchester Schools, will be offered in either money, books, or instruments, at the choice of the successful student, but of course this need not be adhered to in all cases; we simply ask that your assistance and consideration should be given to those who are the future backbone of the profession, and on whose proficiency depends its lasting reputation.

Warrington. Your obedient Servant, THOS. FLETCHER.

[Mr. Fletcher has further received the following promise from Mr. James Wallace of Glasgow :—" I will be exceedingly gratified to give £20, for five years to the successful students in the Glasgow Dental School in operative dentistry, if the Officials of that School think it advantageous as an inducement for proficiency in the practical part of their Profession."]

GAS OPERATIONS

To the Editor of the DENTAL RECORD.

SIR,—One is led to wonder ' What manner of medical man " your correspondent, Mr. Ottley Atkinson is familiar with, when one reads his tirades about the ignorance they display on being called upon to give nitrous oxide gas. It would be ungenerous for me to lay much stress upon a fact which he fails apparently to recognise, that if médical men who have not been trained to administer gas make a mess of it, it is more surprising that dentists who by Mr. Atkinson's showing are trained to it, make a still greater mess of it, and yet such is unfortunately too often the case. Not being "puffed up with pride" I take no delight in revealing the shortcomings of my friends, the dentists, but I can assure your readers that although very many dentists are doubtless as skilled as Mr. Atkinson tells us he is, yet there are very many who habitually break what I have been taught is the first law of anæsthetics, viz., to give enough of the anæsthetic. I have many dental friends who give gas very well, but none of the intelligent members of that profession or of my own would aver that they preferred to give gas and operate single handed.

It is an amusing comment upon Mr. Atkinson's letter to find that all the leading London and Provincial Dental Hospitals seek for the services of medical men as anæsthetists, so that the very dentists whom Mr. Atkinson counsels to give gas for themselves, since medical men are unreliable and unnecessary ! must have received what training in nitrous oxide administration they have had through the kindly offices of the medical men attached to their dental or general hospital. After a pretty large experience of "gas," I am bound to say I regard as utter "fudge" any statement that the operator knows better than the administrator how much gas is required as he knows what he has to do and how long it will require. It is "fudge" for the simple reason that "gas" can only be given to a certain point—when stertor and jactitation appear—and no longer, nor can it be stopped short of that point. Unless the dentist has the faculty of altering the laws of physics and physiology, I fail to see how he will induce his patient to remain unconscious one iota longer than a medical man who administers, even although that functionary may have no idea of how many molars are coming out. It is a significant fact that several if not most of the reputed deaths from nitrous oxide gas have, I believe, taken place in the operating rooms of dentists when they have been operating and administering the gas single handed. I have no desire to push myself into other people's preserves, but I am told Mr. Atkinson's letter needs a reply from

A MEDICAL MAN WHO CAN GIVE GAS.

MONTHLY STATEMENT of operations performed at the two Dental Hospitals in London, and at the Dental Hospital, Manchester, from June 2nd to June 30th, 1890:—

		London.	National	Victoria.
Number of Patients attended ...		——	1910	1463
Extractions	Children under 14 ...	406	183	1535
	Adults	1235	413	
	Under Nitrous Oxide ...	1031	705	120
Gold Stoppings		343	141	23
Other Stoppings...		1144	406	190
Irregularities of the Teeth		80	167	—
Artificial Crowns		12	15	—
Miscellaneous and Dressings		436	223	130
Total		4,687	2,253	1,998

THE DENTAL RECORD.

VOL. X. SEPTEMBER 1st, 1890. No. 9.

THE NEW THEORY OF THE ACTION OF CHLOROFORM.

By Thomas Gaddes, L.D.S., Eng. & Ed.

It has been pointed out in the editorial pages of this Journal, and elsewhere, that an operation with "a small dose of chloroform is a dangerous thing." That statement was based upon certain experiments by Dr. Lauder Brunton, the results of which appeared to be borne out by the clinical experience of many observers, and also by the evidence so frequently obtained at inquests, viz.:—that (by way of showing that death was not due to an incautious overdose) the patient was not fully anæsthetised, or was recovering from the more profound effects of chloroform, when, during the removal of the "last" tooth, or the insertion of the final stitch, death ensued. In such cases it was argued that chloroform was a direct sedative to the action of the heart; that it reduced the excitability of the cardiac (motor) centres of the sympathetic; that, common sensation not being overcome, the "trivial" operation was perceived by the sensory centre in the medulla; that a resulting impulse was transmitted to the adjacent centre of the pneumogastric and, through that nerve, to the heart inhibiting its already impaired action, failure of the heart ensuing. Thus death from shock and syncope was held to take place; and it was further maintained that, had the patient been fully anæsthetised throughout the operation, shock would have been avoided and syncope, at least from that cause, averted. To day that teaching of the physiological action of chloroform has to be, not simply amended but almost entirely reversed. The experiments of the Second Hyderabad Commission give grounds for a different interpretation of the phenomena attending the administration of chloroform from what has hitherto generally been accepted. The results obtained by the First Commission were so much at variance with those acquired by other experimenters that a Second Commission was organised, having among its numbers that distinguished physician and scientist already referred to—Dr. T. Lauder Brunton, F.R.S. The Second Hyderabad Commission confirmed the conclusions arrived at by the preceding one and, furthermore, made several important discoveries, some 500 animals having been killed in the experiments. The report of the commission has not yet been published in a complete form, although important selections from it have at different times appeared in the *Lancet*, to which journal I am indebted for the information which I possess and for the extracts which follow.

These extracts do not by any means cover the whole ground traversed by the experiments. They are, however, sufficient to show that certain hypotheses as to the action and the safety or danger of chloroform are not in accord with the conclusions obtained from the recent and the most elaborate series of experiments ever carried out in that connection. The extracts are arranged in such order as to bear upon the successive stages in which death was supposed to occur in the case depicted above.

"The three series of experiments show that simple chloroform poisoning causes paralysis of the respiratory centre, and then gradual death, the heart being the last organ in the body to die. And, however concentrated the chloroform may be, it never causes sudden death from stoppage of the heart."

"Chloroform, when given continuously by any means which ensures its free dilution with air, causes a gradual fall in the mean blood-pressure, provided the animal's respiration is not impeded in any way, and it continues to breathe quietly without struggling or involuntarily holding of the breath. But it must be clearly understood that such fall of blood-pressure is in no sense a danger, in any case which is fit for an operation, unless it is excessive—that is to say, unless an overdose of chloroform is inhaled.

"That struggling during chloroform inhalation, or anything which interfered with the breathing in any way, such as holding the breath or asphyxia, produced irregularities in the circulation and in the action of the heart.

"Chloroform has no power of increasing the tendency to either shock or syncope during operations. Every operation that ingenuity could suggest, or that has ever been supposed to be dangerous under chloroform, was performed by the Commission in every stage of Chloroformisation, without any effect upon the heart, the pulse, or the blood-pressure.

"That inhibition of the heart's action and slowing of the circulation with rapid fall of pressure, caused by irritation of the vagus, proved to be a safeguard—rather than a danger,—preventing the anæsthetic from being carried too rapidly from the lungs to the nerve centres. That an effect precisely similar to that caused by electrical stimulation of the vagus is produced through the same nerve: (*a*) in the holding of the breath, which occurs in the early stages of chloroform administration; (*b*) in asphyxia; and, (*c*), sometimes after the respiratory centre is paralysed in the later stages of chloroform poisoning."

As soon as this safeguard action of the vagus was demonstrated, it became clear "that chloroform and shock were not associates but incompatibles; and that the supposed capricious action of chloroform upon the heart was due either to the stimulating effect of concentrated vapour upon the nervous system (the vagus), or to the effect of asphyxial blood upon the nerve centres, resulting in the exclusion of the poison from the system, and not the direct effect of the absorbed poison upon the heart or its nerves."

"Though fall of pressure is inseparable from chloroform administration, there is never the least danger if it falls regularly, and if the inhalation is stopped directly the state of the cornea shows that the patient is 'under.' Regularity of the blood-pressure depends entirely upon regularity of the respiration. Any irregularity, therefore, in the fall of blood-pressure during chloroform inhalation, indicates irregularity of, or interference with, the respiration; and, *per contra*, any irregularity of, or interference with the respiration, at once causes irregularity in the fall of blood-pressure; but as long as the respiration is regular and not interfered with, the fall of the blood-pressure will exactly correspond with it, and will cease long before a dangerous point is reached, *if the inhalation is stopped when the cornea becomes insensitive*, or other signs show that the patient is 'under.' If the respiration is kept up without struggling, holding the breath, or asphyxia, chloroform may be given slowly or quickly freely and with perfect confidence, without the slightest risk to the patient.

The Commission has demonstrated that the aim of the surgeon

must be to give chloroform so that the blood-pressure should fall regularly throughout the whole administration, and that the blood-pressure can only be kept free from irregularity by absolute regularity of the breathing. The chloroform must, therefore, be inhaled in such a way that the breathing is natural and regular throughout. Feeling the pulse during chloroform inhalation is no guide whatever either to the blood pressure or to the one thing necessary for safety, which is to keep it regular; and it has been shown above that the pulse is of no value as a sign of approaching danger, since it is only affected dangerously (*a*) when the respiration has been interfered with, or (*b*) by an over dose. Lastly, in order to keep the breathing regular, the whole of the administrator's attention must be concentrated upon this point alone; and it is therefore clear that if, as is now recommended in most of the text books, part of the chloroformist's attention is to be given to the pulse, an important element of danger comes into the administration.

At present, being in the wilds of the Rocky Mountains and amidst scenes of the "far west," I have not any means of referring to the pages of the *Record*, or to other literature bearing upon the subject. But at the earliest moment I hasten to place before the readers of the Journal, with which I was so long and happily associated, this doctrine of the action of chloroform, which, if not entirely new, is different from that which was generally accepted, even by the highest authorities, and also enunciated in the pages of the *Dental Record*. If I remember rightly it was the received opinion in Scotland, as well as that of Sir J. Y. Simpson, Mr. Syme, Sir J. Lister, &c., that death results from failure of respiration and not from syncope, and it was, therefore, of the utmost importance to watch with the greatest care the respiration alone, discarding the pulse, the pupil, &c. This, too, is the lesson urged by the Second Hyderabad Commission.

The question of anæsthesia by chloroform in dental operations has been discussed by the Odontological Society, and some years ago the consensus of opinion was that, owing to the high percentage of fatalities, chloroform should only be administered in exceptionally severe cases (in which nitrous oxide or ether was not suitable), and then, by preference, at the patient's residence. Should the results and recommendations of the Second Hyderabad Commission be proved correct and satisfactory in experience, the data so gathered will necessitate the reconsideration of the question by the dental profession.

Reports of Societies.

ANNUAL GENERAL MEETING OF THE BRITISH DENTAL ASSOCIATION AT EXETER.

THE 10th annual meeting of the above Association was held on the 20th, 21st, 22nd and 23rd of August, in the Art Gallery of the Albert Memorial Museum, Exeter, where a suite of rooms had been set apart and furnished for the use of the members.

There was a large attendance of the members of the Association and the scientific and social sides of the meeting were unanimously voted a great success. Besides the reading of several highly interesting papers, discussions and demonstrations took place and excited much attention. The headquarters of the Association were fixed at the Rougemont Hotel, where commodious rooms were placed at the service of members.

The arrangements for the scientific portion of the programme were excellent, the rooms both at the Albert Memorial Museum and at the County Hospital being both convenient and well fitted up for the requirements of the Association.

On the evening of Wednesday, the 20th, the Worshipful the Mayor of Exeter (MR. T. SNOW) received and welcomed the members of the British Dental Association at the Rougemont Hotel. At 9 a.m. on the 21st, a meeting of the Representative Board took place. At 10.30 a.m., the Annual General Meeting was opened, and Mr. Lee Rymer (the President) gave his valedictory address, vacating the presidential chair in favour of Mr. Browne-Mason, who gave an address. An interesting feature of Thursday's programme, was the presentation of the portrait of Mr. Smith Turner to the Association and of a replica to Mrs. Smith Turner.

In presenting the portrait the PRESIDENT said, Mr. Smith Turner had been a giant as regards the amount of work he had done in the formation of the Dental Association and other important matters. He had always ably and conscientiously performed everything to which he had set his hand. He was one of the first to come forward; he was still at the work, and long might he so continue. (Applause.) Such being the facts, it was no wonder that a spontaneous feeling arose in the minds of the members of the Association that a record of their gratitude should be presented by the Association to Mr. Smith Turner, so that there should be a permanent recognition of his services.

(Applause.) The portrait had been painted by no less capable an artist than Mr. Sidney Hodge, whose fame was well known, and who was a native of Exeter. He was certain they would receive this portrait with the utmost satisfaction. The likeness of their dear old friend was a striking one, and the picture would remain in the custody of the Association for all time, so that those who in the future heard of the gigantic work of Mr. James Smith Turner would be able to look upon his portrait. As they all knew, the great work of Mr. Turner was in regard to the passing of the Dentists' Act, and in the formation of the British Dental Association. In the passing of the Act mentioned, Mr. Turner undertook a work that was astounding. For years night and day that work was in hand, and although he (the President) would not say there were not others who deserved to be thanked for what they had done, he was bound to state that Mr. Smith Turner stood prominently forward as the man who had, above others, interested himself in the proceedings of the Association. (Applause.) The president then accepted the portrait on behalf of the Association, and asked Mr. Smith-Turner to rceive for his family a replica of the painting.

The portrait was an extremely good one, and represented Mr. Turner seated in an armchair. It had a gilt frame, and at the bottom was the following inscription :—"J. Smith Turner, Esq., President of the Representative Board of the British Dental Association. Painted by the direction of the members as a gift to the Association in recognition of his untiring devotion to the welfare of the profession, represented by that body, and as a public expression of the great esteem and high personal regard with which he is held."

Mr. J. Smith Turner, who was received with cheers on rising to receive the replica of the portrait, said it was something strange to him to look back and think how thoughtlessly he had entered upon the work that had been referred to by Mr. Lee Rymer. Had he been able at that time to realise the extent of the work he would, perhaps, have shrunk from it. As it was he undertook it, and he was bound to say that, however hard he might have worked, however constant might have been his application to that work, had it not been for the continued support and encouragement which he had received from others, and more particularly from the high and sagacious intellect of Sir John Tomes, all his efforts would have been unavailing. With regard to the passing of the Dentists' Act, he might say that he was fortunate in finding out those gentlemen who could point him in the right direction, and he might almost have been called a Parliamentary agent. Speaking of that Dentists' Act, and the work he had done in connection with it, he might remind them that he had already had presented to him a time-piece of £70 and a purse of £300, and it was therefore like ancient history in reminding him of that work. Mr. Smith Turner then referred in eulogistic terms to the great assistance rendered him by his wife in all his work, and remarked that if it had not been for that assistance he could never have attended to the inauguration of the Dental Association. In conclusion, he thanked the Committee of the Presentation Fund, and all who had taken part in the presentation.

It was decided, on the suggestion of Mr. Walter Coffin, that subscriptions should be received to provide photogravures or engravings of Mr. Smith Turner's portrait.

On the evening of the 21st a soirée was given in the Museum by the President and the members of the Western Branch of the Association. A most enjoyable time was spent, amusements being provided in the shape of performances of music by the string band of the Plymouth Division, Royal Marines, by permission of the Colonel Commandant Mackay-Heriot; instrumental and vocal music by local amateurs, and dancing. In the East Room of the Museum were a number of valuable exhibits.

On the 22nd August the proceedings commenced at nine o'clock in the Museum, by the annual meeting of the Benevolent Fund.

THE ANNUAL DINNER,

Took place at the Rougemont Hotel on the evening of August 22nd, about 120 gentlemen sitting down. The chair was taken by the President, Mr. J. Browne-Mason.

The Royal Toasts having been duly honoured, the Chairman submitted that of "The Navy, Army and Reserve Forces."

Admiral White, C.B. replied on behalf of the Royal Navy. Colonel Milne-Home undertaking a similar duty for the Army, while Sir J. Shelley responded for the Reserve Forces.

Lord Sidmouth, in a humourous speech, proposed the "British Dental Association," to which toast Mr. J. Smith Turner responded in his usual happy manner.

Mr. Morton Smale who was cordially received, gave the "Medical Profession," and Dr. Woodman replied.

Mr. LEE RYMER proposed "The Visitors," LORD POLTIMORE responding.

Mr. FELIX WEISS, in proposing "The health of the Chairman," said that if there should be any one present who doubted the interest which the Chairman took in the profession, in professional progress, and in seeing that his professional colleagues were well received, the proceedings of the last two days would be a sufficient answer. (Applause.) His address was a very able one, while the reception which the Association had received was one that would not readily be forgotten. In the annals of the British Dental Association, he was fully convinced of this, that when they came to speak of their general meetings, the meeting at Exeter would be remembered as a very memorable one, and as one that had done a great deal of good to the profession at large and to themselves individually. (Applause).

The toast was received with great enthusiasm, the company singing "For he's a jolly good fellow" and giving hearty cheers for Mr. and Mrs. Browne-Mason.

The CHAIRMAN briefly replied, and the proceedings terminated.

On Saturday morning after the demonstrations (to which we refer below) the excursions were undertaken.

The excursions in the afternoon consisted of a visit to the Cathedral, over which building the visitors were personally conducted by the Dean of Exeter; to the Guildhall, where the Town Clerk (Mr. G. R. Shorts) officiated; and to the Rougemont Castle, the ruins of which were described by Mr. Winslow Jones.

At four o'clock an "At Home" was given by the President and Mrs. Browne-Mason at the Victoria Hall. A programme of vocal and instrumental music was carried out.

A more pleasant social gathering could hardly have been arranged, and a more kind and genial a host and hostess would be hard to find.

ADDRESSES, PAPERS AND DISCUSSIONS.

Thursday, 21st.

THE PRESIDENT'S VALEDICTORY ADDRESS

The retiring PRESIDENT (Mr. S. Lee Rymer), discussing matters of special moment to the Profession, alluded to the fact that the crucial question of professional education and examination had of late forced itself much to the front. The weighty opinions of leading men upon the future status of dental surgery as a profession, were of vital moment. There were three sets of opinions existing upon the subject. "(1) That the *status quo*, *i.e.*, the L.D S. diploma, meets all requirements. (2) That a medical qualification ought to be acquired before the L.D.S. is allowed ; and, (3) that Dental Surgery ought to exist as an independent profession. There is nothing new in any of these propositions, and almost all that can be said in favour of or against each has been said over and over again. Nevertheless, the fact remains that each has still its partisans—certainly in different proportions—but in debatable questions of import, the index of mere numbers is not always to be regarded as infallible. The subject under notice, then, having been again broached, I venture, said Mr. Rymer, to offer you a few observations thereon, taking the opinions referred to in inverse order. The independent proposition I know something about, as I was most closely associated with those who espoused it in the year 1856—the period of the first determined movement towards the organisation of dental surgery as a profession. Many prolonged and anxious meetings were then held, the first taking place on September 22nd of the year named, at the London Tavern, in the City of London. At these meetings different schemes were put forward and discussed as to the proper course of action, including the suggested idea of affiliation to the College of Surgeons, the conclusion arrived at being that the profession would best flourish on an independent basis, and the College of Dentists was accordingly proclaimed. This action immediately received a large amount of support, but the promoters had to face serious discouragement from a proposition of others whose professional position entitled them to respect, and whose views, although favourable to reform, were not in accord with an independent organization. Nevertheless, the independent party, believing themselves right, steadily persevered, and if they ultimately failed in obtaining a Charter of Incorporation for the College of Dentists, as they did in fact, it was certainly not on account of lethargy on their part. The other side, as represented by the Odontological Society of London, although numerically small in comparison to the College of Dentists, was highly influential. The bulk of the dental practitioners, of the day remained quiescent. The points at issue between the two active bodies were thoroughly and publicly ventilated for years, and, at last, as everybody knows, the Odontologicals succeeded in their policy, and the Colleges of Surgeons were granted authority to issue diplomas in dental surgery. This act gave the College of Dentists its *coup de grâce*. An independent institution, such as the College of Dentists, could only have lived, under the circumstances thus altered, as an impediment to progress; hence the subsequent fusion with the Odontological side and the general acceptance of the issue by the members of the College, who properly regarded the honour of the profession as above party and a united front as the essential element of success in a calling duly recognised by Parliamentary authority. In passing I should mention that educational requirements were not lost sight of by the College of Dentists during its existence. The Metropolitan School of Dental Science was organised. A curriculum very much in accord with that now in force for the L.D.S., was drafted, and, no doubt, would have been adopted had the College gone on. Two other plans had been submitted for consideration, one being that no curriculum at all should be enforced, and that examination alone should be the test of efficiency; the other, that candidates for admission to the College of Dentists should be in possession of the diploma of membership of the College of Surgeons as a qualification for the special dental examination. Neither proposal met with favour. From what has been announced, it will be gathered that the independent proposition collapsed after years of deliberation and argument, through the preponderating influence of the other side, together with the failure of the mass of dentists to render support at a period when every possible opportunity was afforded for so doing. As to the proposition that a medical qualification ought to be acquired before the L.D.S., is allowed, I have mentioned already that such an idea found exponents amongst certain supporters of the College of Dentists who did not regard it as inconsistent with independent action, although the majority thought otherwise, and so it fell through. The policy of confining the specialty to qualified surgeons, as advocated by others later on, certainly did not include any question of independence. The Association of Surgeons Practising Dental Surgery was started on a hard and fast line on the principle that the practice of dental surgery should be first exclusively confined to surgeons, and without sympathy for outsiders, however eminent. This limited programme failed entirely. It dealt on the wholesale excommunication of all whose names did not appear on the Medical Register. It offended, through its narrowness of conception, the larger number of the best men whose names were enrolled thereon. More in touch with the spirit of the times, other thinkers have advocated that the qualification in dental surgery should be held conjointly with a diploma in general surgery. Few, I apprehend, would object to the expression of such a view; the real point rests in regard to compulsion in the matter. The new regulations of the College of Surgeons of England, which have only come into force during this year, may, at least, be said to encourage the voluntary acquirement of the diploma of membership in conjunction with that of dental surgery. Beyond this it appears to me to be unnecessary to proceed under present conditions. The only proposition of the past which received the necessary support to bring it into being was that which now exists as the recognised license in dental surgery. This qualification has proved of such advantage to the profession of dental surgery as to render it doubtful whether the success of any other policy could have been attended with superior results. The measure of success can scarcely, as yet, be gauged, and the virtue of patience must be exercised as to whether and in what way it can be improved upon in the future. To wait the result of experience is, perhaps, irksome, but the great work of building up a profession upon a lasting basis may not be unduly pressed. A great author—Goethe—has observed: "I cannot but look upon it as one of the greatest misfortunes of our age that it allows nothing to ripen quietly; that the next moment, so to speak, devours the preceding; that no time is allowed for digestion, and that we live from hand to mouth without leisure to bring forth any finished product." The Dentists' Act was a sequence of the institution of the license in dental surgery, as was the establishment and incorporation of this British Dental Association a necessary sequence to the Dentists' Act. Taken altogether, we are, *de facto*, in possession of an organised system of education and examination, of legislative authority and of political action, which is working fairly well. It appears, therefore that the supporters of the *status quo* have a right thus far to claim for it the realisation of practical and beneficial results of a highly important character. If this be so, our duty clearly lies in unitedly and loyally upholding it. Nevertheless, I am convinced there is need for improvement development. The requirements for the L.D.S. diploma, been often said, being equal in degree although differer to those of the M.R.C.S., involve the same amount of and expense, and should, by right, but do not in fac relative privileges. That practical exclusion f highest official positions connected with our sp lot of dental licentiates not possessing while those possessed of the latter *sine* the dental qualification are allowed to register as dentists, and also to be eligible for dental appointments, is, to my mind, altogether anomalous and unfair. The Dentists' Act upon this and other points calls loudly for amendment, so as to remedy defects which have become only too apparent. We may take it for granted, I am sure, that the members of this strong Association will not be wanting in energy to do their part at the proper moment towards securing the just demands of the profession in this matter. The opportunity of amendment may not be far distant ; already the members of our Colleges are claiming a share in the elective rights at present confined to a privileged few, why should not the Licentiate also be included?

ADDRESS OF THE PRESIDENT.

On taking the chair Mr. BROWNE-MASON spoke in favour of the new regulations for the curriculum prescribed by the Royal College of Surgeons of England, for the L. D. S. diploma.

Referring to the question of state regulation of dental surgery in the forces, Mr. Browne-Mason, quoted an author who had written about the Medical Department of the Royal Navy. The writer commenced by pointing out that "no department of the public service has made greater advances during the present century than the medical," and after contrasting the knowledge of the etiology and prevention of diseases shown by the medical service of the Navy at the beginning of the century with the knowledge possessed by the same service at the present date, says, "so great have been these changes, so marked the benefits, that it might almost seem that no further improvements could be made. But is this so? Are we sure that we have done all in our power compatible with the nature of the naval service to prevent disease? Are there no means by which we can raise the standard of health, high as it is, of our seamen, ·ides those already now employed?" He afterwards says, "These ·ons have led me to the conclusion that the teeth of the men worthy of attention than they have hitherto officially Here then we have the words of a distinguished surgeon, and high standing, emphatically pointing out the for some attention to the dental health of our Now as to the attention at present afforded to ·lies in the Royal Navy, he draws a graphic picture in the following words :—" When serving in 1870 on board H.M.S. Warrior, I was one day horrified by a sick-berth steward producing two of Lazenby's pickle bottles, one of which was full, and the other two-thirds full of extracted teeth, which the man said he had extracted in ten months, without the knowledge of the medical officers of the ship, and he was not a little proud of his achievement." Here is a picture of pain and suffering that could be, in a great measure prevented if skilled dental surgeons were attainable at certain periods of the seaman's service. And yet no mention is made of the long list of diseases that are frequently traceable to the absence of teeth, as well as the presence of diseased and imperfect ones, such as chronic dyspepsia with all its attendant maladies, caused by insufficient mastication of food: to which may be added neuralgia, ear-ache, ulcer of the tongue and even epithelioma, odontome, periostitis and necrosis of the maxilla, abscess, salivary fistula and empyema of the antrum, while constipation, diarrhœa, dyspepsia and debility are simple cases, with exceptions, of cause and effect. We know also that remote effects, traceable through reflex irritation of peripheral nerves, consequent on diseased teeth, may be transmitted to both motor and sympathetic fibres, so that mania has been reported as an accompaniment of cutting the wisdom teeth, and paralysis of arm, deafness, epilepsy, and amaurosis have been found consequent on dental diseases, and cured by the removal of the source of the mischief. For the sake of humanity then, how much better would it be for our own soldiers and sailors, if means could be found to remedy this, by instituting a regular examination of their mouths and restoring the ravages made by dental cases before the disease has gone too far. The author of this eminently humane representation to the Naval Authorities, sent in the results of the examination by him of the mouths of 1,022 seamen, while serving at the Royal Naval Barracks at Sheerness, of men of from 20 to 40 years of age ; and an analysis of the tables he made showed that the aggregate of 32,704 teeth that should be present, 1,030 were not cut, of 31,674 remaining to be accounted for no less than 4,929 were either extracted or decayed, being rather more than one-seventh of the total number of teeth, and this, considering the age and quality of the men, is strikingly large, especially when we recall the fact that the men enter the service as boys, on board training ships, and that boys with more than five defective teeth are rejected ; and as a fact, in actual practice it is seldom that a boy passes with more than two or three diseased teeth at the time of entry This amount of disease, therefore, has developed after their admission, and as the age for entry is from 15 to 16 years, those who early show marked tendency to caries of these organs do not get into the service at all. The result of these statistics, which are most exhaustive, and the originals of which are in my possession, is to show that it is the molars, that is to say the most useful teeth, that are chiefly absent or diseased, and without disparaging the examination made by my medical friend, it is possible that, had the examination of these mouths been made by a dental surgeon, more mischief even than he noted would have been apparent. Here we have the strongest possible case for extending to our Navy the means for combating dental diseases. For only remember what a loss of such a percentage of the organs of mastication means to men who need be capable of showing the greatest amount of hardiness, in fact, the *mens sana in corpore sano* in the very highest degree, in order to carry out merely the routine duties of every day work, in every clime, exposed, as they are, to every extreme of weather, from Arctic cold to Equatorial heat. Men, to meet such requirements, should be in the highest condition of physical training, even in times of peace. How much more then is this necessary in time of war? And how can men be in this condition who lack the primary means for the due assimilation of the food for the nourishment of their bodies, especially when, as must frequently be the case in long cruises, that food is of a character to require all the natural apparatus for digestion in good order, to assimilate it at all? The consequences of disease in these organs must be that men are invalided who should not be if we bear in mind the great care that is taken in selecting men of the finest physique at the age best calculated to resist the attack of disease of any kind, that is, between the age of 20 and 40 years. The cost to the nation of turning out an efficient sailor, from the time a boy joins the Navy at one of the training ships at the age of 15, till he passes out two years later to sea-going craft, and becomes at 18 years of age an ordinary seaman—when his education may be considered complete—is not less than £100; so here there would be a great economy in endeavouring to preserve in health such expensive and valuable material as our bluejackets undoubtedly are. In making out a case for the soldier to receive dental attendance, I have not the advantage of access to such a document of the report of the gentlemen I have mentioned, but to begin with, the cost to the country of manufacturing the finished soldier from the recruit is no less than that of turning out an efficient sailor, for, it is allowed, every soldier costs the nation £100, while in the case of cavalry, engineers, and artillerymen, the cost is much more. As far back as 1857, the then Director-General of the Medical Department of the Army, Dr. A. Smith, issued a circular to the Medical-officers of the Service instancing the advances made in conservative Dental Surgery, and bore the necessity of attention to this side of the men's health. I would suggest that in view, of the cost of producing efficient soldiers and sailors for the service of the country, on the ground of economy, to put forward no higher reason, it would repay the nation to add to the staff of the Medical Departments qualified dental surgeons at all Naval stations, at Naval hospitals, flagships, and gunneryships, such as the Excellent and Cambridge, where, in consequence of the men being drafted into them for special training, they are constantly, at intervals, changing the men, who would thus have the opportunity of passing under the observation of the dentists while on board ; and for the soldier in all Army depôts and military centres, and permanent Army hospitals. That this would entail a very slight outlay on the part of the nation, in comparison with the gain that would accrue, I have no sort of doubt ; and the nation would be paid over and over again, by the increased length of time we should find the men serviceable. The statistics of work and costs of the same furnished by the reports of our dental hospitals show at what a comparatively little cost over and above the pay of such officers, such a service could be maintained—for commensurate with the benefits conferred, no medical charities cost so little, there being no expenses for maintenance of patients, and I assert that it would be a national disgrace if such an outlay were grudged by Parliament, even if the reasons for calling it into existence were humanitarian only, instead of being, as they are, eminently utilitarian and economic.

CONSERVATIVE DENTISTRY.

Mr. J. C. Oliver, L.D.S., read a paper on "Conservative Dentistry : Its importance as a National Institution." He said of all the numerous ills that affected civilised nations there was no malady so universal, none that caused such an aggregate amount of suffering, and that so impaired and undermined the health of the people as those diseases of the teeth which, unchecked, ended in their destruction and loss. Could they but estimate the number of teeth annually destroyed by caries, the amount of suffering endured, the injury to health inflicted, they would be astounded at the magnitude of the proportions realised. The loss to the nation which the ravages of dental caries produced in its enfeeblement to the bodies, and the destruction of the happiness of so large a proportion of its population, was a subject which would repay investigation by the State; and seeing that science had discovered the true specific for this disease, the problem of popularising conservative dentistry ought to be regarded as one within the sphere of practical politics. Not that he thought the time had come when they were likely to see State appointments in connection with an Act making compulsory the periodical examination and treatment of the teeth of children. He was prepared, however, to maintain that such a measure would be justified by the beneficial effects that would result therefrom. For the present, however, they must be content with moral suasion, as the means at hand for accomplishing the object of popular education. Mr. Oliver then reviewed the progress of science, and proceeded to show that it should be the work of the British Dental Association to educate the people and assist them to the acquaintance with the subject that was needed. He must distinctly urge that the Association should look beyond its own self-interests and take the people under their protecting care. To this end he would suggest that there should be a Committee appointed by the Association to enquire into the condition and requirements of the people, and see whether measures for their benefit might not be devised. (1.) By establishing a code of dental ethics which might be recognised as a standard for the guidance of dentists in the honourable conduct of their practice; (2.) By issuing a code of instructions for the use of the public in the care and preservation of the teeth; (3.) By instituting a system of instruction for the young of all classes; (4.) By urging the appointment of dental surgeons to public schools; (5.) And by indicating a popular system of Conservative treatment which would be within the reach of the masses.

Discussion :—

Mr. CUNNINGHAM thought that a paper of the kind read by Mr. Oliver, following as it did, the important address of the President, was a matter that did not merely concern the dentists, but was of public interest. Thinking men could not help feeling that the public could derive very much larger benefits from the dentists' labours, if those labours were applied at a different time, he thought the President's address and Mr. Oliver's paper showed that dentists were an earnest body of men associated not only in their own interests as a profession, but for the good of the community. They knew that the best services of the dental profession were not being obtained by the public; and why? Because of the ignorance of the public. It was a fact that dentists, as a profession, were responsible for the ignorance of the public. The public could not educate itself, and he felt that something in this direction should be done by the Association. When they had suggestions thrown out for the appointment of a committee to consider certain specific subjects as suggested by Mr. Oliver, they should not forget that only recently they had such a committee, which was representative of the Association. He believed that something could be done, but for the present it was better that the individual should suffer than the Association.

Mr. Felix Weiss said, what was most needed was a mode by which the public might be able to distinguish between charlatans and *bona fide* practitioners. Some time ago he instituted enquiries, and obtained the services of two ladies, who, at his request, made a point of visiting most of the dentists in London, and also a few of those in the country—men of the advertising class known to be disreputable and obnoxious to the community. He asked the ladies to take particular notice of the literature which the men had for circulation, and he found that in the literature displayed on their tables were sentences which had been written expressly to expose them (the quacks). A great many schemes had been put forward as to how information might be given to the public. It might sound somewhat wild, but he would suggest that they might approach the newspapers, and induce proprietors to exclude all advertisements that were obnoxious.

Mr. W. Mitchell thought it would be advisable to begin at the beginning and educate their patients thoroughly, while they had them in the chair, and they could gradually go out to the general public through those patients.

Mr. Kendrick was sorry that the Association had not seen its way clear to take some steps in the manner indicated by Mr. Oliver. If a phamphlet, had been printed and sent to all medical men whose names were on the Register, giving certain information as to the preservation of teeth, and as to what could be done by dental surgeons in the present day, it would be a great advantage to the public and to the dental profession.

Mr. FOTHERGILL said there were very few medical men in the country who did not know personally the benefits that were to be derived from the assistance of the dental surgeon. They were among constant patients of dental surgeons, and they must know what a very great benefit it was to have their teeth properly attended to. Any attempt like what had been suggested that the Association as a corporate body should act, would be very much like appealing to Government, as people were apt to do for all sorts of evils, and, as they knew, in the majority of cases these appeals ended in failure.

Mr. J. HAY felt that the evil was one that could not be reached unless by carrying out Mr. Oliver's suggestion. He believed the Association, as a body of dental practitioners, speaking for the whole dental community, should adopt some means of bringing to the knowledge of the masses the necessity of their earliest attention to every kind of dental ailment. They would never reach—through the efforts of individual dentists in their own practice—the masses who needed most the information which the Association might be able to put before them. The Association should appoint a committee to examine as to what means they could adopt, as a body, of bringing before every parent in the kingdom, the duty and necessity of urgent attention and care to their children's teeth. He suggested that the Association might bring very powerful influence to bear upon the Board of Education to induce them to adopt a system of careful inspection of all children who attended Board schools. He would have every child who passed into a Board School go under a careful dental inspection, for by these means they would reach immediately a very large body, and obtain an early control over an evil which they wanted to remedy.

Mr. SMITH TURNER said something was in the course of being done in the direction indicated by Mr. Oliver, but he would like to point out that what was done must be done deliberately and systematically; and they must do it in a manner which would not expose them to ridicule, and would not supply the quack and the charlatan with means of taking advantage of the profession.

Mr. MORTON SMALE agreed with Mr. Smith Turner's remarks, and hoped the British Dental Association would never condescend to issue circulars (Hear, hear). They might issue circulars but they could not make people read them, and if they sent them to medical men he was certain they would be put into the waste paper basket.

Mr. OLIVER replied on the whole debate.

HIGHER QUALIFICATION IN DENTAL SURGERY.

Mr. G. G. CAMPION, L.D.S., read a paper on the need of a higher qualification in dental surgery. No one, he imagined, would be hardy enough to maintain that they had as yet arrived at perfection in their system of dental education, but upon the deficiencies which existed in that system and the means whereby they were to be remedied a difference of opinion existed, some contending for a gradual extension on the lines of medical education —an extension ending, perhaps, ultimately in the compulsory acquisition of a medical diploma, while others would embody those parts of medical study which would be of use to a dentist, but which were not now included in the dental curriculum in a separate scheme for a higher dental qualification, retaining the licence in its present form as the minimum qualification in dentistry. Mr. Campion then brought facts forward which pointed, in his opinion, to the latter of these two schemes as affording the better solution of the disquieting problem of the higher education of dentists.

Discussion :—

Mr. MORTON SMALE did not think any man should practise dentistry without a dental diploma. It seemed to him that the desire for a new diploma was a desire that a man might make himself a little taller than his brethren (No, no). That he was not content with the diploma that every other dentist was content with. It was probably an open secret that the College of Surgeons in London, were now considering the desirability of establishing an honours examination. If this examination were established the honours would be only bestowed after additional examination, and only to those who had been marked very high in the first part. His strongest objection to Mr. Campion's proposal was that practically if they multiplied diplomas, they multiplied the letters that were put after a man's name, and they begun to mystify the public and the medical profession. People were beginning to know, and certainly the medical profession were beginning to know, what was the meaning of those three sacred letters L. D. S. (Applause.) It always seemed to him that the multitude of diplomas in the medical profession was a weakness in that profession. They did not want another diploma in dentistry. The suggestion of Mr. Campion seemed to throw a doubt on their own L. D. S., and he would be sorry to see anything passed that would reflect upon that degree. (Hear, hear.) If they wanted a better diploma, he would say, let them make the L. D. S. perfect. (Applause).

The discussion was then adjourned till Friday morning, August 22nd.

At half-past ten o'clock the annual general meeting of the Association was resumed in the Art Gallery, the President in the chair, and the discussion on Mr. G. G. Campion's paper on "A Higher Qualification in Dental Surgery" was continued by—

Mr. CANTON, who said he did not think Mr. Campion had made out sufficient reason or demand for the change proposed. Certainly amongst the dental students in the hospitals in London, he (Mr. Canton) had heard no such demand made.

Mr. REES PRICE said that however desirable the change might be, as suggested by Mr. Campion, he did not think the time was yet ripe for it.

Mr. SMITH TURNER said it was not the number of letters that made the value of the diploma, but it was the knowledge which the profession first gained of the value of the diploma, and by and bye the public. (Hear, hear.) The Association did not want to change the L.D.S.; and no good would come of such a change. (Hear, hear.) The public had scarcely got to know what the degree of L.D.S. meant, and yet Mr. Campion was seeking to cast something else upon it, before it had borne fruit. It would be some time before they could venture upon such a thing, for if they did so now it would make "confusion worse confounded."

Mr. HOPE thought the extolling of the L.D.S. diploma on the one hand, and to a certain extent lowering it on the other, had almost shown that something ought to be done. He felt that, while they were willing to admit that the L.D.S. was almost sufficient—and it ought to be quite sufficient—at the same time the students were given to understand that it was not so. (Hear, hear, and "No, no.")

Mr. SPOKES asked the dentists to make the best of their present opportunities. If, however, there was a need for the L.D.S. to be improved in the direction of Mr. Campion's proposed higher qualification, let it be improved to that extent.

Mr. BOOTH PEARSALL said what they should do in regard to a higher qualification in dental surgery was not to make a new diploma, but to enhance the value of what they had got. (Applause.)

Mr. Rilot submitted that Mr. Campion had not proved his point. With regard to another diploma acting as a stimulus to teaching, he said Mr. Campion must have forgotten that at the last examination in London more than one-half of the men were plucked. (Hear, hear.) That appeared to him (Mr. Rilot) to be sufficient stimulus. (Laughter.) He also failed to see that this extra diploma would grant them any higher professional or social status (Hear, hear.) The whole beauty of the profession was the unity of it. They were one corporate body united in a mystic ring—which was the L.D.S. (Applause.)

Mr. Underwood said there could be only one higher qualification in dental surgery than that now in existence, and that had already been obtained by Mr. Campion, viz., the diploma conferred by his professional friends in their admiration of his abilities.

Mr. Matheson said the question for the members of the Association to consider what would make them better dentists. (Hear, hear.) The question as to the status they were to hold in the eyes of the general public he regarded as entirely secondary They of course, wanted more practical knowledge then they now possessed, but what they wanted more and more was the training in the use of their fingers, and it seemed to him Mr. Campion's suggestion would not help in that direction.

Mr. Headridge said the discussion that had followed the paper read by Mr. Campion proved its value. There were many men who quietly thought that some higher degree beyond the L.D.S. might be given to able men who had done good and practical work, and had shewn extraordinary ability.

Mr. Cunningham said they wanted better teaching, and as for the results of their examinations the teachers ought to assume the responsibility. If they were going to maintain the social position of the L.D.S., the sooner they could identify their examinations with those of the medical students, so far as it was consistent with the practical attainments of the dental profession, then so far they ought to carry it out. He thought that the ideal curriculum of the dental student was the curriculum of the Irish College.

Mr. Coffin thought that something of this kind would take place in the future—viz., that either the L.D.S. would be abolished, and the M.R.C.S. would be the surgical degree, comprising all that a man was required to practice for a speciality in surgery, or that the M.R.C.S. would be abolished, and the L.D.S., with other similar degrees for specialities, would be granted by the College of Surgeons, not as a registrable medical degree, but as a surgical one for the purpose.

Mr. HEPBURN said it appeared to him that the organisation or institution of a higher qualification in dental surgery, instead of drawing them nearer to the medical profession, would have a distinct endency towards separating them from it. (Hear, hear.)

Mr. MUNDELL having referred to the importance of the question raised in the paper.

Mr. F. H. BALKWILL could not see why in the future the medical profession could not see its way to say that a man should go through an examination in what was required for general practice in his special line, and that if he passed he could become a member of the College of Surgeons. But to require a man to have sufficient knowledge to qualify him for general practice, in addition to his speciality, was a great tax upon him. (Hear, hear.).

Mr. CAMPION replied on the whole debate. In the course of his remarks he said his idea was not in any way to supersede the L. D. S. Where he differed from Mr. Morton Smale was that that gentleman would supplement the L. D. S. by the conjoint diploma, whereas he (Mr. Campion) would supplement it by the higher qualification in Dentistry.

MECHANICAL DENTISTRY.

Mr. S. A. COXON, L.D.S.I., read a paper on "The teaching of mechanical dentistry to the coming dental students." Until quite recently the teaching of the present day had a tendency to ignore the necessity of being a thorough dental mechanic. The curriculum specified that the student should be two years with a registered dentist after passing his preliminary examination, but this was in no way a guarantee that he could make a denture. But for all that he would be put to but little further proof as regards his mechanical knowledge when he got to the hospital. There could be but little doubt that a pupil was far better fitted to get on in the surgery when he had been taught the use of his fingers and could handle a file. In the ordinary denture now turned out they saw a piece of vulcanite of uneven thickness, usually over vulcanised, with flat teeth in place of bicuspids and molars, and with thin narrow wires, which do their duty for bands, and the teeth placed with that admirable regularity that gave them the appearance of a row of gate-posts rather than the organs of mastication. Then, with regard to the plate-work they saw the teeth fitting badly to the plate, the backings reaching about half-way up the teeth, and it was only too often that the work of the qualified man and the advertising one were very much on a par. Dentistry had of late made rapid strides, but the mechanical side of their work had stood nearly still, and he feared would do so as long as their pupils were allowed to go into the work room and copy what they saw being done without anyone to instruct them as to the character of the face the teeth were to harmonise with, and why a denture must be strengthened at this place and that, and where the chief strain would occur when it was in the mouth. Therefore, when a pupil entered the workroom everything he did should be carefully overlooked. It was at the beginning that the pupil should be placed on the right path as regards mechanics, and then was the time to instil into him that, before he was able to stop teeth he ought to be proficient in the art of making plates. He hoped in the future to see the examinations in dental mechanics take a more definite form, and that no man who was not a thorough mechanic would be allowed to take his diploma. He did not mean a theoretical examination, but one in which he should sit down and make a denture from start to finish.

THE PRESIDENT said there was no doubt that it was most important that the practitioner of their speciality should be a thoroughly trained dental mechanic as well as a surgeon. (Hear, hear.) In his experience he had found that there was a falling off in the mechanical qualifications of assistants. This was probably, in some degree, due to the introduction of vulcanite.

Mr. BOOTH PEARSALL suggested as a remedy the establishment of a public laboratory and the issue of certificates of efficiency to youths who could pass an examination at a certain time of their pupilage in the mechanical side of their profession. He also advocated the use of better appliances in the workroom, and that great efforts should be made to bring all mechanical apparatus up to modern date.

Mr. HEPBURN said what the reader had complained of applied mainly to the past, but very little to the present, and he hoped it would not apply in the least to the future. Teaching bodies were exerting themselves to organise a system of teaching, but these systems so far as he had been able to see, really were not going to take upon themselves the responsibility of giving complete instruction in dental mechanics. This preliminary instruction must be gained elsewhere, and they must look to the dental practitioners for support in that matter It should be the duty of practitioners to impart to the pupils under their care not only the instruction in the workroom but as far as possible to introduce them into the mysteries of dealing with the mechanical appliances in the mouths of patients. As to how long the student should be allowed to remain at the bench he thought the period of three years fixed by the College of Surgeons should be long enough to help him to understand the practice, and to give him that mechanical aptitude which would make him dexterous in manipulation.

Mr. Coxon, in replying to the discussion, complained that the same pains were not taken to see that a candidate for a diploma was an expert mechanical dentist as that he was well informed in surgical knowledge, whereas he considered that one was as valuable an accomplishment as the other.

CROWNS FOR BICUSPIDS AND MOLARS.

Mr. T. G. Read, L.D.S., Eng., D.M.D. Harv., read a paper on "Some Porcelain and Gold Crowns for Bicuspids and Molars." He said a crown should reduce the chance of destruction of tooth substances to the minimum, be non-irritating to the adjacent parts, natural in appearance, strong enough to resist the strain of mastication, and capable of being quickly constructed with little pain to the patient ; and no crown fulfilled these requirements so well as a cup crown. Mr. Read then described two forms of porcelain and gold cup crowns for bicuspids and molars. There was no discussion on the paper.

A NEW LOW FUSING CONTINUOUS GUM.

Mr. G. Cunningham, M.A., L.D.S., D.M.D., read a paper on a new low fusing continuous gum, which he had previously read before the section of Odontology of the International Medical Congress, Berlin, 1890. He said it would be admitted by almost every dentist that a well-made and properly adapted artificial denture of enamelled platinum, or what was commonly known as continuous gum, was the nearest approach to the perfect substitute for the natural teeth. Yet this almost ideal achievement of the mechanical laboratory, with which the name of John Allen would ever be associated, was, despite improvements both in materials and appearances, possibly even further from being a part of the everyday practice of the ordinary dental laboratory as it was on its introduction some 40 years ago. The subsequent introduction of vulcanite, mainly because of its manipulative facilities, and in spite of its inartistic deficiencies, was a death blow to the general adoption of the more artistic process. The stereotyped sectional gum block of the American, and the improved pink rubbers of the European manufacturers, might be taken as efforts to meet the as yet unsatisfied artistic instinct of the dental mechanic. This strange and somewhat anomalous state of affairs made it worth while to consider in some detail the advantages and alleged disadvantages of continuous gum work, since, without some effectual simplification of the process, it was evident that it would never become part of the everyday practice of the dental laboratory. Firstly, theoretically, continuous gum work possessed capabilities of adaptation of the size, the shape, the colour, the position, and the pitch of the teeth employed far superior to any other known kind of artificial denture except, perhaps, that excellent and nowadays almost old-fashioned method known as English tube work. Practically it did nothing of the kind, mainly from the fact that a proper selection as to shape, size, and colour of the special teeth requisite for the process was not to be found in the average well-equipped dental laboratory, nor, for the matter of that, even in the most important depôts, at any rate on this side of the Atlantic. Secondly, the material of which the continuous form was composed possessed as great capabilities for the restoration of the features to their normal expression as either vulcanite or celluloid, while it far surpassed either of them as a material for producing an artistic imitation of the natural gum. Thirdly, the combination of platinum and fine porcelain constituted a denture, which for cleanliness was unapproached by any other. Fourthly, as to strength, adaptability, and its power of conducting heat, the platinium plate, which was the base of these dentures, possessed all the qualities of gold plate. It must be admitted that the colour of the metallic plate neither pleased the eye of the average dentist, nor that of the average patient, as did the so-called nobler metal. Sentimental though this grievance might be, the colour of platinum was no less a real disadvantage, and paradoxical though the statement might seem, the recent rise in the value of platinum by almost phenomenal leaps and bounds might not be an unmixed disadvantage, since in a few years it will probably be the nobler metal of the two, when this senseless objection to its colour will probably have disappeared. Fifthly, with regard to its durability, it could not be worn out, though it must be admitted that its proper care required more careful treatment than the ordinary dentures, the most frequent injuries being those which occurred out of the mouth. Sixthly, with regard to its capabilities of repair, it certainly was not as easily repaired as, for instance, an ordinary vulcanite denture. There was, however, this additional advantage in favour of continuous gum work that, on proper completion of the repair, the case was again equal to new. Mr. Cunningham then dealt with the alleged disadvantages of continuous gum work, and exhibited specimens of a new enamel, for which he claimed that it was capable of replacing, with advantage to the patient, and with facility to the dentist, and that to a large extent, even in partial dentures, some of the less artistic, ordinary products of the dental laboratory.—There was no discussion on this paper.

CROWN BAR AND BRIDGE WORK.

A discussion on crown bar and bridge work was opened by Mr. Gartrell, and continued by Mr. Lennox, who suggested an exhibition of special appliances or "dodges," as he termed them, in connection with the annual conference of the Association.

Dr. G. W. Mellotte (Ithaca, N.Y.), said he was a firm believer in reasonable bridge work, but a certain amount of work was certainly performed in a manner which none could approve of. It was not clean, and in a short time it had to be removed.

Mr. Cunningham was strongly of opinion that where it was possible removable bridge work was very much better than fixed bridge work.

Dr. Barrett spoke of what had been done in regard to bridge work in America, and said he felt confident that in that country, the amount of evil which had been done by bridge work, far exceeded the good which could be accomplished by it for some time. This was not the fault of the bridge work itself, but of the men who so thoroughly abused it.

The President said in his own practice he had not used any bridge work at all. His idea was that all this work should be carried upon its own foundation without any extensions beyond the root on which it stood, and he confessed when he had to extend beyond that, not to becoming a convert to bridge work. He had been in the habit for many years of fixing crowns upon roots, but mostly in the case of the incisors, and there he had not yet found the necessity for what was a painful eyesore when seen, viz., a gold ferrule or ring, which fitted round the neck of the stump. He had always been in the habit of using the screw pivot. He preferred, if he could, using the ordinary pin-wire. He could fix upon one case now in which he had put in work 27 years ago, and it had not been stirred in any way. As to bars he thought they were very objectionable indeed, because they did not give any masticating surface.

VOTES OF THANKS.

The above discussion concluded the meetings in the Museum.

On the motion of Mr. CUNNINGHAM, a hearty vote of thanks was passed to the readers of papers, and also to the retiring secretary, Mr. Morton Smale, a warm tribute being paid by Mr. Cunningham to that gentleman's untiring energy in the performance of his duties during his many years tenure of office.

DEMONSTRATIONS.

On Saturday, August 23rd, the demonstrations in connection with the annual meeting of the British Dental Association was held at the Devon and Exeter Hospital as follows :—

ANÆSTHETICS.

9 a.m. Dr. Dudley Buxton demonstrated a very useful apparatus which he had had constructed for him for the administration of nitrous oxide. It consisted of a tripod, in which was fixed a steel 50 gallon bottle, containing liquified nitrous oxide. A quieter was attached to this, which, as was seen during the demonstration, effectually suppressed all sound. The gas passing through the quieter traversed a mohair tube of large calibre, and entered a 2 gallon capacity Cattlin's bag. The tube passing from this to the face piece—a Clover's adapted, with Dr. Dudley Buxton's cap expiration valve—is metal and bent into a curve. In the course of this tube is a chamber controlled by a valve easily worked by the fingers. In this metal chamber is placed some material such as morsels of sponge, cotton wool, or asbestos, which can be moistened with perfume, sal volatile, or can be steeped in some antiseptic.

This was useful.

(I.) As making the gas more agreeable to children and nervous people.

(II.) To prevent infection from exhalations from the respiratory tract in phthisis, syphilis, etc., as the cotton-wool filters the air.

(III.) As ensuring cleanliness, and affording a ready means of disinfecting and purifying the apparatus.

Patients who took gas from the apparatus expressed great satisfaction.

II. Dr. Dudley Buxton then explained and illustrated by diagrams the method he adopts in giving gas with ether. A really simple and most effectual apparatus was shown, based upon Clover's original Gas and Ether Apparatus, which was the only one in which the gas was made to pass directly over the ether. By using this method, either gas alone or with ether, or ether with air, or alone, could be used. Dr. Dudley Buxton said that he could make a patient profoundly anæsthetic by its use in from one to one minute and a half.

This apparatus was made by Messrs. Mayer & Meltzer, of London.

III. Referring to Chloroform, the speaker said that although much had recently been said about the supposed safety of that anæsthetic, he was quite sure from his experience, that even when given with the utmost care and skill it was dangerous ; and the arguments based upon experiments upon quadrupeds made in India were not valid for human beings in England.

He spoke very highly of an apparatus he had been using for some time, which had been made for him by Messrs. Krohne & Sesemann, and based upon Dr. Junker's old inhaler.

It consisted of an arrangement whereby air was pumped through chloroform. The current of air was controlled by the rapidity of the action of the hand pump (a ball) and by a stop in the circuit, which could half or quarter the supply. By an arrangement, Mr. Krohne had converted the intermittent into a constant supply of chloroform. A further feature was a flannel mask, replacing the old vulcanite face-piece, which enabled the patient to have plenty of fresh air, and could be replaced after each operation, thus ensuring cleanliness. The apparatus was adapted also for animals, *e.g.*, lambs, calves, horses, etc. ; and Dr. Dudley Buxton urged its employment to spare the sufferings of farm-yard stock under the various necessary operations to which they are subjected.

Mr. Tom Bird, M.R.C.S., demonstrated with gas and ether, next with gas, ether, and air, and afterwards with gas, air, and a new mixture of his own, his object being to produce an anæsthetic which would get rid of the unpleasant and dangerous effects of ether.

The mixture referred to Mr. Bird intends keeping a secret during its experimental stages.

Dr. F. H. Hewitt demonstrated with his modified and improved apparatus for giving nitrous oxide and oxygen gas, the special feature in the improvement being that the oxygen could be cut off, and nitrous oxide only given, if required. The mixture also arranged by this new apparatus was 10 per cent. of oxygen added to the nitrous oxide. The result of the demonstration, was very satisfactory, the patient operated upon being thoroughly under the influence of the mixture ; no blueness of features, perfect tranquility, and no movement of any kind whilst in the operating chair.

At 10 a.m. Mr. Gartrell showed his new improved methods of making removable bridge work, which was greatly admired.

Mr. S. Cooke Parson very successfully fitted a seamless gold collar to a lower bicaspid, and afterwards soldered to it a gold crown.

Mr. R. P. Lennox showed his pneumatic mallet. By means of this contrivance a very rapid blow can be obtained, and at the same time it can be adjusted to a nicety.

Mr. G. Cunningham (Cambridge) showed specimens of his low fusing gum body and enamel, applicable to either English and American teeth. It could be used upon either gold or platinum, one of the special features being that any shade of gum could be obtained.

Mr. Woodruff demonstrated the immediate method of root filling on a suppurating upper bicuspid—first adjusting the rubber dam, then cleaning out débris both in crown and roots, and pumping peroxide of hydrogen up the roots, with cotton-wool in a fine Donaldson's bristle till all bubbling had ceased. He then carefully dried the tooth and roots with hot air and the use of Evans' Root Drier, afterwards working up a solution of guttapercha and chloroform to the ends of the roots and pressing home some solid guttapercha points with warm instruments till the roots were almost filled. He sealed the open ends with an oxyphosphate filling, subsequently making a distinct filling in the crown of the tooth. The peroxide of hydrogen was used in preference to any other antiseptic on account of its chemical action, which indicates by bubbling the presence of pus or sceptic matter.

Mr. Kirby (Bedford) showed his improved electric engine and special automatic regulator.

Dr. Mellotte demonstrated his methods of making dies and counter-dies with moldine fusible metal, &c.

THE DENTAL RECORD, LONDON: SEP. 1, 1890.

DENTAL PROCEEDINGS AT EXETER.

The very successful meeting of the British Dental Association at Exeter calls for some comment. There is a peculiar appropriateness in the report of this meeting appearing in the same issue as the dental students' supplement, as some of the best papers dealt mainly with the various problems of dental education. In a time of activity, of progress more than at any other are the lines of Pope true, "Man never is, but ever to be blessed." The student of five years ago thought himself quite sufficiently blessed in the matter of having enough examination, and showed but little eagerness to assume further test burdens and no anxious craving after more drastic methods for ascertaining the thoroughness of his professional acquirements but *tout cela est chargé*. The budding dentist of to-day is, if we may believe the speakers at the discussions, not only eager for an Honours exam., but keen for more teaching and examining in the matter of mechanical dentistry. The discussion elicited by Mr. Campion's paper was certainly a valuable one and characterised by good taste and candour. Those who spoke were prepared with something to say and said it fearlessly, but did not resent opposition, or attempt that unpleasant sport so prevalent among learned disputants—"jumping upon" their adversaries in debate. Although a report cannot unfortunately do full justice to demonstrations, we give a brief outline of those given at Exeter. These demonstrations, or "clinics," as some of our readers would call them, were certainly of a high order, and owing to the admirable arrangements of the local officers of the Association, were held under unusually favourable circumstances. Such clinics would seem to go far to answer in the affirmative the question, "Are clinics useful?" Busy country practitioners, whether dental or medical, have so few chances of seeing anæsthetics administered according to modern methods that it becomes a matter of real moment to them that those whose experience in chloroform, ether, and gas enables them to speak with authority upon the matter should demonstrate and explain matters anæsthetic. Of course, much must depend upon individual preference, but the experience of the last few years seems to show that whatever be the drawbacks of nitrous oxide as an anæsthetic, it is upon the whole more certain, more reliable, and more effectual than its rivals, at all events, for dental work. Mr. Gastrell's demonstration upon removable bridge work was one of great value, but when so high an average of merit existed among demonstrators, individual comment becomes unnecessary. We can congratulate the Association and its most energetic and kindly local officers upon having scored a decided success in its Annual General Meeting of 1890.

THE STUDENT'S SUPPLEMENT.

Returning to old usage we have appended in a condensed form the information which students, their parents, or those responsible for them require in setting about the commencement of the curriculum for the L.D.S. Possibly a word or two of general guidance may not be amiss, although we may say that, not only are the various secretaries of the examining bodies, but the deans of dental schools are always ready and willing to give courteous and kindly advice as to the best courses for a youth to follow. In many cases parents, &c., find a difficulty in selecting a preliminary examination where there are so many, choice often lies in favour of the easiest test. Against such a choice let us give a word of warning. The successful dentist must for his professional and his personal happiness possess a fair knowledge of the "humanities." General education tells far more in the long run than people imagine, and, things being equal the boy who has the energy and push to pass a good preliminary, such as the London University Matriculation, is far more likely to run a distinguished race in his professional career than the lad who sneaks through one of the less severe tests. As to purely professional schools, whether general or special, little need be said, those of London and the provinces are well known, and the merits and drawbacks are easily learnt from old students. One golden rule is do not decide your school or your hospital in a hurry, hear all sides.

MR. SEWELL'S DENTAL SURGERY.

In reference to the review upon the above volume which appeared in our last issue (Aug. 1st), and to which exception has been taken, we desire to state that the article in question was written in perfect good faith and without any intentional reflection upon Mr. Sewill individually. No personalities were intended, and we should be sorry if anyone were to think otherwise. We consider the book can stand upon its own merits and upon Mr. Sewill's reputation in the fields of literature and dental science. We regret that Mr. Sewill should have considered the review beyond the range of fair criticism, and offer him an apology for any annoyance it may have caused him.

STUDENTS' SUPPLEMENT.

Registration of Dental Students.

The registration of dental students shall be carried on at the Medical Council Office, 299, Oxford Street, W.

Every dental student shall be registered in the manner hereinafter prescribed by the General Medical Council.

No dental student shall be registered until he has passed a preliminary examination, as required by the General Medical Council,* and has produced evidence that he has commenced medical study.

The commencement of the course of professional study recognised by any of the qualifying bodies shall not be reckoned as dating earlier than fifteen days before the date of registration.

Students who commenced their professional education by apprenticeship to dentists entitled to be registered, or by attendance upon professional lectures, before July 22nd, 1878 (when dental education became compulsory, shall not be required to produce evidence of having passed a preliminary education.

Pupils who have been articled to their fathers, or to brothers—with whom money transactions would be nominal—shall, in all other respects, be considered to be in the same position in regard to registration as those pupils provided for in the first part of Section 37 of the *Dentists' Act*, who have paid premiums for instruction.

Candidates for a diploma in dental surgery shall produce certificates of having been engaged during four years in professional studies, and of having received three years' instruction in mechanical dentistry from a registered practitioner.

---

* Exception may be made in the case of a student from any Indian, Colonial, or foreign university or college, who shall have passed the matriculation or other equivalent examination of his university or college, provided such examination fairly represents a standard of general education equivalent to that required in this country.

One year's *bonâ fide* apprenticeship with a registered dental practitioner, after being registered as a dental student, may be counted as one of the four years of professional study.

The three years of instruction in mechanical dentistry, or any part of them, may be taken by the dental student either before or after his registration as a student; but no year of such mechanical instruction shall be counted as one of the four years of professional study unless taken after registration.

The privilege provided by the first clause of Section 37 of the *Dentists' Act*, for persons whose articles of apprenticeship expired before January 1, 1880, shall be extended to all persons whose articles had begun two years before that period.

Forms for registration may be obtained at the office of the General Medical Council. No fee is required for registration as a student.

PRELIMINARY EDUCATION.

Regulations of General Medical Council.

No person shall be allowed to be registered as a medical or a dental student unless he shall have previously passed (at one or more examinations) a preliminary examination in the subjects of General Education as specified in the following List:—

1. English Language, including Grammar and Composition;
2. Latin, including Grammar, Translation from specified authors, and Translation of easy passages not taken from such authors;
3. Elements of Mathematics, comprising (α) Arithmetic, including Vulgar and Decimal Fractions, (β) Algebra, including Simple Equations, (γ) Geometry, including the first book of Euclid, with easy questions on the subject matter of the same;
4. Elementary Mechanics of Solids and Fluids, comprising the Elements of Statics, Dynamics, and Hydrostatics;
5. One of the following optional subjects:—
   (α) Greek; (β) French; (γ) German; (δ) Italian; (ε) any other Modern Language; (ζ) Logic; (η) Botany; (θ) Zoology; (ι) Elementary Chemistry.

List of Examining Bodies whose Examinations fulfil the conditions of the Medical Council as regards preliminary education, and entitle to registration as medical or dental student.*

* Provided that, in all cases, the subject of Mechanics, as set forth in clause 4 be shown to have been included in the Examination.

I.—Universities in the United Kingdom.

Oxford or Cambridge :—

(*a.*) Junior Local Examinations ; Certificate to include Latin and Mathematics, and also one of the following optional subjects, Greek, French, German.

(*b.*) Senior Local Examinations ; Certificate to include Latin and Mathematics.

(*c.*) Responsions. (Oxon.) Higher Local Examinations, (Cantab.)

(*d.*) Moderations. (Oxon.) Previous Examinations, (Cantab.)

(*e.*) Examination for a Degree in Arts.

London :—

(*a.*) Matriculation Examination.

(*b.*) Preliminary Scientific (M.B.) Examination.

(*c.*) Examination for a Degree in Arts or Science.

Durham :—

(*a.*) Examination for Certificate of Proficiency.

(*b.*) Examination for Students at the end of their first year.

(*c.*) Examination for a Degree in Arts.

Victoria University :—

(*a*) Preliminary Examination ; Latin to be one of the subjects.

(*b*) Entrance Examination in Arts, to include all the subjects required.

Universities of Edinburgh, Aberdeen, Glasgow, St. Andrews :—

(*a.*) Local Examination (Junior Certificate) ; Certificate to include English Literature, Arithmetic, Algebra, Geometry, Latin, and also one of the following optional subjects, Greek, French, German, (or all subjects required.)

(*b.*) Local Examinations (Senior Certificate) ; Certificate to include English Literature, Arithmetic, Algebra, Geometry, Latin, and also one of the following optional subjects, Greek, French, German.

(*c.*) Preliminary Examination for Graduation in Science (Edinburgh) or Medicine and Surgery.

(*d.*) Examination for a Degree in Arts.

University of Dublin :—

(*a.*) Public Entrance Examination.

(*b.*) General Examination at end of Senior Freshman year.

(*c.*) Examination for a Degree in Arts.

Queen's University in Ireland:—

(*a.*) Local Examinations for men and women ; Certificate to include all the subjects required by the General Medical Council.

(*b*.) Entrance or Matriculation Examination.

(*c*.) Previous Examination for B.A. Degree.

(*d*.) Examination for a Degree in Arts.

Royal University of Ireland:— Matriculation Examination.

Oxford and Cambridge Schools' Examination Boards:—

Certificate to include the following subjects :—An adequate knowledge of English Grammar and Orthography, as shown in the course of the Examination, to the satisfaction of the Examiners, being held as conforming to the requirements of the Medical Council in regard to those subjects:—

(*a*.) Arithmetic, including Vulgar and Decimal Fractions ;

(*b*.) Algebra, including Simple Equations ;

(*c*.) Geometry, including the first two books of Euclid ;

(*d*.) Latin, including Translation and Grammar ;

(*e*.) Also one of these optional subjects :—Greek, French, German.

II.—OTHER BODIES NAMED IN SCHEDULE (A) TO THE MEDICAL ACT.

Apothecaries' Society of London :—Examination in Arts.

Royal Colleges of Physicians and Surgeons of Edinburgh :—

Preliminary (combined) Examination in General Education.

Faculty of Physicians and Surgeons of Glasgow :—

Preliminary Examination in General Education.

Royal College of Surgeons in Ireland :—

Preliminary Examination ; Certificate to include Mathematics.

III.—EXAMINING BODIES IN THE UNITED KINGDOM, NOT INCLUDED IN SCHEDULE (A) TO THE MEDICAL ACT (1858).

College of Preceptors :—Examination for a First Class Certificate, or Second Class Certificate of First or Second Division, Algebra, Geometry, Latin, and a Modern Language, having been taken.

Queen's College, Belfast ; Queen's College, Cork ; Queen's College, Galway :—Matriculation.

Intermediate Education Board of Ireland :—

Junior Grade Examination
Middle Grade Examination
Senior Grade Examination
} Certificate in each case to include all the subjects required.

St. David's College, Lampeter :—

Responsions Examination, to include all the subjects required.

Educational Institute of Scotland :—

Preliminary Medical Examination.

IV.—CERTAIN INDIAN, COLONIAL AND FOREIGN UNIVERSITIES AND COLLEGES.

Regulations of The Various Examining Bodies for The Diploma in Dental Surgery (L.D.S.)

	Royal College of Surgeons, England.	Royal College of Surgeons, Edinburgh.	Royal College of Surgeons, Ireland.	Faculty of Physicians and Surgeons, Glasgow.
1—Preliminary Examination	Compulsory on all who commenced their Professional Education after July 22nd, 1878. Must be registered as a Dental Student at the Office of the General Medical Council, 299, Oxford St., London, W.	Compulsory on all who commenced their Professional Education after August 1st, 1878.	Compulsory on all, except those who have passed one equivalent examination.	Compulsory on all who commenced the Professional Education after August 1st, 1878.
2—Age at which the Candidate may present himself..................	Twenty-one.	Twenty-one.	Any age, but diploma cannot be granted until he is twenty-one.	Twenty-one.
3—Duration of Professional Education	Four years subsequent to registration.	Four years.	Four years.	Four years.
4—Courses of Lectures, &c., to be attended at a recognised School —				
Anatomy	Two Courses, or one Course and Twenty Lectures on Head and Neck.	One Winter Course.	One Course.	Two Courses, or one Course and twenty Lectures on Head and Neck.
Physiology	One Course. (Six months).	One Course of 50 Lectures.	One Course.	One Six months' Course.

4—COURSES OF LECTURES, &c. *(continued)*—	Royal College of Surgeons, England.	Royal College of Surgeons, Edinburgh.	Royal College of Surgeons, Ireland.	Faculty of Physicians and Surgeons, Glasgow.
Practical Physiology (separate from above)........	Three months' Course.	One Course of 50 Lectures.	One Course.	One Six months' Course.
Surgery..................	Ditto.	One Winter Course.	Ditto.	
Medicine	Ditto.	Ditto.	Ditto.	Ditto.
Chemistry................	Instruction in Chemistry, which must include Practical Chemistry.	Ditto.		Ditto.
Materia Medica	Instruction in Chemistry, Practical Chemistry and Materia Medica need not be taken in the usual period after the Registration.	One three months' Course.	Ditto.	One three months' Course.
Dissections and Demonstrations, or	Three months.	Nine months.	Two Courses.	Nine months'.
Dissections and Anatomy of Head and Neck......		Nine months. One Course of 20 Lectures.		
Midwifery	One Course.	One three months' Course.	One Course.	Twelve Lectures.
Course of Lectures on Surgery	Six months, or one Winter Session.			
One Course of Lectures on Medicine	Six months, or one Winter Session.			
Practice of Surgery, and Clinical Lectures	Two Winter Sessions.	One six months' Course, or two three months' Courses	Two Winter Sessions.	Twenty-four Lectures. Twenty Lectures.
Dental Anatomy and Physiology................	Two Courses.	One Course.	None.	Twelve Lectures on Demonstrations.
Dental Surgery & Pathology	Ditto.	Ditto.	Two Courses.	Twelve Lectures.
Metallurgy (as specially applied in Practical Chemistry	Ditto.	One Course of not less than twelve Lectures.		
Dental Mechanics	Ditto.	One Course	Two Courses.	

4—Courses of Lectures, &c. (*continued*)—	Royal College of Surgeons, England.	Royal College of Surgeons, Edinburgh.	Royal College of Surgeons, Ireland.	Faculty of Physicians and Surgeons, Glasgow.
Practical Instruction in Mechanical Dentistry ..	Three years under a competent Practitioner, eighteen months of which may be previous to Registration.	Three years under a Registered Dental Practitioner.	Three years under a Registered Dental Licentiate.	Three years under a Registered Practitioner.
Practice of Dental Surgery in a recognised Dental Hospital, or in the Dental Department of a recognised General Hospital ..	Two years.	Two years.	Nine months.	Two years.
5—Fee	£10 10s. over and above stamp duty.	£10 10s.	£10 10s.	£10 10s.
6—Least period during which unsuccessful Candidates are referred to their studies	Six months, subject to the decision of the Board.	Three months.	Six months.	Three months.
7—Particulars of Examination	(A) *Written.* On G[illegible]l [illegible] A[illegible]ny a[illegible]d Physiology. G[illegible]al Pathology a[illegible]d Surgery, D[illegible]al A[illegible]-[illegible]ny a[illegible]d Physiology, Dental Pat[illegible]y a[illegible]d Surgery. At the [illegible]al Examina-t[illegible]n [illegible]s may be [illegible]d :	*Written and Oral :* 1st Part—Anatomy, Physiology, Chemistry with Metallurgy.	*Written and Oral :* On all the subjects of the Curriculum.	*Written, Oral, & Practical :* 1st Part—Anatomy, Physiology, Chemistry, and Metallurgy.

8—Courses of Lectures, &c. (*continued*)—	Royal College of Surgeons, England.	Royal College of Surgeons, Edinburgh.	Royal College of Surgeons, Ireland.	Faculty of Physicians and Surgeons, Glasgow.
7.—Particulars of Examination (*continued*)	(*a*) On the treatment of Dental Caries, and any operation to prepare and fill cavities with gold or plastic filling or material, or to do any other operation in Dental Surgery. (Candidates must provide their own instruments.) (*b*) On the Mechanical and Surgical treatment of the various irregularities of the teeth. (*c*) On Mechanical Dentistry. (B) *Oral:* On all subjects in the Curriculum. Preparations, Casts, and Drawings.	2nd Part—Surgery, Medicine, Materia Medica, and Special Subjects of Dental Anatomy and Physiology, Dental Surgery, Pathology, and Dental Mechanics. Registered Dental Practitioners are examined on special subjects only,	Preparations, Microscopes, and other appliances.	2nd Part..Surgery, Medicine, Materia Medica and special Dental subjects. Practical Examination at a Dental Hospital. Candidates are to bring Excavators, Files, and Plugging Instruments.
8—Date of Examination	May and November.	I. Professional Examinations. Tuesday, Oct. 29, 1889. " April 22, 1890.	Quarterly.	1889..October 17..19. 1890..May 1..3. " October 9..11.
9—Modified Conditions of Admission to Examination *sine curriculo:* (*a*) Conditions of eligibility.	Candidates must have been in Practice or have commenced Professional Education prior to September, 1859 (the date of the Dental Charter).	II. Professional Examinations. Following Thursday.	Candidates must be registered Dental Practitioners in practice before 1878.	

9—Courses of Lectures, &c. *continued*—	Royal College of Surgeons, England.	Royal College of Surgeons, Edinburgh.	Royal College of Surgeons, Ireland.	Faculty of Physicians and Surgeons, Glasgow.
(*b*) Certificates, &c., required (*continued*):	[illegible] of [illegible] signed by two [illegible] of the College or two [illegible] of the [illegible]sing Bodies in the [illegible] where the [illegible] was [illegible].		Certificates of moral and professional character, signed by two Registered Medical Practitioners, and by two Registered Dentists.	
[illegible] Conditions of Admission to Examinations..(*contd.*):	[illegible]. Age. [illegible] [illegible]. [illegible] of commencing Dental [illegible]. [illegible] a Member, Licentiate or [illegible] of any [illegible] of [illegible], [illegible] of [illegible], or [illegible], with date of [illegible], &, Of [illegible] [illegible] Societies a [illegible]. [illegible] in Dental [illegible] separately, or if [illegible], in [illegible] with [illegible] [illegible]. [illegible] he has [illegible] Advertisements or Public [illegible]. [illegible] of Professional [illegible].		N[illegible]. Age. [illegible]. [illegible] [illegible]cing [illegible], and [illegible] [illegible] has been [illegible] on in [illegible] with any other [illegible], and if so with [illegible]. Professional status. Particulars of Professional Education.	

9—COURSES OF LECTURES, &c. *continued.*	Royal College of Surgeons, England.	Royal College of Surgeons, Edinburgh.	Royal College of Surgeons, Ireland.	Faculty of Physicians and Surgeons, Glasgow.
(*c*) Mannner of Examination	Same as ordinary Examination.			
Fee....	Ten guineas over and above stamp duty,		£21.	
For further information apply to Secretary.	MR. F. G. HALLETT, Examination Hall, Victoria Embankment, London, W.C.	JAMES ROBERTSON, Soli[illegible], I[illegible] Secretary [illegible]nd [illegible], 1, [illegible]e Square, Edinburgh.	JOHN BRENNEN, Esq., Royal College of Surgeons, Dublin.	ALEX. DUNCAN, Esq., Faculty of Physicians and Surgeons, Glasgow.

SPECIAL (DENTAL) HOSPITALS.

London School of Dental Surgery, Leicester Square.

Consulting Physician.—Sir James Risdon Bennett, F.R.S., M.D.,

Consulting Surgeon.—Mr. Christopher Heath, F.R.C.S.,

Consulting Dental Surgeons.—Mr. Samuel Cartwright, F.R.C.S.; Sir John Tomes, F.R.S., F.R.C.S., L.D.S.,

Dental Surgeons.—Messrs. Storer Bennett; F. Canton; G. Gregson; Claude Rogers; C. E. Truman; R. H. Woodhouse.

Assistant Dental Surgeons.—Messrs. W. Hern; Leonard Matheson; G. W. Parkinson; W. B. Paterson; L. Read; E. Lloyd Williams.

Anæsthetists.—Messrs. G. H. Bailey; T. Bird; Woodhouse Braine; Joseph Mills.

Assistant Anæsthetists.—Drs. Dudley W. Buxton; Frederick W. Hewitt.

Demonstrator of Cohesive Gold Filling.—Mr. J. F. Colyer.

Demonstrator of Non-cohesive Gold filling.—Mr. C. F. Rilot.

Medical Tutor.—Mr. H. Baldwin,

Curator of Mechanical Laboratory.—Mr. H. Lloyd Williams.

Morton Smale, *Dean.*

Lecturers:—*Dental Surgery and Pathology*, Mr. Storer Bennett.

Dental Anatomy and Pathology (Human and Comparative), Mr. Arthur Underwood.

Dental Mechanics, Mr. David Hepburn.

Metallurgy in its application to Dental Purposes.—Professor A. K. Huntingdon (King's College, London), F.I.C., F.C.S., &c.

Mechanical Laboratory.

A mechanical laboratory is now fitted up and opened under the care and superintendence of the lecturer on dental mechanics, and a highly skilled mechanic. Students will be required to take models, manufacture, and fit into the mouth dentures for those patients allotted to them by members of the staff. The actual manufacture to be under the superintendence of the mechanical assistant, while the adapting to the mouth will be supervised by Members of the Staff.

It is intended, in this manner to supply a portion of the Students' Education heretofore unprovided for, and to more perfectly equip him for the exigences of dental practice. It will enable him to be in a better position to meet the requirements of the College of

Surgeons of England with regard to mechanical dentistry, in which subjects the Board of Examiners for the L.D.S. may demand a practical examination from candidates for that diploma.

GENERAL FEE FOR THE SPECIAL LECTURES REQUIRED BY THE CURRICULUM.

Viz., two Courses on Dental Anatomy, two Courses on Dental Surgery, two Courses on Mechanical Dentistry, and one Course of Metallurgy, £15 15s.

Fee for the Two Years' Practice of the Hospital required by the Curriculum, £15 15s.

Total Fee for the Special Lectures and Hospital Practice required by the Curriculum, £31 10s.

Students who perform Operations for Filling Teeth must provide their own Instruments for the same.

Additional Fees for a General Hospital for the two years, to fulfil the requirements of the Curriculum, vary from £40 to £50.

MEDICAL TUTOR.

The medical tutor attends on four days in the week, from 5 to 7 p.m., for two months previous to two of the Annual Examinations.

NATIONAL DENTAL HOSPITAL AND COLLEGE,

GREAT PORTLAND STREET, W.

Consulting Physicians.—B. W. Richardson, M.A., M.D., F.R.S. ; W. H. Broadbent, M.D., F.R.C.P.

Consulting Surgeons.—Sir Spencer Wells Bart., F.R.C.S. ; Christopher Heath, F.R.C.S.,

Consulting Dental Surgeon.—Sir Edwin Saunders, F.R.C.S.

Dental Surgeons.—A. F. Canton ; H. G. Read ; Harry Rose ; Alfred Smith ; F. Henri Weiss ; G. A. Williams.

Assistant Dental Surgeons.—Marcus Davis ; C. W. Glassington ; W. R. Humby ; R. Denison Pedley ; G. Read ; Willoughby Weiss.

Anæsthetists.—Chas. H. Barkley ; Henry Davis ; James Maughan ; S. E. Pedley ; Sidney Spokes.

LECTURERS :—*Dental Anatomy and Physiology.*—Sidney Spokes.

Dental Surgery and Pathology.—Willoughby Weiss.

Dental Mechanics.—Harry Rose.

Dental Metallurgy.—W. Lapraik.

Operative Dental Surgery.—George Cunningham,

Dental Materia Medica.—C. W. Glassington.

Elements of Histology.—James Maughan.

Demonstrator of Dental Mechanics.—W. R. Humby.

Hospital Practice to Registered Practitioners (six months), £7 7s. Ditto (twelve months), £9 9s.

Fee for the two years' Hospital Practice required by the Curriculum, £12 12s. Perpetual Fee, £15 15s.

A laboratory has been arranged for pivot, crown, bar and regulation cases.

Total Fee for the Special Lectures and Hospital Practice required by the Curriculum, £25 4s. Perpetual Fee, £31 10s.

F. HENRI WEISS, *Dean.*

GUY'S HOSPITAL (DENTAL SCHOOL).

Dental Surgeon.—F. Newland-Pedley.

Assistant Dental Surgeons.—Messrs. W. A. Maggs; J. Mansbridge; H. Murray; H. L. Pillin; G. O. Richards; R. W. Rouw.

Anæsthetists.—Drs. F. W. Cock; J. F. Silk; and Shepherd.

LECTURERS:—*Dental Surgery.*—Mr. Newland-Pedley.

Dental Anatomy and Physiology.—Mr. Maggs.

Dental Mechanics.—Mr. Richards.

Metallurgy.—C. E. Groves, F.R.S.

Anæsthetics.—T. Bird.

Dental Microscope.—Mr. Mansbridge.

Tutor.—Mr. Rouw. *Dean.*—Dr. Perry.

FEES:—1. By the payment of £70 on entrance.

2. By two payments of 40 guineas, and 30 guineas at the beginning of the first and second years respectively.

A ticket which gives admission to the special lectures and demonstrations and dental practice only may be obtained for 30 guineas paid on entrance

The inclusive fee for students entering for the M.R.C.S., L.R.C.P., and L.D.S., Eng., is £150 paid in one sum, or 150 guineas paid in three annual instalments at the commencement of each academical year:—First year, £60; second year, £60; third year, £37 10s.

EDINBURGH.

DENTAL HOSPITAL AND SCHOOL.

Consulting Physician.—Alex. Peddie, M.D.

Consulting Surgeon.—Joseph Bell, M.D., F.R.C.S.E.

Consulting Dental Surgeon.—John Smith, M.D., F.R.C.S.E.

Dean and Hon. Treasurer.—W. Bowman Macleod, L.D.S.

Dental Surgeons.—Messrs. Andrew Wilson ; Malcolm Macgregor ; George W. Watson ; J. Stewart Durward ; James Mackintosh ; James Lindsay.

Assistant Dental Surgeons.—William Forrester ; John S. Amoore ; J. Graham Munro ; Wm. Wilson ; John Turner ; David Munroe.

Chloroformists.—R. Stewart ; W. Keiller.

DENTAL SCHOOL (LECTURES.)

Dental Anatomy and Physiology (Human and Comparative).—Mr. Andrew Wilson.

Dental Surgery and Pathology.—Mr. George W. Watson.

Mechanical Dentistry.—Mr. W. Bowman Macleod.

Practical Mechanics.—Assistant Demonstrator, J. Stewart Durward. The demonstrations will be spread over the two years of hospital practice. Students will require to furnish their own hand tools.

General Fee for the Hospital Practice and special Lectures required by the Curriculum.—Hospital Practice, £15 15s. One course each of Dental Anatomy, Dental Surgery, and Mechanical Dentistry and Demonstrations, £9 15s.—£25 10s.

Fees to separate Classes.—Dental Anatomy, Dental Surgery, Mechanical Dentistry, £3 5s. each.

The hospital practice and lectures qualify for the Dental Diploma of the Royal College of Surgeons, Edinburgh, and also for that of the other licensing bodies. Second courses of the lectures, as required by the Royal College of Surgeons of England, £2 4s.

The session 1889-90 opens October 17th, 1889. General fee for the hospital practice and special lectures required, £25 10s.

For Further particulars, apply to the Dean, 5, Lawnston Lane, Edinburgh.

GLASGOW.

DENTAL HOSPITAL AND SCHOOL, 4, CHATHAM PLACE, STERLING ROAD.

Hon. Consulting Physician.—W. T. Gairdner, M.D.

Hon. Consulting Surgeon.—Sir G. H. B. Macleod.

Chloroformists.—Drs. Brown, Campbell and Anderson.

Dental Surgeons.—J. A. Biggs ; W. S. Woodburn ; Rees Price ; James Cumming ; J. R. Brownlie ; J. C. Woodburn, M.D.

Assistant Dental Surgeons.—W. F. Martin ; Alexander White ; James Cameron ; W. Holt Woodburn.

Fee for the two years' practice required by the Curriculum, £12 12s. Fee for each course of lectures, £3 3s.

DENTAL SCHOOL.

Dental Anatomy and Physiology (*Human and Comparative*), by J. Cowan Woodburn.

Dental Surgery and Pathology, by James Rankin Brownlie.

Secretary, D. M. Alexander, Solicitor, 117, Wellington Street, Glasgow, who will forward detailed Prospectus of the School.

BIRMINGHAM SCHOOL OF DENTISTRY, QUEEN'S COLLEGE.

The teaching of Dentistry is now undertaken by the Queen's College acting in association with the Birmingham Dental Hospital, and the Birmingham Clinical Board, so that students may fully qualify themselves for the Dental Diplomas of the Royal Colleges,

LECTURES FOR THE DENTAL CURRICULUM.

Dental Anatomy and Physiology.—J. Humphreys.

Dental Surgery and Pathology.—C. Sims

Dental Metallurgy.—W. A. Tilden, D.Sc., F.R.S.

Dental Mechanics.—W. Elliott.

Dental Tutor.—Frank H. Goffe.

General Subjects.—As taught in Medical Department of Queen's College.

FEES.

A Composition Fee of 60 guineas, payable in one sum or in two sums, viz., 40 guineas at the beginning of the first year and 20 guineas at the beginning of the second year of studentship, admits to the full curriculum required for the Dental Diploma (inclusive of the necessary Hospital Practice).

N.B.—Further particulars may be obtained on application to the Warden at the College, or to the Hno. Secretary of the Dental Board, Queen's College, Mr. J. Humphreys).

BIRMINGHAM DENTAL HOSPITAL.

Hon. Consulting Physician.—Robert M. Simon, M.D.

Hon. Consulting Surgeon.—John St. S. Wilders, M.R.C.S.

Hon. Consulting Dentists :—Thomas R. English; Adams Parker, L.D.S.; Charles Sims, L.D.S.

Hon. Dental Surgeons.—H. Breward Neale; F. E. Huxley; J. Humphreys; F. W. Richards.

Hon. Assistant Dental Surgeons.—F. H. Goffe; Wm. Palethorpe; W. R. Roberts.

Demonstrator in Gold Filling etc.—Mr. W. Palethorpe, L.D.S

DENTAL HOSPITAL OF IRELAND.

25, LINCOLN PLACE, DUBLIN.

Consulting Physicians.—F. R. Cruise, M.D.; John W. Moore, M.D.

Consulting Surgeons.—E. H. Bennett, F.R.C.S.I.; Sir W. Stokes, F.R.C.S.I.

Consulting Dental Surgeons.—R. H. Moore, F.R.C.S.I.; Daniel Corbett, M.R.C.S.E., L.D.S., Eng

Dental Surgeons.—Messrs. Robert Hazelton; W. Booth Pearsall; R. Theodore Stack; A. W. W. Baker; Daniel Corbett; George Wycliffe Yeates; G. M. P. Murray.

Anæsthetists.—Dr. Christopher Gunn; Messrs. John G. Cronyn; John R. Graves.

Pathologist.—William Mallett Purser.

Registrar.—William A. Shea.

In connection with the Dental Hospital of Ireland, the Dental School will be open for the Winter Session on October 7th, 1889.

In addition to Clinical Instruction, courses of lectures will be given at the Hospital in Dental Surgery and Pathology, and in Mechanical Dentistry, by R. Theodore Stack; A. W. W. Baker; W. Booth Pearsall and Daniel Corbett, and at the School of Physic, which is within a few yards of the Hospital, special lectures for dental students will be given in Dental Anatomy, and in Metallurgy by Professor Cunningham and Professor Reynolds. The lectures on dental surgery and mechanical dentistry will be given during the winter, those in dental anatomy and metallurgy during the summer months. Among the advantages of the school is the mechanical laboratory, where every effort is made to assist the student in mechanical dentistry. In addition to practical instruction in the details of gold, dental alloy, vulcanite, celluloid, and continuous gum work, special demonstrations will be given in the mechanical treatment of cleftpalate; in the treatment of dental irregularities, and in the various methods of inserting pivot teeth. Regulations as to fees and other conditions are the same that exist at the Dental Hospital of London, Leicester Square. Any further information can be obtained from the registrar of the hospital, or

R. THEODORE STACK, *Dean.*

THE OWEN'S COLLEGE, MANCHESTER.

DENTAL DEPARTMENT.

Professors and Lecturers.—Anatomy, Professor A. H. Young. Physiology, Professor Wm. Stirling. Medicine, Professor J. E. Morgan ; Professor James Ross. Surgery, Professor A. W. Hare. Clinical Surgery, Messrs. F. A. Heath ; Walter Whitehead ; Thomas Jones ; James Hardie ; F. A. Southam ; G. A. Wright. Chemistry, Professor H. B. Dixon. Materia Medica, Professor D. J. Leech. Dental Surgery, George G. Campion. Dental Anatomy, W. A. Hooton. Dental Mechanics, Thos. Tanner. Dental Metallurgy C. A Burghardt.

The fee for the two years' lectures, &c., required by the dental curriculum of the Colleges of Surgeons is £50, payable in two sums of £25 each at the beginning of the first and second years of studentship.

The two years' general hospital practice is taken at the Royal Infirmary. The fee is £10 10s., and includes that for attendance on the lectures on clinical surgery.

For further particulars with regard to the dental department, application should be made to the Registrar, The Owen's College, Manchester.

THE VICTORIA DENTAL HOSPITAL OF MANCHESTER,

GROSVENOR STREET, ALL SAINTS.

Consulting Physicians.—Sir Wm. Roberts, M.D. ; Messrs. Henry Simpson, M.D. ; J. E. Morgan, M.D. ; D. J. Leech, M.D. ; D. Lloyd Roberts, M.D.

Consulting Surgeons.—Messrs. E. Lund ; F. A. Heath ; W. Whitehead ; T. Jones ; J. Hardie.

Consulting Dental Surgeons.—Messrs. H. Campion ; Parsons Shaw.

Dental Surgeons.—Messrs. H. Planck ; J. Renshaw ; T. Tanner ; J. H. Molloy ; G. O. Whittaker ; W. Dykes ; W. Dougan ; G. Nash Skipp ; G. G. Campion ; W. Sims ; L. Dreschfeld ; W. Headridge ; J. W. Dunkerley ; W. Smithard.

The fee for the two years' hospital practice required by the College of Surgeons is £12 12s.

For further information apply to HENRY PLANCK, *Dean.*

LIVERPOOL DENTAL HOSPITAL, MOUNT PLEASANT.

Consulting Physician.—Thomas Robinson Glynn, M.D.

Consulting Surgeon.—Frank T. Paul, F.R.C.S., Eng.

Consulting Dental Surgeons.—Messrs. C. Alder ; H. C. Quinby ; J. E. Rose ; W. H. Waite.

Honorary Dental Surgeons.—Messrs. R. M. Capon ; E. A. Councell ; R. Edwards ; H. Newton Hindley ; W. Mapplebeck ; W. Matthews ; Thos. Mansell ; J. N. P. Newton ; J. Pidgeon ; M. Quinby ; J. Royston ; G. A. Williams.

Honorary Assistant Dental Surgeons.—Messrs. M. Alexander ; E. A. Davies.

Stipendiary Dental Surgeons.—Messrs. A. B. Dalby ; R. H. Bates ; Charles B. Dobson.

Fees for Hospital Practice, £5 5s. per annum, or a composition fee of £8 8s. for two years' Hospital Practice required for the curriculum to students of the Medical Faculty, University College, Liverpool, and Pupils or apprentices of Registered Dentists.

Further information may be obtained by applying to the Honorary Secretary, W. L. Jackson, Central Buildings, North John Street,

PLYMOUTH DENTAL HOSPITAL (OCTAGON).

Physician.—C. Albert Hingston, M.D.

Surgeons.—Messrs. Christopher Bulteel ; Connel Whipple.

Consulting Dentist.—F. A. Jewers.

Dental Surgeons.—Messrs. W. V. Moore ; F. H. Balkwill ; Ernest E. Jewers ; Ernest Edward Jewers ; Henry William Mayne ; Louis E. Sexton.

Treasurer.—Alfred Payne Balkwill.

Dental School.—Certificates of attendance on the practice of this Dental Dispensary are recognised by the College of Surgeons as qualifying for the Diploma in Dental Surgery. The College also recognises the lectures delivered at the Dispensary.

Pupils of any of the Dental Surgeons of the Plymouth Dental Hospital, or other Dentists holding a Diploma of the College of Surgeons, or Member of the Odontological Society, may attend the Hospital on the day of such practitioner as may agree to accept such pupil or pupils, on the payment of £1 1s. per annum to the Institution.

Lectures.—On Dental Anatomy, by F. H. Balkwill ; on Dental Mechanics, by W. V. Moore. Fee to Lectures, one course, £7 7s. ; fee to Lectures, double course, £12 12s. (required for Diploma); fee to Dental Practice at Hospital, £5 5s. ; fee to entire Dental Curriculum (required for Diploma), 22 guineas.

Further information may be obtained from the Secretary, Mr. E. G. Bennett, at above address.

EXETER DENTAL HOSPITAL.

Consulting Surgeons.—Messrs. A. J Cumming, F.R.C.S., Eng.; James Bankart, M.B., Lond., F.R.C.S., Eng.

Consulting Dental Surgeon.—S. Bevan Fox.

Dental Surgeons.—Messrs. J. T. Browne-Mason; Henry Biging Mason; S. Mundell; T. G. T. Garland; J. M. Ackland.

Honorary Secretary.—George A. Townsend.

Attendance on the practice of this Hospital is recognised by the Royal College of Surgeons of England as qualifying for their Dental Diploma.

Pupils of any member of the staff or other registered Practitioner (being a Life or Annual Governor) are permitted to attend the practice of the Hospital, subject to the approval of the Medical Sub-Committee, on payment of £5 5s. annually to the funds of the Institution. Students attending the practice of the Hospital must consider themselves strictly under the control of the Medical Officers, and must not undertake any operation without the consent of the Dental Surgeon for the day.

MEDICAL SCHOOLS.

BARTHOLOMEW'S HOSPITAL, SMITHFIELD, E.C.

Fee for general subjects for students of dental surgery:—First winter, 31½ guineas; first summer, 31½ guineas; or a single payment of 63 guineas. DR. Norman Moore, *Warden.*

CHARING CROSS HOSPITAL, W.C.

The composition fee for dental students is £42 2s. This may be paid in two instalments of £22 2s. and £20, at the commencement of each winter session respectively. Dr. J. Mitchell Bruce, *Dean.*

GUY'S HOSPITAL, BOROUGH, S.E.

Fee for attendance on the hospital practice and lectures required for the Dental Diploma of the College of Surgeons, 63 guineas, or in two annual instalments of 40 guineas and 23 guineas. The above fee does not include £1 10s. for practical chemistry.

Dr. F. Taylor, *Dean.*

KING'S COLLEGE, STRAND, W.C.

No special arrangements are made for dental students.

Prof Curnow, *Dean.*

LONDON HOSPITAL, MILE END, E.

Composite fee for dental students :—Hospital practice and lectures, £42. This does not include the fee of £2 2s. for practical chemistry.

Munroe Scott, *Warden.*

MIDDLESEX HOSPITAL, BERNERS STREET, W.

Students who intend to become Licentiates in Dental Surgery of the Royal College of Surgeons are admitted to attend the requisite courses of lectures and hospital practice on payment of a fee of 40 guineas, in one sum on entrance, or by instalments of £30 on entrance and £15 at the beginning of the second winter session.

A. Pearce Gould, *Dean.*

ST. GEORGE'S HOSPITAL, GROSVENOR PLACE, S.W.

Fee for general subjects required for the Diploma in Dental Surgery, including practical chemistry, £55 ; payable in two instalments : first year, £30 ; second year, £25. T. T. Whitham, M.D., *Dean.*

ST. MARY'S HOSPITAL, PADDINGTON, W.

Entrance fee to the general hospital practice and lectures required for the examination in dental surgery at the Royal College of Surgeons, England, £55 ; payable in two instalments :—First year, £30 ; second year, £25.

Herbert Page, *Dean.*

ST. THOMAS'S HOSPITAL, ALBERT EMBANKMENT, S.E.

The fee for attendance on the general subjects required of students in dental surgery is, for the two years, £55 ; or by instalments, £50 for the first year, and £10 for the second year. E. Nettleship, *Dean.*

UNIVERSITY COLLEGE, GOWER STREET, W.C.

No special arrangements are made for dental students.

Prof. Marcus Beck, *Dean.*

WESTMINSTER HOSPITAL, BROAD SANCTUARY, S.W.

The fees for the general surgical practice and lectures required for the Dental Diploma of the Royal College of Surgeons may be paid in one of two ways, viz. :—1. In one payment on entrance, £50. 2. In two payments of £32 10s. and £20, to be made respectively at the commencement of each academic year. These payments include the library fee, and entitle the student to attendance on the tutorial classes.

H. B. Donkin, M.B., *Dean.*

SCHOOL OF MEDICINE, SURGEONS' HALL, EDINBURGH.

The fees for the general subjects (including practice at the Royal

Infirmary) required of dental students, according to the curriculum of the Royal College of Surgeons of Edinburgh, amount to £38 10s.

Stevenson Macadam, *Secretary.*

ANDERSON'S COLLEGE, GLASGOW.

The fees for the general subjects required of dental students, as prescribed by the curriculum of the Faculty of Physicians and Surgeons of Glasgow, amount to £25 14s. 6d. And the fees at the dental school for the special portion of the curriculum, including £12 12s. for dental hospital practice, are £23 2s.—total, £48 16s. 6d.

Dr. A. M. Buchanan, *Dean.*

MONTHLY STATEMENT of operations performed at the two Dental Hospitals in London, and a Provincial Hospital, from July 1st to July 31st, 1890:—

		London.	National.	Manchester.
Number of Patients attended		—	1,764	1,143
Extractions	Children under 14	399	241	
	Adults	1,274	293	766
	Under Nitrous Oxide	898	639	173
Gold Fillings		291	127	38
Plastic do.		1,082	398	174
Irregularities of the Teeth		74	185	14
Artificial Crowns		26	21	3
Miscellaneous		403	247	392
Implantations		—	3	—
		4,447	2,154	1,560

GASTROTOMY FOR REMOVAL OF ARTIFICIAL TEETH.—The operation was recently performed in the Portland General Hospital, U.S.A. The same steps were taken as are usually pursued by surgeons at the present day. The abdomen having been opened, the stomach was hooked up out of the wound and sewn carefully to the parietes, and after an interval of some days, to allow of union between the sides of the wound, the stomach was opened and the teeth removed. This certainly is a safer proceeding than to perform the operation at one sitting. In the particular case under notice, a three inch incision into the stomach had been made, the teeth were discovered to be still lodged in the esophagus some three inches from the cardia, and beyond reach. The emergency was met by passing from the mouth a long whalebone threaded with a string attached to a sponge, this was brought through the opening in the stomach, and the sponge acting like a tampon, pushed the teeth on their plate before it.

THE DENTAL RECORD

VOL. X. OCTOBER 1ST, 1890. No. 10.

Original Communications.

THE VALUE OF THE EXAMINATION OF THE TEETH IN ANTHROPOLOGICAL RESEARCH.

By H. LLOYD WILLIAMS, M.R.C.S., L.D.S.

THE following article was almost entirely written as a critique upon Dr. Betty's paper* in the April number of the *Dental Review*. The subject is one which may prove of great importance to the scientific world generally, but it is certain that to the dental profession valuable facts cannot fail to be discovered in such a research as Dr. Betty is pursuing in the Medical Museum at Washington.

In one part of my article a reference is made to Mexico as the country whence material, which may contribute largely to the solution of the question at issue—viz., the ancestry of the Indian tribes—may be found. Morton, when referring to the Toltecan family, which represented the civilization of Central America, refers to two or three conquests by nations less civilized, but who adopted the habits and customs of the vanquished, with possibly some modifications. The question arises—from whence did these nations migrate? Evidence already exists which points to the North or North-west as the direction from which at least one invasion came.

Further, the Anthropological Society of New York has published an account of explorations which were carried on in one of the Southern States, where, after meeting with the skeletons and materials usually found in such excavations of Indian mounds, indications of another and deeper burial place were found; the discoveries here are not yet fully known, but the little which has been described concerning the place seems to point to a period anterior to the Indian mounds referred to in this article.

* "A Critical Examination of the Teeth of several Races, including 150 Mound-builders, selected from the collection of the Army Medical Museum at Washington."—DR. E. G. Betty, D.D.S.—*Dental Review*.

It is a long time since the dental profession has had the pleasure of recording a continuous and vast research undertaken or completed by one of its busy members; the paper under notice betokens such a concentration of energy for a definite end as we have been strangers to for a long period.

The line of research followed lies in the direction taken by the late Mr. Mummery in his classical paper read many years ago before the Odontological Society of Great Britain on "The Relation of Dental Caries to Food and Social Condition."

In the latter paper it is sought, by direct and extensive examination of skulls, to determine the effects of civilization, diet, and climatic conditions upon the teeth.

Following out these indications, the skulls are as clearly classified as the circumstances permitted, the antiquity of the skulls is discussed and approximately determined; the shape is also stated, and the habits of the people deduced from the nature of their implements, etc., where they are pre-historic, and from history or observation in the case of the more recent specimens. The tabulation has not the merit of detailed observation of each individual specimen, but it possesses another advantage which greatly enhances its value, viz., classification into distinct recognized races; the number of skulls belonging to each race examined is given, and the average for that number of cases of caries, irregularity, etc., recorded.

The paper written by Dr. Betty compares favourably with Mr. Mummery's paper in some important matters. Each individual specimen is precisely described in great detail, and it is here that the highest commendation is due to the writer. The information is given under the following headings:—Race, Age, Sex, Lat. and Ant. Post. Diameters of Upper and Lower Jaws, Irregularity, Abscess, Caries, Calculus, Facial Angle, Remarks.

The selection of specimens for examination, so far as the published account has developed it, is open to objections. A series of 100 typical *skulls* without any regard to family or race, was first taken and secondly a series of the best *dentures* the museum afforded, again without regard to race. This will appear to every reader as a preparation for the task which Dr. Betty has undertaken, but it is a preparation which careful readers will not be disposed to neglect.

To derive any benefit from the published tables, the reader must be a most accomplished ethnologist, for to find out the race or family a specimen belongs to will prove to be most perplexing. The reader is told that these matters have been disregarded, because the books for their elucidation are at hand. That the books exist it is not disputed, but that one reader in fifty knows very much of them or possesses them for reference, or even dwells within reach of a library where such books can be obtained, we must be permitted to doubt. It will not take the writer a much longer time to consult authorities and classify his specimens intelligibly, while the gain to his readers will be almost incalculable. The term Indian is acknowledged to be a much abused one, and to merely state that the skull is that of a Hare, Clallam, Tesan, or ancient Pueblo Indian, does not really give us any reliable information regarding the original possessors. It is extremely improbable that even Americans would know to what great division or stock the above specimens, with the exception of the last, belonged, and the rest of the world probably lies in still greater darkness regarding them.

The necessity of such a detailed examination and classification as has been indicated is perceived when it is remembered that perhaps the greatest object to be attained is to observe the effects of the different phases of man's environments in his progress from barbarism to civilization upon his teeth.

In order to elucidate this department of human history, it will be necessary to afford data of known value, in order that new facts may receive due appreciation. The round headed (brachycephalic) skulls are recognized as denoting their possessors as a race intellectually more advanced than the long-headed dolichocephalic, and with a division of a number of skulls into these two classes a certain amount of intelligibility would be gained.

The third series of tables gives the result of the examination of 150 Mound-builders.

With regard to these, Dr. Betty admits that their antiquity is a moot point. A large number of the mounds which have been properly examined do not antedate the European invasion, a certain other number do not differ sufficiently from the former to warrant the conclusion that they are of much earlier origin.

The mounds of Tennessee and Kentucky may be cited as instances to show the difficulty of determining the value to be attached to the skulls that have been discovered in them. The Cherokee nation of Indians once occupied Carolina, Virginia, Tennessee, Kentucky and Alabama; these territories were ceded to Europeans and secured by treaties from time to time. Many mounds have been opened in these parts, and a number of skulls from the Kentucky and Tennessee mounds are included in Dr. Betty's tables. The opinion expressed by those best qualified to judge concerning these mounds is that they are not ancient, in several implements of distinctly European origin, such as sheet copper of different shapes, a sword, &c., have been discovered; others, although nothing could be found in them of European manufacture, depart so little in other characteristics from the former, that capable observers decline to give them a date much if any anterior to the time of the discovery of America.

Dr. Betty's further contributions will be looked forward to with eagerness, and we venture to hope that the next tables will contain the results of the examination of Mexican skulls. It is here possibly that the solution of the complicated question lies. Some light may be thrown upon the relationship of the Toltecan family to the American family of Morton, and thus establish an important link which will serve to elucidate much that is now concealed regarding the latter family. If a sufficient number of skulls of the Toltecan family can be obtained and classified as nearly as possible according to their relative positions in the scale of civilization, and a record of anything in their history or in their country likely to bear upon the matter be added, a very important step will have been taken in the right direction. Even if the determination of the relative positions of the nations comprised in the Toltecan family be the only result, that will be a great work. The determination of the ancestry of the Indian from the contents of the mounds already examined seems to be rather hopeless, still older burial places must exist somewhere and there are already some indications of our being within reach of them.

Whether measurements of the lateral and antero-posterior diameters of the jaws and observations on the teeth will ever form any but accessory aids to the anthropologist is as yet doubtful. Anthropologists do not give these measurements, and take comparatively little notice of the teeth. Dr. Betty seems to entertain the opinion that he may be able to solve or at least contribute largely towards the solution of the question of the ancestry of the American Indian. The possibilities in this direction are entirely in his hands.

If, again, we view the results of the examinations of Dr. Betty as indications from which to deduce conclusions as to the diet, climatic and social conditions of the different tribes examined, and utilize the knowledge which Mr. Mummery's researches have placed at our disposal, we shall not find that much can be stated positively of the environment of a people from observations made upon their teeth.

A very striking fact which Mr. Mummery notices in his examination of British skulls illustrates the above contention. He found two cases of caries among sixty-eight Wiltshire skulls, whereas in about sixty-eight Yorkshire skulls he found twenty-six exhibiting disease. It is further of great interest to find that the Roman skulls in Yorkshire exhibited a much higher percentage of decay than in other parts of England. The ratio in other parts of England was thirty-two per cent.; those found in Yorkshire showed decay in eighteen out of twenty-three skulls.

The nature of the diet, whether animal, fish, or vegetable, or a combination of two or more of these, can be more readily determined. But in all cases where a statement as to the nature of the diet has been ventured upon, other circumstances, particularly the weapons found with or near the skulls, have been taken into consideration, and in this manner a sufficiently accurate knowledge can be obtained.

Dr. Betty is to be congratulated on the work which he has already executed, and we hope that as his work extends and his experience ripens, we shall obtain from him results of great importance.

A NOTE CONCERNING THE ACTION OF CHLOROFORM.

By Dudley Wilmot Buxton, M.D., B.S.Lond.

Member of the Royal College of Physicians, Administrator of Anæsthetists in University College Hospital, the Hospital for Women, Soho Square, and the London Dental Hospital.

The interesting paper from the pen of Mr. Gaddes, which appeared in your issue of September 1st, cannot, I think, be permitted to pass without comment. It is hardly necessary to point out that while everyone feels a debt of gratitude has been incurred through the public spirit of Surgeon-Major Laurie, at whose suggestion his Highness the Nizam of Hyderabad entered upon the enlightened course of subsidising a Commission of Scientists to investigate a physiological problem of the first importance to the suffering human race, yet a large number of persons more or less skilled alike in the science and practice of Anæsthetics are unable to accept as proven the conclusions arrived at by the Commission. Not a little perplexity and misunderstanding will be spared if the history of the subject is more clearly known, and if it be made evident what really was the state of knowledge antecedent to the formation of the first Commission. Again, careful distinction should be made between the physiological work of the Commission, of its kind most excellent, and the theories built up from these experiments. The legend of the Silver Shield bears with striking force upon the matter in hand, for while upon the one hand the Commission may regard the proving of experiments as establishing facts of one kind, viewed from the rigidly impartial view of physiological criticism, these same experiments may lend themselves in other minds to a very different class of facts.

Simpson, disliking the clinging odour of ether in confinements, determined, at the suggestion of Mr. Waldie, of Liverpool, to try the effect of the so-called ' Chloric ether," which he did. In company with Drs. Keith and Duncan, Sir James, then Dr. Simpson, inhaled chloroform, and, profiting by the snoring of one colleague and the involuntary struggles of the other, he decided that chloroform was worthy of extended trial. It was introduced to the profession by him in his historic pamphlet, "Notice of a New Anæsthetic Agent as a Substitute for Sulphuric Ether in Surgery and Midwifery," November, 1847. However, more or less experiment was being made with chloroform in different parts of the world at this time. Flourens, in the March of the same year, had employed "chloric ether" as an anæsthetic for the lower animals, but came to the conclusion that it was too dangerous for general use.

Glover,* as early as 1842, employed chloroform, and found that absolute paralysis of the heart muscle in mammals followed its injection into the jugular vein. Sibson,† again, clearly pointed out that in human beings death from chloroform occurred through heart failure. He wrote: "The heart, influenced by the poison (chloroform), ceased to contract, not from cessation of respiration, for the heart in asphyxia will beat from one to three minutes after respiration has ceased, but from immediate death of the heart." And later on the same author says: "We are obliged, then, to conclude from the experience of these cases that in man the death is usually instantaneous, and due, as every instantaneous death is, to

---

* *Edinburgh Medical and Surgical Journal*, *Vol.* 58.

† *London Medical Gazette*, *Vol.* xiii, 1848.

paralysis of the heart. In animals [? the lower animals] the death is usually due to paralysis of the muscles of respiration," and that is of course the result of paralysis of the respiratory centres in the medulla. But the most thorough investigation of the action of chloroform in its early days is due to Dr. Snow, whose work was so accurate, so careful and thorough, that one finds most modern experimenters merely travelling in his footsteps, amplifying possibly, but not superseding, a physiological investigation worthy of the highest encomium. In 1885, a Commission was appointed in Paris, and it tendered its report to the Society of Emulation, and came to the conclusion (an important one when it be borne in mind that France was then under the influence of Flourens' adverse criticism) that chloroform, when administered to the lower animals, kills them by stopping respiration, and that the heart beats on after respiration has ceased. About this time Mr. Thomas Wakley performed similar experiments in this country, and came to a like conclusion. Thus we see that all these investigations admit that among the lower animals the most usual mode in which death results is through failure of respiration, and that the heart stops subsequently to this. Snow, commencing his research at this stage of our knowledge, showed that what appeared to be a contradiction was in fact a perfectly reconcilable law. Chloroform kills, contends this observer, when its vapour strength in the respired air reaches a certain strength; given to men or the lower animals, if this point is not reached the vital processes remain unimpaired. At the present day this statement requires modification, for there seems to be strong evidence to show that prolonged chloroformization (that is, prolonged contact of chloroform with the tissues) may lead to fatty degeneration, and even bring about post-anæsthetic death from that cause*. But even here Snow seems to have been before us, for he says†: "If animals [? the lower animals] are kept for a very long time under the deep influence of chloroform, they become ultimately exhausted, the circulation and respiration are gradually weakened, and cease nearly together." The experimenters who came to the conclusion that chloroform could not kill directly through the heart had guarded against the use of higher strengths of vapour than formed Snow's safe per-centage, and hence their conclusions were erroneous and amounted in fact only to this: When giving chloro-

* Thiem & Fischer, *Ueber tödliche Nachwirkung des Chloroforms*, 1889.

† *On Anæsthetics*, *p.* 109.

form in such a way as to ensure a strength of less than 5 per cent. animals do not die from primary heart failure. And this is very much what we shall presently see is the contention of the Chloroform Commission of Hyderabad, nor will experts gainsay it, although they demur, and I think justly, when the Commissioners venture to generalize and say: Therefore chloroform never kills primarily through the heart muscle. Snow further showed that high percentages (8 % or 10 %) will even in the lower animals produce primary syncope and death. He makes the following pertinent remark anent deaths of dogs, &c., occurring during experiments. "I have, indeed, been informed of several instances in which animals died in a sudden, and what was thought unaccountable, manner, whilst chloroform was given to prevent pain and struggles which would be occasioned by physiological experiments. In these cases there is no doubt the heart was paralysed, but the experimenters were often too intent on other matters to observe the circumstance." It is curious that the Hyderabad Commissioners state that while their animals never died from primary heart failure, yet, deaths did occur from some unexplained cause. "The fatal result was brought about either by neglecting to watch the condition of the respiration during or after the administration of chloroform, ... or from a reckless administration of chloroform, in the endeavour to check or prevent struggles.* These words would seem to lend themselves to two interpretations, firstly, that the "reckless administration," leads to the use of a high percentage of vapour, which determined primary heart failure; secondly, that the animals died in some cases, from reflex syncope, the result of shock, evinced by their struggles, a contention which would seem to discountenance the view of the Commission, that animals partly anæsthetised feel no shock, and so are not liable to reflex syncope. It is not proposed to go at any great length into the subject, so I must refrain from any attempt at exhaustive quotation from Snow's pregnant remarks, but will sum them in the following quotation.† Speaking of the mode of death in a large number of cases, the particulars of which he gives, he says: "In all the cases in which the symptoms which occurred at the time of death are reported there is every reason to conclude, as shown above, that death took place by cardiac syncope or arrest of the action

* *Lancet*, p. 158, Vol. I., 1890, "Accidental Death"

† Ibid, p. 217.

of the heart. In forty of these cases the symptoms of danger appeared to arise entirely from cardiac syncope, and were not complicated by the overaction of the chloroform on the brain. It was only in four cases that the breathing appeared to be embarrassed and arrested by the effect of chloroform on the brain and medulla oblongata, at the time when the action of the heart was arrested by it ; and only in one of these cases that the breathing was distinctly arrested by the effect of the chloroform, a few seconds before that agent also arrested the action of the heart. * * * Chloroform has the effect of suddenly arresting the action of the heart when it is mixed with the respired air to the extent of 8 or 10 per cent. or upwards ; and we must therefore conclude that in the fatal cases of its inhalation, the air the patients were breathing just before the accidents occurred contained this amount of vapour." Snow's teaching, then, amounted to this—chloroform kills through cardiac syncope, induced by a too concentrated vapour of chloroform, or by an excessive accumulation of chloroform in the blood, giving rise to paralysis of the vital centres in the Medulla Oblongata, and causing cessation of respiration first, and heart failure second, and this may occur even when small doses of chloroform are given when care is not taken to ensure due elimination of the poison. It is obvious that the first cause of death may come into action at any point of time during the administration of chloroform, while the second cause would operate only in the later stages of the anæsthetisation. In 1864 a Committee was appointed by the Royal Medico Chirurgical Society of London to investigate the Physiological action of chloroform, and a number of eminent surgeons and physicians took part part in the work, being assisted by the skill and special knowledge of Mr. Clover.* Its conclusions are thus summarized: "Chloroform at first increases the force of the heart's action, this effect is slight and transient." "When complete anæsthesia is produced by chloroform, the heart in all cases acts with less than its natural force. . . . The strongest doses cf chloroform vapour when admitted freely into the lungs, destroy animal life by arresting the action of the heart." "By moderate doses of chloroform the heart's action is much weakened for some time before death ensues, respiration generally, but not invariably, ceases before the action of the heart, and death is due both to the failure of the heart's action and to that of the respiratory function."

* *See* "*Transac. Roy. Med. Chir. Soc.*" for that year.

Yet another Commission undertook the investigation of the action of anæsthetics in 1880, this time appointed by the British Medical Association.* Mainly experimental in its operations, this Commission accumulated a number of interesting and highly important facts. The experiments were performed by skilled physiologists working in their laboratories with every appliance at hand, so that we may fairly consider the conclusions at which they arrived as worthy of the most careful consideration, if not of credence. The report says: "Chloroform may cause death in dogs, either by primarily paralysing the heart or the respiration." "In most cases, respiration stops before the heart's action." Further, there is the following important statement; "Without going into detail, we may say that it soon became apparent to us that chloroform, administered to dogs and rabbits, has a disastrous effect upon the respiratory centres; it is easy to kill one of these animals by pushing the chloroform until respiration is paralysed. In observing the rate of the heart during these experiments, it could often be determined by auscultation, that its contractions were maintained after respiration had ceased. It was apparent, however, that even when failure of respiration was more directly the cause of death, the heart was, to some extent, simultaneously affected; and there were even cases in which the heart appeared to fail at least as soon, if not before, the breathing." Again, the report runs: "The chief dangers" [of chloroform] "are (i.) sudden stoppage of the heart; (ii.) reduction of the blood pressure; (iii.) alteration of the pulse-respiration ratio and sudden cessation of the respiration. "We showed (see Report, 1880) that chloroform vapour has a paralysing effect upon the muscular tissue of the heart, and, indeed, upon all kinds of protoplasm, when directly applied."

While engaged upon the investigation of the action of chloroform, ether, alcohol, ethidene dichloride, bromide of ethyl, and methylene, upon protoplasm, and especially upon that forming the heart muscle of frogs, I perfused the detached heart with both normal saline and blood solution, in which were varying doses of chloroform, and watched the result. The fluid, of course, circulated freely through the heart, and that organ would beat uniformly for hours unless the chloroform, or what not, was introduced into the circulating medium. When, however,

* *See the Brit. Med. Journ., Dec. 15th*, 1880, *and June 14th*, 1890.

chloroform, even in minute doses, was poured into it, and so reached directly the heart muscle, its beat became less in force and soon ceased. If, however, fresh circulating fluid were then perfused so that the chloroform were washed away, no recovery took place, the heart muscle was permanently damaged. This was a marked contrast to the effect of ether.

The Glasgow Commisson further examined the heart in situ by opening the thorax and maintaining artificial respiration, and found "where chloroform was given, there is a most serious effect upon the heart ; the right ventricle almost immediately becomes distended, the heart presently stops, with the right ventricle engorged with blood." "Ether may be given for an indefinite period, without interference with the heart." Upon the important subject of blood pressure under chloroform, the Report says that "besides the general fall of blood pressure, (which, be it remarked, betokens an incipient vascular failure,) at certain stages of chloroform narcosis, there may be sudden falls in blood pressure, due to interference with the heart's action, and no one can deny that this is a serious state of matters."

The next chapter of our history brings us to the establishment of the first Hyderabad Chloroform Commission. The report of this was not fully published in the English professional journals, and hence some reluctance was expressed as to the acceptance of conclusions based upon premises only imperfectly made known. So to meet this objection the Second Hyderabad Chloroform Commission was, through the generosity of His Highness the Nizam of Hyderabad, established, and Dr. Lauder Brunton was asked by the Editors of the *Lancet* to join it as a representative. This Commission repeated the work done by its predecessor, although upon wider lines. Still its report may be taken as representing the opinions and facts on which these opinions were based, alike of the First and Second Hyderabad Chloroform Commissions.

The main issues to which these Commissions addressed themselves may be stated as follows:—1. How does chloroform kill? (*a*) through respiration failure alone, as taught by Syme and Simpson ; or (*b*) through primary heart failure ; or (*c*) through either of these, according to circumstances. Further attention was directed to subsidiary matters, among which we may note (α) the effect of chloroform upon blood pressure ; (β) effects of shock under chloroform.

The experiments were carefully made upon dogs, goats, monkeys, and other animals, and as a result conclusions were arrived at that these animals died in every case in which they were carefully watched, through failure of respiration, and in no instance was primary heart failure met with. Had the Commissioners stopped here, we should probably have had no occasion to gainsay their "finding," but they did not. They formulated a series of conclusions, applying their facts derived mainly from pariah dogs, not to pariah dogs in the aggregate, but to human beings, and those, by the way, living under the most diverse conditions. Much mischief has already been done by the indiscriminate publication in the professional and lay press, both here and in America, of these "conclusions," without any attempt either to reproduce or examine critically the experiments from which they are supposed to follow. There is a wide gap in the animal scale between pariah dogs and Europeans, and no one conversant with the behaviour of the lower animals under anæsthetics and that of human beings under the same circumstances, would be content to admit that generalizations from one to the other were worthy of more than the most guarded admission.

Again, the conclusions of the Hyderabad Commission are at variance with similar observations made upon the lower animals in this country, and as the experimenters were at least of equal manipulative skill, and possessed of competent physiological knowledge, we are bound to say that the conclusions are of only limited application, and do not apply to less tropical countries. As I have showed above, by quotation from the report, the Commission lost several animals from "accidental deaths," which deaths we may believe were due to heart failure from overdosage.

Again, the evidence brought forward by the Hyderabad Commission concerning chloroform death amounts to this: (i.) when death occurred and the phenomena accompanying it were observed, it was due to paralysis of respiration, and heart failure did not take place until some seconds after cessation of respiration; (ii.) no death among the animals experimented upon was observed to occur from primary heart failure. The animals numbered in all about 500, but many were experimented upon in other ways. Now this is quite in keeping with what other experimentalists have found. Deaths under chloroform are stated to occur about once in every 2,500 or 3,000 persons subjected to the anæsthetic, so that it would not have been any matter of surprise if the Commission had not lost a single animal of their 500 or so, but they did lose them. Again, of the deaths (1 in 3,000 say) a proportion are due to carelessness or ignorant anæsthetising, and some to shock (this the Commission would deny, but, as I shall show later on, their contention falls short of proof), while some are undoubtedly cases in which respiration stops before or simultaneously with the cardiac syncope, so that when all these deductions are made, we shall find the number of instances of primary cardiac syncope per thousand represented by a small fraction. Such being the case—and these facts would certainly be vouched for by anæsthetists of wide experience, such as Snow, Clover, Richardson—we are compelled to regard even positive evidence arrived at by the examination of so few as 500 animals as of slight value, as against evidence furnished by hundreds of thousands of administrations to human beings; and when we come to negative evidence—that the Commission did not meet with a single case among the lower animals of primary cardiac syncope—we are still more strongly impelled to regard the conclusions based upon such evidence as unreliable and wholly unsatisfactory.

There is, however, yet another strong contention to be urged against the results at which the Hyderabad Commissioners arrived, and that is that other observers working in the same lines have arrived at results quite at variance with those obtained in India. It would be out of place here to attempt to explain such discrepancies, by variation in the stamina of the animals used,* the protection of an environing uniformly high temperature, &c., as it is rather the object of the present communication to compare results than to harmonize or explain their divarications.

It has been pointed out above that the Glasgow Commission undoubtedly met with primary heart failure, just as Snow had many years before, and Professor Wood† says, "Chloroform is capable of causing death either by primarily arresting the respiration or primarily stopping the heart. . . ."

The experiments of Prof. McKendrick and Prof. Wood were like those of Surgeon-Major Laurie and Dr. Lauder Brunton, made upon dogs, cats, &c., so that there is no reason to account for their results being so diametrically opposite.

(*To be concluded.*)

---

* Although it is at least interesting in this connection to note that no less an authority than Professor Wood, speaking at the International Congress in London, 1881, stated that he found a great difference obtained in American and English dogs as to their behaviour when experimented upon with drugs.

† International Medical Congress in Berlin, 1890. Address of Anæsthetics, *Brit. Med. Journal*, No. 1,546, p. 386.

EXTRACTS.

THE PREPARATION AND FILLING OF ROOTS AT ONE SITTING.

By E. L. CLIFFORD D.D.S., Chicago.

AN article in "Items of Interest" under the caption, "I do not indorse immediate root filling," reads as follows: "We can never know that incipient abscess is not present, and, if it is, trouble will always follow such an operation. It is to be deplored that this practice is advocated to such an extent in our periodical literature, on account of the danger of leading young men astray. We should be more conservative in our practice. A root may be filled immediately if we have destroyed and removed the pulp ourselves, but, even in those cases, I would prefer to leave it a day or two, to destroy any living tissue that might remain in the canal. For this purpose I know of nothing better than carbolic acid ·95 per cent."

The reason given for the position taken in the above paragraph, and the only reason, is, "We never know that incipient abscess is not present." Well, suppose it is present? What is an "*incipient*" abscess? In medical lexicology I have hunted in vain for an interpretation. The term incipient, I know, is used with freedom by medical writers, and will therefore exonerate the authority quoted from any intention to launch a new word upon our already crowded sea; but as the term has not been thought of sufficient importance to find a place in our special lexicons, I take it for granted that it is used simply in its original and literal meaning. Therefore the term incipient abscess must mean an abscess just beginning, for the word is defined, "beginning, commencing, starting." Now, what has pathology taught us is the beginning of all abscesses? Is it not inflammation? And must not inflammation be preceded by, first irritation, then contraction and dilatation of the vascular surroundings, followed by hyperæmia and more or less complete blood stasis, to be in turn followed by the various steps consequent upon any inflammation; and let us not forget, at this point, that inflammation does not *necessarily* lead downward through the grade of retrograde metamorphosis to finally reach suppuration, atrophy, gangrene, or death. But remember that life is tenacious; that physiological tendencies, with equal fortune, will invariably overcome and overbalance pathological drift, the inclination of all tissues to return to the normal health status being so great. No. "Inflammation ceases to advance just as soon as the irritation is removed, and the blood, circulating through the vessels, restores their walls to a healthy state. When this happens, *recovery* at once begins. The injury to the vessel-walls being slight, and the exudation trifling, the vessels soon begin to perform their normal functions, and what is effused undergoes reabsorption by the lymphatics, or by the blood vessels themselves."

Now, then, this fact established, should the presence of an incipient abscess debar us from finishing our operation, *if* it has been possible to thoroughly clean and sterilize every portion of the pulp canal and dentinal tubuli, and can successfully reach with our filling material the apical foramen. I think not. The position I take in regard to devitalized teeth is, that there is but *one* object to be accomplished in their preservation ; that is to *clean* the roots ; and this I believe can, in a majority of cases, be done (I will not say as well, but better), at one sitting than twenty. In using the word clean, I, of course, use it in its most superlative sense, no half way, or "that is well enough," should ever satisfy the honest operator.

If, then, our sole object is to clean the root, it signifies that the root contains something that is unclean and impure. The question then arises, if this unclean and impure matter is contained in the root in what portion of the root does it find a habitat and a lodgment? Is it in the pulp canal, and the pulp canal *only?* If so, 'twould be an easy matter to purify and clean all roots presenting, at one sitting. But are we not stubbornly met with the fact that the boundary line of this unclean substance, and its effects, reaches farther than the above suggestion, and therefore that our remedies must penetrate farther to be effectual.

Another question would here naturally arise : Can we follow it, and if so, how? Another digression forces itself upon me at this point, but only for a moment, as I will accept it without comment ; that is, to accept the germ theory as an etiological factor in the pathological condition to be overcome. I take it for granted that micro-organisms are accepted as prime movers in all pyogenetic affections, at least until some other theory more plausible is advanced ; and from this bulwark will fire the random shots destined for the field of enquiry upon the ground of progressive surgery. Fermentation and putrefaction having advanced sufficiently, the habitat or lodgment of the micro-organisms has, of course, become too small; their products have generated and produced sufficient gaseous substance to more than fill the cavity of the pulp chamber and canal; consequently a hunt for other quarters is their ultimatum. The nearest and most direct outlet we believe they will take and our minds are at once directed to the dentinal tubuli and apical foramen. The tubuli, having been occupied by animal matter, must certainly come in for their share of fermentation and putrefaction and their results, and must so harbour nests of micro-organisms that might revolt at any moment, declare an insurrection, and proceed to wage a merciless war upon the surrounding tissues. For this reason, it will readily be seen that it is not enough to clean and sterilize the root canal proper, but these tubuli must also be emptied, cleaned, dried, sterilized and filled.

As to how this shall be done: My first thought in the procedure of such an operation is, *thorough dryness and complete* protection from any future inundation of saliva, water, or other septic fluid. To gain this, the rubber dam is brought into play, safely adjusted, and the cavity of decay and pulp chamber relieved of its detritus. Having removed all possible with spoon excavators, and dried as much as possible with bits of amadou, I then saturate the chamber with a *non*-escharotic disinfectant, waiting a few moments, again dry the cavity, and proceed to remove any particles of putrescent pulp within the canal. Should pus already have formed, I use alternately injections of peroxide of hydrogen and an ethereal solution of iodoform, believing that, with these agents, I simplify and render easy what would otherwise be tedious and difficult. I do not know that I have seen a reason given for this alternating of H_2O_2 with iodoform and ether, but, believing that, to be scientific, we should have an end to accomplish in each step taken to re-establish a physiological function, or to eradicate a pathological condition I will try to give you my reasons for each step taken.

First, then, we court perfect dryness. Why? Because moisture, warmth and microbes are the three essentials to septic fermentation. Absence of any *one* of these is sufficient to prevent decomposition.

Second, protection from saliva. Why? First, because it is a liquid, and its presence would thwart our efforts at dryness; next, our scientific researches have shown us that saliva contains and propagates, not only all classes of bacteria now known to us, but most of the fungi as well. Not only benign micro-organisms find a flourishing element in saliva, but most of the pathogenetic species also. In fact, nearly fifty separate and distinct foreign and malignant substances have been extracted from the human saliva, ranging from a simple mucous corpuscle to pus corpuscles and all the malign bacilli known to exist within the animal economy.

Third. Why disinfect the cavity of decay? That you may not push into your pulp chamber, and from thence into and through your root canals, the septic matter you know to exist in that habitat; also on the principle of "an ounce of prevention being worth a pound of cure."

So far we have had a comparatively easy task. We have had only that portion of our root to deal with that we could see or feel. If, however, putrescence has taken place, disintegration has, of course, been established, and it will be impossible to remove the pulp entire, and the process of removing it mechanically is too long and tedious (especially if the case in hand has more than one root). What, then, shall be done? It is my practice, after removing all possible in the manner described above, to saturate the chamber and canal with the volatile extract of eucalyptus (made by Sander & Sons, of Australia; I never use any other), and then drying with amadou, to apply chloroform to saturation. My object in doing this is two fold: First, for its analgesic effect; but mostly as a solvent for the oils and fats left adherent to the walls of the canal, and occupying the spaces of the tubuli.

(Although not pertinent to the subject in hand, I will state that if I were not going to fill at one sitting, and wished to accomplish the same end by prolonged treatment to two or more sittings, I should fill the pulp chamber and canals with Squibbs' carbonate of soda, and leave it for three days. I should thereby saponify these oils, fats and extraneous matter with this alkali, and, at the end of the time named, a little warm water would be all required to wash out and clean the root).

The fatty substance being disposed of, in what condition do we find our organ? Tolerably clean, but we have been compelled to use liquids; therefore we still possess one of the main elements necessary to the growth and propagation of pathogenetic material; *i.e.*, moisture. We insert our cotton, bibulous paper, amadou, and all the other absorbents at our command, but still our work is defective; it is not complete; we have not been thorough, and there is only one element in nature known to me that can be called to our assistance. That element is heat; and although the statement has been made that heat as an antiseptic was useless to the dentist, from the fact that some scientist had discovered that 212° F., and that maintained for 1½ hours, was necessary to destroy microbes without spores, and that the heat must be increased to 284° F., and maintained from 1½ to 3 hours to destroy the spores. I am satisfied in my own mind, and will endeavour to show, that we do not use heat for its direct antiseptic effect; but it is one of our best assistants toward that end. The statement has also been made, that the perfect drying of a root by heat (such, of course, as can be used in the mouth) will not destroy germs or spores. To all this I bow in humble acquiescence. But, acknowledging the fact, is there no other assistance that heat can render us in accomplishing this end? I think so. After drying as well as possible with our absorbents, if we can contrive some method or appliance by which we can carry heat much greater than the normal surroundings of the root into the canal, we certainly can extract from its hiding place all the moisture possible. We certainly know it is a law of physics that no two substances can occupy the same space at the same time. We also know that a superheated instrument, coming in contact with water, will convert it into steam, which is gaseous, and cannot be confined, but must escape; vacuum must be the result. We also know that nature abhors a vacuum, and that these osseous structures, having been deprived of their natural quota of water will seek for and find, if possible, its requisite. Taking advantage of this physical law, we supply the new moisture, first charging that moisture with some element known to be antagonistic to growth and development of pathogenetic elements. I select the ethereal solution of iodoform. The liquid penetrates into all the anfractuosities and diverticula of the bone or abscess; the ether becomes absorbed or evaporated, and the agent is deposited uniformly on the pyogenic membrane, the action of which it modifies, dissolves any oils or fats which may have been left in the tubuli, and leaves the spaces filled with the medicament used. Now, having the root thoroughly saturated with iodine, I promote further evaporation by warmed air, and take a further advantage of our physical law of suction, and compel the dentine to attract chlora-percha solution or oxy-chloride of zinc, whichever material I am using. Of course the less dentine we have in the roots the less disinfecting we are called upon to accomplish; and, if the strength of the organ will permit it, and your sense of touch is sufficiently skilled, I would admit the theory of Dr. Allport, and advise the removal of as much dentine as possible. I should advance, however, in the practice of this theory with caution.

And now to review— are there any impossibilities stated in the foregoing, are there any illogical deductions drawn? You will all recognize the fact that these several steps can be followed in less time, or as much at any rate, as the detailing of them will require, and why shall a patient be required to spend from three days to three weeks in running to our offices when the end can be accomplished in one hour of continuous work. A case in practice comes to mind—a *confrère* resident in one of our suburbs had for a patient a lady about thirty years of age who lived on the west side and consequently a great distance from his office. One of the lower bicuspids had abscessed and the patient had spent her time and money for several months in semi-weekly visits to her dentist with the result that each time the tooth was tightly sealed the inflammation would reappear. The dentist told her that if she had any trouble after his last treatment to call on me. It was only a few days when the patient applied to me with a terrible sore tooth and considerable pain. After getting a full history of the case I removed the dressing in the root, found considerable suppuration, and after washing out as much as possible I filled the canal with carbonate of soda, and dismissed the patient for three days (You will recognize that I was dealing with another man's patient and felt that I would take no risks so I gave two treatments). At the appointed time she returned, when the saponified residue was washed out and a line of treatment similar to what I have detailed above was pursued. The root was filled with oxychloride of zinc and hydronapthol (at that time I had not used chlora-percha) and the crown filled with oxyphosphate, with instructions to return to her dentist at the end of two weeks and have a gold filling inserted.

Another case—A lad about 18 years presented r. l. bicuspid terribly decayed, jaw considerably swollen, but as he lived within a few doors of my office where I could watch him I wanted him for an experimental case. He wanted the tooth extracted. It was in the forenoon and I had a patient in the chair, so I opened into the pulp chamber when his mouth filled with pus and he was to some extent relieved; I told him to call again at 2 o'clock, which he did, when I adjusted the rubber dam, cleaned and filled the roots and crown. It is now about five months and I see the patient often and he is delighted that he did not have the tooth extracted. Now the question may very properly be asked, from what I have stated, if I would advise the filling of *all* roots at one sitting. Judgment must of course be used in any and all operations of surgery, no matter how trivial they may appear. But I am willing to be placed upon record with the statement that the conditions forbidding the procedure are the exception by far and not the rule. I believe the fact is established, and one upon which there is no difference of opinion at this time, that all aseptic canals are ready to be filled. I, also, believe the fact established that all canals possessing an exit through a fistulous opening in the gum may as well be at once cleaned and filled. Thus you will see these two facts would probably embrace three-fourths of all the canals we are called upon to fill, leaving a small minority about which there would be question. In reflecting upon this minority the principal reason, usually given, that would negative our procedure would be the fact of no existing fistula, or what is generally termed a blind abscess. This fact *alone* I cannot accept as reason sufficient for protracted treatment, as experience has shown that (though possibly provoking an acute pericementitis for twelve hours or more) in a vast majority of cases the great tendency of nature to reassert herself and the physiological proclivities being so much greater and overpowering the pathological in her effort to return to health, that victory will at last be proclaimed upon the right side, and a complete subsidence of all outward manifestations will be the result. Should I fear however that the vital energies of my patient may be taxed too greatly, I always anticipate and relieve the immediate pressure by establishing what nature has thus far failed to make, an artificial fistula, and prescribing a few doses of some of our newer anti-neuralgics and analgesics.

From the above, what would we conclude to be the essentials to success in root filling? First, perfect dryness; second, no vacuum; and third, as precautionary and preventive, drainage, as in all surgical cases in other portions of the organism. I can say, with the editor of the *Western Dental Journal*, that immediate root filling should not be practiced unless dryness, which is the first step toward an aseptic condition, can be secured; and this condition I believe can as well be secured in blind abscess as in those with a fistulous opening (hæmorrhage excepted). So much so am I convinced of this fact, that I have reduced the conditions to two that would prevent and forbid an attempt to immediately fill a root presenting for treatment. One of those conditions, and the main one, is the impossibility to dry the whole of the dentine. This will be the case at times in persons of a hæmorrhagic diathesis. The other where the tissues are so swollen and painful as to render it cruel to operate at that time. The treatment I can but regard as philosophical and logical. It is but a sequence of a proved knowledge so beautifully illustrated to our society by Dr. Andrews, of Cambridge, at our recent clinic, that the disease is the result of sepsis, and when the septic condition has been removed, and its place taken by an impermeable and indestructible filling, a certain cure must result, just as certainly as if the canal had been obliterated by the extraction of the tooth. Any remaining products of the once-existing irritant will speedily be absorbed and changed into healthy cicatricial tissue. One condition may exist that would retard and probably prevent a subsidence of all irritation, and that would be the presence of necrotic tissues either in the root or maxilla. In the successful treatment of this condition however, the passage through the root is not essential, and would not debar me from filling the root, as I would continue the necessary treatment through the gum, and expect, in time, a recovery.

The question also arises, if it is deemed hazardous to immediately fill these canals, why is it? What would result? What could result? Well, although the past life of this subject is short, there is hardly any pathological condition that has followed an operation that has not been attributed (not to the filling of the root, not to the existence of an almost foreign substance embedded in the tissues, not simply to dental irritation, but) to *immediate* root filling. A case is reported in the February number of the *Archives*, in which considerable mischief is said to have resulted from *immediate* root filling. The reporter of that article starts out by saying that the patient was served by a *fine* operator, and winds up the facts of his statement with the remark that "the other tooth was *reamed out* and filled." Well, if this reporter has told the whole truth, and nothing but the truth, about the operation, I do not see how any but unfavourable results could be expected. *Reaming* out and *digging* out are certainly not very euphonious terms to the professional ear, and certainly cannot be said to constitute the necessary steps to any surgical precedure; so that, if the statement can be borne out by the facts, the results were certainly not from *immediate* but from *imperfect* root filling, which may have occurred in any case treated for months.

As stated before, almost all varieties of reflex and disseminate neuroses have been attributed to this operation. You all remember a case presented to this society only a few meetings ago, and reported as a result of immediate root filling—a case of alopecia areata. Now, although in the highest degree probable that alterations, and particularly shedding of the hair, may at times be dependent upon nervous influence, yet exact proof of this fact is still wanting. The affection, according to late investigators, is considered as a tropho-neurosis. Experiments have been made, and clinical observations recorded with reference to the influence of disturbances of nutrition, and also of psychoses, upon the condition of the hair; but the data so far obtained is extremely deficient. Joseph has asserted that such a thing as a distinct bundle of trophic nerves does exist, and also that he can produce a circumscribed alopecia in cats by the extirpation of the spinal ganglia of the second pair of nerves of the neck, together with portions of the neighbouring posterior and anterior roots. While these observations thus far made, taken singly, would not be convincing, yet, viewed collectively and in connection with the physiological experiments, we seem to have strong evidence of the tropho-neurotic nature of circumscribed alopecia. Hence it would appear that any irritation reflected to the trophic centres might result in this condition, especially so when we notice that headache is one of the commonest premonitions of alopecia. Cases have also been reported in which heredity was an etiological factor in alopecia areata; and when the neuropathic predisposition is present, very slight influences are enough to cause the appearance of some nervous disease. The most prominent causes however, are the traumatic and the psychical, and it is not astonishing to find the disease following either of these causes, when we reflect that it is only the merging of a hereditary proclivity. The question of age has also entered into the inquiries upon this subject, and 12½ years was found to be the average at which the disease appeared; so it has been suggested that it is in some way connected with the second dentition and puberty; but the fact is not established, and at present we are only certain of one condition dependent upon the trophic nerves, and that is the suspension of their activity, giving rise to subsequent atrophy.

The foregoing may indeed seem a digression to you, but it has proved interesting to me to collect these facts, in order that we might more thoroughly understand the etiology of a pathological condition reported to us as a result of immediate root filling.

I am satisfied the reporter of the case did not intend to convey the impression even that the disturbance was caused by the abstract fact of *immediate* root filling, but that it was the effect of an ill-judged dental operation, resulting in a dental irritation, reflected through the sympathetic ganglia to the trophic centres, and arousing in the case presented, a predisposed hereditary proclivity. I have too exalted an opinion of the diagnostic powers of my friend, not to take this view, especially as I could report another case similar of a young girl who glories in the possession of two bald spots, about the size of a silver dollar, upon the right parietal region, which ceased to enlarge, and again began to be supplied with a new growth of hair after the extraction of an upper molar tooth (which had never been filled) and a few visits to the Sutherland sisters.—*Dental Review.*

ON THE DANGERS ARISING FROM SYPHILIS IN THE PRACTICE OF DENTISTRY.*

By L. Duncan Bulkley, A.M., M.D.,
Attending Physician to the New York Skin and Cancer Hospital, etc.

Happily the recorded instances of the communication of syphilis in connection with the practice of dentistry are relatively few in number when compared with the very numerous cases on record where the disease has been acquired through other innocent channels; for, it must be remarked, the number and variety of modes by which this disease has been spread innocently from one person to another, entirely without sexual transgression, is manifold greater than could be supposed or imagined by one who has not investigated or given some attention to the matter.

The subject of the innocent transmission of syphilis is a very large one, and one to which the public health officials might well direct their attention; but at the present time we can consider only a very small and limited subdivision of it—namely, as the existence of the disease may in any way bring danger through or to any one in the practice of a single branch or speciality in surgery—that of dentistry.

Although, as before stated, the reported instances where syphilis

* Read before the New York Odontological Society.

has been communicated in connection with, or during the operations of, dentistry, are relatively few, nevertheless, there are a sufficient number of cases on record not only to show clearly that this unfortunate accident has repeatedly occurred, and may readily happen, but also to direct our attention to the methods or channels through which this may take place, and so to indicate the means by which the danger may be escaped or avoided. To develop these points will be our task this evening.

It would be quite out of place in this assembly to attempt fully any consideration of syphilis as a disease, or even to give a description of its different manifestations and effects, which are more varied and manifold than those of any other known malady. But before entering upon our subject proper, it may be well to briefly recapitulate the points which are well established in regard to the nature and pathology of syphilis, in order that the real dangers arising from the disease may be better understood, with the reasons therefor.

Syphilis is no longer to be looked upon with the utter abhorrence with which it has been regarded in times past, when it was always believed to be the result of sexual transgressions; it is not, indeed, to be considered always as a venereal disease, for advancing knowledge has revealed, and science recorded, thousands of cases where it has been acquired in scores of ways, where the unfortunate victim was as innocent as is one who catches small-pox, scarlatina, or measles; but, of course, the fact still remains that in the enormous majority of instances syphilis is acquired in sexual intercourse, because here is offered the greatest opportunity for abrasions to occur, through which the poison may gain entrance. But, on the other hand, hundreds, or even thousands, of physicians themselves, and midwives, have contracted syphilis in the practice of their calling; in numbers of instances it has been conveyed in vaccination, tattooing, cupping, and breast-drawing, and, in fine, there is no end to the curious and previously unexpected methods by means of which this disease has been innocently communicated from one person to another.

This innocent transmission of syphilis has also occasionally happened in the practice of the various departments of medicine and surgery. Not only have midwives acquired the disease in the practice of their calling, but several small epidemics are on record where a number of women, and from them their children and others, have acquired syphilis from a chancre on the finger of the woman who had delivered them. The disease has also been communicated in various surgical operations, and a striking illustration is found in the history of Eustachian catheterization, where as many as sixty cases were traced to the practice of one person. Instances will be given later where it has occurred in some of the operations of dentistry.

Syphilis is a well-defined disease, depending always upon the entrance of a definite, specific poison, which has never been perfectly isolated, and of whose exact nature we know nothing. It is most probably due to a micro-organism, but although this has been thought to be discovered on several occasions, it has never been satisfactorily demonstrated, nor have inoculations been made with success by any pure cultivation of the same. It suffices for our purpose, however, to recognize that there is a poison, capable of entering the system, and thereby causing syphilis, which can reproduce or multiply itself there, and again, under proper conditions, communicate the disease to all who are properly and sufficiently exposed to its influence.

The poison always enters the system at some definite point, and at this place, generally within from two to four weeks, a local sore, termed a chancre, develops, which is the first external sign of the syphilitic invasion. This sore presents quite different appearances under different circumstances and in various localities, and time fails to attempt to describe these; their appearances may be learned from many recent text books and journal articles. The only exception to this mode of entrance of the disease is found in the case of hereditary syphilis, where the poison enters with the life, and possibly in some other rare conditions, which need not be entered upon here.

For the entrance of the syphilitic virus a broken epithelial or epidermal surface is necessary, although apparent exceptions to this rule have been occasionally met with. But in some way the poison must come in contact with the absorbing elements of the body—either blood-vessels or lymphatics—and by them be taken into the circulation, where it multiplies and produces lesions in various parts of the body, and then probably increases also in the tissues. When once the virus has gained entrance, the individual is syphilitic, and unless the disease is checked by treatment, it will go on to produce its manifestations, even for many years.

The period during which syphilis is actively inoculable has never been definitely determined, and will probably never be accurately known. It is certainly very contagious, under proper circumstances, during the first year, and also for many months thereafter, and cases are on record where infection has occured from cases many years advanced in syphilis ; indeed, the point or period has never been determined when danger ceases. Although it is questionable if syphilis is often communicated by patients five years after their infection, no prudent man would ever take a shadow of a chance of personal inoculation at this or even at a very much later period. Treatment, of course, greatly modifies the infective power of the disease, and under the fullest possible measure of proper treatment the contagious character of syphilis is greatly lessened, if not entirely destroyed, in some cases, even in the earlier stages of the disease. But all these "ifs" and qualifying statements only show what a dangerous and treacherous affection we have to deal with, and how difficult it is always to be certain of immunity from danger.

The poison of syphilis may be received from four different sources—1, the initial sore or chancre ; 2, from mucous patches ; 3, rom syphilitic ulcerations ; and 4, from the blood. These we will briefly consider in above order.

1. The chancre, or initial sore of syphilis, is occasionally found upon the lips, tongue and other portions of the buccal cavity, but generally the lesion is so marked and painful that the patient avoids the dentist, and there is relatively little danger of infection from this source. But, on the other hand, this danger sometimes occurs, as in the instance of the case which fell under my own observation, about to be described, where the gentleman, supposing that the chancre was only a local sore, due to sharp and rough teeth, went to his own dentist and had them filed off, even when the ulcer was very painful and giving off an abundant, virulently contagious secretion ; so that his dentist must certainly have been exposed to the same. It is well, therefore, in the case of doubtful sores, about the lips, tongue or mouth, either to be assured of their harmless nature or to exercise such precautions as will ensure perfect protection to self and others, which will be considered later.

2. The second source of the contagion of syphilis—namely mucous patches—is far more fruitful of infection, and that against which special care must be exercised. It is to be remembered that at one time or another these lesions appear in a greater or less amount on the buccal mucous membrane of almost every case of syphilis, so that at some moment or other almost every case is capable of communicating the disease from this source of contagion. Mucous patches are slightly raw surfaces, of various sizes and shapes, which are at first elevated slightly, and then may become depressed

by the loss of the epithelial covering. When newly developed, they are of a redder color than the normal mucous membrane, but later may become of a greyish white. They are always superficial lesions, and often do not cause much annoyance, so that the patient may readily attend to all the duties of life, and may go through considerable dental manipulation while having an abundant crop of mucous patches on the tongue, lips, or buccal cavity. The secretion from them is sticky and intensely contagious. It is from these lesions that fresh chancres are most commonly contracted, and it is this secretion which, adhering to instruments and articles of use or convenience—such as cups, spoons, pipes, etc.—commonly gives rise to syphilis in most unexpected manners.

3. Certain deeper ulcerations of syphilis may sometimes give rise to contagion, especially when they occur in the earlier stages of the disease; but practically very few instances of contagion are ever from this source, although this danger should always be guarded against as well.

4. The fourth source of syphilitic infection—namely, the blood—is the least likely to present dangers in connection with dentistry. It is, however, quite possible for blood, which is drawn during an operation or by accident, to communicate syphilis, if it chance to find a proper opportunity to enter another individual. It is just the uncertainty in regard to the possibilities of infection which gives to our subject such great practical interest. In few, if any, of the dozens of methods by which the disease has been innocently transmitted from one person to the other was the possibility of such an accident known, or even suspected, beforehand.

We will now consider some of the observed facts in regard to the communication of syphilis in dentistry, and afterwards examine the modes of transmission and the means of prevention. Our clinical study will naturally divide itself into two lines of thought—(1) in regard to the dangers from syphilis to *patients* undergoing dental operations; and (2) in regard to dangers to the *operator* from the same source.

1. First as to dangers to the *patient* from exposure to the syphilitic poison during dental operations.

Inasmuch as it presents many points of interest relating both to the patient and operator, I may be allowed first to recite the case alluded to, which came under my own observation and treatment, and which first called my attention particularly to the subject.

Mr. X. W., a gentleman of intelligence and position, aged 60 years, came to me September 11, 1884, on account of a sore on the tongue, which he feared to be a cancer. The history was, that some ten weeks before his first visit, he had first noticed a little point of soreness, which had gradually increased in size, in spite of treatment, until latterly it had come to give him considerable annoyance, so that he was conscious of its presence at all times : the true nature of the sore had evidently not been recognized.

On examination, there was found on the right side of the tongue, about an inch from its tip, a hard, inflamed mass, nearly half an inch in diameter, the centre ulcerating and the edges somewhat everted ; it was not painful except when irritating food or drink touched it. The two upper molars were found to have sharp and rough edges, and he had been wearing a red rubber plate until recently. There was a small and painful gland beneath the jaw on that side, slightly enlarged.

Thinking that the ulcer might possibly be due to irritating local causes, he was given a soothing mouth-wash, and an alkali internally. Five days later there was a marked improvement in its condition ; the ulcer had a less angry look, but its edge was more clearly defined as the inflammatory element had somewhat subsided. He had been, of his own accord, to his regular dentist, and had had the roughened teeth made smooth, and had left out his set of artificial teeth.

From a careful second study of the case, I then felt convinced that the sore was a chancre, a primary lesion of syphilis, and he was immediately put on antisyphilitic treatment ; the general eruption and other symptoms which followed a few weeks later rendered the diagnosis certain, together with the remarkable manner in which the sore healed and symptoms vanished under the proper treatment for syphilis.

In searching for the mode by which the syphilitic poison had gained entrance, it was learned that, during the month or so previous to the appearance of the sore upon the tongue, he had, through the persuasion of a friend, been under the care of a dentist of the cheaper, advertising order, who, he had noticed, was not at all cleanly either in his person or with his instruments.—*International Dental Journal.*

(*To be concluded.*)

Dental News.

THE FORMATION OF A DENTAL ASSOCIATION FOR VICTORIA.

Précis of the Preliminary Movements.

THE approval accorded by the Governor in Council under the provisions of the Dentists' Act, 1887, to the regulations submitted by the Dental Board of Victoria for the examination of persons desirous of obtaining certificates of fitness to practice dental surgery or dentistry rendered it imperative that practical means should be adopted for the education of future dental students in Victoria. A number of leading dentists interested themselves in this important matter, and it was decided to hold a general meeting of members of the profession for the consideration of the question.

The meeting was held at the Coffee Palace, Bourke-street, on Wednesday evening, the 7th August, 1889, at eight p.m., when Dr. SPRINGTHORPE was unanimously voted to the chair.

There were also present—Dr. CHEETHAM, Mr. JOHN ILIFFE, Mr. L. J. BLITZ, Mr. L. A. CARTER, D.D.S., Mr. A. R. CLARKE, Mr. E. J. DILLON, Mr. A. L. GEORGE, Mr. F. A. KERNOT, Mr. D. M'GREGOR, Mr. P. M'INTYRE, Mr. H. W. POTTS, Mr. A. REEVE, Mr. GEORGE THOMSON, L.D.S., and a number of other well-known practitioners. Mr. ERNEST JOSKE, LL.B. was appointed hon. secretary.

The meeting was unanimously of opinion that proper teaching should be provided for dental students, in view of the educational curriculum they had now to successfully undergo before they were legally entitled to registration as dentists. After consideration of the question, Mr. Iliffe submitted the following motion :—" That this meeting affirms the necessity of organising a practical scheme of dental education, whereby any dental student, articled pupil, or apprentice, so enrolled, articled, or indentured, after the 10th of May, 1889, may obtain educational facilities which shall enable him to qualify himself in due course for examination and subsequent registration, in pursuance of the regulations of the Dentists Act 1887, relating to the future registration of dentists; and, further, this meeting pledges itself to support such scheme by individual donations and annual subscriptions."

Mr. GEORGE THOMSON, L.D.S., seconded the motion.

Mr. POTTS then placed before the meeting a scheme for the formation of a Dental Association of Victoria. There were, he said,

486 registered dentists in the colony, and he believed that they could be induced to form an association and pay annual subscriptions thereto. A body of united men formed into such an association could go to the Government for a grant to aid the cause of dental education; and he referred to the Working Men's College and the College of Pharmacy, which institutions were liberally supported by the State. Dental education would require that same support which has been accorded to these institutions. He thought that all present should be unanimous in forming one United Dental Association, which would provide for the education of future dental students, and also to support and protect the character, status, and interests of registered dentists; to consider, originate, and promote improvements in the law relating to dentists, and to advance and encourage the study of dentistry and allied subjects by the establishment and maintenance of a Dental College, a Hospital, a Library, a Museum, and the publication of a Dental Journal.

Mr. L. J. BLITZ stated that he would, in order to give the movement a start, make a presentation of a two-story building in Clifton Hill, which would do as a beginning.

The Committee appointed, held two meetings to consider the business entrusted to them, and they came, after the most careful consideration, unanimously to the opinion that it would be advisable to form a Dental Association if it could be established on proper grounds, and if one of its first objects were the establishment of a Dental Hospital, as mentioned in Mr. Iliffe's motion. They accordingly recommended the formation of a Dental Association with the following objects and qualifications for membership, &c.

The objects of the proposed Association to be :—

(*a*) To support and protect the character, status, and interests of registered dentists practising in the colony of Victoria, to suppress malpractice, and to decide all questions of usage in regard to the rights and privileges of dentists.

(*b*) To consider, originate, and promote improvements in the law relating to dentists. and to consider alterations in the law, and to oppose or support the same, and to effect improvements in the administration and practice of dentistry; for the purposes aforesaid to petition Parliament, and to take such other steps and proceedings as may be deemed expedient.

(*c*) To advance and encourage the study of dentistry in all its branches by the establishment and maintenance of a Dental Hospital and College, thereby affording the necessary educational facilities for dental students, in accordance with the regulations relating to education framed under the Dentists Act, 1887.

(*d*) To relieve poor and necessitous persons who are or have been members of the Society, and any other dentists who may, through bodily or mental infirmity, or other misfortune, be incapacitated from carrying on business, and also the wives and families of such persons.

(*e*) To relieve poor and necessitous widows, children, and other relations of deceased members of the Society.

The qualifications for membership to be (as in the British Dental Association)—

(*a*) Every member must be a registered medical practitioner, or a registered dentist of the colony of Victoria, as regards dentists in Victoria; or as regards dentists outside this colony, possess some other qualification, to be afterwards agreed upon.

(*b*) Every member must be of good character.

(*c*) He must not conduct his practice by means of the exhibition of dental specimens, appliances, or apparatus in an open shop, or in a window, or in a show-case exposed for public inspection.

(*d*) He must not conduct his practice by means of public advertisements or circulars describing modes of practice (this is not intended to prohibit advertising name and address), or by means of the publication of a scale of professional charges.

Mode of Election for Membership.—The first members to be those who agree to sign these Articles of Association. First Council.—The first Council to consist of twelve members, to be elected by ballot by those present at the meeting on the 1st October who have signed these articles. Future elections of members of the Association to be (as in the Pharmaceutical Society) by ballot of the Council after twenty-eight days' publicity of nomination. Future Councils to be elected annually by all members of the Association, absent members being entitled to vote.

The powers of the Council to be as specified in the Articles of

Association of the Pharmaceutical Society of Australasia, with the additional object of the foundation and maintenance of a Dental Hospital.

Annual subscription to be one guinea per annum, with an entrance fee of one guinea from members elected six months after the incorporation of the Society. Dental students to be Associates on payment of an annual subscription of 5s.

Honorary and corresponding members to be appointed, general meetings to be held, and a restricted number of calls (if necessary) to be made, as provided for by the rules of the Pharmaceutical Society of Australasia.

The Association to be brought under the Acts of Incorporation Nos. 190 and 764.

The recommendations of the Committee were placed before another general meeting of dentists held on Tuesday evening, the 1st October, 1889 (Dr. Springthorpe in the chair), when they were unanimously adopted, with an addition affirming that advertising "hours of consultation" was unobjectionable. The Association was then formally inaugurated, and its first Council elected by ballot.

Memorandum of Association.

I. The name of the Association is "The Dental Association of Victoria."

II. The Registered Office of the Association is proposed to be situate at Melbourne in the Colony of Victoria.

III. The objects of the proposed Association to be—

(1.) To support and protect the character status and interests of Registered Dentists practising in the colony of Victoria, to suppress malpractice and to decide all questions of usage in regard to the rights and privileges of Dentists.

(2.) To consider, originate and promote improvements in the law relating to Dentists and to consider alterations in the law and to oppose or support the same and to effect improvements in the administration and practice of dentistry, for the purposes aforesaid to petition Parliament and to take such other steps and proceedings as may be deemed expedient.

(3.) To advance and encourage the study of dentistry in all its branches by the establishment and maintenance of a Dental Hospital and College, thereby affording the necessary educational facilities for dental students in accordance with the regulations relating to education framed under the "Dentists Act 1887," and by such other means as the Council may from time to time deem expedient.

(4.) To relieve poor and necessitous persons who are or have been members of the Association and any other Dentists who may through bodily or mental infirmity or other misfortune be incapacitated from carrying on his profession and also the wives and families of such persons.

(5.) To relieve poor and necessitous widows, children, and other relations of deceased members of the Association.

(6.) To invest the moneys of the Association not immediately required upon such securities as may from time to time be determined. To make, accept, endorse and execute promissory notes, bills of exchange and other negotiable instruments. To raise money in such manner as the Association shall think fit, and in particular by the issue of debentures charged upon all or any of the Association's property (both present and future) including its uncalled capital.

(7.) To erect, alter and maintain any buildings necessary or convenient for the purposes of the Association. To purchase, take on lease or in exchange hire or otherwise acquire any real and personal property and any rights or privileges which the Association may think necessary or convenient for the purposes of its business. To sell, improve, manage, develop, lease, mortgage, dispose of or otherwise deal with all or any part of the property of the Association.

(8) To subscribe to become a member of and co-operate with any other Associations whether incorporated or not, whose objects are altogether or in part similar to those of this Association, and to procure from and communicate to any such Association such information as may be likely to forward the objects of the Association.

(9) To do all such other things as are incidental or conducive to the attainment of the above objects.

IV. The income and property of the Association whencesoever derived shall be applied solely towards the promotion of the objects of the Association as set forth in this Memorandum of Association and no portion thereof shall be paid or transferred directly or indirectly by way of dividend bonus or otherwise howsoever by way of profit to the persons who at any time are or have been members of the Association or to any of them or to any person claiming through any of them. Provided that nothing herein contained shall prevent the payment in good faith of remuneration to any officers or servants of the Association or to any member thereof or other person in return for any services actually rendered to the Association.

V. The fourth paragraph of this Memorandum is a condition on which a license is granted by the Attorney-General to the Association in pursuance of Section I. of an Act of the Parliament of Victoria No. 764 being an Act to Provide for the Incorporation of Literary, Scientific and other Associations and Institutions. For the purpose of preventing any evasion of the terms of the said fourth paragraph the Attorney-General may, from time to time on the application of any member of the Association impose further conditions which shall be duly observed by the Association.

VI. If the Association acts in contravention of the fourth paragraph of this Memorandum or of any such further conditions the liability of every member of the Council of the Association shall be unlimited and the liability of every member of the Association who has received any such dividend, bonus or other profit as aforesaid shall likewise be unlimited.

VII. Every member of the Association undertakes to contribute to the assets of the Association in the event of the same being wound up during the time that he is a member or within one year afterwards for payment of the debts and liability of the Association contracted before the time at which he ceases to be a member and of the costs, charges and expenses of winding up the same and for the adjustment of the rights of the contributories amongst themselves such amount as may be required not exceeding five pounds, or in case of his liability becoming unlimited such other amount as may be required in pursuance of the last preceding paragraph of this Memorandum.

VIII. If upon the winding up or dissolution of the Association there remains after the satisfaction of all its debts and liabilities any property whatsoever, the same shall not be paid to or distributed among the members of the Association, but shall be given or transferred to some other institution or institutions having objects similar to the objects of the Association to be determined by the members of the Association at or before the time of dissolution and in default thereof by such Judge of the Supreme Court as may have or acquire jurisdiction in the matter.

REVIEW.

Revue Internationale de Bibliographie Medicale Pharmaceutique et Veterinaire, par Dr. Jules Rouvier, Paris, J. Lechevalier, Rue Racine, and Beyrouth, Syria.

The first issue of this useful work appeared April of this year. A fasciculus of about 300 pp. is promised every three months. Each part contains a carefully compiled list of books, pamphlets and papers, upon some subject falling under one or other of the following headings:—Anatomy, Pathological Anatomy, Anthropology, &c., through the alphabet to Toxicology. In the first fasciculus the important caption—Odontology—was omitted, owing to the hurry incident to getting out the first part of an elaborate reference book of this description. Even in the second part, in which the subject has received attention, we observe many omissions and some errors. For example, Riggs' disease is called "La Maladie de Piggs"; a paper by Mr. Preedy is credited to a hypothetical M. Preredy, while Mr. J. Bland Sutton's well known article on Odontomes, which appeared in the Transactions of the Odontological Society of Great Britain, is stated to have seen the light in the *Journal of Comparative Medicine and Veterinary Archives* of Philadelphia. From the Transactions of the Odonto-Chirurgical Society of Scotland several papers are quoted as if they came from the journals in which they are reprinted, while the original sources are unmentioned. The quotations from the German and French journals are also far from complete. The idea of the book is excellent, and when in future fasciculi greater care is taken to avoid such errors and omissions as are noticed in the issues before us, the work will prove of service to busy practitioners, who desire a ready way of getting at all the literature on any given subject in a short time. At present it would be unsafe to trust to the references, as they are too meagre, and do not cover the ground.

THE DENTAL RECORD, LONDON: OCT. 1, 1890.

How to Deal with Another Man's Patients.

FEW professional men have been so blessed as to have passed through their career without being forced into unpleasantness through misunderstandings arising out of their relations with other men's patients. In many ways this occurs: A. goes away and asks B. to look after casual callers during his (A.'s) absence on a holiday or through illness. Patients, possibly new ones to A., but recommended to his house by other patients, come to B., like him and wish to remain with him, and allege they do not know A. and do not desire to leave B. having once gone to him. Take another case: C. has a misfortune and either gives a patient more pain than he, the patient, thinks necessary and so betakes himself to another dentist D., again recommended by friends. It also happens that some measure is suggested by one dentist which is not to the taste of a patient and so the latter hies him off to get another dentist's opinion, often enough not mentioning names until the opinion is expressed, and if this is unfavourable to the previously proposed operation the patient may elect to remain with No. 2 dentist and forsake No. 1.

Children will often enough lead their parents to change their dentist, because, Mr. So-and-So is so "rough to poor little Willie." A bad smash at one house followed by a successful extraction elsewhere may lead to alienation of patient and dentist, even if the smash was absolutely unavoidable and the lucky extraction the fruit of fortuitous inflammation plus manual dexterity, leaving it an open question which factor played the larger part in the happy result. Under any and all of these circumstances how is the dentist who is appealed to in the second place to act, and what must his demeanour be towards his predecessor whose patients the people were before they came to him? Certainly, no item of professional ethics bristles with more difficulties or presents larger scope for the exercise of tact and judicial honesty. It is too often lost sight of that doctors and dentists alike have no vested interests in their patients, the practice of giving money for the goodwill of a practice gave rise to the idea, but undoubtedly, patients have an absolute right to change their dentist as often as they please, and at the present day they are more than ever disposed to act upon their rights and seek aid in their dental troubles where they consider they can most satisfactorily obtain it. Patient-grabbing is quite another thing to accepting a patient who deliberately selects between A. and B. and prefers B., although, in this case, unless there is a definite cause of complaint against A., it is certainly B.'s duty to point out that the patient being recommended to A. is *ipso facto* his, and to send the person on to A. upon his return to the charge of his practice. Where patient-grabbing comes in is when a dentist asked casually to look in a mouth, volunteers a sneer or faint praise of work already placed in the mouth. In every case it is accepted by professional men as being quite outside the bounds of etiquette to criticise unfavourably the work of another duly qualified practitioner, and the offence is aggravated when the criticism is offered without solicitation. Probably, no better advice upon this most vexed question in professional ethics can be given than that implied in the dictum, "do to others as you would that they should do to you." However, there are very many side issues which need ventilation and being well threshed out, which can very well be done through the columns of our "Correspondence," and we shall be glad if our readers will give their brethren the benefit of their experience upon the matter. Many complain that assistants as "grabbers," and not a few assistants, turn the tables by reporting "sharp practice" by former principals. Even allowing for the Briton's privilege to grumble, we think the question may well be looked at from all points of view.

Affections Likely to Occur in the Alveolar Process.

UNDER this heading Dr. Shurer contributes a short article to the *Dental Register* for May. He considers one of the most important factors in the production of pathological conditions of the alveolar process is a diseased condition of its lining membrane—the periosteum. Speaking of necrosis, he says that there is reason to believe that the process of exfoliation is effected by the action of a corrosive fluid poured out from the fungous granulations of the living bone in contact with the necrosed part. "Necrosis of the alveolar process occurs very frequently while the system is under the influence of mercurial medicines, and during bilious and inflammatory fevers and certain other constitutional diseases, as syphilis, scurvy, smallpox, &c., and may also result from mechanical injuries. In many cases, especially of chronic disease, there is a definite thickening of the alveolar wall at or near its margin, which is clearly the result of exostosis, brought about by irritation in the immediate neighbourhood. In most, if not all, of these cases, the peridental membrane will be found destroyed between this thickened rim and the root of the tooth, and if the gum be slit up and turned back, it is seen that the portion of the alveolus lying next the teeth has been absorbed. We thus have an absorption of the inner portion of the alveolar wall and at the same time a deposit of bone on the outer portion, which causes the gum tissue to be held away from the root of the tooth. This thickening of the rim is very irregular, but seldom fully encircles the teeth. And as the destructive process is going on beneath this thickening of the bone, there will often be found jagged prominences that will interfere with the healing process, unless removed. The destruction of bone in these cases seems to be a process of absorption. A tooth is occasionally slowly forced from its place by a deposit of bony matter at the sides, or, more generally, at the bottom of the socket, causing a gradual displacement of the tooth. The causes are not rightly understood, though it is believed to be due to some irritation of the peridental membrane which seems to be so susceptible to morbid impressions that the pressure of a very conical root may be sufficient to produce this effect, or the pressure of a tooth possessing only a very low degree of vitality.

The writer of the paper connects this class of cases with those in which absence of all pressure causes alveolar exostosis, as, where a tooth has lost its antagonist and becomes elongated in consequence

At the January meeting of the Harvard Odontological Society, Dr. Horatio Meriam brought before the notice of the profession a new set of FILES he had devised FOR FINISHING FILLINGS. They are ten in number, each pattern being admirably adapted to the purpose for which it is intended. They all, except No. 1, have one safe side, and the back is rounded and polished. The rounded back permits of their being run over the gum or rubber dam without chafing, and this is facilitated by coating the back with soap or vaseline. We consider this set of Dr. Meriam's a valuable addition to the dental armamentarium.

In the discussion on Dr, Cooke's paper on "Irregularities" as read before the Harvard Odontological Society, and reported in the *Archives of Dentistry*, some interesting remarks were made. Dr. Clapp, in opening the discussion, said: "We must consider that when the teeth are in place, the hour for the exercise of great skill and judgment is not passed, but has really come, and we must devote fully as much study, as much care, and even more, to retaining the teeth in position as we have done in getting them into place. Dr. Cooke, on being asked what was the most favourable time for extraction of the six year-molars, is reported to have said: "When the second molars are coming through the gum." We are glad to find that this bald and misleading statement was not allowed to pass unchallenged, Dr. Clapp immediately setting Dr. Cooke right by giving it as his experience that "if extraction is to be made to gain room, the best time is when the twelve-year molars are fully occluded, but if the teeth were to be taken out simply because they were badly decayed, and there was no need to gain room, I should prefer to take them out as soon as possible, so that the twelve-year molars might come directly in the place of the six-year molars." We shou'd have thought this elementary principle of treatment was known to every tyro in dentistry, and ought not to have needed reiteration. In the course of the same discussion Dr. Meriam drew notice to the use of china grass line for ligatures. It is also called Ramie or sea-tangle twist. He claims for it that it shrinks considerably, and does not undergo softening in the mouth.

Porcelain Fillings.

In a paper on the above subject read before the Harvard Odontological Society, Dr. H. H. Stoddard reviews very briefly the history of the operation, and the different methods at present in vogue. He then details his own method, which is briefly as follows :—Shape the cavity to general form desired, without undercuts. Take an impression of the cavity and surrounding tooth surface with Ash's modelling compound, used in the form of a pencil. The colour is now selected from the sample colours, each of which corresponds in number to a body of that number. Cast the impression, and, when separated, trim the margin of the cavity in the plaster model, so that it is a trifle larger than the original cavity, to allow for shrinkage of the body in baking. Mix the body of the desired number to the consistency of cream, pack into the cavity in the model, and cover with a thin coating of enamel. Place in the gas furnace and bake about two minutes. This biscuits the filling, so that it may be removed from the plaster, which would melt when exposed to the intense heat of the furnace. Continue the baking for about six minutes. When cool, the porcelain is ground into place, set, and polished. For setting, the writer prefers gutta-percha, when the filling is at the margin of the gum, or in a place that is not self-cleansing ; in other places, cement.

Composition Fees for Dental Students.

We are informed that the fees mentioned in our last issue, both Charing Cross and Middlesex Hospitals, have undergone revision. Thus the Composition Fee for Dental Students at these Hospitals is 54 or 60 guineas, payable in two instalments of 30 guineas each. £12 12s. will be deducted from fees paid by instalments, and £12 12s., less 10 per cent., from fees paid in one sum in the case of Students who produce Certificates on joining the School of previous attendance on Chemistry, Practical Chemistry, and Materia Medica.

An additional reduction of £5 5s. will be made to Dental Students not at present requiring Practical Physiology.

AN ANOMALOUS CASE OF SALIVARY CALCULUS.

By Edmund Owen, F.R.C.S.

A lady recently came under my care for a troublesome but painless swelling of the left cheek. The medical man who sent her to me suggested that it was a case of distention of a greatly dilated parotid duct, possibly caused by a salivary calculus. Unfortunately this gentleman did not accompany her on her visit to me, and on the most careful examination I could detect no calculus, but found the cheek of that side somewhat prominent and unsightly. The lady said that she had been bothered by a swelling in that cheek ever since she was four years old, and that sometimes after a meal it was much more conspicuous than it was at another time. She was determined to have something done for the swelling, and I was content to hold my diagnosis as to the exact nature of the soft tumour in suspense until I could make a thorough exploration, which I did a few days later, Dr. Prickett kindly helping. There was then a rounded doughy swelling of the one cheek, but no calculus was discoverable. Anæsthesia having been produced, and the jaws being separated by Mason's gag, an incision was made through the mucous lining of the mouth and the buccinator, a lobulated piece of yelllow fat at once protruding. Gentle traction being made on this, a lipoma of considerable size readily left its bed between the buccinator and masseter muscles. The cheek was then flat like the other. It seemed as if no further treatment would be required, and nothing more was attempted. Within a few days, however, it became evident that the patient did not share our favourable view of the case. She said that on several occasions the cheek had swollen as badly as ever. Never happening to see the cheek, however, when swollen as she described, I thought it not improbable that her imagination supplied her with such evidence as I failed to discover. She was therefore advised to return home and to apply again should she meet with further inconvenience. In a short while she duly presented herself, and directed attention to a small, hard substance, which shifted its position over the masseter; it was evidently the salivary calculus of which her medical attendant had spoken. An attempt was promptly made to extract it through the mouth by reopening the old wound, but on introducing a pair of forceps the concretion slipped away and so effectually concealed itself that further search for it on that occasion had reluctantly to be abandoned. On a subsequent occasion on which the calculus was discovered I leisurely examined it from the outside of the cheek, and found that the limit of its journey forwards was just beyond the hinder border of the masseter, and that with the slightest touch it slipped back into a dilatation of Stenson's duct, which formed a wide chamber behind the angle and ramus of the jaw. From this pouch the calculus could be swept out by firm pressure. Sometimes it was no easy matter to bring it out again, as it hid itself on the inner aspect of the mandibular angle in the capacious chamber. Having been twice disappointed in the treatment of the case when operating through the buccinator, I determined to cut straight down on to the calculus through the cheek, having chased it forwards and secured it by the finger pressed over the hinder part of the masseter. In this way its extraction proved a simple matter. The skin wound, which was closed with horsehair sutures, healed by first intention, giving no trouble whatever as regards leakage of saliva, and leaving a scar which, from the patient's point of view as well as the surgeon's, is now hardly noticeable. The calculus was a phosphatic concretion of the size and shape of a small date stone.

Remarks.—No one who has carefully dissected the face can fail to have noticed the pad of yellow fat which is lodged between the masseter and buccinator, the little pellets of which obeyed the slightest touch of his forceps. But in the case under consideration the mass of fat far exceeded the normal amount, and when drawn out through the mouth constituted a lipoma of a very respectable size. Moreover, the swelling which had previously disfigured that cheek had so entirely disappeared that I felt justified in saying that the operation would prove entirely successful. Probably the irritation caused by the salivary calculus had brought about an over-nutrition of the fatty pad and so determined its hypertrophy, the other cheek remaining of normal size and appearance. Certainly the removal of the calculus alone would not have restored the symmetry, and had I extracted the concretion on the first occasion I might have hesitated to proceed to the ablation of the buccal lipoma, even if I had made a correct diagnosis of the nature of that swelling. Thus, as possibly not infrequently happens, failure on the part of the surgeon either in the way of diagnosis or treatment, worked for the good of the patient. As regards the removal of the calculus from the outside of the cheek, it is not an operation which one would generally recommend, lest a troublesome salivary fistula should result, but, seeing the perfect way in which the wound healed, the danger of such a contingency is probably over-rated.—*Lancet.*

GOSSIP.

"THE AGE IN WHICH WE HAVE LIVED."—A contemporary, *Iron* very justly says :—"Those of fifty years of age have probably lived in the most important and intellectually progressive period of human history. Within this half century the following inventions and discoveries have either been placed before the world or elaborated :—

Ocean steamships, railways, street tramways, telegraph lines, ocean cables, telephone, phonograph, photography and a score of new methods of picture making, aniline colours, kerosene oil, electric lights, steam fire engines, chemical fire extinguishers ; anæsthetics and painless surgery ; gun-cotton, nitro-glycerine, dynamite, and a host of other explosives ; aluminium, magnesium, and other new metals ; electro-plating, spectrum analysis, and the spectroscope ; audiphone, pneumatic tubes, electric motors, electric railways, electric bells, type-writers, cheap postal system, steam heating, hydraulic elevators, vestibule cars, and cantilever bridges. These are only a few out of a multitude. All positive knowledge of the physical constitution of the planetary and stellar worlds has also been attained within this period."

APHRODISIAC effects from cocaine have, according to the *North Western Lancet*, been reported by several observers, and the possibility of producing strong sexual excitement by the use of a small quantity of the drug should be borne in mind. With male patients this effect is of but little consequence, but where the physician is alone with a female patient the consequences may be embarrassing if nothing worse. A Philadelphia physician reports giving a hypodermic injection of a few drops of a 10 per cent. to remove a small tumor The erotic excitement that followed, led the patient to behave in a most unseemly way, although her usual behaviour was modest and becoming. A St. Paul dentist reports a similar experience, his patient making an indelicate exposure of the person while under the influence of a small injection of cocaine. Dentists should indeed be particularly on their guard, since they use cocaine so often in filling and extracting teeth, and are so frequently alone with their patients.

THE dangers of hypnotism are, according to the *Lancet*, not a few. At Nuremburg a case of some public interest has recently been tried in the police court. A commercial traveller, while in a restaurant, told the waitress to look steadily at the white of his eye and hypnotized her. On the second occasion he repeated the experiment, but this time the sleep was so profound that a medical man had to be called, who had the utmost difficulty in rousing the girl. The commercial traveller was accordingly summoned to appear before the magistrates, and the severe sentence of eight days' imprisonment was passed on him, which will probably be efficient in checking similar performances in that region. In France the practice of hypnotizing people for amusement seems very common, and unpleasant consequences are reported. At a supper party in Paris recently one of the company hypnotized a girl and was unable to rouse her. She was consequently taken to the house of a medical man, and after a time she recovered consciousness. The whole party were taken in custody by the police, and were not released until next day. Even when hypnotism has been practiced by competent medical men for remedial purposes, unpleasant accidents and ulterior consequences have again and again occurred, so much so, that recently an order has been issued by the French Government prohibiting surgeons in the army and navy from practicing it. It ought to be distinctly understood, both by the profession and the public, that hypnotism is not devoid of danger at the time, and not infrequently has permanently impaired the moral and emotional control of patients. A medical man is bound, before recommending hypnotism for a patient, to weigh the question as carefully as he would that of the advisability of administering an anæsthetic.

DENTAL HOSPITAL OF LONDON and LONDON SCHOOL OF DENTAL SURGERY. We understand that the following demonstrations, etc., have been arranged:—Mr. Truman, Mondays, at 12 noon, Oct 6, Dec. 29, May 4; Mr. Woodhouse, Tuesdays at 12, Oct. 14, Jan. 6, May 12; Mr. Gregson, Wednesdays at 12, Oct. 22, Jan. 14, May 20; Mr. Storer Bennett, Thursdays at 12, Oct. 30, Jan. 22, May 28; Mr. Claude Rogers, Fridays at 12, Nov. 7, Jan. 30, June 5; Mr. Canton, Saturdays at 12, Nov. 15, Feb. 7, June 13; Mr. Matheson, Mondays at 12, Nov. 17, Feb. 9, June 15; Mr. Hern, Tuesdays at 12, Nov. 25, Feb. 17, June 23; Mr. Lloyd Williams, Wednesdays at 12, Dec. 3, Feb. 25, July 1; Mr. Parkinson, Thursdays at 12, Dec. 11, Mar. 5, July 9; Mr. Read, Fridays at 12, Dec. 19, Mar. 13, July 17; Mr. Paterson, Saturdays at 12, Dec. 27, March 21, July 25. Subjects will be posted at the hospital one week previously.

MR. DAVID HEPBURN, writing to the *Journal of the British Dental Association*, narrates the following case. A lady of middle age, with an apparently edentulous, but to all appearance healthy and normal upper jaw, has for some years worn an upper suction plate, but always with more or less discomfort and pain, which all ordinary treatment failed to alleviate. On examining the gum recently a minute opening was discovered, this being enlarged and a probe passed, enamel could be distinctly felt. The patient was then placed under an anæsthetic, and with some difficulty a large and well-formed canine tooth was removed from the substance of the bone, After a few weeks the suction plate was re-adjusted, and has since been worn without any discomfort whatever.

Journalistic Memorabilia.

CAMPHO-PHENIQUE.

Dr. J. W. DOWNEY, writing on this antiseptic in *Archives of Dentistry*, says :—Campho-phenique is a germicide and antiseptic Campho-phenique is absolutely free from toxic or caustic properties. Applied to the unbroken skin it produces no sensation whatever On cut surfaces there is a slight burning sensation when first applied, followed by anæsthesia.

Now, which antiseptic is the most agreeable. The brassy metallic taste of the bichloride is intolerable, the taste and smell of carbolic acid and creosote are disagreeable to most people, and the odour and meagre antiseptic properties of iodoform should banish it from the operating-room. Campho-phenique has a pleasant odour and agreeable taste ; this should establish its claim as the most agreeable germicide summing up he says.

1st. That when used pure and undiluted, campho-phenique is one of the most efficient and reliable germicides and antiseptics.

2d. Being non-poisonous and non-irritant, it is perfectly safe.

3d. It is the most agreeable to the patient of any drug of its class.

As to special uses he advises it as a pulp canal dressing in the various pathological conditions, from recent devitalization to alveolar abscess. Here it will take the place of corrosive sublimate, carbolic acid, creosote, oil of cloves, iodoform, or any germicide heretofore used, except peroxide of hydrogen. If thoroughly rubbed on the gum, or injected with a hypodermic syringe, it acts efficiently as a local anæsthetic, not equal, however, to cocaine ; but there are no constitutional effects following its use, and there is no danger of the tissues sloughing. It is quite efficient as an obtunder of sensitive dentine.

The very disagreeable ache which sometimes follows the extraction of abscessed teeth is almost instantly relieved by placing a pledget of absorbent cotton, saturated with campho-phenique, deep in the painful socket.

For chapped hands the following formula is advised :—

℞.—Campho-phenique ... ...
Oil of cade ... ... āā ʒj
Rose cosmoline ... ... ℥j
ᵯ. Sig—Apply frequently.

Campho-phenique should never be mixed with water or glycerine. It will mix in all proportions with alcohol, ether, chloroform, and all fatty substances. In dentistry it will seldom be necessary to dilute it at all.

CORRESPONDENCE.

[We do not hold ourselves responsible in any way for the opinions expressed by our correspondents.]

WHAT CONSTITUTES A RANULA.

To the Editor of the DENTAL RECORD.

Sir.—In the course of a critical review which recently appeared in the *Record*, exception is taken to the view respecting ranula which is adopted in the work under review. Ranula is stated by the reviewer, never to be an obstruction of the duct of a sub-lingual Salivary gland, and never to contain saliva, but, he adds, Ranula has been proved many times to be caused by the enlargement of a sub-lingual mucous gland and in nearly every case the duct can be traced across the ranula, as in another particular. Two cases met with in actual practice are interesting as bearing upon this point. The first was a case the model of which is, I believe, now in the museum of the Odontological Society, where a piece of tartar, shaped like a rough pointed cone, was seen emerging from the common opening of the sub-lingual and sub-maxillary glands, close to the frænulum of the tongue, and the plaster cast (taken by Mr. Gurnell Hammond, the inventor of Hammond's splint) shows this *in situ*. The other case was that of a governess, a patient of my own ; unfortunately I did not see this case, but the moment she described her long sufferings and rapid relief, I said to her, "You have had a ranula," and explained what I meant to her afterwards ; and this was her story. Slowly, after considerable discomfort, the tongue seemed to be raised up on one side, this condition causing pain in mastication, and annoyance even in speaking, etc. The medical man in attendance kept on giving tonics, which naturally gave her no relief whatever ; one day her mouth was suddenly flooded with what she called saliva, tasting very salt—in fact, salty serum I presume—and on spitting this out, she then found what *she* thought was an incisor tooth lying in her mouth, it was about three-quarters of an inch in length, and, under the impression that it was a tooth, she was using some lateral force when it broke in two halves, and much she regretted not having brought it to show me, for she still imagined it was a tooth, and then threw it away. I may add that she was a very intelligent girl, and quite reliable, and never had the remotest idea of "ranula," or anything of the kind. With such cases (and there must surely be many more on record), who can subscribe to the statement that ranula is *never* an obstruction of the duct of a salivary gland? If this is so, how about the escape of these masses of salivary calculus, and the immediate relief following their emergence from the duct? May it not be that we have admittedly the great majority of ranulas caused by the enlargement of sub-mucous glands, with cases of exceptional interest to the dental surgeon, where the duct itself is obstructed by a mass of salivary calculus? Also, as the glands do unquestionably secrete the saliva, why should there *never* be saliva in the salty fluid so freely liberated when the duct (as I maintain does occur occasionally) gets blocked up in the manner described. I should imagine that saliva *and* serous fluid were *both* present in these exceptional cases at least.

Trusting that my remarks may call forth some discussion,

I am Sir, &c.,

Brighton. E. M. TOD.

THE DISCUSSION ON DENTAL EDUCATION.

To the Editor of the DENTAL RECORD.

Sir.—I shall be much obliged if you will allow me to point out an error that appears in your report of the remarks made by me during the discussion of Mr. Campion's paper at Exeter. Your report correctly represents me as saying that what is wanted in the training of students, is a more thorough and extensive "training in the use of their fingers." But then you make me say that I thought "Mr. Campion's suggestion would not help in that direction." What I did say was, that I thought those suggestions "*would* help"; and, indeed, were it not for my strong belief in the value of Mr. Campion's proposals, I should not have troubled you with this letter.

I am, yours truly,

LEONARD MATHESON.

APPOINTMENTS.

HERBERT R. BOWTELL, L.D.S., Eng., has been appointed House Surgeon to the Dental Hospital of London.

WALTER S. HOLFORD, L.R.C.P., Lond., M R.C.S., Eng., has been appointed Assistant House Surgeon to the Dental Hospital of London.

OBITUARY.

We have to announce with much regret the sudden death of William Hy. Woodhouse, L. D.S.I., on the 18th of August, aged sixty years, at his country house, The Hall, East Ilsley, Berks. About a week before his death he took a severe chill, which resulted in congestion of the lungs; his condition gradually became worse until the morning of the 18th, when he peacefully passed away. He leaves a widow and eight children. He was associated in practice for more than thirty years with his brother, A. J. Woodhouse, practising with him. He became a member of the Odontological Society in 1866, being a member of the Council from 1880 to 1881, and for many years he was a constant attendant at the meetings, though he did not take an active part in them.

MONTHLY STATEMENT of operations performed at the two Dental Hospitals in London, and a Provincial Hospital, from July 1st to July 31st, 1890:—

		London.	National.	Manchester.
Number of Patients attended		—	1,764	1,143
Extractions	Children under 14	399	241	
	Adults	1,274	293	766
	Under Nitrous Oxide	898	639	173
Gold Fillings		291	127	38
Plastic do.		1,082	398	174
Irregularities of the Teeth		74	185	14
Artificial Crowns		26	21	3
Miscellaneous		403	247	392
Implantations		—	3	—
		4,447	2,154	1,560

The DENTAL RECORD.

Vol. X. NOVEMBER 1st, 1890. No. 11.

Original Communications.

ALLEGED SWALLOWING OF ARTIFICIAL TEETH.

GASTRALGIA :—EXPLORATORY LAPAROTOMY,

COMPLETE RELIEF FROM SYMPTOMS. *

Under the care of Mr. A. E. BARKER, F.R.C.S., *Surgeon to University College Hospital.*

J. W., a railway labourer, aged 47 years, was admitted into University College Hospital under the care of Mr. A. E. Barker, on the 8th August, 1890. There were no points of interest in the patient's previous history, except that he had hitherto enjoyed excellent health. His father died at sixty of cancer. The symptoms all dated from Easter Monday, April 7th, 1890. Whilst sitting on a platform awaiting the arrival of his train, he dozed, and on waking missed his artificial teeth, which consisted of a plate and a complete upper set. After searching for them he concluded that he must have swallowed them, and for the next day or two experienced a sensation of soreness in the throat and windpipe. About five days later the patient began to suffer from dull-aching pain in the umbilical region, which was aggravated after taking food. From that time onwards the pain persisted, and the increase caused by food was so severe that only milk puddings, occasional small quantities of fish and various forms of liquid nourishment could be taken. There was frequent nausea after food and occasional vomiting. No blood had at any time been noticed in the vomited matter. The only other trouble

* We are indebted for these Notes to Mr. Raymond johnson, M.B., B.S., F.R.C S., Surgical Registrar in University College Hospital.

was obstinate constipation, which necessitated the frequent use of enemata. The patient during the four months which had elapsed since the onset of his illness had lost flesh, and was rendered quite incapable of following his usual occupation.

On admission, the patient had the appearance of a previously well-nourished man much wasted, but was noted as not having the peculiar expression so often seen in cases of severe abdominal disease. It was evident that the patient's subjective symptoms were, if anything, exaggerated by him. The abdomen was quite flat and the lax condition of the abdominal wall allowed very complete examination, but nothing whatever abnormal could be detected. The rectum was examined with negative result. Spoon diet was given, and the bowels were freely opened by enemata. On the third day after admission an œsophageal bougie was easily passed into the stomach, and it was thought that it struck against some thing hard, but on this point there was considerable doubt. On several occasions the stomach was washed out and was found to contain large quantities of acid fermenting fluid. No sarcinæ could be discovered in the fluid. The pain was described as "agonising," and was most severe between the ensiform cartilage and the umbilicus; it was worse in the lying than in the sitting or erect position. Sleep was only obtained by use of opiates. The vomiting occurred usually about ten minutes after food. The following drugs were employed without benefit: creosote, bismuth, hydrocyanic acid, carbonate of soda and gentian. Boric acid, dilute solution of sulphurous acid and solution of bicarbonate of potash were used in succession for washing out the stomach. On August 20th chloroform was given as an aid to abdominal examination, but nothing abnormal could be detected. Meanwhile the patient was emaciating more and more, and on account of increased suffering was urging operation. The severity of the symptoms and the *possible presence of pyloric disease* was now considered sufficient to justify exploratory laparotomy. On August 27th, therefore, the abdomen was opened by Mr. Barker by median incision above the umbilicus. The hand was introduced and the stomach carefully examined. No foreign body could be felt in it nor did the wall of the viscus at any part feel unnaturally thick. The pylorus was found to be perfectly normal as were also all the adjacent structures accessible to the hand. The part of the stomach which could be seen appeared healthy. The incision was closed with seven silk sutures passing through the whole thickness of the abdominal wall, and a dressing of salicylic wool was applied.

During the evening severe abdominal pain was present, but sleep followed a hypodermic injection of morphia. No food was given by the mouth for two days. On the 29th and 30th August sickness followed small quantities of milk and barley water, but did not recur on any subsequent occasion. During convalescence the temperature did not exceed 98·8° and the sutures were removed from the incision on the 11th, a pad of wool being applied with a broad strip of plaster. The diet was steadily increased, so that the patient was taking fish on September 13th and meat a week later. He remained from this time forward quite free from pain and vomiting, relished his food and steadily gained weight. His mental state also was altogether changed, and he became bright and cheerful. He left the Hospital on October 3rd, 36 days after the operation, having put on much flesh and altogether satisfied. The motions had been carefully watched, but no sign of the false teeth could be detected.

Remarks by Mr. Barker :—On first hearing this patient's statement of his case I felt very sceptical as to his having swallowed the artificial teeth, although he himself was evidently convinced that they were in his stomach. It appeared highly improbable that he could have swallowed them during sleep, or, when just awake without knowing more about them than he appeared to know. I thought he was suffering from aggravated dyspepsia. On this hypothesis he was treated for some weeks by dieting, by drugs and, finally by regular washing out of the stomach. There seemed to be no reason why the teeth if they were present should give rise to vomiting and constipation, though they might cause pain. But, when the symptoms persisted in spite of treatment, and *emaciation became extreme*, it was impossible to close one's eyes to the possibility of pyloric obstruction, either the result of ulceration or new growth. This suspicion combined with the patient's urgent requests for operation even more than his conviction of the presence of the teeth, finally determined the question of exploratory operation. The latter was a simple matter and involved but slight risk. The day after I told the patient plainly that I had found nothing, and though he was surprised he seemed well satisfied.

In this case there can be no question, I think, of malingering. All motive in this direction was absent. Moreover a malingerer might complain of pain but would hardly have put up with the restricted dietary, the drugs and the frequent irrigation of the stomach and have clamoured for abdominal section. Again the vomiting and rapid emaciation would be hard to account for on that hypothesis alone.

On the whole I am inclined to attribute all the symptoms subjective and objective to the domination of a great fear. The patient believed that he was in great peril from having swallowed this plate of teeth: his attention was concentrated on his stomach, in which he believed them to lie. His digestion suffered accordingly, and this probably was the cause of the pain complained of, as well as of the vomiting and constipation. The depressing influence of constant apprehension would also probably tend to aggravate his general malnutrition initiated by the stomach neurosis, and so lead to rapid wasting. This again would react on his mental condition and enfeeble his will and thus a vicious circle would be established.

The effect of the operation was simply to relieve him of the incubus of this dominant fear; for, when he was told that his stomach was quite normal and the teeth were nowhere to be found in it he at once brightened up and very soon showed the most unmistakable interest in his food. The rapidity with which he put on flesh was also remarkable. In short his whole condition was changed as well as his demeanour.

ON THE AGENCY OF MICRO-ORGANISMS IN CARIES OF THE TEETH.

By J. Howard Mummery, M.R.C.S., L.D.S.

(A portion of a Paper read before the International Medical Congress, Berlin, 1890)

In opening a discussion on the influence of micro-organisms in caries of the teeth, I think the desired end will be best attained by venturing as little as possible on theoretical ground, and drawing attention especially to the several points which are still debateable—questions on which competent observers hold somewhat different opinions. In order adequately to appreciate these points a brief historical *resumé* of the subject may be advisable.

While the discovery of the association of micro-organisms with caries and the dependence of this disease on their presence and fermentative action is of very recent date, the idea of some organisms being present was held, as is well known, in ancient times. Without dwelling on these early theories, I may allude to the worm hypothesis which held ground for a long period, taking the place of the theory upheld by Hippocrates, that caries, like other diseases, was caused by a bad condition of the humours. Whatever significance we may attach to this ancient worm theory, the first important point which strikes one in this historical aspect, is the question, whether the exploration of our special region (the mouth) may not legitimately claim to have been the means of anticipating, even by centuries, the dawn of bacteriological science, for in the volume of the *Transactions of the Royal Society* for the year 1684, appears a letter, dated September 17th, 1683, from that great pioneer of microscopy, Anthony Leuwenhoeck, of Delft. It is entitled, "Microscopical observations about animals in the scurf of the teeth, the substance called worms in the nose, and the cuticula, consisting of scales."

In this letter he says :—"Though my teeth are kept usually very clean, when I view them in a magnifying glass I find growing between them a little white matter as thick as wetted flour ; in this substance, though I could not perceive any motion, I judged there might probably be living creatures. I, therefore, took some of this flour and mixed it, either with pure rain-water in which there were no animals, or else with some of my spittle, having no animals nor air-bubbles to cause a motion in it ; and then, to my great surprise, perceived that the aforesaid matter contained very many small living animals, which moved themselves very strangely. The largest sort were not numerous, but their motion strong and nimble, darting themselves through the water or spittle as a jack or pike does through the water. The second sort spun about like a top, and were more in number than the first. In the third sort I could not well distinguish the figure, for sometimes it seemed to be an oval, and other times a circle ; these were exceedingly small and so swift that I can compare them to nothing better than a swarm of flies or gnats, flying and turning among one another in a small space.

"Besides these animals there were a great quantity of streaks of threads of different lengths, but of like thickness, lying confusedly together, some bent and others straight. These had no life or motion in them."

There can be little doubt that the last-named streaks were the familiar leptothrix filaments, and, probably, Leuwenhoeck also detected—as suggested by Dr. Miller—the well-known "spirillum sputigenum," which is found in abundance between the teeth near the margin of the gums, and exhibits a very active movement. It is astonishing that, with the imperfect instruments of the day, this great observer should have so anticipated modern scientific discovery. Ficinus, in 1846, describes caries as in part a putrefactive process caused by the presence of infusoria (denticola).

Klenke, in 1850, while agreeing with Ficinus as to the putrefactive variety, describes another form of caries in which a phyto-parasite, which he calls protococcus dentalis, takes a part.

But the first systematic account of the action of micro-organisms in caries is that of Messrs. Leber and Rottenstein, in 1867, when they published their important *Recherches sur la Carie dentaire*, a contribution all the more remarkable when we remember it was published when scarcely any of the great discoveries in bacteriology had been made.

They describe caries as due partly to the action of acids, and partly to the proliferation in the tnbes of the dentine of a definite micro-organism—the leptothrix buccalis; that the growth of this fungus in the substance of the dentine could not take place without a preliminary decalcification of the tissues of the tooth by acid. They found that the tubes of the dentine were dilated and penetrated by granular matter, and, finding that this granular matter stained violet when treated with iodine and acids, they looked upon it as composed of the elements of the leptothrix fungus, which proliferated in the dentinal tubes. They considered that although the preliminary stages were due to the action of acids, the appearances found were not sufficiently accounted for by the action of acids alone, and were due in part to this proliferation of the fungus in the tissues.

They concluded that an acetous fermentation was set np in the mouth with particles of food lodged between the teeth, and in fissures in the enamel, and considered it probable that lactic acid was formed in this fermentation.

Professor Wedl, in his work on "The Pathology of the Teeth," published in Vienna, in 1870, discusses Leber and Rottenstein's views; he considers that the leptothrix described by these authors has no direct connection with the origin of caries. The extension of caries in the dentine he believed to be effected by the acid, and not by the fungus. He says, "The proliferations of the elements of the fungus, without doubt, penetrate and expand the dentinal canals; but, according to my observations, this cannot occur until the decalcification of the dentine is complete, or, at all events, until the first stage of this process. I have never detected a proliferation of fungus in the still hard, carious dentine."

He concludes that "caries of the teeth is a process which has its origin, chiefly, in the abnormal secretions of the gums, and likewise in those of the rest of the oral mucous membrane and of the salivary glands, and commencing at suitable points on the exterior of the tooth, spreads in the direction of the pulp cavity. In consequence of the decomposition of the secretions, acids are formed which extract the calcareous salts from the hard tissues, and give rise to a disintegration of the affected portions of the latter, in which no inflammatory action occurs. The destructive process is promoted essentially by the accumulation of secretions and particles of food, and opportunity is afforded by proliferation of leptothrix buccalis, in the dead and softened dentine."

We meet for some time with no further important researches in this direction. The existence of a micro-organism in caries had been demonstrated, and from the microscopical appearances in carious tissue, it had been assumed that this micro-organism (supposed to be exclusively the leptothrix buccalis) participated in the pathological process; acids produced in or taken into the mouth, having prepared the way for its advance by a preliminary decalcification of the tissue.

At this point in the history of the investigation, the influence of micro-organisms as an agent in the production of caries, was, at all events in England, practically disregarded, notwithstanding the researches of Leber and Rottenstein—the view that held the field at this time being the purely chemical theory of caries.

At the meeting of the International Medical Congress in London, in 1881, Messrs. Underwood and Milles communicated an investigation into the effects of organisms on the teeth and the alveolar portions of the jaws, which, together with the subsequent important researches of Professor Miller, have resulted in placing the facts of the action of micro-organisms in caries on a thoroughly accepted basis.

They considered that "caries is absolutely dependent upon the presence and proliferation of organisms." "That these organisms attack first the organic material, and feeding upon it, create an acid which removes the lime salt, and that all the differences between caries and simple decalcification by acids are due to the presence and operation of germs."

They demonstrated the existence of micrococci and rod-shaped bacteria in the dilated tubes of the dentine, and by submitting healthy teeth to septic and aseptic fluids in flasks, proved that in an aseptic flask caries never occurs, in a septic flask a change, at all events greatly resembling it, frequently does occur. As stated by Mr. Charles Tomes in the discussion on this paper: "In former experiments on the production of artificial caries, germs had not been excluded, and consequently had exerted their full action; but Messrs. Underwood and Milles showed that when they were excluded, caries did not occur, and he considered that this was 'a contribution to our knowledge of the artificial production of caries, which can never be left out of consideration by any snbsequent observer, or writer on the subject.'"

It still remained to be shown what was the acid produced by the micro-organisms, and in what way it was formed in the mouth. The first place in this investigation belongs to Professor Miller, of Berlin, who, bringing a sound knowledge of chemistry to bear upon his researches, conducted a series of important experiments, which have done a great deal to clear up this portion of the subject, and to establish it upon a thoroughly scientific basis.

He found that fresh saliva mixed with sugar or starch invariably became acid in four or five hours—whether the experiment was performed in the mouth by means of a small tube attached to a tooth, or out of the mouth, the mixture being kept at blood temperature; when the saliva was subjected to a temperature of 100° before mixing with the starch, no acid was produced. When the starch alone was submitted to a much higher temperature than this, acid was still produced, showing that the ferment was in the saliva, and not in the starch. By other experiments it was proved that the ptyalin of the saliva was not the cause of the acid reaction. By inoculating a sterilized solution of saliva and starch with carious dentine, or with saliva taken direct from the mouth, acid fermentation was produced, proving the existence in the mouth and in carious dentine, of an organized ferment capable of producing an acid reaction. By control experiments it was proved that sterilized cultivation tubes *invariably* became acid when inoculated direct from the mouth, the uninfected tubes remaining neutral. It was also shown by conducting similar experiments without the access of air, that, given the necessary food, this action can go on in the deeper layers of the dentine excluded from the air—in other words, that some of the organisms found in caries were anærobic. Other experiments tended to show, that by the use of strong antiseptics in the mouth, conbined with careful cleansing with tooth brush and silk, the amount of acid produced in specimens of saliva, tested, could be greatly reduced.

All the cultures made, showed under the microscope a fungus, as either micrococci, diplococci, bacteria, bacilli, or thread forms. Dr. Miller described all these forms as sometimes found on a single thread, which he considered to prove the genetic connection of the forms. He also concluded that it was only from carbohydrates, especially sugar, that this fungus appears to be able to produce acids in any considerable quantity at all. He finds, furthermore, that the "great majority of the fungi found in the human mouth are capable of producing acid from cane or grape sugar. In nearly all cases investigated this acid appeared to be lactic."

One link in the chain of evidence was, however, still wanting—could caries be produced out of the mouth artifically, imitating the conditions found in the mouth as nearly as possible? Dr. Miller answers this question in the affirmative, and has been able to produce artificial caries which is indistinguishable from natural caries under the microscope.

Messrs. Underwood and Milles, in a further communication contributed to the Odontological Society in 1884, described some experiments on the production of artificial caries in which the results obtained were not identical with Dr. Miller's.

In their first experiment, malic and butyric acids were present in a flask with an infusion of meat and saliva, fragments of dentine were exposed to this fluid; but the change produced was only quite superficial, although the tubes were enlarged and contained a material that stained readily. It has been suggested, that in this experiment the necessary food of the micro-organisms was absent, for albuminous substances, such as meat, when decomposed in the mouth do not produce acids. They required starch or sugar as the material from which to form the acid.

In their second experiment, in which putrefactive changes in the materials were allowed to go on for a considerable period, scarcely any perceptible change took place. It has been since suggested as an explanation of this result, that putrefaction causes an alkaline reaction, and interferes with the acid-forming properties of the micro-organisms; an instance of putrefaction interfering with caries is seen in those cases in which a growth of suppurating gum has partially filled a large carious cavity, the caries is often arrested and the reaction at the margin is found to be alkaline.

In a third experiment, in which fragments of dentine were exposed in a flask to a mixture of saliva and bread, a change was produced in the dentine, but Messrs. Underwood and Milles considered this change to be a very weak caries, if caries at all. In connection with this experiment it may be remarked that if the mixture was not often renewed the micro-organisms might soon be devitalized by their own products, so that while we should obtain decalcification, there would be no infiltration with micro-organisms. They came to the conclusion, as the result of these experiments, that the process to be effectual must be carried on in a living mouth, probably because that is the only situation in which the special germs are really active.

The researches, thus described, enable us to formulate a definite explanation of caries in relation to micro-organisms. It is now well established, as first stated by Messrs. Leber and Rottenstein, and confirmed by Messrs. Underwood and Milles, Miller, and other observers, that in all cases of caries, micro-organisms are present, and without their presence caries never takes place.

The phenomena in dental caries may be divided into two stages; the first being a process of partial decalcification, and the second a stage of digestion and solution of the tissue. The first stage of caries consists in a partial decalcification of the tooth substance by acids, these acids being formed in the mouth by a process of fermentation; this fermentation being the result of the action of micro-organisms on the sugar present in the mouth, either taken in as such, or as starch which is converted by the ptyalin of the saliva into sugar Prolonged contact of the micro-organisms with the teeth is necessary to the first stage of caries, either by the lodgment of particles between the teeth, or in fissures or depressions in their substance.

In the second stage of caries, such decalcification having occurred, the micro-organisms are able to penetrate the softened tissue, and feeding upon the sugar present in solution, form fresh acid in its substance, and especially in the tubules of the dentine, proliferate freely, expanding and dilating the tubes until they break into one another, destroying the matrix and causing complete disintegration of the tissue. According to Dr. Miller, several germs of the mouth possess the power of dissolving albuminous substances and changing them into a soluble modification, and he therefore considers the second stage of caries to be a digestion process ; the cartilage of the tooth being dissolved by a ferment similar to pepsin, just as albumen is by the pepsin of the fluid of the stomach. The same observer has never found a putrefactive organism in the deeper portions of carious dentine, and he does not consider putrefactive changes at all *essential* to caries. "The presence of putrefactive organisms, while it would accelerate the second stage of caries, could only retard the first." The acid formed in this fermentative process, appears from the investigations before described to be in most cases lactic acid. The power of forming lactic acid from carbohydrates appertains to a large number of species of bacteria (Flügge).

It is well known that the growth of the bacteria is injuriously affected by the products of their own tissue change. Lactic acid, in the lactic acid fermentation, is injurious even in the amount of 0·8 per cent. (Flügge). In experiments with lactic acid bacteria it has been found necessary, when the formation of lactic acid has reached this proportion, to neutralize the acid with chalk. There is evidence, that in carious teeth the lime salts liberated form with the acid a lactate of lime, thus taking up the excess of acid formed and allowing the fermentation to go on unimpeded, the micro-organisms being set free from its inhibitory effects.

MICROSCOPICAL APPEARANCES IN CARIES.

We have to consider the microscopical appearances in enamel, in cementum, and in dentine :—

In Enamel.—The enamel loses its transparency and the prisms are seen to be separated from one another ; the elements of the fungus are only seen in the spaces formed by this disintegration, as there are no channels in its substance along which they can penetrate, its structure, in fact, does not admit of the proliferation of micro-organisms in the tissue. A dark colouration of the enamel is generally to be noticed.

Dr. Abbott, in a paper published in the *Dental Cosmos*, in 1879, in describing the decalcified portion of carious enamel, speaks of the readily stained masses of softened substance as protoplasmic bodies "embryonic corpuscles," which the change in the enamel, caused by caries, has brought into view. He considers this, as also a similar appearance in carious dentine, to be evidence of a high vitality in the tissues.

Other observers consider that these are irregular masses of germs mixed with the detritus of the decayed tooth, that not being homogeneous they take up the colouring matter unequally at different parts and produce a false appearance of cells (Miller).

Caries in Cement.—When caries extends to the cementum, the organisms are found in the lacunæ and extending along the canaliculi.

According to the observations of Dr. Miller, the Sharpey's fibres in the cement become infiltrated with germs and dilated and the tissue lying between them dissolved.

Caries in Dentine.—The structure of dentine is eminently suitable for the proliferation of micro-organisms, and it is in this tissue, accordingly, that their effects can be best studied. If we examine with a low power a longitudinal section of carious dentine in a tooth, in which the decay has commenced from a fissure in the crown, and which has been treated with fuchsine or gentian violet, it is noticeable at once that the stained portion has more or less the appearance of a cone, the most deeply stained part forming the base of the cone, corresponding to that portion of the dentine which formed the floor of the cavity of decay, and that the apex of the cone is directed towards the pulp cavity of the tooth.

On examination with a higher power, it is seen that the micro-organisms, usually either micrococci or rod-shaped bacteria, penetrate freely along the tubes of the dentine, in the more superficial portions being crowded together, and in the deeper layer of the tissue filling the tubes less completely, in some cases being reduced to a single line. The base of the cone is seen to be formed by the extension of the micro-organisms in a lateral direction along the fine terminal branches of the tubuli. The tubes are seen to be expanded at intervals into irregular globular or oval shaped spaces filled with micro-organisms; in many cases large cavities appearing where these have become confluent. These cavities breaking into one another, the whole tissue of the dentine becomes broken down and gradually destroyed. We frequently see groups of canals filled with organisms lying in the spaces of the dentine apparently free from infection, in other cases, the matrix seems to have disappeared and the whole of the dentine in the part examined is found to be a mass of micro-organisms. Leptothrix threads are especially noticeable on the margins of the preparations, where their invasion of the decalcified tissue is marked by bundles of threads penetrating for some distance into the dentine.

Specimens are met with where the leptothrix threads penetrate the tubes to a considerable depth, some specimens showing leptothrix threads throughout, to the exclusion of other forms. Mixed with the leptothrix filaments are often seen small round points which may easily be mistaken for micrococci; these are cross sections of the leptothrix threads and may be seen by altering the focus of the objective. Cocci and short rod-shaped bacteria are, however, the forms of micro-organisms usually found in the deeper layers of the dentine. In many specimens some tubes are found filled with micrococci, others in their neighbourhood filled with bacilli, and according to the observations of Dr. Miller, single tubes are found in which both micrococci and rod-shaped bacteria are seen. Inter-globular spaces, so often found in teeth immediately beneath the enamel, play an important part in caries by increasing the porosity of the dentine and leading to its rapid disintegration in a lateral direction; being one reason of the undermining of the enamel so common in caries commencing at the masticating surface.

Dr. Miller describes germs as penetrating into the inter-globular spaces, but in the many specimens I have examined, showing these spaces, I have never seen them occupied by stained micro-organisms, those contained in the tubes seeming to be arrested at the inter-globular spaces, and it does not appear as if they proliferated within them. Some specimens show a curious traverse splitting of the matrix at right angles to the tubes, oval spaces being formed having a very characteristic appearance.

Mr. C. Pound, of the Bacteriological Laboratory at King's College, London, who has cut and examined a great number of specimens of carious dentine, says, he has always found these oval spaces in teeth with dead pulps, and recognises a dead tooth by this particular appearance. I do not know how far this observation has been corroborated by other observers.

According to Dr. Miller there is always present in carious dentine, a zone of softened tissue in advance of the line of micro-organisms, separating the healthy from the infected tissue, this zone not corresponding in outline with that of the area infected. Messrs. Underwood and Milles, however, failed to detect any softening in tissue not attacked by micro-organisms, any tissue that was penetrated in the least degree by a sharp point, exhibiting these organisms under the microscope. They also inoculated nutrient gelatine with portions of the dentine taken from the extreme limits of the softened part, and found that an abundant growth of micro-organisms took place.

They therefore came to the conclusion that although, as these organisms secreted an acid capable of softening dentine, one would *à priori* expect to find a softened zone, it was very difficult to demonstrate, and if present, it existed to a microscopical extent only. In his latest work, Dr. Miller mentions as evidence of the existence of this zone, the fact that longitudinal sections of carious dentine stained with fuchsine, show large unstained portions of the tissue at the sides of the preparation. These specimens are evidently softened sufficiently to cut, although they contain no germs. The germs spread more quickly in the direction of the canals than sideways, as in this direction they can only make way through the narrow transverse branches of the tubuli, but the decalcifying acids can infiltrate the tissue in this direction with ease.

The same observer states that germs are able to penetrate into the tubuli of the normal tooth. The diameter of a tubule being larger than that of a micrococcus, there is no mechanical impediment to the penetration of germs, and with a high magnifying power a small number are sometimes seen, an advance guard, so to speak, which have penetrated into the normal tooth structure, without causing any changes in it. In absorbing milk-teeth germs are frequently seen to have penetrated into the open tubes for a short distance (Miller).

An appearance is often met with in longitudinal sections of carious teeth, the cause of which is not understood with any certainty. Short disconnected rods are seen, some lying scattered about in all directions, and others still within the tubes, lying at different angles to one another, like a pile of bricks in the act of falling. It is possible that these are casts of the tubes, especially as they disappear on the addition of dilute sulphuric acid. (Miller.) "They may on the other hand be portions of the consolidated fibrils, or of the sheath of Neumann which has broken up in this manner." (Tomes.)

In transverse sections the tubes are seen cut across and crowded with micro-organisms, and largely increased in diameter at the expense of the matrix. In many parts three or four tubes have run together, the matrix and parietes of the tube being destroyed.

There are some appearances in cross section which are difficult to explain. When several of these expanded canals approach one another they exhibit prismatic or angular forms, the intertubular substance having disappeared, but the limiting wall remaining intact. It is difficult to account for the disappearance of the matrix unless, as suggested by Dr. Miller, the germs form a pepsin-like diffusible element, which dissolves the intermediate substance, while Neumann's sheath is still intact.

Transverse sections also exhibit a peculiar condition, which has been described as the tobacco pipe appearance. Rounded masses of apparently homogeneous substance, which stains deeply, are seen to occupy the much expanded tubes, and in some specimens, micro-organisms in fine thread form, are seen running between and around them, leaving a clear circle of tissue uninvaded by the threads. This latter appearance is seen more frequently at the margins of the preparations where leptothrix forms are most abundant. It seems to be a kind of secondary encroachment of these thread forms on the matrix.

The Micro-organisms concerned in Caries.

According to Leber and Rottenstein the leptothrix buccalis, which is found abundantly in the mouth in the form of long thin threads and felted masses, is the principal organism concerned in dental caries.

This was disputed by later observers, although Dr. Miller, in a paper in the *Independent Practitioner*, speaks of a fungus which appeared as either micrococci, diplococci, bacteria, bacilli, or thread forms, and describes all these forms as sometimes found on a single thread, which he considered to prove their genetic connection But he nevertheless admits, that while there occur in the mouth both monomorphous and pleomorphous forms, stable forms, and forms that exhibit different transition stages, the majority of the micro-organisms found in caries are monomorphous.

Dr. Flügge (*Micro-Organisms*, English Edition, p. 393) says:—"It is evident that the designation leptothrix cannot be employed as a generic term, for the most various kinds of bacilli may produce these thread-like formations, and the threads which occur in the buccal secretions and in the deposit on the teeth, are probably nothing more than the thread form of various well-known, or still unknown and widely distributed bacilli.

"It is possible, for example, that bacillus butyricus not uncommonly takes part in the formation of leptothrix in the mouth; it is probable, however, that many other bacilli, more especially anærobic bacilli do the same."

He points out that leptothrix threads do not appear to belong to one individual species, showing variations in thickness, flexibility, &c., and that the bacilli which have been isolated from the mouth by cultivation are not the forms which produce the leptothrix; or may it not be possible that the same micro-organism which would produce threads in the mouth might fail to do so under changed and artificial conditions?

Recently Dr. Kreibohm (*Centralblatt f. Bacter.* vii, 1890) came to the conclusion, both from microscopical examination and from cultivation, that leptothrix merely represents a peculiar phase of growth of different schizomycetes; he found four forms to develope leptothrix, two of which were bacilli, and two short bacteria.

Dr. Miller in his last work says, "In short, the name leptothrix buccalis, does not apply to any germ with distinctive characteristics, and the name does deserve to be retained, since it has only been the expression of a confused and erroneous view."

Of twenty-two kinds of germs from the mouth isolated by Dr. Miller in 1885, ten were in the form of cocci (showing very different dimensions), five appear as shorter, six as longer staffs. One species formed spirilla, another grew out into long threads. Of thirty species cultivated subsequently, eighteen were cocci, eleven staffs, one formed threads. In fluids, three grew to long connected or unconnected threads, one formed spirilla, eight were motile, fourteen motionless. He could only discover spore formation in three, the others seemed to propagate themselves by transverse division.

They showed great variations in their relation to oxygen, ten only grew while there was free entrance of air, four grew better when exposed to the air, but could grow without it, eight seemed to grow well whether with or without oxygen. Eight produce colouring matter in gelatine cultures some days old, forming brick-yellow masses, such as may be seen occasionally on the buccal surface of teeth which are not kept well cleaned, the colouring matter being in the protoplasm or cell membrane, the cultivation medium not being coloured.

In the pigmentation which occurs in caries the germs remain colourless, while the tooth itself is coloured. These colours are not seen in early stages of caries, but only when it is far advanced, and usually when it is of a slow or chronic nature. Organic substances decomposed by micro-organisms assume a dark colour, and in experiments, which Professor Miller has made on this point, he has detected iron in these discoloured teeth

He says, "Whether in caries of the dentine and enamel, the iron salt is formed in sufficiently large quantities, for the discolourisation to be ascribed to that source has not yet been decisively ascertained."

Of the germs especially characterized by the formation of lactic acid in the mouth Dr. Miller has separated by cultivation twelve. He finds that "a great majority of the fungi found in the human mouth are capable of producing acid from cane or grape sugar, and it is probable that with very few exceptions, all can, when the proper conditions are presented to them."

He finds also that "the same fungus may produce an acid reaction in one substratum and an alkaline in another," and says, "In such a case we undoubtedly have two distinct processes going on, first, the nutrition of the organism accompanied by the appearance of alkaline products; secondly, its fermentative action, accompanied by acid products." He further points out that "under the various conditions and with the numerous fungi present in the human mouth the reaction may occasionally be neutral or alkaline, and this would give a temporary check to the advance of the caries." He considers that many of these fungi have a peptonizing action and that a number both possess this action, and are both capable of producing acid by fermentation of carbohydrates, and thus may be capable of producing the phenomena of caries in the mouth.

MM. Galippe and Vignal claim to have isolated six kinds of micro-organisms taken from the tubules of dentine. They thus continue :—Among these six kinds we have always met with four in every one of the eighteen we have examined. We have met with another kind eight times, and with a sixth five times. (1) The first kind constantly met with is a short, thick bacillus, not forming chains. (2) The second kind is a bacillus, which is about twice as long as it is broad. (3) The third kind is a bacillus, which is very like the preceding one in appearance, except that it has no constriction. (4) The fourth kind is a very short, very thin bacillus, nearly as broad as long; at first it would be taken for a coccus. (5) The micro-organism, which we have met with eight times, is a bacillus, which is rounded off at its ends. (6) The micro-organism, which we have met with only five times, is a rather large coccus. *Dental Record* Vol. IX. 1889.

The micro-organisms owe their rapid development to the secretions, deposits, &c., of the oral cavity, and not until the tissue of the tooth has undergone a certain change, first decalcification, second peptonization, can they adapt it to their nourishmeut. The decalcification is produced chiefly by acid, resulting from the action of the organisms upon certain carbohydrates in the human mouth, while the peptonization is produced either by the direct action of the protoplasm of the organisms upon the decalcified dentine, or by the action of a ferment which they produce. In the study and separation of the different germs in the mouth, the mass of material has been so great and the opportunities for error so varied, that it has been found impossible, with few exceptions, to classify them or decide their conditions of life. There is still an immense amount of work to be done in this direction, and this can only be accomplished by investigators who will take up the study of separate species and work out their individual life history.

Our more complete knowledge of the morbid changes in dental caries throws great light upon the predisposing and exciting causes of the disease. Sugar being the food of these acid-forming micro-organisms, all foods containing sugar, or starch, which is converted into sugar in the mouth, tend to increase the liability to decay of the teeth.

Some interesting observations of Dr. Miller's on this point show that the acids formed in the mouth by cooked starch are at least as destructive to the teeth as those formed by sugar. Saliva containing starch shows at blood temperature acid reaction in as short a time as that containing sugar, and in equal quantity. He points out that starch and starch-containing substances are more hurtful than sugar, because sugar, being easily soluble, soon flows away and is thus rendered harmless. Starch clings longer to the teeth and thus exercises a more enduring action than sugar. This is confirmed by the observations of Hesse on decay in bakers' teeth. Vegetables seem to be less fermentable in the raw state than when cooked, hence the cooking of food would seem to have an injurious effect in causing caries. Meat when decomposed in the mouth does not produce acid, and the observations of my father and others, on the agency of the food in the causation of caries, show that races whose food is confined almost exclusively to meat show a very low percentage of decay. Dr. Black's researches, however, point to a different conclusion, he says (Article on "Etiology of Caries, American System of Dentistry," vol. 1, p. 730) :—"Races of men who have eaten largely of acid fruits have had less decay of the teeth than those who have been debarred by their position or climate from the use of such articles of food. Generally those tribes that have subsisted largely on meat and grain have suffered more from caries than those that have had a more exclusively vegetable and fruit diet."

From the conditions of fermentation in the mouth, one would certainly expect to find more caries in vegetable and starch eaters generally, than in flesh eaters, but as Dr. Black says, "Our knowledge is too meagre to warrant any lengthy discussion on this point."

An irritated condition of the gum, giving rise to an acid secretion, is supposed by several writers to be a cause of caries, but this is disputed by Dr. Miller, who points out that in pyorrhœa alveolaris, where an irritated condition of the gum exists for months, caries seldom occurs, and where decay does occur in cases where there is considerable congestion and separation of the gum at the neck of the tooth, it may be explained by the lodgment of food.

Among the predisposing causes of caries, defective structure holds the first place; deep fissures and cavities in the enamel, imperfections in the dentine, especially interglobular spaces (increasing the porosity of the tissue) irregular position of teeth leading to the retention of food, are other predisposing causes. Many diseases which give rise to an acid reaction in the mouth must be included among these, especially also diseases giving rise to dryness, *e.g.*, typhoid fever.

A predisposition to decay of the teeth is said to be inherited. Dr. Miller considers that this is only possible in so far as the inheritance of ill-developed and irregularly placed teeth is possible.

The surgical treatment of dental caries by the thorough removal of the diseased tissue, the treatment of the cavity with an antiseptic, and the insertion of a material which by its density and applicability to the walls of the cavity shall thoroughly exclude the germs, is, so far as our present knowledge goes, the most complete cure for the disease.

We can scarcely maintain, however, that with the most careful manipulation every germ is removed, but any that are left under a tight fitting plug are cut off from their food supply and their further growth prevented, seeing that they are probably incapable of attacking dentine in the absence of carbohydrate.

The incorporation of antiseptic materials in fillings has lately received some attention, and perhaps more may yet be done in this direction. Whatever the care taken by operator we must all now and then meet with those most unsatisfactory cases where in spite of the most careful treatment decay rapidly progresses and filling seems to be only a partially successful mode of treatment. In such cases there is no doubt usually an undue porosity of the tissues of the tooth.

As to means of prevention, germicides, which can be used in the mouth of such a strength that they are not injurious to the system, have no very great penetrating power. The fermentative action of the micro-organisms at the bottom of cavities and fissures in the tooth is not interfered with by any mouth wash. In the mouth the difficulty of applying any thorough antiseptic treatment is very great, we may seal up a disinfectant in a pulp cavity very effectually, but it is impossible to obtain any prolonged and complete disinfection in the cavity of the mouth, such as is necessary for the prevention of caries. Thorough cleansing of the teeth is the most effectual means of preventing decay, and the experiment of Dr. Miller's above referred to, shows that by the use of antiseptic mouth washes, combined with thorough cleansing with tooth brush and silk, the amount of acid produced in the mouth may be very greatly reduced.

A NOTE CONCERNING THE ACTION OF CHLOROFORM.

By Dudley Wilmot Buxton, M.D., B.S.Lond.

Member of the Royal College of Physicians, Administrator of Anæsthetists in University College Hospital, the Hospital for Women, Soho Square, and the London Dental Hospital

(*Continued from page* 449).

We are now in a position to examine in more detail the work of the Chloroform Commission, not because its experiments present any great novelty or reveal any unfamiliar facts, but because the systematic record of its proceedings presents to us a convenient centre about which to collect the knowledge obtained during the past few years in this country, on the Continent, and the United States. Part II.* deals with experiments made, of which no graphic record was taken. 268 dogs and 31 monkeys were killed with chloroform which was given, under various circumstances, such as fasting after heavy meals, in different postures, with and without inhalers. The animals all died from stopping of respiration, and, according to the report, an interval of time, varying from two to six minutes elapsed before cardiac movements ceased. Slow and prolonged chloroformisation, asphyxial conditions, and struggling seemed to lessen the interval between the cessation of breathing and stopping of the heart's movements. The method of testing the failure of respiration is not mentioned; auscultation, and, in some cases, the placing of a needle in the heart muscle, was used to test cardiac action; while, in cases of doubt, the chest was laid open. Attempts at resuscitation were made after natural respiration had failed; but, as a rule, failed when resorted to after an interval of 60 seconds, being usually successful after 30 seconds' interval. The figures are: In forty-four cases, successful, after an average of 28·2 seconds after respiration had failed; thirty-eight cases, unsuccessful, after an average of 31·5 seconds. These facts are highly significant. We shall see that chloroform acts directly upon the heart-muscle, and up to a certain point this action can be carried without grave results; beyond that point one of two things happens: failure gradually results whether respiration goes on or not, or the heart remains able to maintain the circulation, so long as a low tension persists, but as soon as reaction occurs, and the general vascular tone revives, the greater stress laid

---

* *Lancet, Jan.* 18, 1890.

upon the heart leads to the utter extinction of its action, and cardiac syncope takes place. The occurrence of death in this last way accounts for fatalities, common enough, occurring as the patient, after a surgical operation, is beginning to come round. The animals in which the respiration failed before the heart were, none the less killed by heart-syncope, for, whereas the respiratory failure resulted from poisoning of the respiratory centres in the medulla concurrent, action upon the heart-muscle was going on, and, although perfect artificial respiration was performed, the heart-muscle, being poisoned, failed. To understand this, one has to be familiar with the following facts, which are daily noted in the physiological laboratory: that artificial respiration will keep a dog or monkey alive for hours, if the heart be not poisoned by chloroform, even when the medullary centres are quite inactive; and, secondly, that dogs, especially, are difficult to save when once breathing has ceased, even though prompt resort be had to artificial respiration.

Again, the animals subjected to slow and prolonged chloroformisation, and those which struggled, incurred cardiac syncope most rapidly. Here, again, we find evidence of my contention. The prolonged action of the chloroform upon the heart led to the pathological changes which give rise to syncope while, in the struggling animals, a greater strain was imposed upon an already enfeebled heart, and hence early syncope obtained.

Turning to the experiments, the results of which were recorded by apparatus, we are informed that, in a certain number of cases, "the animal died accidentally before it was ready to be attached to the manometer" (used for taking blood pressure curves). These deaths, as was noticed above, may or may not have been due to primary heart failure.

The objects kept in view during these experiments were five n number:—

I.—To test suitability and safety of chloroform as an anæsthetic. To establish some comparison, experiments were made with ether and the A.C.E mixture (presumably that of the Medico-Chirurgical Society Committee on Chloroform, 1864); but as the commission themselves admit the experiments were insufficient to afford a complete exposition of the action of these drugs, as a matter of fact the ether and A.C.E. experiments may be disregarded, for they are not only too few to be of the least value but were conducted in a very unsatisfactory manner.

II.—The effect of pushing the anæsthetics (*a.*) to a dangerous degree, (*b.*) until failure of respiration, (*c.*) to death.

III.—Modification in symptoms caused by anæsthetics when complicated by asphyxia ; by pressure of other drugs, the alkaloids, &c. These last experiments do not concern us.

IV.—To test the alleged liability to primary syncope, to secondary syncope, to reflex syncope through shock : the effect of fatty heart ; hæmorrhage, &c.

V.—To test the effect of the anæsthetics on various animals, especially monkeys, as being the closest allied to human beings.

In eight experiments, animals were anæsthetised until death took place. The open method was employed and the anæsthetic pushed until respiration failed. It was noticed in these cases that the heart's action stopped about 3 min. 27·5 sec., on an average, after failure of respiration.

It will be noted that the animals were treated as human beings are treated, and it is not surprising they died in the most usual way, namely, from respiratory failure. All who have, like myself, had abundant opportunities of studying the behaviour of dogs and monkeys under chloroform will recognise that the phenomena, somewhat elaborated by the commission, are very familiar, and even the relation of respiration to circulation will appear less novel than the report would seem to imply must be the case. In these experiments blood pressure fell, the heart, after primary stimulation, became feeble, the systolic contraction of the ventricles being gradually lessened.

(*To be concluded.*)

"A NEW LOW-FUSING CONTINUOUS GUM."

By George Cunningham, M.A.Cantab , L.D.S.Eng., D.M.D.

Abstract of a paper read before the International Medical Congress, Berlin, 1890.

A reference to the formulæ for continuous gum work, as given in vol. II of the American System of Dental Surgery, shows that they consist of ingredients of very different degrees of fusibility, and it seems to me that such ingredients as cryolite, Bohemian glass, and flint glass are added for the purpose of reducing the fusibility of the more refractory ingredients, such as silica or quartz, kaolin and spar. I therefore instituted a series of experiments, the very opposite, that is, adding the more refractory substances to give stamina and cohesion to glass as a basis. With the help and assistance of Mr. Harry Powell, of the White Friars Glass Works, I succeeded in producing a body of enamel capable of fusing at a relatively low temperature, and by which, just as we match teeth, it will be almost as easy to match the varying colours of gum. The new materials can be fused on copper, dental alloy, and gold, but it was soon found that platinum was the only material practically available, for two reasons. Firstly:—on heating, chemical change, causing discoloration, took place between the ingredients of the enamel and metallic base, except in the case of platinum and pure gold, and though this might possibly be obviated by using a glass which did not contain silicate of lead, it was considered advisable to keep to flint glass as a basis on the score of its strength and practical insolubility in the mouth. This discoloration seems to be due to an oxidising of the metal under the influence of heat, and the metallic oxide thus formed, imparting its color to the vitreous enamel. Secondly:—the coefficient of expansion of platinum and glass being the same, platinum must possess obvious advantages, especially as to adhesion, over any other material. If it be desired to give the denture the more acceptable appearance of gold it may be done by sweating a piece of pure gold and pure platinum together, and rolling them out in the mills to the desired gauge, the enamel is fused upon the platinum surface, leaving an exposed surface of pure gold. On dental alloy, the enamel simply flakes off as the specimen cools.

The method of use is briefly described as follows:—The teeth are mounted as usual in wax, the case is then set teeth downwards on a base of plaster, sand and fire clay, equal parts, the investment being carried over so as to embrace the tops of the teeth, and thus to hold them in position. The wax is then removed in the usual way, and the body built up around the teeth. Although the enamel seems to adhere with tolerable firmness to the smooth platinum plate, it is better to increase its attachment by either stippling the plate or forming a boundary for the material by means either of a turned-up edge, or soldering to the plate a ring of triangular platinum wire with pure gold. For full, but especially for partial dentures, both upper and lower, this new material seems to afford a great and important sphere of usefulness for the excellent English tube work. The plate is struck up in platinum, and instead of gold, platinum pins are mounted in the usual way, only soldered with pure gold. No fine fitting of the teeth to the plate is necessary, as the body does that more effectually than the most expert manipulator of the corundum wheel. The use of sulphur cement, and the working loose of the teeth is also obviated, since they are held firmly in position by the body and the enamel. The general excellence of ordinary tube work is further improved by the filling up of all spaces where the food might lodge, without impairing in any way the utility and strength of the older method ; the artistic coloring of the restored gum is a great advance on the often unsightly long rooted tube teeth. With regard to firing, I use at present a platinum muffle adapted to the ordinary small Fletcher's muffle furnace.* This is simply an ordinary draught gas and air furnace, and the whole process of firing can be accomplished in about a quarter of an hour, though it is sometimes advisable to take a little longer time. In regard to annealing, I have so far found little difference in cases which have been slowly or quickly annealed. Some dentists and experts have predicted that this material will not last in the mouth. The almost universal receptacle for fluids of all kinds, whether acids or alkalies, is a bottle made of flint or other glass. To all practical intents and purposes, this new continuous gum is flint glass, and, therefore I think that the acknowledged fractional solubility of flint glass in weak alkaline solutions will not prove a serious drawback to the employment of the process. With regard to the production of different colours, a very considerable modification of each colour from a darker to a lighter shade may be obtained by means of rubbing down with a muller, or ground glass, or the gum given a mottled appearance in other ways. In conclusion, although I do not claim this new material to be superior to continuous gum work as at present used by experts, yet it is capable of replacing with advantage to the patient, and with facility to the dentist some of the less artistic ordinary products of the dental laboratory.

---

* A special muffle and furnace is being designed.

EXTRACTS

ON THE DANGERS ARISING FROM SYPHILIS IN THE PRACTICE OF DENTISTRY.

By L. Duncan Bulkley, A.M., M.D.,

Attending Physician to the New York Skin and Cancer Hospital, etc.

(*Continued from page* 464.)

He could not locate the exact date of the injury to the tongue by the dental instruments, but work had been done in that locality, and he remembered the instrument occasionally slipping, as will often happen, inflicting injury to the soft parts. He was a married man with a family, and was very desirous of learning how he had become infected; he had certainly not been exposed in sexual intercourse, nor in any other manner which we could discover.

The interesting points in the case are: First, that while the proof is not absolute that he was infected in the dentist's chair, still the circumstantial evidence is so strong that little, if any, doubt can be entertained that the poison came through this channel. The habits and ways of the particular dentist were such that poisonous material from the mouth of a previous syphilitic patient could readily have been transferred on instruments or otherwise to the wound made in the tongue, either by the sharp teeth or by a slip of an instrument. The second interesting point is that this patient, before the true nature of the disease was ascertained, had been to his own regular dentist for smoothing the teeth, and so had certainly exposed him, and others through him, to the poison, which was secreted freely from the raw surface of the chancre.

The earliest recorded cases of the transmission of syphilis in dental operations are in connection with the transplantation of teeth, during the last quarter of the eighteenth century.

Sir William Watson* published a case of this description, and John Hunter† relates two similar cases about which there can be no doubt. J. C. Lettsom‡ also recorded three cases: of these one was personal, one seen by a Dr. Hamilton, and the third occurred in

---

* Watson, "Transactions of College Surgeons," 1785, iii. p. 328.

† Hunter, "Treatise on the Venereal Disease," 1st Engl. ed., 1786; 1st Amer. ed., Phil., 1818, p. 362.

‡ Lettsom, *Transactions, Lond. Med. Soc.*, vol. i. 1787, p. 137.

America, having been observed by Kühn in Philadelphia; these gentlemen furnished notes of the cases to Dr. Lettsom. This mode of transmission does not occur again in literature, to the knowledge of the writer, although Gibier* says that "Cases have been recently related." In view, however, of a recent revival of the operation of tooth transplantation, or implantation, it is quite possible that the future may furnish fresh instances of this mode of the innocent acquiring of syphilis.

From this period no other causes of the transmission of syphilis through dental procedures are found recorded for nearly a century; indeed, not until the advent of modern operative dentistry and active medical observation.

The first case met with is one reported by Dr. C. W. Dulles,† of Philadelphia, and which was also seen by the late Dr. Maury. The patient, a female domestic, of excellent character, developed a chancre of the lip two weeks after a visit to a dentist; on that occasion he extracted a tooth, and later did some cleansing of the teeth. Although no confirmation was obtained, it seemed reasonable to suppose that the operation of extraction was in some way responsible for inoculation.

Dr. F. N. Otis‡ also mentions a chancre of the lip which occurred in a gentleman "about three weeks after a morning spent in a dentist's chair."

Lancereaux§ relates a similar case of chancre of the lower lip in a women, after extraction of a tooth and other dental work, and Giovannini,|| of Bologna, has reported a chancre of the lip apparently from a dentist's instrument.

Leloir¶ mentions having seen a man with chancre of the gum, in whom the infection seemed to have taken place in consequence of cleaning and filling a cavity in a tooth with soiled instruments. Lydston** has likewise reported the case of a woman with syphilis,

---

* Gibier, "Ann. de Dermatt. et de Syph.," 1882, p. 129.

† Dulles, *Phil. Med. and Surg. Reporter*, Jan., 1878.

‡ Otis, "Lectures on Syphilis," New York, 1881, p. 102.

§ Lancereaux, "Proc. Acad. de Méd. de Paris," *Union Méd.*, 1889, xlviii. p. 655.

|| Giovannini, "La Sperimentale," 1889, p. 262.

¶ Leloir, "Leçon sur la Syphilis," 1886, p. 62.

** Lydston, *Journ. Amer. Med Assoc.*, 1886, vi. p. 654.

in whom the chancre on the gum, below the lower middle incisors, appeared to be the result of some cleaning and repairing of the teeth done three weeks previously; the glands beneath the jaw were enlarged, beginning a week or more after the appearance of the sore on the gum.

Roddick,* of Montreal, has recorded a case of more than usual interest, where the primary syphilitic sore on the gum was undoubtedly the result of inoculation by means of dental forceps used in extracting a tooth; it is worth mentioning somewhat in detail. The patient was the wife of a physician, aged about thirty, and the mother of healthy children. She had always been in excellent health until about a year previous to her visit, when she had a tooth extracted, the operation being difficult and accompanied by considerable laceration of the gum. The wound showed no tendency to heal, but became sloughy and indurated. Within a few weeks the glands beneath the jaw were found to be enlarged, and shortly an erythematous rash covered the body and extremities, followed later by a papular and squamous eruption, and sore throat and alopecia were soon added, to complete the picture of constitutional syphilis. Careful investigation failed to reveal any other source of contagion than the dental operation; the husband was entirely free from disease, and Dr. Roddick, who is an exceptionally careful man, and thoroughly qualified to judge, concluded that "in all probability the instrument used by the dentist was made the vehicle of contagion by being brought in contact with a mucous patch in the mouth of a syphilitic person previously operated upon."

2. Dangers to the *dental operator* from exposure to the syphilitic poison.

In the second division of this portion of our subject, namely, the dangers from syphilis to the operator in dental procedures, the number of instances on record is fewer, but they are very striking and well authenticated.

The first instance discovered was that of a dentist who reported his own case.† The inoculation took place on the middle finger of the left hand, above the nail, which was followed by constitutional syphilis. He could not trace the infection to any particular patient,

---

* Roddick, *Montreal Med. Journ.*, August, 1888, p. 93.

† *Boston Med. and Surg. Journ.*, vol. lviii. p. 38.

but there could be no doubt that the poison came from mucous patches in some one's mouth, which lodged in one of the little cracks which so commonly come about the root of the nail.

Bumstead,* when speaking of the digital inoculation of accoucheurs, says that he has "known dentists to suffer in the same manner."

Neumann† knew of a dentist who tore his hand on a sharp tooth while operating on a syphilitic patient, which injury was followed by severe syphilis.

Jonathan Hutchinson,‡ in his excellent little clinical work on Syphilis, gives a plate of a well-marked circular indurated chancre on the pulp of the finger of a dentist, which had been produced by a scratch on a patient's tooth.

Dr. Otis has, recently, in a personal communication to me, related the following case, which is of peculiar interest, as it illustrates a method of infection in dentists which has not been previously noted. Mr. C., a dentist in large practice, applied for treatment with a chancre on the lips, accompanied with a general syphilitic eruption; his wife also contracted a chancre on the lip from him, with subsequent general syphilis. The infection was traced to a patient whom he had operated upon, who had in the mouth a suspicious sore, claimed to be a "canker sore," but found afterwards to be syphilitic. The dentist was in the habit of occasionally holding instruments between the lips while operating, and the poison was conveyed thus to his lips by an instrument infected from the patient.

Although the number of these recorded instances of syphilis communicated in dentistry, which I have been able to find, after a very careful study of the subject during several years past, is relatively small, it is yet quite sufficient to establish the fact that such infection does occasionally take place, and to place us on our guard against such accidents in future. Undoubtedly but few of the cases occurring have ever found their way into print, and it is possible that when special attention has been called to the subject many more of them will be recognised and reported.

Having now considered the clinical basis on which rest the grounds for believing that there are dangers arising from syphilis

---

* Bumstead, "Venereal Diseases," edition of 1879, p. 432.

† Neumann, *Allg. Wien Med. Zeitung*, 1884, p. 61.

‡ Hutchinson, "Syphilis," London, 1887, plate ii., Fig. 2, p. 96.

in the practice of dentistry, we will examine the modes in which this accident can arise, and then consider the means for preventing the occurrence of this sad event.

Two methods of the non-venereal transmission of syphilitic virus are recognised, namely: First, the *direct*, and second, the *indirect*.

1. *Direct syphilitic inoculation.*—In the first instance the poison is transferred directly from one individual to another, either through already existing wounds or in those occasioned at the time. The number of recorded cases of the communication of syphilis by kissing is now very great; hundreds can be found in literature, and I myself have seen over thirty cases of chancre of the lips. Infants at the breast of syphilitic nurses frequently acquire the disease, and breast-drawing by adults has given rise to numberless cases. In several series of instances syphilis has been both acquired and given by the application of the tongue to the eye to remove foreign particles and to heal disease; the poison has also been acquired and given in the process of wound-sucking, and other more rare modes of transmission which have been reported could be enumerated did time permit.

The particular method which is, perhaps, of most interest to us in the present connection is that of tooth wounds. The number of cases of this class which are on record is very great. Nearly all of them are from bites, usually intentional, and details of these need not be presented here. There are also a number where the infection has taken place from a blow on the mouth, the knuckles being wounded by the teeth. The first of these tooth-wound cases was observed near the beginning of the century by Boyer* but not reported until 1840 by his son. Since that time a number of observers have recorded cases, some of whom have each seen several. Thus, Gamberini† saw three cases, C. Pellizzari‡ three cases, Van Harlingen § five cases, Lavergne and Perrin || five cases, Lesage ¶

* Boyer, *Gaz. Méd. de Paris*; Behrend's "Syphilidology," 1841, iii. p. 322.

† Gamberini, "Gior. ital. d. mal. ven.," 1878, p. 365.

‡ Pellizzari, "Gior. ital. d. mal. ven." 1882.

§ Van Harlingen, *Phil. Med. Times*, 1884-85, xv. p. 80.

|| Lavergne et Perrin, "Ann. de Derm. et de Syph.," 1884, 2d. Series, v. p. 332.

¶ Lesage, "Chancre par morsure," *These de Paris*, 1885.

three cases, Finger * four cases, and Jonathan Hutchinson † three or four cases.

In this connection may also be mentioned the fact that surgeons have repeatedly been inoculated in wounds occurring accidentally during operations on syphilitics, as also in other wounds when examining those with the disease.

When we consider the relatively large number of physicians and surgeons who have become thus accidentally inoculated in the discharge of professional duties (and I myself have seen at least seven or eight cases), the only wonder is that the accident does not occur oftener to dentists, whose fingers are continually bathed in the buccal secretions, often from mouths with active and intensely contagious syphilitic lesions.

Syphilis is rarely communicated to the patient in dental operations by the direct or immediate method of contact, although the cases of the communication of syphilis by tooth transplantation, already referred to, were probably by the direct method, the poison being undoubtedly carried directly in the transplanted tooth from a syphilitic to a healthy person, as the tooth was then inserted quickly after its removal.

It would also be possible for a dentist with an unrecognised chancre on the finger, in an early stage, to communicate the poison directly to a patient's mouth, as in the case of midwives, already mentioned; but no such instance has been found in literature.

2. *Indirect Syphilitic inoculation.*—The second, indirect or mediate, method of contagion is that which usually takes place in cases where the disease is transmitted during the operations of dentistry, and, indeed, in a very large proportion of the cases of syphilis innocently acquired.

Time and space would fail to tell of even a small share of the methods of mediate contagion of syphilis which are scattered throughout literature, but a brief statement of some of the principal modes by which it has been observed to be conveyed innocently from one person to another may aid us in understanding how the accident can occur in connection with dental operations.

(*To be concluded.*)

---

* Finger, "Die ven, Krankheiten," 1886, p. 14.

† jonathan Hutchinson, "Syphilis," London, 1887.

THE DENTAL RECORD, LONDON: NOV. 1, 1890.

Ambidexterity.

THERE are perhaps few accomplishments so useful to a dentist as the power of employing at will the left as well as the right hand. And yet comparatively few persons acquire the facility of using the hands inter-changeably. It is a very curious circumstance that the neglected use of the left member seems to be the result of a widespread aversion to the practice of replacing it for its neighbour. We go a long way back in history, when we attempt to discover a period when the hands were regarded as of equal value. The very words *right* and *left*, and their analogues in the dead and continental languages, imply something underhanded in connection with those who work with the left, but uprightness, probity and straightforwardness when the right hand is employed. Dexterity suggests aptitude and skilled performance of some delicate manipulation, whilst the sinister action connotes, it may be skill, but brought to bear in a way that is not for the benefit of the persons concerned. A left-handed blow is a blow in the dark, and many are the curious charms, invocations to evil spirits, which constitute a large portion of the folk lore in the less civilised villages in the United Kingdoms containing directions where the word "left" appears figuring in a truly sinister way. However, it would seem that prejudice enters in no small measure into the causation of the disrepute into which the left hand has fallen. The majority of individuals are content to employ half their faculties and half their manual possibilities. Custom, it would appear, has induced mankind to favor the "right" and neglect the "left," a neglect which has resulted in a less skill and adroitness in that hand; hence has arisen clumsiness, ineptitude, or even manipulative failure, and from these of course, obloquy. How far nature has given us a bias towards adroitness, that is right-handed action, is a moot point, for children as a rule employ one or the other hand, apparently as the fancy dictates, until taught by the minatory slaps from the guardians of their tender years. Indeed, the frequency with which children evince ambidexterity encourages the belief that this faculty is almost inherent in the average individual. Many of our readers may remember how strongly the late Charles Reade, the novelist, insisted upon this. Even if the natural state of affairs is that the majority of mankind are born, grow up and die right-handed, there can be very little doubt that careful training, more especially during youth, can accomplish almost perfect ambidexterity. The degree of success in any given case will of course depend upon the general handiness of the individual. The average man bungles at threading a needle, a feat which is accomplished without apparent effort by the most unneat-handed of Phyllises. Here education and use come in, and it is the object of the present article to insist upon the value to dentists of educating the left hand to do what the right hand is capable of doing. The enormous power of substitution in nature cannot but prove to us that we are dependent upon one set of members only so far as we neglect making use of auxiliaries. Handless monsters acquire a nicety of touch and facility of use with the toes, which carries them to the fore front of skilled workers with paint brush, pencil, etc. Persons afflicted with writers' cramp, and those who have, through accident, lost the use of their right hand, soon acquire the art of writing and drawing, and general manipulation with their left. The spur which necessity brings to bear in these cases would not be needed were a commonsense view of the matter taken by mankind at large, and the young of either sex duly instructed in the use of both hands. We do not for the moment wish to imply that ambidexterity may not be acquired in later life, and would urge our readers, as far as possible, to cultivate the left hand, unless they should be what is called "left handed," for then the right hand should receive its share of the useful, if irksome, training. None but those who have tried it will be able to appreciate the usefulness of ambidexterity in dentistry. It enables difficult manipulations to be performed with increased facility, and forms the means of lessening the labour and relieving the monotony of prolonged operations.

Dr. W. D. Miller upon the Action of Antiseptics on the Pulp.

Dr. W. D. Miller, who was recently in London on his way back to Berlin from America, kindly consented to give some account of the experiments he has been conducting with reference to the action of certain antiseptic substances upon the pulp. Accordingly, on the 20th ult. he took Dr. Cunningham's place in the Operative Dental Surgery Class at the National Dental Hospital, and several gentlemen unconnected with the school also availed themselves of the opportunity to be present. Although the lecturer had none of his original preparations with him he was able to make use of some photographs of them which were already in England, and these were thrown upon a screen with an oxyhydrogen lantern by Messrs. Mummery and Cunningham. By the same process some of the actual culture plates were also exhibited.

Dr. Miller has experimented with a large number of substances which have been supposed to exert an antiseptic action. Without going through the whole list, we may say that the two practical points laid before the audience were the inability of iodoform to render aseptic and the satisfactory results obtained with corrosive sublimate.

One of the modes of experiment consists in putting the pulp of a calf's tooth into a small glass tube, drawn out to a fine point at one end to represent the apical foramen. The pulp, over an inch in length, is then inoculated at this point, whilst the supposed antiseptic is applied to the surface at the top, which is then closed with wax, and the whole placed in a much larger tube containing agar-agar at the bottom; the point of the smaller tube extends into this well below the surface. The test-tube is kept in an incubator, and the condition of the pulp can be kept under observation. After a period, varying from a few days to many weeks, the small tube is opened and the pulp transferred to a plate of agar-agar. The value of the antiseptic used will be made manifest according as the absence or growth of bacteria is observed.

Dr. Miller holds strongly that some such method as this is necessary in order to determine the real action of antiseptics, and that it is impossible to rely upon the statements of practitioners as to results obtained with patients. A photograph was shown of a pulp which had been actually rolled in iodoform, but which was seen to be covered with bacteria; whilst another, treated with sublimate, remained quite sterile, and showed its borders clearly defined. With regard to the latter, it was said that if a small quantity of the sublimate, in powder, be applied to a pulp, it will penetrate the whole substance within forty-eight hours, and turn it into a stiff mass, which does not undergo decomposition.

Dr. Miller also took the opportunity of showing upon the screen a section of dentine in which artificial caries had been produced, and at the close of the lecture replied to various criticisms and questions.

The Mechanical Workroom of the Dental Hospital of London.

THE winter session commences with an entry of 35 students. The entry last summer being 14, makes 49 new students during the past year.

The authorities, having in view the best possible professional education of the dental student, have, during the summer, caused to be constructed a very good workroom, or rather series of three rooms, well fitted in every particular with the most improved apparatus for mechanical dentistry.

Mr. A. J. Watts has been appointed superintendent demonstrator, and will be in attendance from 9 to 6 daily, to superintend all work done in that department. In order that the work may be completed independently of weather, the rooms are fitted with the electric light, and we already hear talk about the desirability of using that light for the whole hospital. (We hope this may soon be accomplished.)

The new rooms were formally opened on Oct. 20th, and work will really commence on Nov. 1st.

The Dental Hospital of London is to be congratulated on having taken the bull by the horns and fearlessly set to work to solve a very difficult question. We have seen and carefully considered the regulations made by the executive to prevent abuse by patients of the charitable supply of artificial work, and we believe that they solve the question most successfully of how to prevent undeserving claimants obtaining benefits from the hospital. There appears to be a great future before such an undertaking, for it supplies a first-rate school within which means are afforded to educate the dental mechanic of the future, while the opportunities for experience offered to the students of the hospital should be eagerly sought by all those whose heart is in their work.

The students of the hospital wishing to use the new rooms and gain the experience to be had in the matter of making and filling in of dentures will, we understand, be appointed "dental appliance dressers," each surgeon and assistant surgeon being supplied with such dressers, and they will construct and follow the denture under the supervision of the officer of the day.

CORRESPONDENCE.

[We do not hold ourselves responsible in any way for the opinions expressed by our correspondents.]

"HOW TO DEAL WITH ANOTHER MAN'S PATIENTS."

To the Editor of "THE DENTAL RECORD."

SIR,—In compliance with the desire expressed by the writer, that this subject be "thrashed out through the columns of our Correspondence," I venture to take up my pen, and my very first observation would be that we can best deal with such a question by looking at it from the opposite point of view, "How *not* to deal," &c.

I think we will concede that the men whose lives are actuated more by principle than self-interest hardly need any code of ethics.

To all such, actuated by broad and generous—not to say lofty views—there can never be the slightest temptation; and, I venture to say, that some of the noble men whose lives have been devoted to the furtherance of the good of their profession—nay, even the silent ones, backward ever in pushing forward—gentlemen in virtue of their professional conduct, for all that—would equally read with surprise that it was thought necessary to frame a code for the use of professional men.

Perhaps they are old fogeys who have started with "Love thy neighbour as thyself" as the keynote of life—but surely, to all such the need of a sermon on "Man's duty to his neighbour," in the form of ghostly tracts on professional conduct (misconduct, rather!) "turned by application to a libel" (as Hood has it about religious tracts)—is not very obvious.

It is the writer's good fortune to have been associated with a few of the very best men in the profession, at a time when professional habits were still forming, and he has ever observed that modesty not assurance, honour not greed, marked them with the stamp of gentlemen in dealing with their professional brethren.

I remember one of them—now abroad—laughingly saying, that, when called on to give an adverse opinion, it was well to bear in mind the quaint observation of a "junior," who, it appears, once had to submit to the process at the hands of his senior (and I think before the patient), and who afterwards remarked to a friend: "By Jove! he kicked me into the cellar so politely and kindly, that I felt as if he was leading me upstairs to the drawing room."

I commend this story to all who wish to know how to do an unpleasant professional duty when it is *forced* upon them.

The writer observes that, "it is accepted by professional men as being quite outside the bounds of etiquette to criticise unfavourably the work of another duly qualified practitioner."

I can't help a smile when I read this in the light of the Scriptural words, "Do good unto all men—especially to those who are of the household of the faith." In *our* case, "especially to duly qualified practitioners."

Well, it is not a bad way, perhaps, to put it, but fancy how diluted and watery "Love thy neighbour," especially &c., would sound, "as thyself," brings it *home* to all men worthy of the name.

For even the so-called quack may be a capital operator, or do very excellent mechanical work. I have been asked my opinion in such a case, and, *once* at the risk of offending against professional feeling, I said, "The work is very well done indeed."

Sometimes this is hard to do, when, as in the instance I allude to the practitioner was a "Yankee," advertising right and left, and no doubt making capital, by running down his English professional brother, in order to praise *Self*—and practising but a few yards off. I was asked to speak, and—the patient returned to Mr. Yankee to have the rest of the work completed. Perhaps I went rather too far in this, but a patient of mine begged me for her sake to see the case, trusting absolutely in my verdict. Had I "damned with faint praise," I could have "grabbed" that patient who was paying *full* fees, but I simply spoke out: "I don't much like the man, but his work is very well done; go back and let him finish your teeth—since you have no objection to his fees." And I have *never* regretted my action.

Let us, however, be practical, and see how it looks when a duly qualified practitioner so lowers himself, and alas, one hears of some sad sinners—successful sinners, too—who, apparently, have more work to do than they can well accomplish, and whose cry like that of the horse-leech seems to be ever the same, Give! Give!!

From practitioners who have suffered at their hands, and from patients who have successfully evaded their wiles, the writer has heard some sickening details of "how not to do it." Here is a case.

A lady presented herself, an old tooth having given away and required filling.

D. Q. P. (duly qualified practicioner) begins a systematic examination. "Very bad work here; this filling also very roughly done; that one abominable"; and so on.

Patient (a woman in a thousand) sat tight, and only said, "Will you kindly attend to the broken down tooth first." This finished, paid her guinea, and went to her family dentist whenever she returned home. Family dentist of excellent and deserved repute, being invited to look round, found everything in order. Patient, to his surprise, renewed her request, and in amazement the request was complied with increased vigilance in the second inspection. "I find, as I before said, that you can go on for six or twelve months in perfect safety." And then, to his horror, the patient related how this usurious "brother" (save the mark) wanted to remove all *his* fillings in order to make money, knowing that he could only achieve this by first ruining the reputation of a highly respectable practitioner. This is no fable, but true, and I only wish we dared publish the name of *that* professional charlatan, as a warning to evil doers.

This is a glaring case, one of many told of the very practitioner, who has acquired quite a reputation by reason of the scorn with which he treats the work of others, when addressing the bewildered patients—who seem to swallow all that sort of nonsense only too greedily, regarding it as a proof of *skill*, instead of *cunning*.

In its lesser forms it is only less objectionable, that is all. Now, where self-interest is clearly and wholly absent, and where a man's life is spent in the opposite direction, I admit that even such a practitioner may be placed in a very awkward predicament, occasionally.

Mr. A., for instance, is a D. Q. P., but he has the misfortune to be losing his sight, or his health has given way, and he can't bring himself to abandon his work; for, blind as he is, or weak as he may be, he *has* to win the bread by which his family lives. A patient of our own, an old friend as well as patient, goes to him when away from home, and returns to *you*, and in that full confidence which she reposes in your simple word, frankly tells you that, being in the town of ——, and feeling something wrong, she went to Mr. A.; "but since he filled my teeth I never feel quite comfortable, and can no longer use my tooth-pick, whilst the gums feel sore and inflamed."

You examine. An old amalgam filling had tumbled out of a distal cavity in the first left lower molar, exposing decay in the anterior surface of the second molar: both had been cut away, but the two were filled with Sullivan's amalgam *as one*, and this big black bridge of solid metal presses hard on the gum, and is, all round, very bad work. If asked, "Is it all right? Is the work such as *you* approve of?" What can one say, where truth itself is a libel?

I merely quote this as a sample. Again, a man may be a drunkard, and still a D. Q. P., and a patient may have the misfortune to consult *him* when he is in his cups, with the inevitable result, "Smash! likewise crash!" I ask (I do not in *any* case wish to lay down the law), is it unfair to condemn the unprofessional conduct of *such* practitioners when we are consulted, and *paid* for giving a professional opinion. I have never, so far as I know, been in such a fix, but I can imagine it all the same, and what I seem to see is the plain fact that "you can't put honourable principles into the heart of a knave," and that the only way in which the professional etiquette of the rising generation and of all future generations is to be raised: is by their teachers, and heads of the profession generally, showing them a high example, and instilling into their young minds the utter meanness, shabbiness, and degradation of all such practices, and the value of *character* in professional life.

Those who have high instincts in youth will never forsake them in after years in order to fill their pockets, or add to their reputations, by running down the work of *any honest brother* doing his *best* according to his lights.

The young man fresh from the irons is apt to scorn the work of, perhaps, his own father. When old age or infirmity comes to *him*, how will *he* like it? Therefore, even *prudence* would suggest modesty in lieu of self-sufficiency.

As for fixed "Codes of Etiquette," they are impracticable, but they are also useless, seeing that where most needed, they are tossed aside unread, and in no case can they be *enforced*. "By what *compulsion* shall I, tell me that?" You may look as long and as longingly as you like at a sow's ear. You "gets no farder" in the direction of fashioning silk purses out of its structure.

Every man can be in virtue of his actions, a *gentleman*, and he who is *this*, requires no code of professional etiquette to guide him in his life

It is melancholy, but the fact, that as the jostling crowd thickens, the temptation increases to push your brother to the wall in order to get past him. Thackeray saw all this when he wrote :—

> "Who misses or who wins the prize,
> Go lose, or conquer as you can,
> But if you fail, or if you rise,
> Be each—pray God—a gentleman."

Is *this* not "the little leaven which leaveneth the whole lump?"

If the inculcation of principles like this won't stir the soul to honourable deeds, will dry "codes" succeed? Let us live—*and let live*.

I am, &c., A "D. Q. P."

[D. Q. P. is in error if he supposes we advocated the codification of a system of dental ethics; we advocated the discussion of how to deal with recognised difficulties which often occur between professional men as regards patients. He has missed the spirit of our remark, that professional etiquette demands reticence about the work of another professional. When the work has been scamped, and the patient applies to the other practitioner for an opinion, he may be compelled to blame; but as a rule the difficulty is easily met by tact, without a whole-hearted damnatory criticism of work, which may be badly done through the patient's own wilfulness—through no fault of the dentist.—Ed.]

To the Editor of the Dental Record.

Sir,—Many will have been glad to read your Editorial remarks with regard to the treatment of another man's patients, and some, I hope, will appreciate the invitation to your "Correspondence" columns. Most will agree that one duly qualified practitioner must not criticise unfavourably the work of another, especially if not invited. May we not go still further and formulate a reply when we *are* asked? If a reply of praise be not available, would not it be honourable to the professional brother and at the same time not dishonest to the patient, to say that inasmuch as one had not the opportunity of judging of all the conditions antecedent to the treatment, it is impossible to pronounce a trustworthy opinion? This, said without a sneer, would not damn with faint praise, and would be a properly scientific position to assume. With regard to the more difficult cases where there is reason to believe the patient has suffered at the hands of a quack, and may do so again, it is equally right to be cautious. A conscientious practitioner may feel it his duty to advise and warn for the future, but it will be well if he can do this without referring too much to the past. If he be a wise man he will not play too strongly for his own hand; such conduct will easily be seen through, and the effect of his sermon will recoil upon himself. It may be a pity the public are so ignorant. The process of education must be gradual; we can only assist. *Caveat emptor* is still a legal maxim.

I am, Sir, &c., SIGMA.

WHAT CONSTITUTES A RANULA?

To the Editor of the Dental Record.

Sir,—Mr. Tod hopes for discussion upon this point. Is it not a question of nomenclature? Mr. Tod wishes to include cases of salivary calculus under the generic term "Ranula," whilst modern opinion would restrict the term to an abnormal condition found in association with sub-mucous glands. It seems to me that Mr. Tod might next ask, "May we no longer call any swelling in the floor of the mouth Ranula?"

I shall look forward with interest to the reply of the reviewer. I can imagine Mr. Tod making to him a statement something like this : " Every man is a hero. Most are so to the outside world, but (in cases of exceptional interest) a few are so only to their valets." Your reviewer may reply, " I do not admit every man is a hero. When a man is a true hero he will be accepted as such by the outside world, but when he is admitted to be a hero only by his own valet, the term loses its meaning."

I am, Sir, &c., PERPETUAL STUDENT.

[As our correspondent justly remarks, the question of what constitutes a Ranula is one of nomenclature, but the nomenclature of the best authorities — such as Rechlinghausen — confines the term to cysts arising behind an inflammatory constriction of the tube of a sublingual gland. Cases such as those quoted by Mr. Tod are most exceptional, and belong rather to the class of pathological curios, than to those to which our reviewer referred.—ED.]

Journalistic Memorabilia.

THE PLACE OF CEMENTS IN DENTAL THERAPEUTICS.

UNDER this caption Mr. A. H. THOMPSON, D.D.S., writing in the *Dental Review*, says : "The first prime quality of the zinc phosphate cements is that of clinging to the tooth substance. This tenacious attachment necessarily forms a closer and better contact than is possible with any other filling material. The contact of all other materials is a mere mechanical juxtaposition which cannot be air-tight and only approximately moisture tight. Capillary attraction will draw in moisture around all mechanical fillings that depend solely upon manipulation for such a contact, except, perhaps, those of the very finest workmanship, but there are very few fillings that attain this ideal perfection. Then again, as moisture comes also from the tubuli of the dentine, drawn by capillary attraction, it follows that mere mechanical exclusion can never be absolute. With the phosphate cements, however, the principle of adhesive contact, by which the filling becomes as one piece with the tooth substance to which it clings, the exclusion of moisture and the consequent prevention of caries is absolute. Not only is the external moisture perfectly excluded and capillary flow prevented, but the very orifices of the tubuli are closed and moisture even from that quarter shut out. No other materials which we use for filling possess this invaluable quality in the slightest degree, and its great value will be apparent as we describe the situations in which the cements ought to be employed. This is seen first in their use in lining large cavities and strengthening weak walls. It is a good rule in practice that all cavities, where depth will permit it at all, should have a layer of cement in the deeper portions. After preparing the cavity—leaving the softened dentine over the pulp in deep cavities—cement is carefully placed in contact with all the inside while in a sticky, clinging condition, and the cavity nearly filled with it. After hardening, the cement is cut out to sufficient depth to retain the metal filling and the margins carefully finished. In teeth of soft structure the cement lining will ensure their better preservation, for it is a well-known fact that in such teeth caries will nearly always return under the metal fillings. Gold cannot be condensed against the walls sufficiently well to exclude moisture and the dentine itself is like a sponge, while amalgam, when it prevents caries at all, does it by hardening these soft tissues by impregnating them with the salts of its decomposition and consequent discoloration of the tooth. In such teeth, better preservation is insured by lining with cement and thereby excluding moisture from all sources by absolute adhesive contact. This is accomplished by filling the cavity to the enamel margins with cement and allowing the metal to come in contact with that tissue only. The contour of the tooth can often be preserved by filling overhangs of enamel with cement, which will strongly support such weak walls and thus reduce the size of the exposed filling. Thus the labial walls of proximate cavities in the anterior and buccal teeth should be lined with white cement to support and retain the tooth substance and give the tooth a lighter colour. The corners of incisors which are weak and thin can be preserved in this way, the gold being carried round the enamel to bind it in. This makes a much more artistic operation than the old system of cutting away all weak walls and exposing a mass of gold. In the molars also, deep overhangs can be supported with cement, and the natural face of the tooth be preserved for the more effective performance of the functions of mastication. Not only is this hardening treatment indicated in the soft and structureless teeth of many adults, but it is especially applicable for the filling of the permanent teeth during childhood and adolescence when the dental tissues are soft and immature. The teeth are much less dense and solid at eruption in childhood than after the maturity of the individual, the teeth naturally partake of the nature of the other bony tissues and solidity during the growing years, becoming more dense as age progresses. For this reason there are few cases in which the teeth are sufficiently dense to allow of being filled with gold with any hope of permanence, before puberty. Occasionally small fillings of gold can be made on the grinding surfaces in dense teeth at an early age with a prospect of durability, but rarely large fillings in any position. How often have we seen large fillings fail in the proximate surfaces when put in for children, and how seldom do they succeed? Then again we must consider the danger of subjecting children to prolonged operations; and that each succeeding generation as it appears in the families of our *clientele* is less able to endure nervous fatigue or shock. Therefore we contend that the permanent teeth should be filled with phosphate cement during childhood and adolescence that the teeth may be hardened both by nature and art, and that children may be saved suffering. Of course there are exceptions when small gold or amalgam fillings may be put in with safety, but it is very rare that the teeth in childhood should be filled with gold. The first molars for instance, which nearly always decay early, and sometimes the incisors, should be filled with cement and renewed when necessary until the teeth become sufficiently hard and the child becomes sufficiently strong to endure a permanent operation. As soon as possible the molars should be filled with amalgam which can remain until after full maturity, when it can be replaced with gold. Then again, the durable cements are especially valuable for filling the deciduous teeth in young children. With the little three and four-year-olds, perfect cleansing and preparations of the cavity is rarely practicable, and often quite impossible. Cement can then be used with good results until the sensitiveness of the tooth is overcome and the confidence of the little one gained so that a better cement or amalgam filling can be made. The soft and porous nature of the deciduous teeth indicate the use of cements, especially as it is always necessary to leave as much tooth substance as possible in the direction of the pulp, for this organ is certain to perish sooner or later under large fillings in these teeth. Cement linings are necessary under large amalgam fillings to support the soft and frail walls and protect the pulp. When the pulp dies and the tooth becomes a shell, cement makes a better root filling than anything else, and supports the frail tooth as no other filling can. The tooth can then be finished with amalgam or crowned, for it is imperatively necessary for the child's health that the baby molars should be preserved for mastication until the first permanent molars are all in place, at least. Children are better chewers than adults. When the teeth of the aged have become soft and often extensively carious, and when the individual is unable to endure severe or long operations, the cements are the best of filling materials. They answer an excellent purpose in the preservation of senile teeth, and are readily renewed without severity on the aged patient, when they do waste away. With invalids who cannot endure any painful or protracted operations—and whose teeth are often unfit for good fillings of metal—cement answers the best purpose for tiding over the time until the patient and the teeth are in better condition. If both do not recover, it is best to renew the cement as it may wear or dissolve away. During pregnancy and lactation it should be used also until the teeth recover their normal tone and the patient her wasted strength, for metal fillings are contra-indicated at this time. Another important use of cements is in the treatment of sensitive dentine as a temporary filling material. For this it is absolutely unequalled for safety and efficiency. A sensitive cavity can be filled for one or two weeks and the sensitiveness reduced so much, in most cases, as to permit of comfortable and thorough operating. Occasionally the pain persists, especially in nervous subjects or in buccal cavities, and the cement will need to be renewed, but it will pay to do this two or three times for the comfort of the patient and the safety of the pulp. Excessive sensitiveness should always be allayed, not only for the comfort of the patient, but for the safety of the tooth and pulp, for there is danger in the irritable condition of the dental tissues If there is forced preparation and filling of the cavity when great sensitiveness exists, with or without obtundants, there is likely to be annoying after-sensitiveness to thermal changes and the constant shocking will ultimately result in congestion and death of the pulp. This is a result that occurs too often as a sequel of the forced filling of sensitive teeth, for the danger is ignored in theory and practice. It may be said, that no tooth which has been filled when very sensitive and remains tender afterward, is in good condition or that the pulp is safe. Even if the sensitiveness is temporarily allayed by obtundants it will return when it recovers from the effects of the anæsthetic, and the tooth will be sensible to thermal changes. Therefore it is the best practice to permanently allay sensitiveness of the dentine and this can be done effectively and safely by the use of zinc phosphate cement, which accomplishes this probably by the exclusion of air and other irritants, the prevention of thermal shock, the neutralizing of the product of carious fermentation and the impregnation of the dentine by the cement and subsequent hardening. The permanent operation can afterward be performed with comfort to the patient, with safety to the tooth and satisfactory thoroughness to the operator. Devitalization does not follow except when the pulp is in such a condition as to render its death probable under any filling. Aching pulps are sometimes, though rarely, preserved alive permanently under favorable conditions in favorable organisations, and the zinc phosphates do not show a larger percentage of dead pulps than any other material. The precaution should, of course, be taken in exposure of the pulp, and even in very deep cavities, to interpose a a protecting cover of carbolized paper, or film of gutta-percha, to prevent irritation, for no one claims that it would be safe to stop an exposed pulp with a dab of zinc phosphate or any other irritant. If perfectly protected the pulp is as safe under cement as under any filling. But after the pulp is dead, comes the last use of the cements to be enumerated—that of filling pulp canals. A mixture of oxy-chloride of zinc and iodoform, in the writer's practice, has had no failures. The reason for preferring the oxy-chloride to the oxy-phosphate is obvious, in that the chloride being a powerful coagulant as well as an antiseptic, places the contents of the tubuli and the stump of the pulp at the foramen, in the best condition to resist decomposition. Then the iodoform is present to destroy any septic poisons that might arise—especially the ptomaines, for which it has a special affinity.

GOSSIP.

Mr. Morton Smale, writing to the *British Medical Journal*, says :—" It is felt by many that the time has arrived when the dental profession should be represented on the General Medical Council, and I venture to lay before your readers the reasons upon which this conclusion has been arrived at, with the view of raising a discussion on the question. I trust that what follows will not be taken as a reflection on the General Medical Council, for, as a profession, we are much indebted to that body for the way they have aided us in the past. It may not be generally known that the Dentists' Act is administered, and a register of dental practitioners and students kept by the General Medical Council; that the Council consists of about thirty members, but that the dental profession has no representative. When, from time to time, matters of dental interest arise there is no one on the Council with special knowledge who could be considered an authority upon such matters, and a judicial body of such high authority can hardly be expected to seek outside opinion. If it be admitted that such an alteration in the constitution of the Council is desirable, there are two ways in which it may be effected. (1.) The Privy Council, as soon as a vacancy occurs amongst the Crown nominees, can nominate a dentist to fill such vacancy. (2.) At the next period of election, the medical profession might select a dentist as one of the direct representatives. It is hardly an excessive demand that in the Council there should be an individual who, because he is a member of the dental profession, would be likely to have a more intimate knowledge of matters relating to the administration of the Dentists' Act, and be able to advise on the important matter of dental education. Such a candidate would be none the less able to consult with his colleagues on matters of general medical interest, as he should be on both the *Medical* and *Dentists' Registers* Our desire would be that such a candidate should be nominated by, and receive the support of, the whole medical profession at the next election."

Charing Cross Hospital Medical School.—The first entrance scholarship of 100 guineas has been awarded to Mr. Molloy, and the second of 50 guineas to Mr. J. R. Langley.

National Dental Hospital and College.—The Annual Distribution of Prizes and Dinner for past and present Students, will take place at the Holborn Restaurant, on Friday, November 21st. when Dr. Benjamin Ward Richardson, F.R.S., will take the chair.

Royal College of Surgeons' Examination. — The next Examination for the L.D.S.Eng. will take place at the Examination Hall, Embankment, commencing: the written, Monday, November 3rd; the practical, Tuesday, 4th, and Thursday, 6th; and the oral on Wednesday, 5th, and Friday, 7th.

Guy's Hospital Dental School.—The number of new entries for October has been eleven, and there are now twenty-two dental students in the school. Additional operating-chairs have been provided, and there are more patients requiring conservative treatment than can be attended to. At the present time there is an average of about ten gas cases daily.

The Past and Present Students' Dinner of the London Dental Hospital.—This dinner is planned to take place at the Holborn Restaurant, on November 29th. Dr. Joseph Walker will take the chair.

Dental Hospital of London.—Sir Edwin Saunders has, we are informed, accepted the Treasurership of the Dental Hospital of London, in the place of the late R. C. L. Bevan, Esq.

NOTICE OF SOCIETIES.

ODONTOLOGICAL SOCIETY OF GREAT BRITAIN,

40, Leicester Square, W.C.

The next Meeting of the above Society will take place on November 3rd, at 8 p.m., when papers will be read by

(1) Mr. Leonard Matheson, on "Some Practical Points in the Relation of the Upper to the Lower Teeth"; and by

(2) Mr. Storer Bennett, "A Description of some Interesting Specimens of Comparative Pathology at present in the Museum";

and Casual Communications by Mr. John Ackery and others.

The Chair will be taken at 8 p.m. The Council meets at 7 p.m.

E. G. Betts,
John Ackery, } *Hon Secs.*

THE DENTAL RECORD.

VOL. X. DECEMBER 1ST, 1890. No. 12.

Original Communications.

THE EFFECTS OF MERCURY ON THE TEETH.

By E. D. MAPOTHER, M.D., F.R.C.S.I.

IT is difficult to over-estimate the importance to dentists of questions bearing upon the prophylaxis of diseases of the teeth, so that no excuse is needful when such as that involved in the title of this paper is taken for discussion.

A large experience of the use of mercury in the treatment of syphilis, and of psoriasis and some other skin diseases, convinces me that its power of injuring the teeth has been greatly over-rated.

A hundred years ago it was given so rapidly and in such large doses, especially by quacks, that dire results were reported, and this most potent of remedies fell into undeserved disrepute. However, so recently as 1862, Professor Laycock taught: "It is a question how far the administration of mercury in early childhood or even to the parents during impregnation or growth of the ovum affects the form and development of the teeth." The male parent cannot have been meant, for no one could believe that the spermatozoon, wondrous as are its influences on the offspring, carried enough of the metal to harm the second set of teeth. From the mother the fœtus could scarcely receive, or still less could the infant store enough to interfere with the stages of dental development, the final one, that of calcification, not beginning until the sixth month in the first permanent molar.

As an example of the rapid change of scientific opinion, the following seems most noteworthy. The Government Committee on Venereal Diseases, 1864, having been instructed to inquire into "the best antidotes to injurious mercurial action," reported that any reference to the subject was almost unnecessary, and the voluminous evidence offered to it does not allude to the point.

With regard to idiosyncrasy, I have never met a severe case of mercurial stomatitis which could be thus entirely accounted for. There had existed some discoverable cause, such as great debility, or undetected albuminuria in the general system, or some faulty condition of the teeth.

Irregularity and crowding of the teeth, giving rise to chronic gingivitis, and erosion, caries and encrustation of them, so soon encourage salivation, no matter how carefully the drug is given, that in all cases where delay is permissible, the dental surgeon should treat these conditions before a mercurial course is commenced. If severe salivation ensues from these exciting conditions, the physiological and curative effects of mercury have not been produced, yet the drug must be discontinued, and in acute diseases recovery is retarded and even loss of life may result.

My practice, therefore, not having afforded opportunities of witnessing the destructive results occasionally reported, most of the observations which follow refer to the cases of mirror-makers, whose sanitary conditions I have extensively inquired into. By them minute particles of the metal or its oxide are inhaled, and the gums and teeth suffer sooner and more surely than after administration by the skin or stomach. The edges of the gums swell and separate from the necks of the teeth, then they become spongy and hæmorrhagic. Between their everted ulcerated surfaces and the conical roots, pouches are formed, which lodge, especially in the case of the lower teeth, many products which tend to destroy the alveolo-dental membrane, the ligament of the gomphosis joint, which at the neck is especially vascular. The teeth then gradually loosen and fall out. After this, these reckless artizans follow their pernicious occupations, for the mouth gives them no further trouble. The same is recorded as to quicksilver miners.

It is very hard to produce salivation in the elderly, who are wanting in teeth, and, as all know, in the infant or young child, and the reason appears to be that the unbroken surface of the gum does not allow the access of air to, or the evolution of some gas, possibly chlorine or hydrochloric acid, from the mercurial compound. Amongst the many syphilitic infants for whom I have prescribed mercurial inunction I have never seen any stomatitis, the liver and bowels only having shown signs of its action; besides, it is undoubted that mercury may act directly on the sympathetic system and produce salivation without any local irritation. Light also appears to be promotive of such chemical change, for the effects are never so marked round the posterior teeth.

It is not fully determined in what exact form mercury circulates in the blood: that it is as a chloride, with sodium also as a base, is generally believed. By this compound, after undergoing some chemical change, the albuminoids of the tissues round the teeth would be destroyed, the vessels of the inner surface of the gums would bleed, and the cementum would die from want of vascular supply, and then blacken, as does a piece of dead bone exposed to the air. Reducing agents, such as sugar, change mercuric into mercurous salts: chlorine or hydrochloric acid would be set free, and either of these may be the destructive agent. If a ferment, which is likely to be present, were added to the latter, a digestive fluid capable of dissolving cementum would be afforded.

The whitish sticky stuff about the roots of the teeth during salivation is an albuminous substance undergoing decomposition and thereby emitting much fœtor.

It has been said that a single dose of mercury has produced toothache, but I can find no authority for the statement and no evidence whether it resulted from the drug injuring the nerve when falling into a carious cavity, or brought to it through the circulation.

Enamel, with its ninety-seven per cent. of earthy matter, cannot be susceptible of injury by mercury, and it is also proof against the attacks of bacilli, which undoubtedly can feed on the gelatin of the cementum and dentine. There is much reason to suppose that these destroyers give rise to the evolution of some acid, probably lactic, which acts on the lime salts. The indestructibility of enamel is well exemplified in the teeth of the mastodon, which have been buried for thousands of years.

There are some who believe that the loss of teeth, together with necrosis of the corresponding part of the alveolar process, which is occasionally, but rarely, seen amongst mirror-makers, is the result of merely the anæmia which mercury produces, and which firstly shows itself in the pale bloodless gum. The similar mischief, which is sometimes seen in the course of the eruptive fevers of children, has also been attributed to the poor condition of the blood; but more probably the specific poison has attacked the teeth because they are part of the dermal system. If a dose of mercury had been given, the opponents of that remedy would lay the blame on it.

It may not be out of place to mention that the French process of making mirrors by the precipitation of silver is entirely harmless, and an article at least as good and as cheap is obtained. If our workmen are still to use mercury, their factories should be provided with every possible means of allowing the particles and vapours to escape, and they should be compelled to change their clothing after work, and to take daily baths. The skin can, if urged into complete activity, eliminate much of the poison. In the many cases of mercurial stomatitis among mirror-makers, and the very few resulting from the use of the medicine which I have seen, stoppage of the exciting cause, free exposure to air, and the frequent giving of albuminous foods, have rapidly produced amendment.

As to the local treatment of the diseased gums, it is difficult to speak with confidence until the chemical changes which occur in them shall be absolutely determined. Good effects follow the application with a very soft brush, firstly, of white of egg to neutralise the mercuric salt, and secondly, the washing of the mouth with a solution of common salt to remove it. Chlorate of potash is also a valuable remedy as a wash, in tablets slowly dissolved, or given internally. It is asserted that if used freely in the last-named way while mercury is being given, the gums never become affected.

Touching the hæmorrhagic surface of the gums with a pencil of nitrate of silver certainly checks oozing, and causes them to renew their normal hold on the neck.

To return to preventive measures, when mercury is used therapeutically, inunction or the pill form is far safer than fumigation, which really admits it, not by the unbroken cuticle, but by the mouth, much in the same way as when the injuries to mirror-makers arise. This is the main point in the administration of mercury at Aix-la-Chapelle, for by ventilation of the rooms, open air exercise, ablution of the body and cleansing the mouth every two hours, the slightest salivation is avoided. Alum is there the favourite drug for local application. Although I do not believe the teeth suffer from the mercury in Stedman's powders and such nostrums, their use ought to be deprecated by every practitioner.

With regard to the mercury contained in amalgam fillings and vulcanite plates, no remarks are needed, as Sir John Tomes and a Committee of the Odontological Society in 1877 proved it to have been wholly guiltless of having caused salivation.

NATIONAL HEALTH.

By W. Rushton, L.D.S. Eng.

Those who have read the speech upon the above subject delivered by Sir Spencer Wells at the opening of the Session at Owens' College must agree that it is a masterly treatment of the subject.* Beginning by looking backward, the speaker touched upon the advances made in surgery during the last half century, and then proceeded "to show what sanitary administration and recent advances in medical science and practice (curative and preventive) have done for the English nation, not only by lowering the death rate, and thus increasing the number of the population, but by raising the standard of the people, replacing a feeble and sickly race by one strong and healthy, and so improving the weak and incompetent that they may become healthy, vigorous, useful workers for the commonwealth, not part of a nation of invalids."

The speaker then went on to show how the condition of National Heath could be greatly modified by legislative means, bringing in evidence the tables of annual mortality in England and Wales before and after the passing of the Acts of 1872 and 1875 for the improvement of public health, the tables for the four decades 1841-80 being respectively per thousand 22·4, 22·2, 22·5, and 21·2, while for the last ten years 1881-90 the average per thousand is 17·9, a remarkable drop. But, although the average for the whole country has been so far satisfactorily reduced, in looking at some individual towns Sir Spencer Wells showed some startling figures as to the death rates recorded in the second quarter of 1890, and, although exception may be taken to the method of simply taking one quarter instead of a more extended period, yet the lecturer seemed to think that it was sufficient to point out the tremendous difference existing

* "National Health," a lecture delivered at the opening of the session of the Medical Department of the Owens' College, Manchester, by Sir Spencer Wells, Bart.

in towns, some of which, though similar in size, population, and unhealthy manufactures, yet have the greatest disparity in the size of the death rate, as, for example, Birmingham, which has only a little over 18 per thousand, while Manchester has an average of close upon 30.

Of large towns Nottingham heads the list with 14 to 15, Birkenhead is 16 to 17, while her large sister on the north side of the Mersey is 21 to 22. The Lancashire and Yorkshire manufacturing towns have an average of about 25, while London comes near the head of the list with 17 to 18, while that of one of her parishes, Hampstead, was only 10·5 for 1889.

The lecturer then asked the question, "Why does this disparity exist?" And, of course, the only answer was "neglect of sanitary laws." He then went on to prove that so far from increase of population being a burden to the state, it is, or ought to be, the most precious capital the state possesses, provided it is healthy. Therefore, it rests with all who have the good of the country and their fellow creatures at heart, to do their best to work to this end, especially those who are engaged in the healing art.

We, as dentists, see a very great deal of the misery and disease produced or aggravated by the neglect of the teeth, and Mr. Oliver in his paper at Exeter did not overshoot the mark when he said that, "Of all the ills that affected *civilised* nations (the *italics* are mine, W.R.) there was no malady so universal, none that caused such an aggregate amount of suffering and that so impaired and undermined the health of the people, as those diseases of the teeth which, unchecked, ended in their destruction and loss." *

That this view is in the main correct, has been recognized years ago by our nostrum manufacturers, those patent medicines advertised for the relief and cure of toothache, neuralgia, and dyspepsia having a fabulous scale, but to have the same fact recognised by the state (before it is obliged) is a very different thing, and, therefore, it behoves us to work with the end in view, namely, the compulsory examination and treatment of children's teeth and also of those of civil and military servants (in the lower ranks), because granting

---

* Paper, by J. C. Oliver, L.D.S. Eng., delivered at the annual meeting of the British Dental Association, 1890, on "Conservative Dentistry, its importance as a National Institution."

the fact that each man is so much state capital (the average is about £159 per head),* it stands to reason that if that capital is unfit to be employed to its full value the state is a loser to that amount.

The state can only be moved by public opinion, and the public can only be instructed in dental matters by dentists in their public capacity in connection with charitable institutions, and in their private capacity by instructing their patients in the chair, not in an aggressive or self-laudatory spirit, but by tempering zeal with discretion. When we reflect upon the fact that a company of empirics pervades the country, and are looked upon as prophets and carried like Elijah in his flaming chariot to the heaven of wealth and favour by the breath of an ignorant applauding public, we may well think that something ought to be done to instruct that public more in the care of their teeth. The National Health Society has done good work, and that work is increasing. Let them, instead of wedging the subject of teeth into a lecture dealing with a dozen other matters, employ lecturers well versed in their specialty to speak to the people on this important subject. This would be a step in the right direction. Meanwhile, let each one do his little to instruct his patients and friends in a little common sense care of those useful organs, which seem to be deteriorating with such appalling rapidity.

A NOTE CONCERNING THE ACTION OF CHLOROFORM.

By Dudley Wilmot Buxton, M.D., B.S.Lond.

Member of the Royal College of Physicians, Administrator of Anæsthetics in University College Hospital, the Hospital for Women Soho Square, and the London Dental Hospital.

(*Concluded from page* 507.)

The effect upon the heart of artificial respiration was experimented upon in the second series of cases. The average time elapsing between cessation of natural breathing and the failure of the heart was, in these experiments, $3\frac{40}{60}$ minutes (in one case 13 minutes), and artificial respiration when commenced 52 seconds after the natural respiration had ceased (37 cases) resuscitation was effected.

* "William Farr, the highest authority on vital statistics, has calculated that the *minimum* value of the population of the United Kingdom, men, women and children is £159 a head, that is the value interest in them as a productive money-earning race." Sir S. Wells.

When tried in 46 cases after cessation of pulse, *i.e.*, 3 min. 5 sec. before cardiac stoppage (taking the average) it failed in 17, succeeded in 29. When tried after cessation of cardiac movements it failed. The results are easily understood when we recognise a fact, which it would appear the Commission does not accept, that the actual heart muscle is itself affected. McWilliam* has shown that chloroform produces a dilatation of the heart due to relaxation of its muscle. Indeed, as we know, both voluntary and involuntary muscles are rendered flaccid and relaxed by chloroform, it is not surprising to learn that the heart muscle also relaxes and dilatation results. When, however, only a small dose of chloroform is given, dilatation is followed upon withdrawal of the anæsthetic by contraction. But if a larger dose is taken the heart muscle fails to recover itself, its action becomes weaker and weaker, and finally ceases. In cases when artificial respiration is successful as a means of resuscitation, the dose of chloroform taken is only such a one as permits of the heart's regaining its tone, *i.e.*, dilatation is succeeded by contraction. When, on the other hand, where artificial respiration fails to restore vital processes, the heart has dilated beyond the point when contraction can subsequently occur; the dose of chloroform has been too large. What is especially noticeable, both in these cases and those met with in actual practice, is that individuals differ so largely in their power of resisting or recovering from the chloroform cardiac syncope. But when we remember that the tonus of the heart muscle is itself subject to wide vicissitudes, depending upon the health or disease of the individual at the time, one readily understands how it is that a fatal dilatation of the myocardium may occur at one time and not at another.

Experimenting upon dogs to investigate the question, whether reflex inhibition of the heart's action can be produced under chloroform by "shock," the Commission formulated the deduction that no such reflex inhibition of the heart's action occurs. They add, "it is impossible to produce syncope from chloroform in dogs." Even accepting the experiments as sufficiently numerous to be of much value, I can only say that the Cmmission's results differ from those of other observers and from my own experience. I have insisted both in this paper and elsewhere that dogs show great immunity from primary syncope, the result of reflex cardiac inhibition; indeed, we

* See *British Medical Journal*, 1890, vol. ii., pp. 831, 948, &c.

find that shock is revealed far more in highly organised than in lowly organised animals. The more complex is the nervous system the greater is its liability to suffer from shock. In the animal kingdom mutilations of the most severe character are sustained without the individuals being apparently any the worse, but such an immunity is enjoyed less and less as we ascend in the animal scale, until we reach man in whom, as is well known, severe pain or even subjective emotions are capable of producing syncope. In dogs, cats, and monkeys, whether under chloroform, or not, a true faint is rarely met with as the result of a fright, or reflexly through irritation of a nerve, and so far the results arrived at by the Commission would seem to tally with my own; but only so far, for we now know that the heart is always directly affected by chloroform, the effect revealing itself in dilatation to which syncope must eventually succeed should the continuance of the anæsthetic be carried beyond the point of final resiliency of the muscle. In man, however, reflex inhibition must be accepted as a proved fact, and my own experience in the matter leads me to assume a dogmatic position, for I have again and again witnessed profound interference both with circulation and respiration caused by reflexes when a patient was under chloroform. Dragging upon the spermatic cord, its division in castration, manipulation of pelvic, or abdominal viscera in laparotomies, section of the optic nerve in enucleation, all give evidence of shock under chloroform and cannot fail to impress any careful observer with the grave danger to the heart when insufficient of the anæsthetic has been administered. In dental operations again, where the shock occasioned by laceration of branches of the fifth pair of nerves is out of proportion to the severity of the undertaking, there is an especial danger of primary cardiac failure through reflex inhibition. In the space at my command it is impossible to attempt to traverse all the issues entered upon by the Hyderabad Commission, but upon the two main practical points to which I have addressed myself, viz., the Commission's contention that chloroform kills, not through the heart but through the respiration, and that shock does not, through reflex action, interfere with the heart under chloroform, I think we are bound to say that the Commission have failed to substantiate their position. And further, I would add that the so-called "conclusions" do not without grave reservation apply to human beings, while any attempt to make such an application is likely to lead to the most calamitous results by inducing a false confidence in the supposititious safety of the heart under chloroform, and by leading to a studied neglect of the signs of cardiac failure during administration of that anæsthetic. Much space and argument have been devoted by the Commission in the attempt to prove that the fall of blood pressure and weakened cardiac action from chloroform are themselves protective, inasmuch as they prevent a rapid circulation of the anæsthetic. Such a theory, however, must fall completely to the ground when it is recognised that the heart muscle and the arterial system are not a rigid series of tubes which can be regulated by a mechanism producing slowing or acceleration of their contraction, but are highly organised muscular tissue actually and directly affected by the chloroform circulating in the blood, and only capable of sustaining that injurious action to a certain point. The fall of blood pressure and the lessened cardiac action are phenomena of cardiac dilatation, and even if their occurrence prevented a fresh take in of chloroform they would, at the same time prevent a speedy elimination of the drug, such as would be necessary to ensure the after contraction of the heart muscle and maintenance of circulation. The indictment against chloroform, as it reads at present, is at least so severe as to make one regard it as an agent too capable of producing dangerous cardiac derangement, to be used save by those trained in its administration, and under circumstances when other anæsthetics cannot be used.

But when we find that even in the hands of the most skilled and wary chloroform kills, and, further, when we are assured upon very high authority that this lethal power of chloroform is due to changes in the heart muscle visible to the eye and demonstrable to all, we are led to still further narrow the field of its use, and to say that chloroform should only be employed when other anæsthetics are unable to be exhibited, and when all precautions against a fatality have been taken. Much capital has been made by those who appear to regard any animadversion upon chloroform as a personal reflection upon themselves, out of the supposed dangers of ether. In one of the less known medical journals a considerable stir was recently made about ether deaths, and "the many dangers of ether" were therein vaguely cited. A prolonged use of ether and chloroform has led me to the following conclusions:—

I. Ether is incomparably less dangerous. Among the many cases one meets with in hospital, especially where the patient, broken down by illness, privation, or debauchery, has to take an anæsthetic and manifests alarming symptoms, hovers as it were upon the confines of death, most perils arise during the administration of chloroform. And, further, when such occurrences take place under ether the recovery is less tardy and less doubtful than under chloroform.

II. The after effects of ether are not what they are so often represented to be. Bronchitis, pneumonia, or nephritis are most rare. I cannot recall one in my own practice, and when they do occur they are generally due to excessive and reckless use of the anæsthetic.

III. Chloroform is incontestably the less disagreeable anæsthetic to take, and this has led some persons to use it as an introductory inhalation to ether, but the practice I believe is dangerous because the heart, weakened and relaxed by the chloroform, is less able with impunity to react to the stimulus of the ether. But the objectionable character of the ether is readily overcome when it is administered in combination with and succession to nitrous oxide, after the admirable method which we owe to the late Mr. Clover. This method also reduces the consumption of ether from a half-a-pint or more to one or two ounces for the duration of an ordinary operation. The importance of this becomes readily apparent when we remember that the lung and kidney trouble, to which reference is made above is dependent largely upon the quantity of ether which the patient inhales.

IV. It is easier to administer chloroform than ether, although anyone who will devote a very short time to the subject will readily enough master the use of Clover's small portable regulating inhaler, But, again, if it is easier to administer chloroform, it is still easier to kill with the use of this agent. In working with chloroform the point when urgent danger commences may be overlooked, but the contrary is the case with ether.

In conclusion, I may be permitted to say in what cases chloroform may be used. Accepting ether as our routine anæsthetic, except, of course, in dental surgery, in which nitrous oxide takes the first place, I should restrict chloroform to cases of prolonged operations about the jaw, tongue, mouth, larynx, and trachea. In exceptional cases, operations for abdominal, thoracic, brain surgery may require chloroform, but I am dealing here rather with routine than exceptional cases. When chloroform has to be given, I believe free and even dilution of its vapour is of more importance than dribbling out the anæsthetic drop by drop, and so prolonging the period of "going off" and that of struggling. With care, the open method (that used by Sir Joseph Lister) answers well, but when, as in most of the operations named, the lint or towel is in the way of the operator, I find the use of the apparatus made by Krohne and Sesemann,* and modified from Dr. Junker's original model, secures a fairly uniform dilution and is handy and easily worked.

Summing up, it is asked, shall we retract our belief that chloroform is not a safe and appropriate anæsthetic for the minor operations of surgery, such, for example, as those of dental surgery? I would reply, in the negative, because, as I have striven to show, not one iota of fresh evidence has been advanced by the recent experimental investigations into the action of chloroform showing its safety, while much has now accumulated proving its extreme danger as compared with other anæsthetics. Of course, it may be said one death in three thousand is at worst a small mortality, and this is so; but while one would let a patient incur that risk for a major operation, which would itself suggest to the patient the idea of risk, one should, I submit, hesitate before permitting the patient to incur the risk when presenting himself for an operation such as tooth extraction, which he and the rest of the world regard as a matter entailing no appreciable degree of danger.

REPORTS OF SOCIETIES.

ODONTOLOGICAL SOCIETY OF GREAT BRITAIN.

The ordinary Monthly Meetings of the above Society, adjourned from June last, were resumed on 3rd November, the President, Mr. Felix Weiss, L.D.S.Eng., being in the chair. There was a good average attendance of members.

The minutes of the previous Meeting having been read and confirmed, Messrs. J. F. Colyer, M.R.C.S., L.D.S.Eng., and G. W. Bateman, L.D.S., were admitted members of the society and signed the obligation book. Mr. J. H. Badcock, L.D.S.Eng., 140, Harley Street, W., was nominated for membership.

---

* Shown at the Annual General Meeting of the British Dental Association at Exeter, 1890.

THE LIBRARIAN, MR. ASHLEY GIBBINGS, reported the receipt ot the new edition of Mr. Henry Sewill's "Dental Surgery," as also the reports of various scientific societies, and a drawing of the trigeminal nerve, together with a chart.

THE CURATOR, MR. STORER BENNETT, stated that he had received on behalf of the Society a humorous sketch in colours of the extraction of a tooth by means of a key, such as was commonly used years ago. The sketch was the gift of Mr. William Merson, of Bournemouth. Mr. A. H. Farebrother, a student, had presented the skull of a bushman which had been discovered in Africa. The specimen was interesting because it contained on the right side the sockets of three incisors, on the left side there were the normal number.

THE PRESIDENT thought the frontal elevation of the skull rather higher than one would expect in a bushman, it seemed to him to suggest the possibility of European origin.

MR. ROBERT. H. WOODHOUSE presented to the Museum a necklace composed of human teeth, and in doing so remarked that it had been brought from Central Africa by the Emin Pasha Relief Expedition. It had been taken from the neck of a native killed in the skirmish in which Lieutenant Stairs was wounded. With the necklace Mr. Woodhouse presented a letter from Mr. H. M. Stanley explaining where the necklace came from. Mr. Woodhouse pointed out that the necklace consisted of thirty-four teeth, two of them being temporary ones, one, a lower wisdom tooth, gave evidence of extensive caries. The teeth were got out by burning the skull, the single-fanged ones were pulled out and the others were broken out apparently by great violence. He mentioned that he had been anxious to obtain some skulls from Africa from Mr. Stanley, and asked him particularly if he had any pigmies' skulls. Mr. Stanley replied that he only brought home two, and these had been sent to Natural History Museum, South Kensington. Mr. Woodhouse stated that Mr. Stanley had told him that in one place there were on each side of the road in the position corresponding to the curb in the streets of civilised cities, continuous rows of skulls, half a mile in length, whose owners had all died a violent death. Mr. Woodhouse was rather surprised to hear from Mr. Stanley how great an amount of caries existed in the teeth of the native Africans. The great explorer mentioned that he and his subordinates were called upon to extract some 400 or 500 teeth. Mr. Woodhouse added that the teeth in the necklace came from a region never hitherto reached by a white man, but the caries he had spoken of existed amongst the tribes of the extreme western and extreme eastern coasts, and these tribes had doubtless been in contact with some form of civilisation for some hundreds of years.

THE PRESIDENT remarked that they were very much obliged to Mr. Woodhouse for the necklace, more particularly as it was accompanied by a letter from a man of such large experience as Mr. Stanley. He added that he had been told that it was quite a common thing among savage tribes for the victors to extract all the teeth of the slain and wear them as a kind of trophy.

MR. CHAS. VINCENT COTTERELL showed and explained a small device which he had designed, and had been using for some time, the object of which was to keep the rubber dam from the nose. In filling anterior cavities and other operations he had found it of great advantage. In several cases where building up centrals or laterals with cohesive gold had to be done he had noticed a tendency of the gold to peel or not to adhere, and it occurred to him that it was due to the breath of the patient. The nose-guard was designed to obviate this. It was made in four sizes.

MR. J. ACKERY adverted to a case of "absence of lower incisors" reported by himself some two or three months previously. He stated at the time that these cases were rare. His object in alluding to it was to modify the statement which, it seemed, he was a little premature in making. The gentleman who first challenged his accuracy had been kind enough to show him several models of a similar condition, and some of them were on the table:—1. A case in which two incisors were missing in both the upper and lower jaw. 2. Two cases in which two lower incisors were missing. 3. One lower incisor missing from the temporary dentition He also had a model showing extensive erosion or abrasion of incisor, canine, and bicuspid teeth, which he thought would be interesting. The condition was not in any sense due to the attrition of the lower teeth, because the measurement of extreme anterior upper and lower teeth was three-eighths of an inch when the jaws were closed. The patient was a male aged 35. The mouth was what might be called a distinctly clean mouth, nor was the patient in the habit of using a hard brush. With this model Mr Ackery passed round a model of the mouth of a brother of the patient showing erosion in the most natural position, viz., the lower incisors; the dentine had suffered, if possible, more than the enamel. In connection with this he also passed round a pair of lower teeth which he had extracted from a man aged 56, showing erosion on the lingual surface.

Mr. R. H. Woodhouse said that he should like to ask Mr. Ackery if these teeth were at all sensitive. He had himself noticed three or four cases in which patients had come suffering obscure pain, and on examination he had found that there had been a nerve perishing from the attrition of the teeth. He did not gather from Mr. Ackery's remarks whether the patient had suffered any severe pain or not.

Mr. W. H. Coffin.—Of course Mr. Ackery looked for the black membrane of erosion ?

Mr. James Stocken stated that a short time ago he had a case under observation in which the labial surfaces of the incisor teeth were eroded throughout the whole surface, and in that case there was no sensitiveness. The erosion had gone so far as to produce quite a knife-edge to the teeth. In one or two cases he had tested the saliva, and had found it decidedly acid.

Mr. J. Ackery, in reply to Mr. Woodhouse, said that in his cases there was absolutely no sensitiveness of the teeth. The patient did not complain of any, and when questioned on the subject, he did not even seem to regard the condition of his teeth as in any way peculiar. It would be noticed he had lost the first upper right molar, and the tooth he consulted Mr. Ackery about was the *second* upper right molar. In reply to Mr. Coffin, ne might say that the teeth were so stained, that it was impossible to detect the dark film which Mr. Hutchinson had taught them to expect in cases of erosion.

Mr. Leonard Matheson then read a paper on—

"Some Practical Points Involved in the Relation of the Upper to the Lower Teeth."

Mr. Matheson grouped his remarks under the following heads : —(1.) The articulation of the teeth in relation to the etiology and treatment of approximal decay. (2.) Irregularities of articulation as productive of pathological conditions of the alveolo-dental periosteum. (3.) The "bite," as affecting certain modes of treatment adopted in the correction of irregularities. Speaking under the first head, he stated that the "bite" held an important place as a factor in the production of approximal decay, for owing to its action, food became wedged into approximal spaces, and by decomposition, promoted decay. Sometimes the very beginning of decay was due to this cause, and even in the larger number of cases where the actual inception of disease occurred before there was any interspace to admit of the lodgment of food, yet when once the coronal wall of the cavity gave way, allowing food to enter in appreciable quantity, the rate of decay was generally much accelerated, and its ravages made to extend rapidly over the whole approximal surface. In those instances where the lodgment of food was the primary cause of decay, the space which admitted the food was due to one of three things, either to simple want of contact in two neighbouring teeth otherwise normal, or to a flat instead of a contour filling having been employed on one or both sides of the space, or to the injudicious use of contour instead of flat fillings. Much might be done in the way of operative interference to limit or prevent the action of this predisposing cause to caries, by contour fillings on the one hand, and judiciously shaped spaces on the other; the use of both methods being demanded by the varying conditions met with.

In dealing with approximal cavities, one's aim must be as far as possible to achieve three things, viz.:—(1.) To prevent the recurrence of decay. (2.) To render the tooth under treatment useful in mastication. (3.) To protect the gum from irritation. To the question, in what circumstances did contour filling accomplish these things better than any other method? the answer was simple, viz.: when by contouring the filling could be brought into *close* contact with the adjoining tooth. Apart from the question of appearance, the whole value of a contour filling lay in its knuckling up to the neighbouring tooth so as to entirely prevent the lodgment of food between the two neighbours, this lodgment being the fruitful source of recurrence of decay, irritation of the gums, and inability to properly masticate. Contour filling was called for then, when the tooth to be treated was standing so close to its neighbour that a reasonable amount of contouring would restore the normal relation of the two. This could be done in the majority of instances, but the minority consisted of not a few cases in which the diseased tooth stood so apart from its neighbour that a restoration of its normal contour did *not* restore the normal relation of the two teeth. In these circumstances, contouring was bad practice, and recourse must be had to flat fillings and judicious shaping of surfaces forming the mesial and distal walls of the space. Broadly speaking, this shaping consisted in making the walls boldly divergent, and very smooth and straight. Sometimes, in order to render the space as non-retentive, and at the same time sacrifice as little tooth substance as possible, the original space might be deliberately increased by means of gutta percha or wool and mastic before finally shaping and filling. As to the value of such spaces, it could not be denied that, properly made and used only where contouring was inadmissible, they conduced to the comfort and safety of both teeth and gums. It could not however be too strongly maintained that between full contour and wide space there was no middle course, though which to adopt was by no means easy in every case to determine. Desiring to speak without bias, Mr. Matheson was inclined to say, "When in doubt play contour."

It did not infrequently happen that one had to deal with teeth, the relation of which to their neighbour and to the bite necessitated their restoration in contour, but in which disease was so very extensive as to render the wisdom of contour filling questionable. In such cases, the use of all gold collar crowns was invaluable, or in the case of bicuspids, all gold, faced with porcelain. The particular advantage of this form of crown lay in the fact that it could be contoured out in any direction or to any extent, so that it knuckled tightly against the adjoining teeth, and antagonized exactly with its opponents ; whilst the collar gave a security and finish which could be obtained by no other method, and produced, if properly adjusted, absolutely *no* irritation of the gum after the day of insertion. Mr. Matheson's own experience of this method had tended to convince him that perfect adaptation of the collar could only be obtained by fitting it to the root in the mouth—he had no faith in the use of a model for fine fitting. As to the modelling of the articulating surface, there was no question in his mind, that the best way was to strike it upon a cast obtained from a wax model, built up and carved for each case, rather than by the use of the die plates sold for the purpose, which made each crown a stereotyped and inartistic copy of every other. Partial gold crowns rendered excellent service where the amount of sound tissue was such as not to warrant its removal for the sake of inserting a complete crown, while at the same time the carious cavity was so far spreading as to make the security and durability of a larger filling quite a question of chances.

Under the second head, Mr. Matheson referred to the periosteal mischief set up by fillings insufficiently cut down to articulate accurately with antagonizing teeth. The inflammatory disturbance varied in intensity; fully pronounced periostitis was rare, more commonly the condition was one of irritation rather than inflammation. A curious point, in many cases, was the sensitiveness to thermal irritants, such as generally characterised irritation of the pulp. Similar symptoms to those named were due, not only to badly finished fillings, but also to a disarrangement in the articulation of one or more teeth produced by the forward pressure of an erupting wisdom tooth. In like manner, the eruption of the second, and even the first permanent molars, in some few instances, produced similar results, as did also the extraction of teeth.

Coming to the last division of his paper, Mr. Matheson limited his remarks to the consideration of the removal of molars or bicuspids for the relief of a general overcrowding of the arch as a whole. Having discussed and defended judicious extraction as against retention of the full number of teeth, he then dealt with the question as to which teeth to remove. Agreeing that the four first molars were the best to get rid of as a rule, he pointed out that many cases, for reasons mainly concerned with the "bite," indicated one of the bicuspids as the tooth to be sacrificed. Bearing in mind the value of the first molar as the chief grinding tooth, the comparative condition of molars and bicuspids ought to be most carefully examined and weighed at the time extraction is decided on. Should the loss of the first molars, after due consideration of all the circumstances, be finally determined on, it was nevertheless generally of the utmost importance that these teeth should be patched up, kept comfortable, and if possible retained until the second molars were quite erupted, and this for three reasons: first, that if the extraction were done at an earlier date the health of the patient would be seriously endangered by inability to masticate properly; second, that the second molars tilt less the later the extraction of the others takes place; and third, that early extraction may injuriously affect the position of the incisors by leaving them and only partially erupted biscupids to bear all the strain of the "bite."

With reference to "Raising the bite," made necessary in those cases of irregularity where projecting incisors are kept in their abnormal position by the close contact of the lowers, the methods for accomplishing this would vary in detail according to the circumstances of the individual case in hand, but a typical appliance for the purpose, was a simple vulcanite plate made to cover the palate *without* capping any of the teeth. This being worn for some time would prevent the lower incisors from rising any more, their tips being made to impinge against the vulcanite, whilst it allowed of the molars lengthening.

"Jumping" the bite. This unscientific but useful term had been applied to an operation which, when it could be accomplished, was a very pretty one, and one which helped very materially to improve certain mouths. By its means such a sudden alteration is made in the whole articulation, as to justify the use of the word "jumping." Its peculiarity consisted in this, that whilst nearly every other regulating operation aimed simply at altering the position of the teeth in relation to the jaw which carried them, this operation altered the relation existing between the jaws themselves. In other words, the bite is "jumped" by the lower jaw suddenly, in the course of a few days, being made to close upon the upper, in a manner entirely and markedly different to that in which it has been accustomed to close. The operation would be called for in cases where the upper incisors project, where the lowers bite far behind them, and where, besides these conditions, the bicuspids and molars interarticulate abnormally, the lowers closing too far back, by the whole width of a tooth ; the chin being consequently very retreating and the whole facial expression weak and foolish. What had to be done here if possible, independently of some retraction of the upper incisors, was an alteration in the position of the lower jaw, so that the chin might be brought bodily forward. This desirable end might be attained by various means. Having referred to a most interesting case communicated by Dr. Bogue and printed in the *Dental Cosmos* for May, 1887, Mr. Matheson mentioned a somewhat similar case recently occurring in his own practice. Having drawn back some prominent upper incisors in a case with a markedly retreating chin, and desiring to keep them in position, he attached a retaining wire to gold caps made to fit the second upper bicuspids—the first molars being gone, and the second scarcely long enough to furnish a secure hold. In order to prevent the bicuspids themselves being brought forward, instead of the incisors being held back, he furnished the caps with tiny inclined planes, directed downwards and backwards for the lower bicuspids to bite against. In a week's time he saw the patient, and was not a little pleased to find that not only had the end he had in view been accomplished, but the lower jaw had come right forward by the width of a tooth, and the retreating chin offended the eye no longer.

It might be observed that in both cases the movement of the lower teeth was due, not to any active mechanical interference with them, but to a spontaneous action on the part of the lower maxilla, when once it was set free from the abnormal position that it was locked in by the bite."

Discussion on Mr. Matheson's Paper.

Mr. Ashley Gibbings desired to ask Mr. Matheson if he had seen any jumping of the bite result from the extraction of six-year old molars. He had a case in hand in which the history showed that when the first molar was extracted, the bite was normal. The lower jaw then commenced to move forward. The patient was now using an apparatus capping the molars, and wearing an inclined plane, so as to hold the jaw back and move it to the right side. The girl was now over fifteen years of age, and Mr. Gibbings was glad to say the bite had improved immensely, The upper canine was now biting, whereas before it was one-sixth of an inch in front of the lower canine. He would add that he had just put in a fresh apparatus, capping the lower teeth, to keep the jaws in position and induce the lower molars to grow down, as they were not in position with the uppers.

Mr. Walter H. Coffin felt that it would be unnecessary to assure Mr. Matheson that if there were any paucity of debate it would not be due to any poverty in his admirable paper but rather that his views had been put forward with such lucidity and reasonableness as to leave it a matter of difficulty to say anything at the moment in discussion. With regard to jumping of the bite, Mr. Coffin thought that the cases were exceptional in which it took place to the extent of the whole width of a tooth. In many cases a jumping of the bite could be produced, and occurred in a manner which need not necessitate the movement in the teeth of either jaw to this extent. Where teeth are biting abnormally, or on their cusps in one place and others are normal, a judicious extraction may produce what must be termed a partial jumping of the bite, and a perfect interlocking of the jaws. The hints which Mr. Matheson had given, both as to the extraction or retention of first molars, were valuable, and he had put forward very forcibly the arguments for their retention, at least up to a certain age. His hints also on contouring must place his paper amongst the most useful contributed to the society.

Mr. JAMES STOCKEN said that the indebtedness which he personally felt to Mr. Matheson for his paper would doubtless be general. He was quite satisfied that is was wrong to extract the six-year old molars before the twelve-year old had developed: if that were done a tilting resulted and that approximation with the upper jaw which was so desirable, was not obtained. He had only just received a case which was fairly represented in the diagrams (prepared by Mr. Matheson and exhibited on the walls). The lower jaw was projecting at least half an inch. The case had been treated in Paris, and the patient—a young lady—had come to him to take up the case again. He could not help thinking that the treatment of jumping was in this case just the one he should adopt. He had not quite clearly grasped Mr. Matheson's method, and would be glad if in replying he would explain it more fully.

Mr. LEONARD MATHESON said, in reference to Mr Gibbings' remarks, it would seem as if possibly his case might have been one of those in which the premature extraction of the first molar did the harm. He would like to know from Mr. Gibbings if the second molars had come through at the time, when the patient was eleven years of age; he should imagine not. If not, it was probably due to the premature extraction to which he had alluded. The lower incisors easily thrust themselves forward and push the upper incisors out. As regards jumping, he quite admitted, and gladly admitted, that there was a partial as well as a complete jumping of the bite. The two instances he mentioned were only given as striking examples of what might be done, he repeated, what *might* be done, because it was more or less a matter of chance in these cases; the dentist was not always the prime mover. In reply to Mr. Stocken he would say that he should always look at the position of the canines to see if the upper canines might be very close together, and in the second place, if they were widely enough expanded from the lower jaw to come forward, he should do what he did in his own case: he put a gold cap on the upper bicuspid with an inclined plane backward and downward, so that the lower cusp was urged forward.

Mr. STORER BENNETT, being called upon by the President at this point to speak upon the subject for which he was announced, said that he would very willingly defer his remarks in order that Mr. Matheson's important paper might be fully discussed. The paper was on a practical subject, and if the discussion were now stopped it would not be resumed, whereas his own remarks would be on a scientific subject which would very well keep.

Mr. WM. HERN (continuing the discussion) would only occupy the time of the Society very briefly. There were but two points to which he desired to draw attention. First, with regard to contour fillings, the gist of Mr. Matheson's advocacy was *for* contouring: when, however, a cavity was suitable for a contour filling it would be advisable to get a previous separation which would give room for knuckling back; as soon as the tooth was filled it would knuckle back to its position. Without a previous separation the tooth would be a constant source of annoyance to the patient. With reference to the jumping of the bite, both those cases mentioned had been where the lower jaw had come forward easily in relation to the upper teeth. Cases in which patients deliberately protruded the jaw would be known to everyone, and it should be borne in mind that it was almost impossible to retract. The lower teeth would come forward in a very short space of time, and the glenoid cavity would adapt itself to a forward, while it would not adapt itself to a backward, movement.

Mr. WALTER H. COFFIN would like to ask a question, viz., when a case of approximal filling presented itself, and there was hesitation as to whether a permanent (flat or wedged) or contour filling should be adopted, he would like to know if Mr. Matheson had tried the method of inserting what was known as a "chewing bar." This bar was inserted between approximal cavities with a view of affording protection to the gum. He had seen cases of several years' standing where patients had expressed the greatest satisfaction with this method, but he had not himself had the courage or audacity to adopt it.

Mr. C. ROBBINS remarked that he had been brought up to believe flat fillings and V-shaped spaces between the teeth very heterodox, and until about eighteen months ago he had only adopted them with great caution. He was very glad to hear Mr. Matheson clear these points up. Where the contour was so exaggerated, of the two he preferred the V-shaped spaces, opened a little larger on the lingual than the buccal aspect. He would like to say one word in reference to jumping the bite. He had recently had a case in which the patient was fifteen or sixteen. The mother urged him to push out an instanding lateral, which he did partially by expanding the arch. He got the teeth into a pretty position, but to his dismay the lateral would keep going in; he afterwards found this was due to a cusp to cusp bite, which, opening the mouth, prevented a lower tooth from keeping the lateral in its proper position. A little grinding with stones and sand paper remedied this and made the occlusion so perfect that it was a pleasant surprise.

Dr. Field, referring to contouring, said, ought they not to ask themselves the question, "What do we understand by contouring? Is it restoring the tooth to its normal contour, or is it bringing out these large spaces so as to knuckle up?" If it was to restore the contour he might say that he had never seen a prejudicial result from the adoption of the method, perhaps with one exception, viz., those normally dirty mouths where neither contouring nor flat filling could be successful. In all cases he was inclined to contouring for the best results. In regard to the chewing bar he would give his experience: the patients were delighted with it as an aid to mastication, but he had seen very poor general results: it necessitated too much destruction of good tooth substance, and without great care on the part of the patient the cervical margin of the teeth was apt to be undermined. The teeth were injured when the other end of the bar was put on by a cap, and when it was put in by a mortice the movement took place which undermined the teeth.

Mr. Leonard Matheson, in reply, said that he was very glad that Mr. Hern had called attention to the importance of previous separation before contour filling. With regard to the chewing bar he had had no experience with it, and he felt they were much indebted to Dr. Field for having brought forward his experience on the matter, as it would be a guide to them. His only experience was in the case of an old gentleman who had extensive approximal decay between the second and third molar on both sides. The teeth were very long, the food lodged up there, and it would have been quite impossible to make a contour filling in such a position. He therefore, thought the best plan with an aged man was to bridge across the cavity, and put over tith a cap of gold having a pin going down the middle into the mass of gutta-percha. He believed that on a former occasion Mr. Hepburn had suggested this plan. He would like to say that Mr. Robbins need not have apologized for grinding the teeth, that was very often the best practice and would sometimes save a regulation case. With regard to restoring the contour again he desired to say that even in restoring the natural contour it was often necessary to make large spaces. In such cases as where one got a small cavity at a cervical edge, and extending on each side of that a white film, where it is extremely difficult to make satisfactory fillings, there he should feel it the best plan to boldly cut away sound tooth substance, that he was aware would be bold and what Mr. Coffin would call audacious.

Mr. Storer Bennett, having been called upon for his paper, suggested that the meeting be now adjourned. This course would enable him to complete some photographs which he desired to show in connection with the paper.

After the usual votes of thanks and announcements for next meeting the suggestion was acted upon.

The National Dental Hospital and College.

The Past and Present Students' dinner of the above institution took place at the Holborn Restaurant on the 21st ult. Dr. B. W. Richardson, F.R.S., presided, and was supported by Messrs. H. Morris, G. Gregson, J. Smith Turner, Morton Smale, Felix Weiss, Dr. Dudley Buxton, and a number of the staff.

Dr. Richardson distributed the prizes. The successful students were introduced by the Dean, who, in some prefatory remarks, referred to the fact that two additional prizes appeared in the Honours List for the first time. These were, the prize of three guineas given by Messrs. Ash for the best thesis on some dental subject, to be selected by themselves, and an entrance exhibition of £15. The latter, the Dean observed, was the first exhibition instituted at any dental hospital in this country, so far as he was aware. In introducing Messrs. Moore and Bascombe, the Dean called attention to the fact that, together, they had monopolised most of the prizes.

HONOURS LIST.

Bronze Medals.—Dental Anatomy, Mr. Moore; Dental Surgery, Mr Bascombe; Dental Mechanics, Mr. Moore; Metallurgy, Mr. Bascombe; Operative Dental Surgery, Mr. Moore; Dental Materia Medica, Mr. Moore; the "Rymer" Gold Medal for General Proficiency, Mr. Moore; the "Ash" Prize of three guineas for the best thesis on "Hæmorrhage after Tooth Extraction," Mr. Arnold Prager; the Entrance Exhibition of the value of £15, Mr. McFarline; Students' Society Prize, Mr. Haycroft; Mechanical Work, Mr. Keele.

Certificates.—Dental Anatomy, Mr. Cutts; Dental Surgery, Mr. Burbery Rowe; Dental Mechanics, Mr. Prager; Metallurgy, Messrs. Johnson and Keele; Operative Dental Surgery, Mr. Bascombe; Dental Materia Medica, Mr. Prager; Elements of Histology, Mr. Bascombe.

After the usual loyal toasts,

The CHAIRMAN proposed "The Hospital and Staff," and said that, among the friends and students of the school, there was not one who could propose it with greater pleasure than himself, for he knew of its birth, and assisted in bringing it into existence. Some generation ago there was a college existing in the metropolis called the College of Dentists, and he had the honour of being called upon to deliver the first course of lectures. He delivered and afterwards published them. At the end of the session, the President, Mr. Peter Matthews, entertained him, Mr. Kimpton, Mr. Lee Rymer, Mr. Harding, Mr. Robinson, and many more, at supper, and it was upon that occasion he suggested the foundation of a dental school, which resulted in the formation of the Metropolitan School of Dental Science, now known as the National Dental Hospital and School, In that school he had the pleasure of being among the first of the lecturers, which included the names of Mr. (now Sir) Spencer Wells. Prof. Wood, Mr. Holmes, and Mr. Perkins. They formed that school, and he believed it was just thirty-three years ago since he had the honour of giving the address, and then, in the evening presiding at the dinner. After the lapse of a generation, he was so fortunate as to be again presiding. Soon after that the Dental Hospital of London was started, and Mr. Gregson (sitting next him) was among its first teachers. For some years a keen rivalry existed between the two institutions, but they were now, happily, running side by side in friendship. Well, the school had originated in small beginnings, and had gone on steadily maintaining and adding to its reputation. That morning he had had the pleasure of being taken over the old place by the Dean, and he found great improvements, great advancements, and everything required for teaching dental science, but the most joyous thing of all that he had heard was the projected new building. But let them not be in a hurry to leave the old place—there was always something exceedingly pleasant in holding on to old places. When they had their new building, it would be like starting a new school—perhaps it would not be a better one It would probably be attended by a larger number, and would have more experienced teachers, for teaching was of that nature. that it had a continual and progressive development. In conclusion, he asked them with warm hearts to drink in remembrance of the old and in anticipation of the coming time. He gave them the toast of "The Hospital and Staff," coupled with the names of the Dean and Mr. Roughton.

The Dean, in responding, said that the hospital itself was an institution which endeavoured to attract the public within its walls, so as to supply the material which was best suited for the instruction of the future generation of practitioners, and the interest of those conducting such an institution was centred in organising it in such a way that the teaching might be successfully carried out and might result in the greatest possible relief to the suffering poor. Some critics had said that the school and the hospital must be antagonistic to each other, but this did not seem quite true. If the demands upon a student were such that they were called upon to work too rapidly and scamp their instruction, then he would say that the charity was detrimental to the school; but so long as the number of students and patients was relatively balanced, the hospital and school would be mutually beneficial; indeed, the former was necessary to supply the material for the latter, With reference to the history of the hospital, which was generally well known he would make but one remark, viz., that until dental education became compulsory its presence was hardly necessary, and it and the sister hospital were rivals. With the Act of 1878, that condition of things ceased. The scourge of dental disease was such that 90 per cent. of the population passed through the hands of the dentist, and he believed that, at the present time, half-a-dozen dental hospitals in the metropolis would not be too many. With reference to the recent examinations, without trenching on Mr. Roughton's ground, he might venture to give expression to a feeling of pride at the success of the students. The examination of the Royal College of Surgeons, as was well known, was a searching, he might say, a vexatious one. A man was called upon to be examined in anatomy, physiology, surgery, materia medica, dental mechanics, &c. With the present multiplicity of subjects, it was impossible for a candidate to know in what branch of a subject he would be examined. From fourteen years' experience, he was strongly of opinion that the examination should be divided. If they were to be examined in anatomy and surgery, let it be thorough. He hoped the authorities would, before long, see their way to put an end to the present confusion. In conclusion, he begged to thank them for the kind way in which the toast had been proposed and received.

Mr. Roughton also replied.

Dr. Maughan proposed "The Past and Present Students," and said, with reference to the relation of the staff to the students, it was the object of the former to turn out men into the world who would be honest and true, and who would do their work conscientiously. The staff supplied the necessaries to make the craft seaworthy, and it was for the student to take every care that he availed himself of the equipment offered before he was finally launched on the sea of life by the Royal College of Surgeons.

Mr. Rushton, in replying, referred to the change in the examination since the previous distribution of prizes by the inclusion of dental mechanics—a change, in his opinion, greatly for the better. No dentist, he contended, could be thoroughly efficient in his profession who was not fully competent in the workshop as well as in the surgery.

Mr. Bascombe briefly replied on behalf of the present students.

Mr. Alfred Smith proposed "The Visitors," and said that this annual festive gathering was looked forward to with the most enjoyable anticipations, as affording a pleasant opportunity for past and present students and their teachers to meet each other, but to none was a more hearty welcome accorded than to their visitors. He concluded by reading a letter of regret from Sir Spencer Wells, and mentioned the absence of other visitors who were expected.

Mr. Morton Smale, in responding for the visitors, remarked upon the kind way in which Mr. Weiss had spoken of the school at Leicester Square, and said that it was a source of great gratification to him to be included among the friends of the National Dental Hospital, for his feelings for the hospital and school were of the most cordial character. He hoped that the days of rivalry between the two schools had for ever gone; there was no reason why rivalry should exist, for they were working for a common object, and there was ample room for both. Touching upon the question of a dental representative on the General Medical Council, he urged its importance, and pointed out that the object might be helped forward in this way: there was not a single student who had not a medical friend, and each medical man had three votes. Let them all obtain promises for at least one of these three votes for Mr Charles Tomes at the next election.

Dr. Geo. Cunningham proposed the health of the Chairman, warmly eulogising his labours in the medical profession and the dental branch of it, in science, in literature, and as a social reformer.

The Chairman, in acknowledging the toast, gave a few interesting reminiscences of his life and the friends he had made in the various fields in which he had laboured. He spoke of his sense of gratitude for unbroken health, happiness of temperament, and many circumstances of his past career, especially for the close ties and many friends he had in connection with the National Dental Hospital.

An excellent selection of instrumental music was well rendered by the Bijou Orchestra during the dinner, the vocal part of the programme being entrusted to Messrs. Hodges, Strong, Parkin, and Vernon Taylor.

Mr. W. H. Thomas presided at the piano.

The Dental Hospital of London, Annual Dinner.

The staff and students are to be congratulated upon having given their guests a most delightful evening on the 29th ultimo at the Holborn Restaurant. The speeches were light, effective, and neither too long nor too numerous; the toast list having been judiciously curtailed. The music was excellent and all the more enjoyable because it was chiefly provided by the "dentals," such well-known names as Mr. David Hepburn, Mr. Wheatley, Mr. Alfred Smith, and Mr. Barrett being contributors to the musical programme. Among the many good things was an original transcendental ditty, collabo rated by two distinguished dentals, we believe, specially for the occasion. Rendered by Mr. Alf. Smith in his best style it "brought down the house"; our limited space prevents our giving more than a verse or so :—

I'm now become of such repute, so crammed with useless knowledge,
I really think my gifts would suit an examiner at the College.
I'd question on neuralgic pain, on Koch's tuberculosis,
The convolutions of the brain, the bacillus of exostosis.

* * * * *

I'd also set a paper on the origin of caries,
The cure in labyrinthodon of pyorrhœa alveolaris,
How creosote reacts with starch, eruption in Bos taurus,
And how to treat a V-shaped arch in the young Icthyosaurus.

Mr. Sholto's clever parody on "Sally in our Alley" and "The Magpie," given with all the art and finish of Corney Grain, were also highly appreciated.

Dr. Joseph Walker presided, and was supported by Drs. Wilks, W. J. Collins, and Messrs. Christopher Heath, Silbey, Pearce Gould, Hy. Morris, Hy. Power, Andrew Clark, Stanley Boyd, Scott-Thomson, De Haviland Hall, S. J. Hutchinson, and a numerous company.

After the toast of "The Queen and Royal Family" the Chairman proposed "The Past and Present Students." He was glad to say he had nothing but congratulation to offer them, and, thanks to the efforts of Sir John Tomes and the acumen of Mr. Jas. Smith-Turner, he could address them as members of one commonwealth; through them the profession enjoyed an inheritance, the importance of which it was impossible to estimate; an inheritance absolutely closed to all comers except through four portals: one for England, two for Scotland, and one for Ireland. What other profession, he asked, was so safely guarded at the present moment as theirs? There was one only, and that the Navy; the Navy was bound to have apprentices, who were bound to serve five years, and had to present themselves for periodical examination. In order to keep their inheritance let them put their shoulders together and preserve a united front, let them send their best men, those who held their profession in the highest possible estimation, to the examining boards. They had one other protection, viz., the General Medical Council, which possessed the power of maintaining the standard of everyone of these Boards. In advocating clinics he claimed Sir John Tomes as the originator of dental clinics in this country. In espousing the cause of benevolence the Chairman remarked that it was a regrettable fact that of the 976 registered dental surgeons only 54 were found on the regular subscription lists. In conclusion, he referred to the increasing number of students, the general prosperity of the school, and the high estimation in which the Dean and staff were held. He coupled with the toast the names of Mr. W. A. Maggs for the past students, and Mr. W. May, Mr. Coysh, and Mr. Gask for the present students.

Mr. W. A. Maggs, in responding, felt the difficulty of adequately representing the sentiments of so many men as had passed through the school, but thought he would have their unanimous support in expressing their sense of indebtedness for the instruction which enabled them to carry on the profession of their adoption.

Mr. W. May, in reply, spoke of the congenial nature of a student's work, his pleasant companionships, agreeable associations, and students' meetings, making their student career a happy dream far too short.

Mr. Coysh having also briefly replied,

Mr. Gask was called upon, and said, "It would ever be their endeavour to uphold the honour and traditions of an institution on whose foundation stones were graven some of the most revered names of their profession; the names of those who had been mainly instrumental in making their profession what it was; of those who stood at the vessel's helm in those dark hours, in the grey beginning of things, and who, loosening her from her moorings by a barren and pestilential shore, directed her bow toward the open sea, that she—

"In healthier climes might live a more regenerate life."

Dr. Samuel Wilks then rose to propose "The Hospital and School." Those who knew him, knew that he had a great objection to "specialism" in medicine; but in surgery, the manual skill and dexterity demanded, could only be obtained by long and patient training, such as could not be given to the whole field of surgery, and necessitated specialism; from this point of view, dentistry was more differentiated than any other, and must be put at the head of the profession as a specialism. When he spoke well of dentistry, he did so for a particular reason : the great advance of late years is, in what is called conservative surgery, and he was under the impression that long before the surgeon commenced conservatism, the dentist did it ; he looked upon it as one of the highest arts of the present day, this conservation of the organs of the body. The man who preserved an old tooth was better than the man who put in a new one. He had always heard and felt that dentists were the leaders in this great department of conservative surgery. If the dentist could do so much for those who could afford it, what a boon was a hospital which gave the poor access to the same advantages ! In alluding to the extent to which sentiment influenced the direction of charity Dr. Wilks said that he once asked a wealthy old lady where all her money was going to, and she replied "Lifeboats and Idiot Asylums." Would not some of the money be more wisely spent in the support of such institutions as the Dental Hospital of London ? Referring to the relation of hospitals to schools, he maintained that they were mutually necessary and beneficial to each other. In conclusion, Dr. Wilks remarked that he had heard that 26 good reasons could be given in favor of artificial teeth, to these he could add one or two which he had not heard before ; in the first place, a man who had no teeth couldn't eat, and he therefore drank the more, but an artificial denture restored his powers of mastication, and so it obviated the necessity of so much drink : hence Dr. Wilks claimed for the profession a greater influence in the cause of temperance than all the teetotal institutions in the country. An old lady of his acquaintance gave another reason : she was able once more to bite her nails, a luxury she had not enjoyed for many a long day (laughter). He begged to give them the toast of "The Hospital and School," coupled with the names of Mr. Septimus Sibley and Mr. Morton Smale.

Mr. SIBLEY briefly replied, and said that he was happy to be able to assure them that the object of the toast was in a most flourishing condition, full of health and activity.

Mr. MORTON SMALE, who was received with prolonged cheers, having expressed his hearty thanks for the enthusiastic reception given to the toast, referred with satisfaction to the large number of reporters present, and hoped that they would make the public understand that the L.D.S. was the only criterion of fitness for a dental surgeon, and that these letters did not necessarily mean L.S.D.

Mr. Smale spoke strongly in support of the admission of a dental represectative upon the General Medical Council.

Mr. Frederick Canton, in a few well chosen sentences, proposed "The Visitors," coupled with the name of Dr. W. J. Collins.

Dr. W. J. Collins, in acknowledging the toast, spoke warmly in favour of direct representation for the Dental Profession on the General Medical Council. It had now attained to such a position that it was entitled to ask it as a right. He based his argument on the broad ground that representation should go with taxation; that a distinct and separate register entitled it to a distinct and direct representative.

Mr. David Hepburn, in proposing the health of the Chairman said, they had in the chair a gentleman who was associated with the early beginnings of the hospital; a gentleman who was appointed as one of its first assistant surgeons. Dr. Walker would feel some sense of gratification when looking round upon the large gathering, and contrasting the growth of the Hospital with what it was in those early days, in knowing that it was in no small measure due to himself. It was the fashion to enlarge upon the virtues of a chairman, he would take but one of Dr. Walker's virtues; his peculiar distinctive quality was the wonderful energy he threw into every undertaking—for the younger men it was really an example to follow. He would now pass on to Dr. Walker's faults, for he would not be human if he were perfect, and Dr. Walker was very human. Well, he only knew of one fault, and that was the fault of never growing old. When they went back into antiquity for their Chairman they expected to find silvery hair and a little becoming decrepitude, but in Dr. Walker they found the brightest, and liveliest, and best type of what a dental surgeon should be. That was the only fault he knew of; if he knew of any other he would enlarge upon it.

Dr. Walker expressed his heartfelt acknowledgements. He was more than repaid to know that what little he had done, or tried to do, was appreciated, and that he had many friends in the profession.

EXTRACTS.

ON THE DANGERS ARISING FROM SYPHILIS IN THE PRACTICE OF DENTISTRY.

BY L. DUNCAN BULKLEY, A.M., M.D.,

Attending Physician to the New York Skin and Cancer Hospital, etc.

(*Concluded from page* 515.)

As is well known, various household utensils, such as cups and drinking-vessels, spoons, tobacco-pipes, etc., have been the means of spreading the disease to hundreds of cases. The glass-blower's pipe has also caused a number of small epidemics, and cases have been traced to the assayer's blow-pipe, whistles, musical instruments, toys, pencils, pins, tack-nails, thread, paper-money, coin held in the mouth, &c. Of instruments used about the mouth, laryngoscopes and tongue-depressors are peculiarly liable to transmit the disease, but the only instance found is a case reported by Jumon,* where a paper-cutter used to depress the tongue gave rise to syphilis. The cases traced to the use of the Eustachian catheter have been already mentioned.

Syphilis has also been conveyed by means of various fabrics, and a number of striking instances are on record where towels and napkins have transmitted the disease. An interesting case is given by Leloir,† where syphilis was communicated by means of a handkerchief.

Of peculiar interest are the cases on record, of which there are a number, where the disease has been transmitted by means of a tooth-brush. This was first observed by Blumenbach ‡ in the last century, and later by Baxter,§ and also by Bumstead‖ and Taylor,‖ and more recently Haslund ¶ has reported a similar case. Knight,** has also recorded a case, seen by Bumstead, where a lady received a chancre of the tonsil apparently by means of tooth-powder, her syphilitic nephew dipping his brush into her box when cleaning his teeth.

---

* Jumon, *Thèse de Paris*, "Syph. ignoræ," 1880.

† Leloir, Leçons sur la Syph," Paris, 1886, p. 60.

‡ Blumenbach, "Bibliothek für Aerzten," iii. p. 197.

§ Baxter, *Lancet*, May 31, 1879.

‖ Bumstead and Taylor, "Path. and Treat. of Ven. Dis.," Phila. 1879, p. 432.

¶ Haslund, *Monatshefte für prakt. Dermat.*, 1885, p. 456.

** Knight, *New York Med. Journ.*, 1884, p. 662.

It is understood, of course, in all these instances that the various objects served as a medium to convey the dried syphilitic secretion which adhered to them directly to the tissues of the individual who became infected, and it is readily seen how, unless precautions are exercised, the various implements and articles used in connection with dentistry may very easily become likewise the bearers of syphilitic virus.

It is not possible always to determine exactly upon which instrument, or in what manner, the poison is conveyed, but the preceding instances which have been cited show, on good authority, that the infection did take place in some way in connection with and in consequence of dental operations.

The agents and objects which may become the conveyors of the poison are as numerous as the implements and articles which may come in contact with the mouth in dental manipulation. For conveniences these may perhaps be grouped in three or four classes, as follow: 1, instruments proper; 2, napkins; 3, rubber dams, wedges, dental floss, etc.; and, 4, plaster, rubber, etc., used in connection with the making of artificial teeth and sets.

Among instruments the only one plainly shown to have communicated the disease is the forceps, in the case related by Dr. Roddick, in which the site of the extracted tooth, where the gum was torn by the forceps, became a syphilitic ulcer, the seat of the chancre or primary sore of syphilis. But it is readily seen that the instruments used in excavating and plugging may also become infected, while there is peculiar danger in such instruments as files, burrs, and drills, where there are many depressions difficult of cleansing which may receive and retain the virus. Napkins and towels may convey the poison, as has been shown, while rubber dams, if used a second time, would very readly give infection from their prolonged contact with the soft parts. The same is true of wedges, a portion of which is often used for different patients, as also, thread, ribbon, or dental floss passed between the teeth. The different workmen in a furrier's shop were once infected* from a thread passed between them and bitten off. My scanty knowledge of the process of taking casts and preparing and fitting artificial teeth does not permit me to speak in regard to any dangers arising

---

* *Arch. f. Derm. u. Syph.*, viii., 660.

from this, but I should judge that possibly accidental infection might occur in this line of work, perhaps quite as unexpectedly as it has happened in connection with other branches of dental practice.

We come, finally to the most practical and important part of our subject,—namely, the prophylaxis, or prevention of the occurrence of this most unfortunate accident, the transmission of syphilis in the practice of dentistry. It may be somewhat out of place in the presence of this Society, including, as it does, many of the best elements of the dental profession in this city, to urge the simple matters of precaution about to be mentioned; but, as some may not heretofore have recognised the immense importance of the matter, it is best to err on the safe side, and to present briefly and clearly the precautions which seem to be indicated from what we know of the nature and virulence of the poison of syphilis.

As before mentioned, the virus or contagious element comes in liquid form from a chancre or a moist, exuding surface, or, more rarely, with the blood itself, from a fresh wound. The secretion is very sticky and adherent, and when dried on an article forms a delicate coat, which could hardly be perceived. Nothing is known in regard to the viability of the virus, or the length of time during which it may retain its actively contagious character, but from many instances in the various conditions of life and in medical experience, it would seem that, under proper circumstances, it retains its vitality and activity for some considerable period longer than that possessed by the somewhat similar virus of vaccine. Days, weeks, or perhaps months after an instrument or article has become infected, it may again give off the poison and produce inoculation. Simple washing will not destroy the poison, although it may so dilute it that it becomes innocuous.

There are, however, several elements which are destructive to the life of the syphilitic poison, and these are heat and cold and the so-called disinfectants, antiseptics, or germicides. Cold can hardly be utilized practically, as a sufficiently low temperature for a requisite length of time would be difficult to maintain. Heat, however, may readily be employed in a thoroughly efficient manner, and is undoubtedly the very best means for destroying contagious principles. Inasmuch as dry heat, as in a flame, would injure instruments, as to their temper, the desired results are best obtained by means of moist heat, obtained in boiling water. Instruments and other articles placed in a vessel, and then subjected to vigorous boiling for half an hour or so, may be considered absolutely freed from any power of conveying contagious matter.

Various chemical substances are also capable of destroying the virus when efficiently used ; prominent among these stand bichloride of mercury and carbolic acid. The mercurial salt has its disadvantages, both from its poisonous nature when in strong solution, and also from its corroding action on some metals. Carbolic acid, therefore, remains as the best of the two ; and, indeed, when properly used, answers all the requirements of the case. But one must not be deceived by the odour, and be led to use a too weak solution, for it is questionable how serviceable the high dilutions used in antiseptic surgery are in overcoming such a poison as syphilis. The strong acid certainly destroys it, and a safe method is to dip the instruments in a ninety-five-per-cent. solution, wiping or scrubbing them afterwards. A much weaker strength, possibly even a ten-per-cent. solution, would probably be effective if they were left a considerable time in it and then thoroughly washed. I will not take your time in discussing other disinfectants, but only wish to impress the fact that not only for ordinary cleanliness, but also and particularly to avoid the possible danger of infection, too great care can hardly be spent in rendering instruments and everything pertaining to dental practice is absolutely clean as thought and labour can possibly make them.

Files and burrs are particularly liable to catch and hold the poison of syphilis in their fine serrations, and as they are also peculiarly liable to wound the soft parts they may readily become means of contagion. Also the various articles connected with polishing the teeth are dangerous, if not properly cared for. I well remember more than one dentist, in times past, polishing my own teeth with a bit of wood dipped in pumice-stone, which wood had evidently been used for former patients. Rubber dams and wedges can, of course, be readily disinfected in strong carbolic solutions, and napkins are rendered aseptic by boiling.

In regard to the personal prophylaxis of the dentist against acquiring syphilis in dentistry little need be said. The careful guarding of fresh wounds and thorough cleansing of the hands, and immediate sucking of any wound made during operations, will generally suffice to prevent the untoward event. "Forewarned, forearmed" applies well in regard to all the dangers from syphilis in dentistry. If the danger is thoroughly well known and appreciated, half the battle is won.

The question here arises, how far the dentist should be acquainted with syphilis, so as to be able to recognize it and avoid its dangers? Undoubtedly it would be most desirable that this knowledge should be obtained; but, unfortunately, a practical acquaintance with syphilis is somewhat difficult to obtain, except after considerable clinical experience in this branch of medicine. But it would certainly,be extremely desirable that the mouth lesions should be known to dentists so as to be recognized, and this would be a fitting subject for the consideration of instructors in dental colleges.

A word may be added in regard to the duty of the physician in charge of syphilitic cases, when the patient may desire dental wrok to be performed. Should he prevent the patient from having the work done, and from thus exposing others, or should he acquaint the dentist with the diagnosis of the case and warn him against contaminating himself and others? The latter question involves an ethical point as to how far the medical adviser is right in revealing the nature of a patient's disease to others, and is a difficult one to answer; for professional relations require secrecy, especially in such a complaint. But, on the other hand, it cannot be right to wittingly expose others to the poison of syphilis. My practice has been to warn the patient earnestly of the danger, and, as far as in my power, to prevent his having dental work done while in th infective period, and especially while there were mouth lesions present, frequently examining the mouth for this purpose. If he failed to heed my instructions I should feel justified in warning his dentist.—*International Dental Journal.*

TANNIC ACID: ITS INTERNAL ADMINISTRATION FOR HÆMORRHAGE AFTER TOOTH EXTRACTION.

By Dr. W. L. Roberts, Weymouth, Mass.

Tannic acid, as we all know, has a yellowish-white color and strongly astringent taste. It is decomposed and entirely dissipated when thrown on red-hot iron. It is very soluble in water and less so in alcohol and ether. Its solution reddens litmus and produces with solution of gelatin a white flocculent precipitate, and with solution of the alkaloids white precipitates, and is very soluble in acetic acid. Dose from three to ten grains.

Very little has ever been written, and less said, upon the internal administration of this most valuable adjunct to our list of hæmostatics.

The most of us do at times have those perplexing cases of hæmorrhage after extraction which are very hard to control, and necessarily resort to numerous devices to bring about the desired results, all or a portion of which are very disagreeable to both dentist and patient.

Tannic acid, administered internally in proper doses, will stop I believe, any case of hæmorrhage caused by tooth extraction, in from thirty minutes' to one and one-half hours' time. The manner and results of administering this very simple remedy I will illustrate by one case in practice.

I was called, March 25th, 1885, at 8 p.m., to check hæmorrhage from the lower gum of a lady, caused by the removal of eight badly-decayed and broken-down teeth. They were removed while patient was under nitrous oxide gas, with no more laceration of the gums than generally occurs. Patient did not bleed very profusely at the time, but as she was of a hæmorrhagic diathesis I kept her there until it had entirely ceased, with instructions to call me at once if there was a return of the hæmorrhage to any great extent. As she lived some distance away, and being at home alone, I did not hear from her until about 7 p.m., when her husband came to me with the information that his wife was bleeding to death. I immediately went to their residence and found the patient in a bad state indeed. Pulse was very weak, and she looked about ready to expire, but there was life, and, upon enquiry, I found that she had expectorated nearly one quart of blood. Upon examination I found blood oozing from all portions of the gum. I immediately placed three grains of tannic acid in one third glass of water and gave her two teaspoonfuls every five minutes until she had taken three doses, then two teaspoonfuls every fifteen minutes ; after the second dose the flow had diminished to such an extent that I left them with instructions to administer the same amount every half-hour, which they did, and were only obliged to give two doses before it ceased entirely, with no return.

I have used tannic acid for the past five years, whenever occasion presented, with the same good results, in fact it has never failed me.

Now what is its physiological action? From experiments on animals with very large doses, it appears that this acid renders the gastric mucous membrane pale and lustreless and coagulates its mucus. Injected into the blood-vessels it coagulates the albumen of the blood. To the former of these actions, as well as to its inherent astringency, must be attributed the dryness and sense of constriction which it produces in the mouth and fauces.

We are told that tannic acid is not absorbed and does not circulate as such, but is converted into gallic acid. It is true that in this form alone it is found in the blood and urine. Indeed, it could not remain in the blood without coagulating it, as experiments on animals demonstrate; but as gallic acid is not an astringent, it is difficult, while admitting the conversion of the one acid into the other, to explain the therapeutic operation of the latter.

Several theories have been proposed for this purpose, but, as far as I can find, all of them are unsatisfactory.

Lewin has shown that the coagulum of albuminous substances formed by tannic acid, if made slightly neutral, loses its coagulating power. Thus an albuminate of tannin formed in the blood is dissolved again in an excess of that alkaline liquid. A small portion of tannin escapes neutralization and is discharged with the urine unchanged, and hence, according to Lewin, tannin, as such, may exert its power in all parts of the system. It would appear, also, that the hæmostatic and analogous qualities of tannic acid are due not to an action upon the blood, but upon the blood-vessels, by which they become contracted and the flow of blood through them is checked.

We also see in nervous patients frequent anomalies of the vaso-motor and trophic functions, but up to the present time we know comparatively little that is certain as to the precise nature of their occurrence.

Physiology distinguishes two varieties of vaso-motor nerves,—the vaso-constrictors and the vaso-dilators; but since experiments have detected the latter variety in only a few places, for example, in the chorda tympani, the nervi erigentes, and the sciatic, they have not acquired a very great significance in human pathology. We are at present much more disposed to refer every abnormal constriction of the vessels to an irritation, and every abnormal dilatation of the vessels to a paralysis, of the vaso-constrictor nerves, although perhaps pathological conditions of irritation of the vaso-dilators may not be at all rare. In regard to the precise anatomical course of the vaso-motor nerves, it is necessary to state that vaso-motor irritations may certainly proceed from the cerebrum, as is shown by the well-known symptoms of blushing and pallor from mental emotions. In experiments on dogs Eulenburg and Landois have succeeded in producing a fall of temperature on the opposite side by irritating certain portions of the cortex in the immediate vicinity of the motor centres, and by extirpation of the same parts they have produced a rise in temperature. It is now known with certainty that there is an important vaso-motor centre in the medulla oblongata, the irritation of which, directly or reflexly, is followed by an almost universal vascular constriction, and its destruction by an almost universal vascular dilatation. We must probably seek the further course of the vaso-motor nerves largely in the lateral columns, from which they pass out chiefly by the anterior roots; but there are also experimental data suggesting the presence of vaso-motor nerves in the posterior roots. It is not known with certainty whether there is any decussation of the vaso-motor fibres, or, if there is, where it occurs. The larger part of the vaso-motor nerves collect, at any rate, in the principal trunks of the sympathetic, from which, as is well known, the separate plexuses that surround the vessels arise. It is probable, however, that there is in part a direct passage of vaso-motor fibres from the cord into the peripheral nerves. There are also ganglia in the walls of the blood-vessels themselves that are capable of maintaining the tone of the circulation in the absence of the central force or influence, but under ordinary conditions these minor ganglia are denominated and controlled by the one central power which unifies the whole system and renders it complete.

But, be it as it may, tannic acid, administered internally in proper doses, does stop the flow of blood from ruptured blood vessels, and is a hæmostatic that I wish to commend to the careful consideration of all, for by looking deeper into this subject we shall all be benefited and perhaps add one more drug to our list.—*International Dental Journal.*

THE DENTAL RECORD, LONDON: DEC. 1, 1890.

The L.D.S. Examination of the Royal College of Surgeons of England.

THE millenium of dental examinations has not arrived, it is true, but anyone who reads carefully the report which we have purposely obtained of the recent test imposed upon L.D.S. men at the Examination Hall will admit that some marked progress has been made. Reformers, when they turn their attention to test examinations, very often content themselves with "piling up the agony," by imposing still severer burdens upon the shoulders of budding practitioners, mistaking severity for thoroughness. Two of the most experienced examiners in science have told the writer again and again that they could estimate the relative merits of candidates far more readily by easy than by severe "papers," and it is commonly admitted that men come to grief far more over answering questions about simple every-day operations and points in practice than over abstruse matters upon which they are primed with information to the bursting point from the most recent manual or vest-pocket crib dealing with the matter. The crammed student will probably rattle off seven or eight theories about the etiology of pyorrhœa alveolaris, but is floored when requested to write out a prescription for a mouth wash, or asked the reason for not operating upon both sides of a mouth on one day. But the L.D.S. examination, as at present conducted, works upon sound lines. It aims at estimating practical knowledge by practical tests. Occupying five days, it commenced with the papers, which we print below, and for these six hours were allowed.

On the second day 20 students were taken to the Dental Hospital of London, and there made to fill teeth from 1 p.m. to 4.30 p.m., while the time from 5 to 8 p.m. was devoted to regulation and other cases including mechanical dentistry.

The third day was given up to viva voce interrogation, which was, as far as one can judge, both thorough and fair in its character, although perhaps more severe than has heretofore been deemed necessary.

The last two days were devoted to practical work for the remaining batches of students and to viva voce questions. This seems to us to be a tolerably searching examination, and he must be a lucky fellow who "scrapes" through without being really "posted" in his work. To the man who can thoroughly satisfy the examiners in the various stages of this test, much praise will be due, and everyone having so meritoriously acquitted himself cannot help feeling proud, and justly proud, of the letters L.D.S. Eng., to which he has so well earned the right.

The thoroughness of the L.D.S., and the enforced efficiency of the men who compete for it, certainly suggest to the mind of the thoughtful whether any further degree or diploma is really a desideratum. It may be that the more vigorous and busy of our schools, sons of dental Anakim, may strive for further distinction, and yearn for an honors examination, or an arrangement of names in the order of their merit, but the suggestion, as far as a fresh degree goes, has lost much of its force when the standard of the general examination is so materially raised, and has taken the position itself of practically an honors examination, intended, some would say, for duly qualified surgeons who aim at specialising practice as dental surgeons. However, we are not here concerned with any such position. We have simply to deal with the L.D.S. Eng., as it at present exists, and we venture to affirm, without fear of contradiction, that it presents a thorough, fair, and most practical examination for dentists, and that those who are able to obtain it, may well be proud of the diploma they hold and the school which taught them so well as to ensure their success.

Representation of Dentists upon the General Medical Council.

Our contemporary the *Lancet* traverses Mr. Smale's arguments, which we published last month in the following words. "But, first, let us see if any particular hardship has existed," *i.e.*, in the now representation of the dental profession upon the Council, " If so, it has not been alleged. It is true that at the last meeting serious complaints from the dentists were received by the Council. But they were carefully examined, and, we believe, practically met. Mr. Smale himself allows that the profession is greatly indebted to the Council for its administration of the Dentists' Act in the past. We do not doubt that any representations made to the Council as at present constituted from the registered dentists will always meet with impartial and attentive consideration. So much for the proposition as it stands by itself; but if it be considered in what it it implies, we feel the more need to be chary in accepting it. If dentists are to be conceded a special representative, why not ophthalmic surgeons? Indeed, it is clear that as an eye is more than a tooth, so the claim of the latter to special representation exceeds that of dentists. If a Midwives' Bill should pass, are we to be told then that the midwives must have a seat in the Council? We shall not push this objection into the region of the ridiculous, but it might easily be so pressed. We have said enough to show that Mr. Smale's proposition is not to be accepted hastily. Specialism, it must be remembered, is a defect. It is an incompleteness. A dentist ministers only to a bit of the human body. It is not desirable to specialise in the General Medical Council. It would not even be good for dentists, whose best interests are seived when they are kept up to full professional standards of knowledge and of conduct. The direct representation of the profession is already too slight to expect that the profession would give up one of its representatives to this speciality and another to that. Moreover, the law requires that direct representatives be registered medical practitioners. The only other source to which the dentists can look is the Crown. But its representation has been shorn already, and it is not very likely to initiate a representation of specialties which are best controlled by men who view special practice from the broader standpoints of medicine, surgery, and midwifery. Of course, there are men on the dental register who are also on the medical register eligible in point of law, and equally so in point of breadth of knowledge and of training. But they cannot feel themselves unrepresented in the existing Council; they are medical practitioners and dentists. And the more of such the better."

The *Lancet's* position, although many will admit the two-sidedness of the question under discussion, will not be held to be impregnable. At least neither Mr. Smith Turner nor Mr. Morton Smith are inclined to admit as much, for they frankly deal with the *Lancet's* arguments and certainly state a strong case. Mr. Smale writes :—

"The position occupied by the dentist is an unique one, and his specialty has no analogue, for he has his separate Act and Register, the sums paid for registration to the General Medical Council being kept as a separate dental fund. He also has a special curriculum and diploma, and, while all may agree with you that specialism is a defect, it must be agreed that dentistry is a specialty that is necessary for the general welfare, and in no branch of the medical profession is the student at the end of his career so well equipped in his own department as is the dental student. In the future some of the business that the Council must consider will be of purely a dental character, and inasmuch as the sittings of the Council cost £1 2s. a minute, it is desirable, to save the expenditure of the Dentists' Fund, which necessarily is a small one, that some body, cognisant with the needs and requirements of dentists, shonld have a seat upon that Council to direct the discussion of a subject with which most of the members are not familiar, and thus save both time and money. It is desirable that this question should be discussed upon its merits rather than in relation to the manner in which the General Medical Council has so far administered the Dentists' Act. Is it possible to find gentlemen who will adequately represent both the dental and medical profession?" This question both Mr. Smith Turner and Mr. Smale answer in the affirmative, and oddly enough both mention the same three as possible men, any of whom would be competent, representatively, alike of the dental and medical professions: Dr. John Smith, of Edinburgh, a past President of the Royal College of Surgeons; Dr. Theodore Stack, of Dublin, a Member of the Council of the Royal College of Surgeons in Ireland; and Mr. C. S. Tomes, F.R.S., of London.

ROYAL COLLEGE OF SURGEONS OF ENGLAND.

EXAMINATION FOR L.D.S.

November 3rd, 1890.—2 to 4 o'clock, P.M.

ANATOMY AND PHYSIOLOGY.*—1. Describe the structures which form the soft palate, give its nerve and blood supply. 2. Describe the mechanism of ordinary respiration, and state briefly the changes which the blood and the air undergo respectively.

SURGERY AND PATHOLOGY.*—3. Give an account of the process of healing of (*a*) a simple incised wound, and (*b*) a lacerated and contused wound. 4. Describe the principal manifestations of Constitutional Syphilis found in the mouth.

November 3rd, 1890.—5 to 8 o'clock P.M.

DENTAL ANATOMY AND PHYSIOLOGY.†—1. Compare the jaws and teeth of man and the Anthropoid Apes. What inferences can be drawn from the teeth as to food appropriate? 2. Contrast dentine as to structure and chemical composition, with bone. 3. At what stage of development have the several permanent teeth arrived at the age of 6 years; and what is their position in relation to the roots of the temporary teeth?

DENTAL SURGERY AND PATHOLOGY.†—1. What are the causes, other than septic matter in the pulp-chamber, that give rise to inflammation of the alveolo-dental periosteum? Give the treatment appropriate in each case. 2. Mention the drugs to be used in treating the following conditions:—(*a*) Sensitive dentine at neck of tooth. (*b*) Sensitive dentine in carious cavity. (*c*) Exposed pulp —previously painless; ditto, painful. (*d*) Decomposed pulp. (*e*) Ulceration of tongue due to ragged teeth. (*f*) Ulcerative Stomatitis. What quantities would you use and what precautions would you observe? 3. By what appliances would you treat a fracture of the lower jaw in the Canine region:—(*a*) Most of the teeth standing and uninjured. (*b*) Few firm teeth remaining. (*c*) An edentulous jaw.

VIVA VOCE AND PRATICAL EXAMINATION.—On the second day one student had to put a gold filliing in the mesial surface of an upper left central, after which he was taken to the work-room and set to work to repair a vulcanite upper plate broken right across the centre; before he had finished it he was sent upstairs and two regulation cases shown to him, the treatment of which was asked. On the third day, at the examination hall, he was at one of the tables and was shown microscope specimens, (*a*) a developing tooth germ, (*b*) a section of dentine and cement, and asked the different structures; he was then given a jaw with holes by the side of the teeth and asked what they were for. After-

---

* The candidate is required to answer at least one of the two questions, both on Anatomy and Physiology, and on Surgery and Pathology, unless he is entitled by the regulations to exemption from any of those subjects.

† The candidate is required to answer at least two of the three questions, both on Dental Anatomy and Physiology, and on Dental Surgery and Pathology.

wards asked what was the "gubernaculum," what was the structure of the gum, and how did it differ from ordinary mucous membrane. At another table he was shown an articulated model of an open bite, asked what it was and what was the cause and treatment Also asked the nature, cause, symptoms, and treatment of antral abscess. In Dental Anatomy another candidate had shown to him a transverse section of cementum and dentine (with interglobular spaces) to spot. He was also questioned on the growth of the lower jaw, functions of the teeth, and was shown skulls of bears and tigers, showing a carnivorous type of dentition, and had to describe a carnassial tooth. In Dental Surgery he was asked to discuss the treatment of inflamed pulp, the part played by micro-organisms in caries. He had to give an opinion on some models of irregularity, and to give treatment of abscess bursting externally.

In General Anatomy he was taken over the base of the skull, the tongue (muscles, nerve supply, ducts, &c.), the soft palate, deep dissection of the neck.

In General Surgery he was shown a pickled specimen of enlarged tonsils and was asked cause, symptoms, and treatment; also had ranula, cause symptoms, diagnosis and treatment, and ditto of nævi.

For the practical work he was required to insert a gold filling in an upper lateral. The mechanical part consisted of a vulcanite on gold repair, *i.e.*, he had to back a tooth, fit it to the model, solder a flange on to the backing, fit this to the plate and there rivet it.

DENTAL ANATOMY.—Microscopic subjects to spot: 1. Dentine and cementum. 2. Interglobular spaces and Sharpey's fibres. 3. Dentine and enamel.

QUESTIONS:—Structure of cementum. Differences cementum and bone characteristics of (1) rodent dentition, and (2) carnivorous dentition. Differences—felidæ and arctoidea.

GENERAL ANATOMY:—Bones—Occipital, Temporal, Sup. Maxillary.

DISSECTIONS:—Pterygo-maxillary regions. Pharynx and Larynx. Tongue. Side of the neck.

GENERAL SURGERY: — Dislocation in general. Dislocation of lower jaw—causes, symptoms, treatment. Fistula—definition, treatment of salivary fistula. Cleft Palate—causes, similar instances of non-union in other parts of body, operation of staphyloraphy, time of operation, with reasons.

DENTAL SURGERY:—Questions: Uses of the elevator, causes of closures of jaws, extraction complicated with closure, dangers of extraction, treatment of fractured root, salivary fistula. Causes and treatment: two modes of irregularities, treatment required, supernumerary teeth.

MECHANICAL WORK:—Solder a pivot. Let down and solder a flat tooth to a gold plate. Let down tube teeth and solder the pins for them in the plate. Repair a cracked gold plate by rivetting a piece of plate on either side of the crack. Repair broken vulcanite pieces. Flask a full upper already set up in wax. Add a tooth to a gold plate with vulcanite on it, by rivetting and not soldering. Cut a clasp off a plate and re-solder it on.

CORRESPONDENCE.

[We do not hold ourselves responsible in any way for the opinions expressed by our correspondents.]

"AMBIDEXTERITY."

To the Editor of "THE DENTAL RECORD."

SIR,—This, although of the utmost value both to the operator and the mechanician, is not at all a simple matter. Until a few years ago I was myself ambidexterous to a fair extent, but for most purposes I selected one hand in preference to the other; for any heavy work, except using the hammer, I always selected the left hand, and also for manipulations requiring extreme delicacy and steadiness, but writing with ease with the left hand was out of all question, and there was always a selection, one hand doing some things better than the other. Some years ago I met with an accident which prevented my using the left hand for some months, and I have never been able to use it in the same manner since: the power of changing instruments from one hand to the other is gone apparently for ever.

A friend, who is the most perfectly ambidexterous man I have ever met with, draws with a pencil equally well with both hands, but instinctively selects the left for a hammer or a file, either hand for a knife, the right hand only for writing and for picking up anything he has dropped, and this selection is invariable. The fact that he is a first-rate draughtsman with either hand shows plainly that he is perfectly ambidexterous, but even in his case there is almost invariably a selection of one hand only for certain special work, as there was in my own. I have known writers who used the left hand, but with one single exception I never met with a left-hand writer who could use the right: it has been an acquirement from absolute necessity, and the writing was inferior and not so quickly done.

The true value of ambidexterity lies in the power to do certain work with the hand most convenient for the special purpose; it is neither necessary nor desirable that both hands should do everything equally well, for the very simple reason that if the work were divided each hand would only get half the training, and the results would, as a rule, be inferior. The whole thing is simply a matter of training, and any one may with reasonable perseverance train each hand specially for the work best suited for it; this is true ambidexterity and the only form which is of any real value.

Yours obediently, THOMAS FLETCHER.

MR. A. HILL'S HISTORY OF DENTAL REFORM.

To the Editor of "THE DENTAL RECORD."

DEAR SIR,—In the year 1877 the late Mr. Alfred Hill published, through Messrs. Trübner & Co., a history of Dental Reform embracing the principal events of the twenty years prior to that date. Since the death of the author, Messrs. Trübner have generously placed the remaining volumes in stock at the disposal of Mrs. Hill. Messrs. Ash and the Dental Manufacturing Company have undertaken to distribute these volumes free of charge to the widow, and copies may be had on application, price 5s. each, just one-half of the publishing price. I sincerely hope that all who wish to have at hand a record of the progress of our profession during twenty eventful years of its history will secure to themselves this interesting work, which in all likelihood will soon be out of print. The insertion of this letter in your next issue will greatly oblige

Yours truly,

JAMES SMITH TURNER.

12, George Street, Hanover Square, W.

GOSSIP.

WE understand that three gentlemen, who were referred to their studies at a recent examination for the L.D.S.Eng., have since been successful in obtaining the L.D.S.Glasgow, but, nevertheless, they again presented themselves for the L.D.S.Eng. at the recent examination in London.

MR. HILL'S HISTORY OF DENTAL REFORM.

WE have had to deplore more than once that the dentists who are yearly being started into the profession from our schools know so little of the inspiriting history of their "young profession." They are ignorant of the stress and toil in which their Act and their Register were won, and so are callous and shortsighted in dental politics of to-day. In Mr. Hill's valuable little book they will find an unvarnished tale, and one which they should read, mark, learn, and inwardly digest. We publish in another column a letter from Mr. James Smith-Turner, in which he tells us that the remaining volumes of the edition are to be disposed of for the benefit of Mrs Hill. The profession owes a debt of gratitude to the deceased gentleman, and can now recognise their appreciation of his labours by promoting the sale of the work.

Lightning Source UK Ltd.
Milton Keynes UK
UKHW021328100219
336936UK00006B/522/P

9 780365 295969